Liver Transplantation

Bijan Eghtesad • Marina Berenguer
Nazia Selzner • Koji Hashimoto
Editors

Liver Transplantation

What Every Hepatologist and Gastroenterologist Needs to Know

Springer

Editors
Bijan Eghtesad
Liver Transplantation and Hepatobiliary Surgery Desk A100
Cleveland Clinic
Cleveland, OH, USA

Nazia Selzner
Director Liver Transplantation
University of Toronto
Toronto, Canada

Marina Berenguer
La Fe University Hospital
Dept of Hepatology and Liver Transplant
Valencia, Spain

Koji Hashimoto
Liver Transplant and Hepatobiliary Surgery
Desk A-120
Cleveland Clinic
Cleveland, OH, USA

ISBN 978-3-032-07071-5 ISBN 978-3-032-07072-2 (eBook)
https://doi.org/10.1007/978-3-032-07072-2

This Springer imprint is published by the registered company Springer Nature Switzerland AG
The registered company address is: Gewerbestrasse 11, 6330 Cham, Switzerland

Preface

Liver Transplantation: What Every Hepatologist and Gastroenterologist Needs to Know

This book is a comprehensive overview of the whole spectrum of liver transplantation from pretransplant assessment including indication for liver transplantation, timing of referral, medical evaluation to surgical aspects: transplant procedure, living vs. deceased donation, machine perfusion, and posttransplant care. Sections include management of critically ill patients with end-stage liver failure, acute or chronic, and patients with other co-existing end-stage organ failures. Perioperative management, early surgical complications, and management of combined liver with other grafts are discussed. Most importantly, dedicated sections to posttransplant management of liver transplant recipients cover all questions raised by non-transplant providers, including community hepatologists and gastroenterologists. These include immunosuppression therapy, management of rejection, infection, disease recurrence, and posttransplant malignancies.

This book is the perfect reference for non-transplant providers who require a comprehensive, clinically relevant, step-by-step guide for managing patients with end-stage liver cirrhosis, covering all spectrum of liver transplantation, and who wish to provide care to these patient population pre and post transplantation.

Cleveland, OH, USA — Bijan Eghtesad
Valencia, Spain — Marina Berenguer
Toronto, Canada — Nazia Selzner
Cleveland, OH, USA — Koji Hashimoto

Contents

Part I Pre-transplant Period

1 **Indications for Liver Transplantation** . . . 3
Fei-Pi Lin, Alex Miller, Andy Wu, Abidemi Akinrinmade, and Naudia Jonassaint

2 **Pathophysiology of End-Stage Liver Disease** . . . 23
Claire Francoz

3 **Candidate Evaluation for Liver Transplantation** . . . 31
Laia Aceituno Sierra, Vishan Seetahal, and Cynthia Tsien

4 **Management of Portal Hypertension** . . . 51
Nicolas Chong Lugon and Guadalupe Garcia-Tsao

5 **Management of Critically Sick Patient with End-Stage Liver Disease (Acute Liver Failure and Acute-on-Chronic Liver Failure)** . . . 63
Julie Gorham and Thierry Gustot

6 **Kidney in Liver Transplant Candidates (Pre-transplant Evaluation)** . . . 79
Sapna V. Shah, Fadi A. Tohme, and Mitra K. Nadim

7 **Cardiopulmonary Issues in Patients with End-Stage Liver Disease** . . . 91
Elena Gavrila, Lisa B. VanWagner, and Dempsey L. Hughes

8 **Pre-transplant Infectious Problems** . . . 113
Carmen Vinaixa Aunés and Rosa Blanes-Hernández

9 **Liver Transplantation for Malignancies** . . . 123
Christian T. J. Magyar, Luckshi Rajendran, Laia Aceituno, Owen Jones, Anudari Zorigtbaatar, and Gonzalo Sapisochin

10 **Metabolic Liver Diseases and Their Management** . . . 139
Lindsey Creech and Manhal Izzy

11 Role of Social Workers in the Evaluation of Candidates for Liver Transplantation 151
Sonali Pendharkar

12 Evaluation of Living Donors for Liver Transplantation 163
Taylor M. Coe and Anand Ghanekar

Part II Transplant Process

13 The Liver Transplant Procedure 173
John J. Fung, Arielle Cimeno, Bijan Eghtesad, John LaMattina, and Rolf Barth

14 Deceased Donation and Liver Transplantation 203
Alicia Pérez-Blanco, Eduardo Miñambres, and Beatriz Domínguez-Gil

15 Liver Transplantation from Partial Livers: Living Donor, Split and Reduced-Size Transplantation 221
Sadhana Shankar, Ashwin Rammohan, and Mohamed Rela

16 Machine Perfusion in Liver Transplantation 241
Chase J. Wehrle, Rebecca Panconesi, and Andrea Schlegel

17 Histocompatibility Tests for Liver Transplantation: An Immunological Aspect 253
Qignyong Xu and Adriana Zeevi

18 Combined Organ Transplantation 263
Sangeeta Satish and Alejandro Pita

Part III Post-transplant Care

19 Interpretation of Blood Work After Liver Transplantation 281
William Carey

20 Immunosuppression and Treatment of Rejection After Liver Transplantation 289
Geoff McCaughan

21 The Role of the Clinical Transplant Coordinator in Liver Transplantation 299
Stacy Acevedo and Sandra Chicko

22 Post-transplant Liver Pathology 307
Nigar Anjuman Khurram

23 Early and Late Complications of Liver Transplantation 325
Alyssa Justus and James J. Pomposelli

24 Infection After Liver Transplantation 343
Anita R. Modi and Christine E. Koval

25 Role of the Interventional Radiologist in Caring for Patients with Complications After Orthotopic Liver Transplant 363
Anouva Kalra-Lall, Dhruv Patel, Anvit Kalra-Lall, and Sameer Gadani

26 Abdominal Imaging Post-Liver Transplantation 385
Xiaoyang Liu, Christie Cheng, Martin O'Malley, and Korosh Khalili

27 The Role of Interventional Endoscopy Post Transplantation 399
Mohamed Tausif Siddiqui and John Vargo

28 Disease Recurrence After Liver Transplantation 413
Marina Berenguer and Marta Tejedor

29 Post-transplant Metabolic Complications: A Contemporary Overview 435
Marius Vögelin and Nazia Selzner

30 Post-liver Transplant Malignancies 447
Maryam Sadat Aleali and Kymberly D. Watt

Index 465

Contributors

Laia Aceituno Sierra Multi-Organ Transplant Program, University Health Network, Toronto, Canada

Department of Medicine, Faculty of Medicine, Universitat Autònoma de Barcelona, Barcelona, Spain

Department of Medicine (Gastroenterology and Hepatology), University of Toronto, Toronto, ON, Canada

Stacy Acevedo University of Pittsburgh Medical Center, Pittsburgh, PA, USA

Abidemi Akinrinmade University of Pittsburgh School of Medicine, University of Pittsburgh Medical Center, Pittsburgh, PA, USA

Maryam Sadat Aleali Department of Internal Medicine, Division of Gastroenterology & Hepatology, Mayo Clinic, Rochester, MN, USA

Carmen Vinaixa Aunés Hepatology Unit, Digestive Diseases Department, Hospital Universitario y Politécnico La Fe, Valencia, Spain

CIBERehd, Instituto de Salud Carlos III, Madrid, Spain

Rolf Barth University of Chicago, Department of Surgery, Chicago, IL, USA

Marina Berenguer Hepatology and Liver Transplantation Unit, Hospital Universitario la Fe—IIS La Fe Valencia, CiberEHD and University of Valencia, Valencia, Spain

Rosa Blanes-Hernández Infectious Diseases Unit, Internal Medicine Department, Hospital Universitario y Politécnico La Fe, Valencia, Spain

William Carey Cleveland Clinic Lerner College of Medicine of Case Western Reserve University School of Medicine, Cleveland, OH, USA

Christie Cheng Department of Medical Imaging, University Medical Imaging Toronto, University Health Network, University of Toronto, Toronto, ON, Canada

Sandra Chicko University of Pittsburgh, Thomas E. Starzl Transplantation Institute, Pittsburgh, PA, USA

Arielle Cimeno Department of Surgery, University of Chicago, Chicago, IL, USA

Taylor M. Coe, MD Department of Surgery, University of Toronto, Toronto, Canada

Lindsey Creech Department of Medicine, The University of Florida, Gainesville, FL, USA

Beatriz Domínguez-Gil Organización Nacional de Trasplantes, Madrid, Spain

Bijan Eghtesad Cleveland Clinic, Digestive Disease and Surgery Institute, Cleveland, OH, USA

Claire Francoz Liver ICU and Transplantation, Hopital Beaujon, Clichy, France

John J. Fung University of Chicago, Department of Surgery, Chicago, IL, USA

Sameer Gadani Cleveland Clinic Foundation, Section of Interventional Radiology, Cleveland, OH, USA

Guadalupe Garcia-Tsao Yale University, Digestive Diseases Section, New Haven, CT, USA

Veterans Administration Healthcare System, Digestive Diseases Section, West Haven, CT, USA

Elena Gavrila Department of Internal Medicine, University of Texas Southwestern Medical Center, Dallas, TX, USA

Anand Ghanekar, MD, PhD Department of Surgery, University of Toronto, Toronto, Canada

Julie Gorham Intensive Care Unit, H.U.B. Hôpital Erasme, Brussels, Belgium

Thierry Gustot Department of Transplantation, H.U.B. Hôpital Erasme, Brussels, Belgium

Liver Transplant Unit, Department of Gastroenterology, Hepato-Pancreatology and Digestive Oncology, H.U.B. Hôpital Erasme, Brussels, Belgium

Laboratory of Experimental Gastroenterology, Université Libre de Bruxelles, Brussels, Belgium

Inserm Unité 1149, Centre de Recherche sur l'inflammation (CRI), Paris, France

UMR S_1149, Université Paris Diderot, Paris, France

EASL CLIF Consortium, European Foundation of Chronic Liver Failure (EF-Clif), Barcelona, Spain

Dempsey L. Hughes Department of Medicine, Division of Gastroenterology and Hepatology, Northwestern University Feinberg School of Medicine, Chicago, IL, USA

Manhal Izzy Vanderbilt University Medical Center, Division of Gastroenterology, Hepatology, and Nutrition, Nashville, TN, USA

Naudia Jonassaint University of Pittsburgh School of Medicine, University of Pittsburgh Medical Center, Pittsburgh, PA, USA

Owen Jones Department of Surgery, University of Toronto, Toronto, ON, Canada

HPB Surgical Oncology, University Health Network, Toronto, ON, Canada

Multi-Organ Transplant Program, University Health Network, Toronto, Canada

Alyssa Justus Department of Surgery, University of New Mexico School of Medicine, Albuquerque, NM, USA

Anouva Kalra-Lall Cleveland Clinic Foundation, Section of Interventional Radiology, Cleveland, OH, USA

Anvit Kalra-Lall Cleveland Clinic Foundation, Section of Interventional Radiology, Cleveland, OH, USA

Korosh Khalili Department of Medical Imaging, University Medical Imaging Toronto, University Health Network, University of Toronto, Toronto, ON, Canada

Nigar Anjuman Khurram University of Pittsburgh, Department of Pathology at the Thomas Starzl Institute of Transplantation, Pittsburgh, PA, USA

Christine E. Koval Cleveland Clinic Foundation, Cleveland, OH, USA

John LaMattina Department of Surgery, University of Chicago, Chicago, IL, USA

Fei-Pi Lin University of Pittsburgh School of Medicine, University of Pittsburgh Medical Center, Pittsburgh, PA, USA

Xiaoyang Liu Department of Medical Imaging, University Medical Imaging Toronto, University Health Network, University of Toronto, Toronto, ON, Canada

Nicolas Chong Lugon Yale University, Digestive Diseases Section, New Haven, CT, USA

Veterans Administration Healthcare System, Digestive Diseases Section, West Haven, CT, USA

Christian T. J. Magyar Department of Surgery, University of Toronto, Toronto, ON, Canada

HPB Surgical Oncology, University Health Network, Toronto, ON, Canada

Multi-Organ Transplant Program, University Health Network, Toronto, Canada

Department of Visceral Surgery and Medicine, Inselspital, Bern University Hospital, University of Bern, Bern, Switzerland

Geoff McCaughan Royal Prince Alfred Hospital, Centenary Institute, University of Sydney, Sydney, Australia

Alex Miller University of Pittsburgh School of Medicine, University of Pittsburgh Medical Cente, Pittsburgh, PA, USA

Eduardo Miñambres Transplant Coordination Unit & Service of Intensive Care, University Hospital Marqués de Valdecilla-IDIVAL. School of Medicine, Universidad de Cantabria, Santander, Spain

Anita R. Modi Cleveland Clinic Foundation, Cleveland, OH, USA

Mitra K. Nadim Division of Nephrology and Hypertension, Keck School of Medicine, University of Southern California, Los Angeles, CA, USA

Martin O'Malley Department of Medical Imaging, University Medical Imaging Toronto, University Health Network, University of Toronto, Toronto, ON, Canada

Rebecca Panconesi Department of Inflammation and Immunity, Lerner Research Institute, Cleveland, OH, USA

Dhruv Patel Cleveland Clinic Foundation, Section of Interventional Radiology, Cleveland, OH, USA

Sonali Pendharkar University Health Network, Toronto, Canada

Alicia Pérez-Blanco Organización Nacional de Trasplantes, Madrid, Spain

Alejandro Pita Department of General Surgery, Digestive Disease and Surgery Institute, Cleveland Clinic, Cleveland, OH, USA

James J. Pomposelli Tufts Medical Center, Boston, MA, USA

Luckshi Rajendran Department of Surgery, University of Toronto, Toronto, ON, Canada

HPB Surgical Oncology, University Health Network, Toronto, ON, Canada

Multi-Organ Transplant Program, University Health Network, Toronto, Canada

Ashwin Rammohan The Institute of Liver Disease & Transplantation, Dr. Rela Institute & Medical Centre, Bharath Institute of Higher Education & Research, Chennai, India

Mohamed Rela The Institute of Liver Disease & Transplantation, Dr. Rela Institute & Medical Centre, Bharath Institute of Higher Education & Research, Chennai, India

Gonzalo Sapisochin Department of Surgery, University of Toronto, Toronto, ON, Canada

HPB Surgical Oncology, University Health Network, Toronto, ON, Canada

Multi-Organ Transplant Program, University Health Network, Toronto, Canada

Department of Medicine, Faculty of Medicine, Universitat Autònoma de Barcelona, Barcelona, Spain

Sangeeta Satish Department of General Surgery, Digestive Disease and Surgery Institute, Cleveland Clinic, Cleveland, OH, USA

Andrea Schlegel Transplantation Center, Cleveland Clinic, Cleveland, OH, USA

Department of Inflammation and Immunity, Lerner Research Institute, Cleveland, OH, USA

Vishan Seetahal Multi-Organ Transplant, Toronto General Hospital, University Health Network, Toronto, ON, CanadaDepartment of Medicine (Gastroenterology and Hepatology), University of Toronto, Toronto, ON, Canada

Nazia Selzner Department of Medicine, Division of Gastroenterology, University Health Network, University of Toronto, Toronto, ON, Canada

Sapna V. Shah Division of Nephrology and Hypertension, Keck School of Medicine, University of Southern California, Los Angeles, CA, USA

Sadhana Shankar The Institute of Liver Disease & Transplantation, Dr. Rela Institute & Medical Centre, Bharath Institute of Higher Education & Research, Chennai, India

Mohamed Tausif Siddiqui Department of Gastroenterology, Hepatology and Nutrition, Digestive Disease Institute, Cleveland Clinic, Cleveland, OH, USA

Marta Tejedor Division of Gastroenterology and Hepatology, University of Iowa Healthcare, Iowa City, IA, USA

Fadi A. Tohme Division of Nephrology and Hypertension, Keck School of Medicine, University of Southern California, Los Angeles, CA, USA

Division of Pulmonary and Critical Care, Keck School of Medicine, University of Southern California, Los Angeles, CA, USA

Cynthia Tsien Multi-Organ Transplant, Toronto General Hospital, University Health Network, Toronto, ON, Canada

Department of Medicine (Gastroenterology and Hepatology), University of Toronto, Toronto, ON, Canada

Lisa B. VanWagner Department of Internal Medicine, Division of Digestive and Liver Diseases, University of Texas Southwestern Medical Center, Dallas, TX, USA

John Vargo Department of Gastroenterology, Hepatology and Nutrition, Digestive Disease Institute, Cleveland Clinic, Cleveland, OH, USA

Marius Vögelin Department of Medicine, Division of Gastroenterology, University Health Network, University of Toronto, Toronto, ON, Canada

Kymberly D. Watt Department of Internal Medicine, Division of Gastroenterology & Hepatology, Mayo Clinic, Rochester, MN, USA

Chase J. Wehrle Transplantation Center, Cleveland Clinic, Cleveland, OH, USA

Andy Wu University of Pittsburgh School of Medicine, University of Pittsburgh Medical Center, Pittsburgh, PA, USA

Qignyong Xu Department of Pathology, University of Pittsburgh, Pittsburgh, PA, USA

Adriana Zeevi Department of Pathology, University of Pittsburgh, Pittsburgh, PA, USA

Anudari Zorigtbaatar Department of Surgery, University of Toronto, Toronto, ON, Canada

HPB Surgical Oncology, University Health Network, Toronto, ON, Canada

Multi-Organ Transplant Program, University Health Network, Toronto, Canada

Part I

Pre-transplant Period

Indications for Liver Transplantation 1

Fei-Pi Lin, Alex Miller, Andy Wu, Abidemi Akinrinmade, and Naudia Jonassaint

Introduction

Liver transplantation has transformed the treatment landscape for patients with end-stage liver disease and various life-threatening malignancies. Transplantation provides those with end-stage liver disease with a curative option and offers life-prolonging therapy for carefully selected patients with cancer. The indications for liver transplantation encompass four major categories that are commonly encountered in gastroenterology practice: acute liver failure, complications of decompensated cirrhosis, metabolic liver disease, and systemic complications of chronic liver disease. In addition, less commonly encountered are the oncologic indications for liver transplantation. Lastly, a discussion around transplantation for severe acute alcoholic hepatitis, which has been a growing indication for transplantation over the last decade. Fundamental to transplantation is a basic understanding of its indications, which remains essential to optimize timely referral.

Timing of Referral for Liver Transplantation

The timing of transplant referral varies significantly by disease category. For example, acute liver failure demands immediate referral given its unpredictable course and high mortality rate without transplantation. In contrast, for patients with cirrhosis, the decision to refer requires careful clinical judgment. Importantly, in cirrhosis, the presence of cirrhosis alone does not constitute an indication for

F.-P. Lin · A. Miller · A. Wu · A. Akinrinmade · N. Jonassaint (✉)
University of Pittsburgh School of Medicine, University of Pittsburgh Medical Center, Pittsburgh, PA, USA
e-mail: Lin-linf3@upmc.edu; Miller-milleraj24@upmc.edu; Wu-wuay@upmc.edu; Akinrinmade-akinrina@upstate.edu; naudia.l.jonassaint@emory.edu

B. Eghtesad et al. (eds.), *Liver Transplantation*,
https://doi.org/10.1007/978-3-032-07072-2_1

transplantation. Rather, transplantation should be considered when patients develop complications of cirrhosis—ascites, hepatic encephalopathy, and variceal bleeding—that prove refractory to medical management.

The timing of liver transplant referral is largely based on disease severity and potential survival benefit. The measure of the severity of illness historically relied heavily on subjective criteria [1]. A transformative change occurred in 2000 with the implementation of the Final Rule, which mandated the development of an objective scoring system to ensure equitable organ allocation [2]. The Model for End-Stage Liver Disease (MELD) score, initially developed to predict mortality following transjugular intrahepatic portosystemic shunt (TIPS) placement, emerged as the standard [3]. The score's superior ability to predict disease severity and survival led to its adoption for organ allocation in 2002. Since then, the MELD score has undergone several refinements to enhance its predictive accuracy [4]] [5]. These iterations reflect an ongoing commitment to refining the objective assessment of liver disease severity while promoting equitable access to lifesaving transplantation.

With the MELD score came an objective means of assessing disease severity, and with that, the ability to measure who most benefits from transplantation. As liver disease worsens, the MELD score typically rises. Merion's study [6] demonstrated a clear survival benefit following transplantation for those with MELD scores above 15. This paper was critical in providing the needed guidance for when transplantation was advantageous to patients. Nevertheless, while for the majority of patients with end-stage liver disease, the MELD score is a good surrogate for disease severity, insome cases particularly with cholestatic liver diseases [7, 8], the severity of illness is sometimes not captured by the scoring system or the presence of decompensation. Therefore, while the MELD score provides an excellent initial framework for timing of referral in patients with cirrhosis, the decision must ultimately incorporate both the objective MELD score and presence of clinical symptoms, which diminish the patient's overall quality of life.

Acute Liver Failure

The triage of acute liver failure (ALF) represents one of the most critical decisions in hepatology. ALF differs from acute liver injury based on key features: the presence of encephalopathy in patients without pre-existing liver disease, illness duration under 26 weeks, and coagulopathy (INR $\geq$1.5) resulting from massive hepatocellular destruction [9–11]. Given the condition's potential for rapid deterioration and its high mortality rate, immediate transfer to a liver transplant center is imperative for patients meeting ALF criteria.

Etiology The etiology of ALF differs by geographic region. In developed countries, approximately 80% of cases are from acetaminophen toxicity, drug-induced liver injury (DILI), ischemia, hepatitis B, and autoimmune hepatitis. Conversely, in developing nations, viral hepatitis, particularly hepatitis A, B, and E, predominate as the primary causative agents [12]. This etiological distinction significantly influences both management approaches and outcomes, underscoring the importance of early recognition and appropriate triage in this critical condition.

Clinical Prognostication in ALF In the management of ALF, accurate prognostication is crucial for optimizing patient outcomes. Acetaminophen toxicity represents the leading cause of ALF in developed nations and many patients have the potential for spontaneous recovery with supportive care alone. This recovery potential must be carefully weighed against the significant implications of liver transplantation and lifelong immunosuppression. The grade of hepatic encephalopathy (HE) serves as a key prognostic indicator, with survival rates of 65–70% in patients with grade I-II encephalopathy, dropping dramatically to less than 20% in those with grade IV encephalopathy [13, 14]. Among the various prognostic scoring systems, the Kings College Criteria (KCC) remains the most widely utilized tool, particularly for acetaminophen-induced ALF, owing to its simplicity in bedside assessment [14].

Evidence suggests that while KCC demonstrates superior accuracy in predicting hospital mortality for acetaminophen-related cases, the MELD score may be more reliable for non-acetaminophen etiologies [14]. Although alternative scoring systems such as Clichy, APACHE II, and the Acute Liver Failure Study Group Index have demonstrated potentially improved predictive capabilities, KCC has maintained its popularity as prognostic tools in clinical practice due utility and ease of use [14–20].

In the context of acute liver failure, the single most critical decision remains early transfer to a liver transplantation center. The unpredictable trajectory and potential for rapid clinical deterioration in ALF demand immediate access to transplant capabilities. This urgency stems from the potentially narrow window of opportunity where emergent liver transplantation can prove lifesaving, making the timing of transfer a pivotal determinant in patient outcomes. Given these high stakes, delaying transfer to a transplant center could irreversibly compromise a patient's chance for survival, even in cases where the patient initially appears stable.

Complications of Decompensated Cirrhosis

Decompensated liver disease remains the predominant indication for liver transplantation worldwide, although the underlying etiology varies significantly by geographic region. In the United States, the landscape of liver transplantation has undergone a dramatic shift following the introduction of direct-acting antivirals for hepatitis C. Currently, alcohol-related liver disease and metabolic associated steatotic liver disease (MASLD) have emerged as the leading indications for transplantation in the United States, reflecting changing patterns of liver disease in Western nations [21–24]. In contrast, hepatitis B virus infection continues to be a primary driver of liver transplantation globally [25].

The onset of decompensation represents a seminal event in the natural history of liver disease, fundamentally altering both prognosis and management approaches [26]. Each year, approximately 11% of patients with cirrhosis will experience decompensation, marked by the development of ascites, variceal hemorrhage, or hepatic encephalopathy. This transition dramatically impacts survival, with median life expectancy decreasing from 12 years in compensated cirrhosis to less than 2 years following decompensation, with each additional decompensating event further reducing survival [26]. However, while decompensation often signals the need to consider liver transplantation, it is crucial to recognize that some patients can return to a compensated state with appropriate medical intervention. Specific examples include abstinence in alcohol-related liver disease, antiviral therapy in viral hepatitis, and immunosuppression in autoimmune hepatitis. Furthermore, advances in interventional procedures, particularly transjugular intrahepatic portosystemic shunt (TIPS), have emerged as powerful tools in managing refractory ascites and variceal bleeding [27–30] and improving transplant-free survival [31, 32]. Therefore, while liver transplantation evaluation should be considered when decompensation occurs, clinicians should thoroughly explore the therapeutic options in their treatment arsenal that might offer benefit and potentially delay or obviate the need for transplantation.

Ascites Ascites often represents the first clinical manifestation of decompensated liver disease, signaling the onset of clinically significant portal hypertension alongside other potential complications such as variceal hemorrhage and hepatic encephalopathy [33]. The development of ascites marks a critical prognostic threshold, with five-year survival rates dramatically declining from 80% to 30% after its appearance [34]. The pathogenesis of ascites involves a complex interplay of multiple mechanisms, including sodium retention, arterial underfilling, and portal hypertension, necessitating a multifaceted therapeutic approach [35, 36]. When evaluating patients with new-onset ascites, establishing its hepatic origin through diagnostic paracentesis is crucial, with a serum albumin-ascites gradient greater than 1.1 and total protein less than 2.5 g/dL confirming portal hypertension as the underlying cause [37]. Following diagnosis, management follows a stepwise approach, progressing from dietary sodium restriction and diuretics to more invasive interventions such as large-volume paracentesis or transjugular intrahepatic portosystemic shunt (TIPS) in refractory cases. The development of ascites should prompt early consideration of liver transplant evaluation, particularly in cases that prove difficult to manage with conventional therapy.

Dietary sodium restriction forms the cornerstone of ascites management, with patients prescribed a daily sodium intake of 2 grams (88 mmol/day). While sodium restriction is the first and possibly most essential piece of education, anecdotally, this step is often missed. The initiation should happen in parallel with sodium restriction to be most effective. While early studies supported initiating monotherapy with aldosterone antagonists for the first occurrence of ascites [38], practical experience has led to a common approach of starting combination diuretic therapy using a 1:2.5 ratio of loop diuretics to aldosterone antagonists (typically furosemide 40 mg and spironolactone 100 mg daily) to prevent hyperkalemia. In cases of tense ascites, large-volume paracentesis should be performed as the initial intervention followed by diuretic initiation. Importantly, when paracentesis volume exceeds 5 liters, albumin infusion at 6–8 grams per liter of fluid removed is crucial to prevent post-paracentesis circulatory dysfunction (PPCD) [39, 40]. For patients with refractory ascites despite optimal medical management, TIPS represents a valuable therapeutic option. Selection of patients with MELD scores ≤18 and without contraindications can achieve significant survival benefit from TIPS placement [41, 42]. Although TIPS may temporarily eliminate the need for transplantation in some patients, a subset will continue to experience refractory ascites, ultimately requiring transplantation as their definitive treatment. Therefore, while implementing therapeutic interventions for ascites, clinicians should simultaneously consider liver transplantation evaluation.

Hepatorenal Syndrome When faced with acute kidney injury (AKI) in the setting of ascites, hepatorenal syndrome (HRS) must be on the differential. Acute kidney injury (AKI) in cirrhosis, defined as an increase in serum creatinine ≥0.3 mg/dL within 48 h or an increase in serum creatinine of ≥50% [43], is a serious complication in patients with decompensated cirrhosis and ascites. While HRS must be on the differential for patient with ascites and AKI, the initial diagnostic approach should mirror that of patients without liver disease, recognizing that prerenal injury and acute tubular necrosis remain the most common etiologies in both populations [36, 44, 45]. Evaluation should include thorough clinical assessment, urinalysis, and urine sediment examination, complemented by a detailed review of potential contributing factors such as dehydration, diuretic use, contrast exposure, medications, and urinary obstruction. When intravascular depletion is suspected, an albumin challenge (1 g/kg for 2 days) represents the initial therapeutic step after addressing modifiable risk factors [46]. If creatinine fails to improve following albumin administration and alternative causes of AKI have been excluded, the diagnosis of HRS-AKI (formerly HRS type 1) should be considered [44]. At this point, vasoconstrictor therapy with either terlipressin or norepinephrine, in combination with albumin, becomes the standard of care. Treatment should continue until creatinine returns to baseline or for up to 14 days. Importantly, terlipressin should be avoided in patients with significant cardiopulmonary disease [47]. In settings where terlipressin is unavailable or contraindicated, the combination of midodrine and octreotide offers an alternative, albeit less effective option. While vasoconstrictor therapy can be highly effective [44], it is crucial to recognize these interventions as temporary bridges to liver transplantation rather than definitive treatments.

Variceal Bleeding Variceal hemorrhage represents a critical, life-threatening manifestation of decompensated liver disease, carrying substantial mortality [48]. Successful management requires a coordinated, time-sensitive approach beginning with prompt resuscitation and early endoscopic intervention, which should be performed within 12 h of presentation. The comprehensive treatment strategy includes prophylactic antibiotics (ceftriaxone 1 g daily for up to 5 days) and vasoactive medications (octreotide, terlipressin, or somatostatin for 2–5 days), alongside endoscopic variceal ligation as the primary therapeutic intervention [49–55]. In cases where endoscopic management fails, or when temporary bridging is needed, balloon tamponade or preferably expandable esophageal stents [56] can be employed while preparing for transjugular intrahepatic portosystemic shunt (TIPS) placement in select patients. Notably, preemptive TIPS (within 72 h of initial endoscopy) should be considered in high-risk patients, defined as those with Child's B score 8–9 with active bleeding during endoscopy or Child's C score 10–13, regardless of initial endoscopic success [57–59]. For patients who do not meet the requirements for preemptive TIPS, secondary prophylaxis combining nonselective beta-blockers with scheduled endoscopic band ligation represents the standard of care [60, 61]. Importantly, given the severity of liver dysfunction that variceal bleeding represents, parallel evaluation for liver transplantation should be initiated while optimizing medical management, recognizing that this complication may signal the need for definitive therapy with transplantation.

Hepatic Encephalopathy Hepatic encephalopathy (HE) represents a significant manifestation of decompensated liver disease, affecting 30–40% of patients during their clinical course [62]. The clinical presentation of HE encompasses a broad spectrum of neurologic and psychiatric manifestations, with family members and close contacts often providing the most valuable insights into subtle changes from the patient's baseline mental status. While ammonia levels, CT, and MRI may be included in the initial evaluation of mental status changes, these tests alone are neither diagnostic nor prognostic in HE and one should guard against making clinical decisions based on ammonia levels. Once HE is identified, the cornerstone of management involves identifying and addressing precipitating factors, including medication effects, non-adherence to treatments for HE, infection, dehydration, and bleeding, with approximately 90% of cases responding to correction of these underlying triggers [63]. Lactulose, a nonabsorbable disaccharide, serves as the first-line therapeutic agent, but persistent symptoms despite lactulose therapy should prompt further investigation for precipitating factors [64]. For patients with recurrent HE, the addition of rifaximin to lactulose therapy is recommended [65]. Lastly, in cases refractory to conventional treatment, contrast-enhanced imaging should be performed to evaluate for large portosystemic shunts that may contribute to persistent symptoms. Given the profound impact of recurrent HE on quality of life and its debilitating nature, liver transplantation should be considered for patients with symptoms that persist despite optimal medical management.

Metabolic Liver Diseases

Inborn errors of metabolism (IEM) represent a heterogeneous group of disorders that disrupt critical cellular metabolic pathways [66], potentially leading to severe illness or death. These conditions encompass disorders affecting amino acid, carbohydrate, and lipid metabolism; metal handling; and mitochondrial hepatopathies [66]. A hallmark feature of many IEMs, particularly urea cycle disorders (UCD), is hyperammonemia, which can result in devastating neurological damage or death due to increased intracranial pressure and herniation. Liver transplantation plays a crucial role in these disorders by restoring normal urea cycle activity, effectively providing a metabolic cure [67]. While IEM were traditionally considered pediatric conditions, it is important to recognize that UCDs can be unmasked in adults during periods of metabolic stress [68, 69]. Modern diagnostic approaches have evolved to include targeted genetic testing and whole exome sequencing as part of the standard evaluation process [70]. Encouragingly, studies demonstrate excellent post-transplant survival outcomes for these patients, highlighting liver transplantation as a definitive therapeutic option for patients with IEM [70].

While a full review of the metabolic disorders is beyond the scope of this chapter, Wilson disease (WD) is an important metabolic disease that manifests as acute liver failure in adults and requires rapid recognition and diagnosis. WD is a disorder of copper transport and excretion that results in pathological copper accumulation. While chronic WD can be effectively managed with copper chelation therapy or zinc salts, its acute presentation demands immediate recognition and rapid transplant evaluation. The acute presentation demonstrates a characteristic constellation of findings: severe coagulopathy, Coombs-negative hemolytic anemia, modestly elevated aminotransferases (typically <2000 IU/L), paradoxically low alkaline phosphatase [71], and rapidly progressive renal failure [72–75]. Korman [76] established highly specific diagnostic criteria for WD: an alkaline phosphatase to bilirubin ratio < 4 (94% sensitive, 96% specific) and an AST/ALT ratio > 2.2 (94% sensitive, 86% specific), with the presence of both criteria yielding 100% sensitivity and specificity in the studied population [76]. Acute liver failure due to WD carries a devastating mortality rate of 80–99% without transplantation [77]. This high mortality rate underscores the critical importance of early recognition and immediate referral to a transplant center when acute WD is suspected.

Oncologic Indications for Transplantation

Hepatocellular Carcinoma Hepatocellular carcinoma (HCC), accounts for approximately 80% of primary liver cancers and ranks among the top three causes of cancer-related deaths worldwide [78]. Given that HCC develops most commonly in the setting of cirrhosis, current practice guidelines from the American Association for the Study of Liver Disease (AASLD) [79] recommend regular surveillance with ultrasound every 6 months, along with alpha-fetoprotein (AFP) measurement, for patients with cirrhosis. While HCC can occur in non-cirrhotic livers, screening is currently only recommended for patients with chronic hepatitis B in the absence of cirrhosis. The treatment and prognosis for patients with HCC depends primarily on tumor burden (size and number), location, and presence of extrahepatic spread [80]. Liver transplantation, while a potentially curative treatment option according to the Barcelona Clinic Liver Cancer (BCLC) criteria [80], is typically reserved for patients who are not candidates for surgical resection due to their underlying liver dysfunction or tumor characteristics.

For patients ineligible for surgical resection, liver transplantation represents a compelling therapeutic option, offering the unique advantage of simultaneously treating both the cancer and the underlying chronic liver disease [81]. The Milan criteria [82] for liver transplantation in HCC patients, established nearly three decades ago, continues to serve as the gold standard for transplantation in HCC at many transplant centers around the world. These criteria specify eligibility as: single tumor ≤5 cm or up to 3 tumors each with diameter ≼ 3 cm with no vascular invasion and/or extrahepatic spread [82]. While various expanded criteria have been proposed [78], the challenge remains balancing broader inclusion with acceptable post-transplant outcomes. Treatment decisions ultimately require a coordinated multidisciplinary approach, incorporating expertise from transplant surgery, hepatology, interventional radiology, oncology, and radiation oncology to determine the most durable therapeutic strategy for each patient.

Hilar Cholangiocarcinoma Cholangiocarcinoma (CCA), the second most common primary hepatobiliary malignancy after HCC, comprising three distinct types: hilar, intrahepatic, and distal. Among these, hilar CCA (hCCA, also known as Klatskin tumor) accounts for approximately two-thirds of all cases and along with intrahepatic CCA, has emerged as amenable to transplantation in select patients. While potentially curative, surgical resection is achievable in only 25–40% of patients [83, 84]. A significant breakthrough in the treatment of hCCA came when Sudan [85] and colleagues first explored neoadjuvant chemoradiation, leading to the Mayo Clinic's development of a standardized pre-transplant protocol in 2002. Studies demonstrated [86] that for carefully selected patients with early-stage disease (stages I and II) durable survival could be achieved through a combined approach of neoadjuvant chemoradiation followed by transplantation. Transplanted patients achieved survival rates of 92%, 82%, and 82% at 1, 3, and 5 years respectively, substantially surpassing the rates of 82%, 48%, and 21% observed in patients treated with resection alone [86]. Therefore, select patients with unresectable hilar cholangiocarcinoma should be considered for liver transplantation.

Intrahepatic Cholangiocarcinoma Historically, intrahepatic cholangiocarcinoma (iCCA) has been considered a contraindication to liver transplantation at most centers, due to poor post-transplant outcomes demonstrated in early studies [87]. However, more recent retrospective analyses of incidental iCCA discovered in liver explants have revealed more promising results [88]. These studies demonstrated overall 5-year post-transplant survival rates exceeding 50%, with particularly favorable outcomes in patients with small tumors (<2 cm), who achieved an impressive 73% disease-free survival rate—significantly better than those with more advanced disease (tumors >2 cm or multifocal disease) [88]. Unlike hepatocellular carcinoma and hCCA, iCCA do not qualify for MELD exception points in the current organ allocation system. Nonetheless, the allocation system remains iterative and iCCA is under consideration for MELD exception points. In the interim, living donor liver transplantation (LDLT) as an early intervention for carefully selected iCCA patients who might achieve durable survival with transplantation and remains an option at some transplant centers.

Metastatic Colorectal Cancer The history of liver transplantation for colorectal liver metastasis (CLM) reflects an evolution in transplant oncology. Originally attempted during the earliest days of liver transplantation, the approach was abandoned due to poor outcomes [89, 90] before being successfully revisited decades later. The 2013 SECA trial [91] marked a turning point in this field, demonstrating promising outcomes in a prospective study of carefully selected patients. Among 21 patients without extrahepatic disease, the trial reported 1-, 3-, and 5-year survival rates of 95%, 68%, and 60% respectively, with a median survival of 27 months [91]. While post-transplant disease recurrence occurred early (median 6 months), patients with exclusively extrahepatic recurrence, primarily pulmonary metastases, achieved 5-year survival rates of 72%, notably, without any standardized protocol for neoadjuvant or adjuvant chemotherapy [91]. The growing evidence supporting liver transplantation for CLM reveals superior survival compared to standard chemotherapy alone. Although prospective data comparing transplantation with modern chemotherapeutic agents and multimodal treatments are still pending, current literature suggests clear benefits of liver transplantation for carefully selected CLM patients [91].

Metastatic Neuroendocrine Tumor Metastatic neuroendocrine tumor (NET) represents an established indication for liver transplantation. While surgical resection remains the first-line treatment for patients with liver metastases from neuroendocrine tumors, particularly in cases of solitary lesions or unilobar disease, curative resection is achievable in only approximately 20% of patients due to the frequently diffuse nature of metastases at diagnosis [92]. Liver transplantation emerges as a viable option when metastases are unresectable, prove unresponsive to medical or interventional treatments, or cause life-threatening hormonal symptoms [93]. Although no prospective randomized trials have definitively demonstrated the superiority of liver transplantation over resection or non-surgical treatments, orthotopic liver transplantation (OLT) for metastatic neuroendocrine tumors has shown promising results, with documented survival rates of 71%, 55%, and 44% at 1, 3, and 5 years, respectively [94]. However, transplantation is typically reserved for cases where all other treatment modalities have been exhausted, and careful patient selection following UNOS criteria is essential to optimize outcomes [95].

Systemic Complications of Chronic Liver Disease

Hepatopulmonary Syndrome Hepatopulmonary syndrome (HPS) represents an important complication of chronic liver disease and is the most common cause of respiratory insufficiency, characterized by intrapulmonary vascular dilatation leading to impaired gas exchange and hypoxemia [96]. Screening for HPS should be performed in all liver transplant candidates presenting with dyspnea or oxygen saturation below 96% [97], as early recognition is crucial given the associated twofold increase in mortality. The clinical presentation includes distinctive features such as cyanosis, clubbing, and the pathognomonic finding of platypnea-orthodeoxia [98], where breathlessness and oxygen desaturation paradoxically worsen when moving from a supine to upright position. While the diagnosis can be challenging in the setting of concurrent pulmonary conditions, contrast-enhanced echocardiography serves as the primary diagnostic tool. During this test, agitated saline is injected, and the appearance of microbubbles in the left heart three or more beats after reaching the right heart confirms the diagnosis; this finding occurs because the pathologically dilated pulmonary vasculature allows microbubbles to traverse the pulmonary circulation. Although supplemental oxygen can provide symptomatic relief for affected patients, liver transplantation remains the only definitive therapeutic intervention. Patients who meet certain criteria: (1) presence of ascites, varices, splenomegaly or thrombocytopenia, (2) shunt on contrast ECHO or lung scan, (3) PaO_2 less than 60 mmHg on room air within 30 days of request and (4) no clinically significant underlying pulmonary disease are eligible for MELD exception points. Carefully selected patients with HPS have excellent survival with 75–88% 5-year post transplant survival [97].

Portopulmonary Syndrome Portopulmonary hypertension (PoPH), occurring in 2–9% of patients with portal hypertension [99], represents a distinct form of pulmonary arterial hypertension characterized by complex pathophysiology involving hyperdynamic flow, increased venous congestion, and pulmonary arterial bed obstruction or constriction. Most patients are initially identified through elevated pulmonary arterial systolic pressures on routine echocardiography, despite being largely asymptomatic, leading to confirmatory right heart catheterization. Diagnostic criteria include mean pulmonary artery pressure (mPAP) >25 mmHg, elevated pulmonary vascular resistance (PVR) >240 dynes.s.cm, and pulmonary capillary wedge pressure <15 mmHg. Interestingly, while the severity of liver disease (measured by MELD score or portal pressures) does not correlate with the initial clinical severity of PoPH [97, 100], the MELD score remains a crucial predictor of survival in these patients [101]. Management mirrors that of other forms of pulmonary arterial hypertension with the use of phosphodiesterase inhibitors (sildenafil, tadalafil), endothelin receptor antagonists (bosentan, ambrisentan), and parenteral prostacyclins (epoprostenol, treprostinil). Liver transplantation represents a viable option for selected patients with PoPH, with MELD exception points available for qualifying candidates. Importantly, post-transplant outcomes in patients with well-controlled hemodynamics are superior to those of non-transplanted PoPH patients and comparable to outcomes following transplantation for other indications [102, 103].

Other Indications

Severe Acute Alcoholic Hepatitis

In the management of severe acute alcoholic hepatitis (SAH), liver transplantation has emerged as a lifesaving intervention for carefully selected patients who fail to respond to medical therapy and face imminent mortality. While historically, a 6-month abstinence period (the "6-month rule") was strictly enforced before considering transplantation, this paradigm has evolved significantly following Mathurin's landmark study [104], which demonstrated remarkably improved survival rates with early liver transplantation (77% versus 23% in matched controls). Despite the controversial nature of allocating scarce organs to patients with alcoholic liver disease, particularly given the acute presentation without prolonged sobriety, the compelling survival benefit has led to increasing acceptance of early transplantation. Patients with SAH often receive high priority status for transplantation due to their critical condition and poor short-term prognosis without intervention. Subsequent research following Mathurin landmark study (2011), demonstrated that carefully selected SAH patients who undergo liver transplantation achieve post-transplant survival rates comparable to those transplanted for other etiologies [105–108], providing strong evidence to support this approach in appropriate candidates despite the ethical complexities surrounding organ allocation.

Liver transplantation has transformed the treatment of end-stage liver disease, metabolic disorders, and select malignancies, offering both curative and life-prolonging options. The timing of transplant referral varies significantly by indication, from immediate referral in acute liver failure to more nuanced decision-making in chronic liver disease, where medically refractory symptoms should guide the timing of referral. While the Model for End-Stage Liver Disease (MELD) score provides an objective framework for transplant prioritization, certain conditions warrant special consideration through MELD exceptions when the score doesn't fully capture disease severity, including those with cholestatic liver disease. Decompensation of chronic liver disease represents a critical turning point in disease progression, and when symptoms prove refractory to medical management, transplantation should be considered. The field has evolved to encompass transplant oncology, with liver transplantation now complementing traditional treatments for hepatocellular carcinoma, cholangiocarcinoma, and metastatic colorectal cancer. Regardless of indication, successful outcomes in liver transplantation depend on appropriate patient selection and timely referral.

Clinical Pearls

Timing and Referral

- Presence of cirrhosis alone is not an indication for transplantation—decompensation should drive referral
- MELD is a good surrogate for liver disease and is used for organ allocation
- MELD score greater or equal to 15 is a key threshold for transplant referral due to demonstrated survival benefit
- While the natural history of most patients' disease will be well represented by the MELD score, some conditions (i.e., cholestatic diseases) and patient's severity of illness will not represented by the score; those patients should be referred despite low MELD

Acute Liver Failure

- Three cardinal features: encephalopathy, illness duration <26 weeks, and INR ≥ 1.5 in absence of chronic liver disease
- Presence of hepatic encephalopathy is the most important clinical hallmark of the disease presentation
- King's College Criteria remains the most practical prognostic tool for acetaminophen-induced cases
- MELD score may be more reliable for non-acetaminophen cases
- Requires immediate transfer to transplant center

Wilson Disease

- Key diagnostic features: low alkaline phosphatase, Coombs-negative hemolytic anemia, modest transaminase elevation, and renal failure
- Diagnostic criteria: alkaline phosphatase/bilirubin ratio <4 and AST/ALT ratio >2.2
- 80–99% mortality without transplantation in acute presentation
- Requires immediate transplant evaluation when suspected

Decompensation Management

- Once patient decompensate, survival drops from 12 years to <2 years
- Some patients can return to a compensated state with specific interventions (abstinence, antivirals, immunosuppression)
- TIPS should be considered for variceal bleeding and ascites not responsive to medical therapy and with MELD ≤ 18

Ascites Management

- Paracentesis with SAAG >1.1 and total protein <2.5 confirms portal HTN as the cause
- Start with sodium restriction at 2 g/day immediately
- In addition to salt restriction, diuretics in 1:2.5 ratio (furosemide:spironolactone) should be initiated
- In tense ascites, paracentesis is first-line therapy
- Give albumin (6-8 g/L) for paracentesis >5 L
- Consider TIPS for refractory cases if MELD $\leq$18
- Patient refractory to medical management should be referred for transplantation

Hepatorenal Syndrome (HRS)

- HRS is a diagnosis of exclusion
- Should be consider in patient with ascites and AKI once other etiologies are ruled out
- Start with albumin challenge (1 g/kg for 2 days)
- HRS can be effectively treated with vasoconstrictor therapy plus albumin
- Avoid terlipressin in patients with significant cardiopulmonary disease

Variceal Bleeding

- Early resuscitation and endoscopic intervention (within 12 h) are essential
- Use prophylactic antibiotics (ceftriaxone) and vasoactive medications (octreotide, terlipressin, somatostatin) is the standard of care
- Consider Early TIPS (within 72 h) for high-risk patients (i.e., Child's B 7–9 with active bleeding or Child's C 10–13) regardless of initial endoscopic success
- Secondary prophylaxis with B-blockers and scheduled endoscopic band ligation (ideally every 2–4 weeks) for those not in the high risk group
- Variceal bleeding signals severe liver dysfunction; LT evaluation should be initiated alongside medical management

Hepatic Encephalopathy

- Ammonia levels, CT, and MRI are not diagnostic or prognostic
- Treat underlying precipitating factors (e.g., infections, dehydration, bleeding, med nonadherence)
- Lactulose is first line therapy; rifaximin is added for recurrent cases
- LT should be considered for severe or recurrent HE impacting QoL

Table 1.1 King's College criteria

Indicators of poor prognosis. Patients who meet criteria may benefit from liver transplant	
Acetaminophen Induced Acute Liver Failure (APAP ALF)	Non-acetaminophen Induced Acute Liver Failure (non-APAP ALF)
Consider referring patients with the following criteria for liver transplantation:	Consider referring patients with the following criteria for liver transplantation:
Arterial pH < 7.3 OR Grade III or IV hepatic encephalopathy AND INR > 6.5 AND Creatinine >3.4 mg/dL	INR > 6.5 OR Three of the following: Age < 10 or > 40 Seven days or more between onset of jaundice and encephalopathy Unfavorable etiology (non-A, non-B hepatitis, drug induced, Wilson) INR >3.5 Serum bilirubin >18 mg/dL

Malignancy

- Milan criteria for HCC: one lesion ≤5 cm, 2–3 tumors none >3 cm, no vascular or extrahepatic spread
- Cholangiocarcinoma requires neoadjuvant chemoradiation before transplant in selected patients
- Small (<2 cm) intrahepatic cholangiocarcinoma has good post-transplant outcomese
- Metastatic neuroendocrine tumors have a favorable post-transplant survival

Other Indications

- Early liver transplantation for severe alcoholic hepatitis can be considered in select patients with good social support
- All patient with dyspnea and/or O_2 saturation < 96% should be screened for HPS
- PoPH is confirmed on right heart cath: mPAP >25 mmHg, PVR > 240 dynes.s.cm and PCWP <15 mmHg
- MELD exceptions exist for certain conditions that are not captured well by the MELD scoring system (Table 1.1)

References

1. Brown RS Jr, Kumar KS, Russo MW, Kinkhabwala M, Rudow DL, Harren P, et al. Model for end-stage liver disease and Child-Turcotte-Pugh score as predictors of pretransplantation disease severity, posttransplantation outcome, and resource utilization in United Network for Organ Sharing status 2A patients. Liver Transpl. 2002;8(3):278–84.

2. Organ Procurement and Transplantation Network. Health Resources and Services Administration, HHS. Final rule. Fed Regist. 1999;64(202):56650–61.
3. Malinchoc M, Kamath PS, Gordon FD, Peine CJ, Rank J, ter Borg PC. A model to predict poor survival in patients undergoing transjugular intrahepatic portosystemic shunts. Hepatology. 2000;31(4):864–71.
4. Kim WR, Biggins SW, Kremers WK, Wiesner RH, Kamath PS, Benson JT, et al. Hyponatremia and mortality among patients on the liver-transplant waiting list. N Engl J Med. 2008;359(10):1018–26.
5. Kim WR, Mannalithara A, Heimbach JK, Kamath PS, Asrani SK, Biggins SW, et al. MELD 3.0: the model for end-stage liver disease updated for the modern era. Gastroenterology. 2021;161(6):1887–95 e4.
6. Merion RM, Schaubel DE, Dykstra DM, Freeman RB, Port FK, Wolfe RA. The survival benefit of liver transplantation. Am J Transplant. 2005;5(2):307–13.
7. Goldberg D, French B, Thomasson A, Reddy KR, Halpern SD. Waitlist survival of patients with primary sclerosing cholangitis in the model for end-stage liver disease era. Liver Transpl. 2011;17(11):1355–63.
8. Johannes Klose MAK, Metz C, Lehner F, Manns MP, Klempnauer J, Hoppe N, Schrem H, Kaltenborn A. Outcome stagnation of liver transplantation for primary sclerosing cholangitis in the Model for End-Stage Liver Disease era. Langenbeck's Arch Surg. 2014;399:1021–9.
9. European Association for the Study of the Liver, Electronic address EEE, Clinical practice guidelines p, Wendon J, Panel M, Cordoba J, Dhawan A, et al. EASL clinical practical guidelines on the management of acute (fulminant) liver failure. J Hepatol. 2017;66(5):1047–81.
10. Maiwall R, Kulkarni AV, Arab JP, Piano S. Acute liver failure. Lancet. 2024;404(10454):789–802.
11. Shingina A, Mukhtar N, Wakim-Fleming J, Alqahtani S, Wong RJ, Limketkai BN, et al. Acute Liver Failure Guidelines. Am J Gastroenterol. 2023;118(7):1128–53.
12. Stravitz RT, Lee WM. Acute liver failure. Lancet. 2019;394(10201):869–81.
13. O'Grady JG, Alexander GJ, Hayllar KM, Williams R. Early indicators of prognosis in fulminant hepatic failure. Gastroenterology. 1989;97(2):439–45.
14. McPhail MJ, Farne H, Senvar N, Wendon JA, Bernal W. Ability of King's College criteria and model for end-stage liver disease scores to predict mortality of patients with acute liver failure: a meta-analysis. Clin Gastroenterol Hepatol. 2016;14(4):516–25 e5; quiz e43-e45.
15. Kulkarni AV, Gustot T, Reddy KR. Liver transplantation for acute liver failure and acute-on-chronic liver failure. Am J Transplant. 2024;24:1950.
16. Rutherford A, King LY, Hynan LS, Vedvyas C, Lin W, Lee WM, et al. Development of an accurate index for predicting outcomes of patients with acute liver failure. Gastroenterology. 2012;143(5):1237–43.
17. Bernuau J, Goudeau A, Poynard T, Dubois F, Lesage G, Yvonnet B, et al. Multivariate analysis of prognostic factors in fulminant hepatitis B. Hepatology. 1986;6(4):648–51.
18. Gill RQ, Sterling RK. Acute liver failure. J Clin Gastroenterol. 2001;33(3):191–8.
19. Mitchell I, Bihari D, Chang R, Wendon J, Williams R. Earlier identification of patients at risk from acetaminophen-induced acute liver failure. Crit Care Med. 1998;26(2):279–84.
20. Knaus WA, Wagner DP, Draper EA, Zimmerman JE, Bergner M, Bastos PG, et al. The APACHE III prognostic system. Risk prediction of hospital mortality for critically Ill hospitalized adults. Chest. 1991;100(6):1619–36.
21. Younossi ZM, Blissett D, Blissett R, Henry L, Stepanova M, Younossi Y, et al. The economic and clinical burden of nonalcoholic fatty liver disease in the United States and Europe. Hepatology. 2016;64(5):1577–86.
22. Younossi ZM, Stepanova M, Al Shabeeb R, Eberly KE, Shah D, Nguyen V, et al. The changing epidemiology of adult liver transplantation in the United States in 2013-2022: the dominance of metabolic dysfunction-associated steatotic liver disease and alcohol-associated liver disease. Hepatol Commun. 2024;8(1):e0352.
23. Wong RJ, Singal AK. Trends in liver disease etiology among adults awaiting liver transplantation in the United States, 2014–2019. JAMA Netw Open. 2020;3(2):e1920294.

24. Wong T, Dang K, Ladhani S, Singal AK, Wong RJ. Prevalence of alcoholic fatty liver disease among adults in the United States, 2001–2016. JAMA. 2019;321(17):1723–5.
25. Terrault NA, Francoz C, Berenguer M, Charlton M, Heimbach J. Liver transplantation 2023: status report, current and future challenges. Clin Gastroenterol Hepatol. 2023;21(8):2150–66.
26. D'Amico G, Garcia-Tsao G, Pagliaro L. Natural history and prognostic indicators of survival in cirrhosis: a systematic review of 118 studies. J Hepatol. 2006;44(1):217–31.
27. Skeens J, Semba C, Dake M. Transjugular intrahepatic portosystemic shunts. Annu Rev Med. 1995;46:95–102.
28. Colombato L. The role of transjugular intrahepatic portosystemic shunt (TIPS) in the management of portal hypertension. J Clin Gastroenterol. 2007;41(Suppl 3):S344–51.
29. Ong JP, Sands M, Younossi ZM. Transjugular intrahepatic portosystemic shunts (TIPS): a decade later. J Clin Gastroenterol. 2000;30(1):14–28.
30. Boyer TD. Transjugular intrahepatic portosystemic shunt: current status. Gastroenterology. 2003;124(6):1700–10.
31. Larrue H, D'Amico G, Olivas P, Lv Y, Bucsics T, Rudler M, et al. TIPS prevents further decompensation and improves survival in patients with cirrhosis and portal hypertension in an individual patient data meta-analysis. J Hepatol. 2023;79(3):692–703.
32. Bai M, Qi XS, Yang ZP, Yang M, Fan DM, Han GH. TIPS improves liver transplantation-free survival in cirrhotic patients with refractory ascites: an updated meta-analysis. World J Gastroenterol. 2014;20(10):2704–14.
33. Harrison PM. Management of patients with decompensated cirrhosis. Clin Med (Lond). 2015;15(2):201–3.
34. Pant C, Jani BS, Desai M, Deshpande A, Pandya P, Taylor R, et al. Hepatorenal syndrome in hospitalized patients with chronic liver disease: results from the Nationwide Inpatient Sample 2002–2012. J Investig Med. 2016;64(1):33–8.
35. Bernardi M, Moreau R, Angeli P, Schnabl B, Arroyo V. Mechanisms of decompensation and organ failure in cirrhosis: from peripheral arterial vasodilation to systemic inflammation hypothesis. J Hepatol. 2015;63(5):1272–84.
36. Angeli P, Gines P, Wong F, Bernardi M, Boyer TD, Gerbes A, et al. Diagnosis and management of acute kidney injury in patients with cirrhosis: revised consensus recommendations of the International Club of Ascites. J Hepatol. 2015;62(4):968–74.
37. Runyon BA, Montano AA, Akriviadis EA, Antillon MR, Irving MA, McHutchison JG. The serum-ascites albumin gradient is superior to the exudate-transudate concept in the differential diagnosis of ascites. Ann Intern Med. 1992;117(3):215–20.
38. Gatta A, Angeli P, Caregaro L, Menon F, Sacerdoti D, Merkel C. A pathophysiological interpretation of unresponsiveness to spironolactone in a stepped-care approach to the diuretic treatment of ascites in nonazotemic cirrhotic patients. Hepatology. 1991;14(2):231–6.
39. Runyon BA, Committee APG. Management of adult patients with ascites due to cirrhosis: an update. Hepatology. 2009;49(6):2087–107.
40. European Association for the Study of the L. EASL clinical practice guidelines on the management of ascites, spontaneous bacterial peritonitis, and hepatorenal syndrome in cirrhosis. J Hepatol. 2010;53(3):397–417.
41. Salerno F, Merli M, Riggio O, Cazzaniga M, Valeriano V, Pozzi M, et al. Randomized controlled study of TIPS versus paracentesis plus albumin in cirrhosis with severe ascites. Hepatology. 2004;40(3):629–35.
42. Narahara Y, Kanazawa H, Fukuda T, Matsushita Y, Harimoto H, Kidokoro H, et al. Transjugular intrahepatic portosystemic shunt versus paracentesis plus albumin in patients with refractory ascites who have good hepatic and renal function: a prospective randomized trial. J Gastroenterol. 2011;46(1):78–85.
43. Russ KB, Stevens TM, Singal AK. Acute kidney injury in patients with cirrhosis. J Clin Transl Hepatol. 2015;3(3):195–204.
44. Gines P, Sola E, Angeli P, Wong F, Nadim MK, Kamath PS. Hepatorenal syndrome. Nat Rev Dis Primers. 2018;4(1):23.

45. MacDonald AJ, Nadim MK, Durand F, Karvellas CJ. Acute kidney injury in cirrhosis: implications for liver transplantation. Curr Opin Crit Care. 2019;25(2):171–8.
46. Biggins SW, Angeli P, Garcia-Tsao G, Gines P, Ling SC, Nadim MK, et al. Diagnosis, evaluation, and Management of Ascites, spontaneous bacterial peritonitis and Hepatorenal syndrome: 2021 practice guidance by the American Association for the Study of Liver Diseases. Hepatology. 2021;74(2):1014–48.
47. Wong F, Pappas SC, Curry MP, Reddy KR, Rubin RA, Porayko MK, et al. Terlipressin plus albumin for the treatment of type 1 Hepatorenal syndrome. N Engl J Med. 2021;384(9):818–28.
48. Zhao JR, Wang GC, Hu JH, Zhang CQ. Risk factors for early rebleeding and mortality in acute variceal hemorrhage. World J Gastroenterol. 2014;20(47):17941–8.
49. Garcia-Tsao G, Abraldes JG, Berzigotti A, Bosch J. Portal hypertensive bleeding in cirrhosis: risk stratification, diagnosis, and management: 2016 practice guidance by the American Association for the study of liver diseases. Hepatology. 2017;65(1):310–35.
50. Seo YS, Park SY, Kim MY, Kim JH, Park JY, Yim HJ, et al. Lack of difference among terlipressin, somatostatin, and octreotide in the control of acute gastroesophageal variceal hemorrhage. Hepatology. 2014;60(3):954–63.
51. Wells M, Chande N, Adams P, Beaton M, Levstik M, Boyce E, et al. Meta-analysis: vasoactive medications for the management of acute variceal bleeds. Aliment Pharmacol Ther. 2012;35(11):1267–78.
52. Amitrano L, Guardascione MA, Manguso F, Bennato R, Bove A, DeNucci C, et al. The effectiveness of current acute variceal bleed treatments in unselected cirrhotic patients: refining short-term prognosis and risk factors. Am J Gastroenterol. 2012;107(12):1872–8.
53. Bernard B, Grange JD, Khac EN, Amiot X, Opolon P, Poynard T. Antibiotic prophylaxis for the prevention of bacterial infections in cirrhotic patients with gastrointestinal bleeding: a meta-analysis. Hepatology. 1999;29(6):1655–61.
54. Chavez-Tapia NC, Barrientos-Gutierrez T, Tellez-Avila F, Soares-Weiser K, Mendez-Sanchez N, Gluud C, et al. Meta-analysis: antibiotic prophylaxis for cirrhotic patients with upper gastrointestinal bleeding – an updated Cochrane review. Aliment Pharmacol Ther. 2011;34(5):509–18.
55. Fernandez J, Ruiz del Arbol L, Gomez C, Durandez R, Serradilla R, Guarner C, et al. Norfloxacin vs ceftriaxone in the prophylaxis of infections in patients with advanced cirrhosis and hemorrhage. Gastroenterology. 2006;131(4):1049–56; quiz 285.
56. Escorsell A, Pavel O, Cardenas A, Morillas R, Llop E, Villanueva C, et al. Esophageal balloon tamponade versus esophageal stent in controlling acute refractory variceal bleeding: a multicenter randomized, controlled trial. Hepatology. 2016;63(6):1957–67.
57. de Franchis R, Bosch J, Garcia-Tsao G, Reiberger T, Ripoll C, Baveno VIIF. Baveno VII – renewing consensus in portal hypertension. J Hepatol. 2022;76(4):959–74.
58. Boike JR, Thornburg BG, Asrani SK, Fallon MB, Fortune BE, Izzy MJ, et al. North American practice-based recommendations for Transjugular intrahepatic portosystemic shunts in portal hypertension. Clin Gastroenterol Hepatol. 2022;20(8):1636–62 e36.
59. Garcia-Pagan JC, Caca K, Bureau C, Laleman W, Appenrodt B, Luca A, et al. Early use of TIPS in patients with cirrhosis and variceal bleeding. N Engl J Med. 2010;362(25):2370–9.
60. Cheung J, Zeman M, van Zanten SV, Tandon P. Systematic review: secondary prevention with band ligation, pharmacotherapy or combination therapy after bleeding from oesophageal varices. Aliment Pharmacol Ther. 2009;30(6):577–88.
61. Gonzalez R, Zamora J, Gomez-Camarero J, Molinero LM, Banares R, Albillos A. Meta-analysis: combination endoscopic and drug therapy to prevent variceal rebleeding in cirrhosis. Ann Intern Med. 2008;149(2):109–22.
62. Amodio P, Del Piccolo F, Petteno E, Mapelli D, Angeli P, Iemmolo R, et al. Prevalence and prognostic value of quantified electroencephalogram (EEG) alterations in cirrhotic patients. J Hepatol. 2001;35(1):37–45.
63. Strauss E, Tramote R, Silva EP, Caly WR, Honain NZ, Maffei RA, et al. Double-blind randomized clinical trial comparing neomycin and placebo in the treatment of exogenous hepatic encephalopathy. Hepato-Gastroenterology. 1992;39(6):542–5.

64. Vilstrup H, Amodio P, Bajaj J, Cordoba J, Ferenci P, Mullen KD, et al. Hepatic encephalopathy in chronic liver disease: 2014 Practice Guideline by the American Association for the Study of Liver Diseases and the European Association for the Study of the Liver. Hepatology. 2014;60(2):715–35.
65. Bass NM, Mullen KD, Sanyal A, Poordad F, Neff G, Leevy CB, et al. Rifaximin treatment in hepatic encephalopathy. N Engl J Med. 2010;362(12):1071–81.
66. Oishi K, Arnon R, Wasserstein MP, Diaz GA. Liver transplantation for pediatric inherited metabolic disorders: considerations for indications, complications, and perioperative management. Pediatr Transplant. 2016;20(6):756–69.
67. Squires RH, Ng V, Romero R, Ekong U, Hardikar W, Emre S, et al. Evaluation of the pediatric patient for liver transplantation: 2014 practice guideline by the American Association for the Study of Liver Diseases, American Society of Transplantation and the North American Society for Pediatric Gastroenterology, Hepatology, and Nutrition. J Pediatr Gastroenterol Nutr. 2014;59(1):112–31.
68. Blair NF, Cremer PD, Tchan MC. Urea cycle disorders: a life-threatening yet treatable cause of metabolic encephalopathy in adults. Pract Neurol. 2015;15(1):45–8.
69. Stepien KM, Geberhiwot T, Hendriksz CJ, Treacy EP. Challenges in diagnosing and managing adult patients with urea cycle disorders. J Inherit Metab Dis. 2019;42(6):1136–46.
70. Vittorio J. CAQ corner: pediatric indications for liver transplantation. Liver Transpl. 2022;28(7):1245–53.
71. Shaver WA, Bhatt H, Combes B. Low serum alkaline phosphatase activity in Wilson's disease. Hepatology. 1986;6(5):859–63.
72. Roche-Sicot J, Benhamou JP. Acute intravascular hemolysis and acute liver failure associated as a first manifestation of Wilson's disease. Ann Intern Med. 1977;86(3):301–3.
73. Hamlyn AN, Gollan JL, Douglas AP, Sherlock S. Fulminant Wilson's disease with haemolysis and renal failure: copper studies and assessment of dialysis regimens. Br Med J. 1977;2(6088):660–3.
74. McCullough AJ, Fleming CR, Thistle JL, Baldus WP, Ludwig J, McCall JT, et al. Diagnosis of Wilson's disease presenting as fulminant hepatic failure. Gastroenterology. 1983;84(1):161–7.
75. Ferlan-Marolt V, Stepec S. Fulminant Wilsonian hepatitis unmasked by disease progression: report of a case and review of the literature. Dig Dis Sci. 1999;44(5):1054–8.
76. Korman JD, Volenberg I, Balko J, Webster J, Schiodt FV, Squires RH Jr, et al. Screening for Wilson disease in acute liver failure: a comparison of currently available diagnostic tests. Hepatology. 2008;48(4):1167–74.
77. Schilsky ML, Scheinberg IH, Sternlieb I. Liver transplantation for Wilson's disease: indications and outcome. Hepatology. 1994;19(3):583–7.
78. Moghe A, Ganesh S, Humar A, Molinari M, Jonassaint N. Expanding donor selection and recipient indications for living donor liver transplantation. Clin Liver Dis. 2021;25(1):121–35.
79. Singal AG, Llovet JM, Yarchoan M, Mehta N, Heimbach JK, Dawson LA, et al. AASLD practice guidance on prevention, diagnosis, and treatment of hepatocellular carcinoma. Hepatology. 2023;78(6):1922–65.
80. Reig M, Forner A, Rimola J, Ferrer-Fabrega J, Burrel M, Garcia-Criado A, et al. BCLC strategy for prognosis prediction and treatment recommendation: the 2022 update. J Hepatol. 2022;76(3):681–93.
81. Mahmud N, Hoteit MA, Goldberg DS. Risk factors and center-level variation in hepatocellular carcinoma under-staging for liver transplantation. Liver Transpl. 2020;26(8):977–88.
82. Mazzaferro V, Regalia E, Doci R, Andreola S, Pulvirenti A, Bozzetti F, et al. Liver transplantation for the treatment of small hepatocellular carcinomas in patients with cirrhosis. N Engl J Med. 1996;334(11):693–9.
83. DeOliveira ML, Cunningham SC, Cameron JL, Kamangar F, Winter JM, Lillemoe KD, et al. Cholangiocarcinoma: thirty-one-year experience with 564 patients at a single institution. Ann Surg. 2007;245(5):755–62.

84. Kimura N, Young AL, Toyoki Y, Wyatt JI, Toogood GJ, Hidalgo E, et al. Radical operation for hilar cholangiocarcinoma in comparable eastern and Western centers: outcome analysis and prognostic factors. Surgery. 2017;162(3):500–14.
85. Sudan D, DeRoover A, Chinnakotla S, Fox I, Shaw B Jr, McCashland T, et al. Radiochemotherapy and transplantation allow long-term survival for nonresectable hilar cholangiocarcinoma. Am J Transplant. 2002;2(8):774–9.
86. Rea DJ, Heimbach JK, Rosen CB, Haddock MG, Alberts SR, Kremers WK, et al. Liver transplantation with neoadjuvant chemoradiation is more effective than resection for hilar cholangiocarcinoma. Ann Surg. 2005;242(3):451–8; discussion 8–61.
87. Robles R, Figueras J, Turrion VS, Margarit C, Moya A, Varo E, et al. Liver transplantation for peripheral cholangiocarcinoma: Spanish experience. Transplant Proc. 2003;35(5):1823–4.
88. Sapisochin G, Rodriguez de Lope C, Gastaca M, Ortiz de Urbina J, Suarez MA, Santoyo J, et al. "Very early" intrahepatic cholangiocarcinoma in cirrhotic patients: should liver transplantation be reconsidered in these patients? Am J Transplant. 2014;14(3):660–7.
89. Foss A, Adam R, Dueland S. Liver transplantation for colorectal liver metastases: revisiting the concept. Transpl Int. 2010;23(7):679–85.
90. Hoti E, Adam R. Liver transplantation for primary and metastatic liver cancers. Transpl Int. 2008;21(12):1107–17.
91. Hagness M, Foss A, Egge TS, Dueland S. Patterns of recurrence after liver transplantation for nonresectable liver metastases from colorectal cancer. Ann Surg Oncol. 2014;21(4):1323–9.
92. Coppa J, Pulvirenti A, Schiavo M, Romito R, Collini P, Di Bartolomeo M, et al. Resection versus transplantation for liver metastases from neuroendocrine tumors. Transplant Proc. 2001;33(1–2):1537–9.
93. Blonski WC, Reddy KR, Shaked A, Siegelman E, Metz DC. Liver transplantation for metastatic neuroendocrine tumor: a case report and review of the literature. World J Gastroenterol. 2005;11(48):7676–83.
94. Mathe Z, Tagkalos E, Paul A, Molmenti EP, Kobori L, Fouzas I, et al. Liver transplantation for hepatic metastases of neuroendocrine pancreatic tumors: a survival-based analysis. Transplantation. 2011;91(5):575–82.
95. Organ Procurement and Transplantation Network. Guidance to Liver Transplant Programs and the Nationaal Liver Review Board for: Adult MELD Exception Review United Network of Organ Sharing. 2021. https://optn.transplant.hrsa.gov/media/2847/liver_guidance_adult_meld_201706.pdf.
96. Fuhrmann V, Krowka M. Hepatopulmonary syndrome. J Hepatol. 2018;69(3):744–5.
97. Krowka MJ, Fallon MB, Kawut SM, Fuhrmann V, Heimbach JK, Ramsay MA, et al. International Liver Transplant Society Practice Guidelines: diagnosis and management of hepatopulmonary syndrome and portopulmonary hypertension. Transplantation. 2016;100(7):1440–52.
98. Gomez FP, Martinez-Palli G, Barbera JA, Roca J, Navasa M, Rodriguez-Roisin R. Gas exchange mechanism of orthodeoxia in hepatopulmonary syndrome. Hepatology. 2004;40(3):660–6.
99. Krowka MJ. Portopulmonary hypertension. Semin Respir Crit Care Med. 2012;33(1):17–25.
100. Sithamparanathan S, Nair A, Thirugnanasothy L, Coghlan JG, Condliffe R, Dimopoulos K, et al. Survival in portopulmonary hypertension: outcomes of the United Kingdom National Pulmonary Arterial Hypertension Registry. J Heart Lung Transplant. 2017;36(7):770–9.
101. DuBrock HM, Goldberg DS, Sussman NL, Bartolome SD, Kadry Z, Salgia RJ, et al. Predictors of waitlist mortality in Portopulmonary hypertension. Transplantation. 2017;101(7):1609–15.
102. Salgia RJ, Goodrich NP, Simpson H, Merion RM, Sharma P. Outcomes of liver transplantation for Porto-pulmonary hypertension in model for end-stage liver disease era. Dig Dis Sci. 2014;59(8):1976–82.
103. Verma S, Hand F, Armstrong MJ, de Vos M, Thorburn D, Pan T, et al. Portopulmonary hypertension: still an appropriate consideration for liver transplantation? Liver Transpl. 2016;22(12):1637–42.

104. Mathurin P, Moreno C, Samuel D, Dumortier J, Salleron J, Durand F, et al. Early liver transplantation for severe alcoholic hepatitis. N Engl J Med. 2011;365(19):1790–800.
105. Lee BP, Mehta N, Platt L, Gurakar A, Rice JP, Lucey MR, et al. Outcomes of early liver transplantation for patients with severe alcoholic hepatitis. Gastroenterology. 2018;155(2):422–30 e1.
106. Weeks SR, Sun Z, McCaul ME, Zhu H, Anders RA, Philosophe B, et al. Liver transplantation for severe alcoholic hepatitis, updated lessons from the world's largest series. J Am Coll Surg. 2018;226(4):549–57.
107. Lee BP, Chen PH, Haugen C, Hernaez R, Gurakar A, Philosophe B, et al. Three-year results of a pilot program in early liver transplantation for severe alcoholic hepatitis. Ann Surg. 2017;265(1):20–9.
108. Im GY, Kim-Schluger L, Shenoy A, Schubert E, Goel A, Friedman SL, et al. Early Liver Transplantation for Severe Alcoholic Hepatitis in the United States–a single-center experience. Am J Transplant. 2016;16(3):841–9.

Pathophysiology of End-Stage Liver Disease

2

Claire Francoz

The clinical manifestations of end-stage liver disease are the consequence of liver failure and portal hypertension. Several organs or systems may be involved. It is important to note that the complications of cirrhosis are independent of the cause of the disease. Knowing the pathophysiology of each organ damage is important for guiding treatment. Interestingly, most complications of cirrhosis are completely reversible after liver transplantation.

Cirrhosis and Portal Hypertension

Cirrhosis is characterized by fibrosis and nodule formation of the liver, secondary to a chronic injury, which leads to alteration of the normal lobular organization of the liver. These architectural changes are accompanied by capillarization of the sinusoids and the formation of intrahepatic shunts [1]. In addition to this mechanical component, there is an increase in intrahepatic vasoconstriction due to the dysfunction of hepatic endothelial cells through the transformation of stellate cells into contractile myofibroblasts. These functional and structural abnormalities result in increased intrahepatic resistance to portal venous flow [2].

This increased resistance favours the development of portosystemic collateral circulation and splanchnic and systemic arterial vasodilatation, which in turn activates the vasoconstrictor systems (sympathetic nervous system and renin-angiotensin-aldosterone system) responsible for water retention and increased plasma volume. These hemodynamic and volemic changes also result in increased portal flow and worsening portal hypertension (despite the development of collaterals), sustained by the systemic inflammation observed in decompensated cirrhosis. This systemic inflammation is the consequence of microbiota changes and increased

C. Francoz (✉)
Liver ICU and Transplantation, Hopital Beaujon, Clichy, France

B. Eghtesad et al. (eds.), *Liver Transplantation*,
https://doi.org/10.1007/978-3-032-07072-2_2

intestinal bacterial translocation observed during cirrhosis. These changes are more pronounced the more severe the cirrhosis. The resident microbiota normally acts as a protective barrier against pathogenic bacteria. In cirrhosis, there is an imbalance between indigenous and non-indigenous (potentially pathogenic) species. Decreased intestinal motility is the main factor favouring microbial overgrowth. The mechanisms contributing to this reduction in intestinal motility are manifold and not yet fully understood. In addition to this reduced intestinal mobility, there is also an increase in intestinal permeability. In addition, qualitative changes in the local immune surveillance system (lymphoid tissue associated with the mucosa) contribute to a reduction in symbiotic homeostasis. Architectural changes associated with fibrosis affect the reticuloendothelial system that normally guarantees homeostasis between the host and the microbiome; Küpffer cells are less numerous and less functional, and hepatocyte synthesis of tolerogenic proteins is diminished. In the Acute-on-Chronic Liver Failure (ACLF) stage, a form of immune paralysis is observed, similar to that seen in sepsis. This immune paralysis is correlated with the more frequent occurrence of bacterial infections, the main "trigger" for acute decompensation and a major risk factor for mortality [3]. Bacterial translocation is involved in hepatic sinusoidal vasoconstriction and increased intrahepatic vascular resistance, as well as splanchnic and systemic arterial vasodilation via increased synthesis of TNF-α, a potent activator of inducible NO synthase. Lower systemic vascular resistance leads to increased portal flow, shear stress, and hepatic endothelial dysfunction. Bacterial translocation promotes the generation of microthrombi in portal venules, which contribute to parenchymal extinction and aggravate portal hypertension.

Consequences of Portal Hypertension and Systemic Inflammation: Extrahepatic Organ/System Dysfunction

Circulatory Dysfunction

End-stage cirrhosis is associated with low mean arterial pressure, an increase in heart rate, and cardiac output. This hyperkinetic syndrome becomes more severe as the disease progresses. It results from both splanchnic and systemic vasodilatation, which are responsible for effective hypovolemia. In response to hypovolemia, there is an activation of vasoconstrictive systems (angiotensin-aldosterone system, sympathetic nervous system, and antidiuretic hormone) which help to maintain euvolemia by retaining water and salt. Consequences are ascites, hyponatremia, and, in cases of extreme activation, acute kidney injury (AKI).

Acute Kidney Injury (AKI)

Several mechanisms contribute to the development of AKI in patients with cirrhosis, including circulatory changes, intrinsic kidney factors and systemic inflammation [4, 5]. At the early stage, decreased systemic vascular resistance results in a mild reduction in mean arterial pressure, which is balanced by increased cardiac output that maintains adequate kidney perfusion. At this stage, glomerular filtration rate (GFR) is preserved. In more advanced stages, systemic vasodilation increases, leading to a state of decrease in effective blood volume that induces systemic vasoconstriction systems, namely the renin-angiotensin-aldosterone system (RAAS), sympathetic nervous system (SNS) arginine vasopressin (AVP) and renal sodium and water retention. This stage is characterized by a switch from preserved to reduced kidney blood flow. At the most advanced stages of cirrhosis, renal vasoconstriction can no longer be balanced by increased cardiac output, and renal blood flow markedly decreases [6]. In addition to changes in systemic hemodynamics, alterations of intrarenal hemodynamic along with abnormal autoregulation of renal blood flow contribute to decreased GFR. [7] Decreased cardiac output, characterizing the so-called "cirrhotic cardiomyopathy" may contribute to decreased renal perfusion and altered GFR. [6] However, circulatory changes associated with portal hypertension and kidney factors do not explain per se all the changes observed during HRS and other causes of AKI.

Recently, the concept of systemic inflammation in multiorgan disease has emerged and challenged the vasodilation theory. [8] Sepsis is a common trigger of AKI in patients with cirrhosis. In patients without cirrhosis, hemodynamic changes and inflammatory response are clearly involved in the mechanisms leading to sepsis-associated AKI. [9] In severe sepsis, AKI may develop in the absence of decreased renal blood flow [10–12]. In patients with preserved renal blood flow, intrarenal microvascular changes resulting in decreased GFR may include an imbalance between preglomerular and postglomerular resistance (which corresponds to both preglomerular and postglomerular vascular tone) as well as impaired renal microcirculation affecting tubular and glomerular function [12]. Finally, it has been hypothesized that sepsis could lead to intrarenal redistribution of blood flow out of the cortex thus inducing corticomedullary junction ischemia with subsequent tubular injury [12]. In most clinical situations, hemodynamic changes are associated with systemic and/or renal inflammatory responses leading to microcirculatory changes and a significant reduction of perfused capillaries.

Even in the absence of overt bacterial infection, cirrhosis is characterized by a state of systemic inflammation, correlated to the severity of liver disease and portal hypertension. [8] Translocation of bacteria and/or pathogen-associated molecular patterns (PAMPs) from the lumen of the gut to the bloodstream is probably the main mechanism leading to inflammation. Translocation induces a wide spectrum of genes encoding molecules responsible for inflammation via specific receptors called pattern recognition receptors (PPR) [8]. Pro-inflammatory mediators may then extend to the systemic circulation and peripheral organs leading to extra hepatic organ dysfunction, including the kidney. For instance, patients with bacterial translocation have increased levels of pro-inflammatory cytokines (tumor necrosis factor-α [TNF-α] and interleukin-6 [IL-6]) as well as increased levels of vasoactive factors (such as NO) as compared to patients without translocation [13, 14]. A substantial proportion of patients with HRS have bacterial infection as a precipitating factor and/or systemic inflammatory response syndrome (SIRS) [15]. However, about 30% of patients with HRS have SIRS without documented bacterial infection [15].

Toll-like receptor 4 (TLR4) is the main PPR that has been studied in this field. In an experimental model of cirrhosis, inflammatory insult induced by lipopolysaccharide resulted in increased expression of TLR4 in proximal renal tubules and eventually, tubular cell injury [16]. In experimental models, digestive decontamination reduces expression of TLR4 and protects against tubular damage [16]. A similar overexpression of tubular TLR4 has been described in patients with cirrhosis and renal dysfunction [17]. Interestingly, a subset of patients with a diagnosis of HRS showed both overexpression of TLR4 in tubular cells and evidence of tubular cell damage. These findings suggest that a diagnosis of HRS does not exclude some degree of structural changes.

Overall, the pathophysiology of AKI in decompensated cirrhosis is complex with various factors being involved, including hypovolemia, administration of nephrotoxic agents, infection, and/or SIRS that may precipitate renal hypoperfusion and intrarenal circulatory changes, which are a hallmark of cirrhosis-associated AKI, regardless of the etiology.

Cirrhotic Cardiomyopathy

In patients with cirrhosis, a specific type of cardiac dysfunction occurring independently of the aetiology of liver disease has been termed cirrhotic cardiomyopathy (CCM). It combines structural and functional abnormalities of the myocardium in the absence of underlying heart disease. CCM is characterized by a combination of systolic dysfunction, impaired diastolic relaxation and electrophysiological disturbances such as prolonged QTC interval. Systolic dysfunction is defined by a blunted increase in cardiac output on exercise or pharmacological stimuli, and a resting ejection fraction <55%. Diastolic dysfunction is defined as a E/A ratio <1.0, a prolonged deceleration time (>200 ms), and a prolonged isovolumetric relaxation time (>80 ms). In addition, supportive criteria include electrophysiological abnormalities (prolonged QTC interval), heart chamber alterations (enlarged left atrium and myocardial hypertrophy), and humoral changes (elevated B-type natriuretic peptide, atrial natriuretic peptide, and hs-Troponin-1) [18, 19]. Pathophysiology is related to an inflammatory phenotype and protein/lipid/carbohydrate synthetic/metabolic defects [20]. Cirrhotic cardiomyopathy may be present in up 50% of patients with cirrhosis and seem independently of other complications of cirrhosis. It may be implicated in complications such as the development of hepatorenal syndrome. Cardiodepression during inflammatory conditions such as bacterial infection may contribute to the pathogenesis of acute kidney injury and acute-on-chronic liver failure. The reversibility of CCM after liver transplantation has not been yet investigated and so far, there is no specific treatment.

Hepatic Encephalopathy

Hepatic encephalopathy (HE) is a neuropsychiatric disorder of cirrhosis that can present with a wide range of symptoms, the most severe stage being coma. Although it is a frequent complication of cirrhosis, alternative or associated diagnoses must always be sought (in particular septic, metabolic, toxic/drug-induced encephalopathy, alcohol withdrawal, stroke, intracranial lesion, psychiatric pathology). The pathophysiological mechanisms of HE are multiple and as yet incompletely understood [21].

Ammonia has long been regarded as the key metabolic factor in the development of HE. In the presence of liver failure, decreased utilization of ammonia as a substrate in the hepatic urea cycle and portosystemic shunting lead to the accumulation of ammonia in the systemic circulation, which readily crosses the blood–brain barrier. Cerebral ammonia detoxification occurs via glutamine synthetase, exclusively expressed in cerebral astrocytes, in the formation of glutamine, which is an important precursor of the main excitatory and inhibitory neurotransmitters: glutamate and gamma-hydroxybutyric acid (GABA), respectively. Astrocytic glutamine accumulation exerts an osmotic effect resulting in swelling and cytotoxic oedema, which leads to increased brain water worsening HE. Hyperammonemia and subsequent glutamine accumulation induce changes in cerebral neurotransmission. Acute hyperammonaemia leads to excessive glutamate-induced N-Methyl-D-aspartic acid (NMDA)-receptor activation, which can cause neuronal death. Blockade of the NMDA receptor has been shown to be protective in this context. Also noted is an increase in "GABAergic tone," with an observed clinical response to flumazenil, a $GABA_A$ receptor antagonist.

In addition to hyperammonemia, inflammation plays a major role in HE. Potential pathophysiological mechanisms explaining the susceptibility to developing HE during episodes of infection include cerebral hyperaemia with increased brain ammonia delivery, astroglial oxidative stress with microglial activation and neuronal dysfunction, and innate immune system dysfunction arising from systemic inflammation and circulating endotoxemia. Finally, changes in the gut microbiota and dysbiosis in patients with liver cirrhosis are central to bacterial translocation, endotoxemia, and systemic inflammation and can result in the development of HE.

Coagulopathy

During cirrhosis, the usual laboratory tests assessing primary haemostasis (platelet count) and coagulation (prothrombin time) usually show abnormalities which, in the absence of liver disease, would put the patient at risk of bleeding. In fact, cirrhosis is a procoagulant state; cirrhotic patients are not protected against the risk of deep vein thrombosis or pulmonary embolism [22], and portal vein thrombosis is an event that occurs in 10–15% of patients undergoing liver transplantation [23].

Thrombocytopenia is common and can be explained by several mechanisms: splenic sequestration linked to portal hypertension, increased immunological platelet destruction and reduced thrombopoietin synthesis. In parallel with the severity of cirrhosis, von Willebrand factor levels increase, as do von Willebrand factor multimers, which improve platelet adhesion. Primary haemostasis is thus preserved. Occasionally, bleeding time is prolonged, reflecting impaired platelet function, but its impact on bleeding is debated. Despite the decrease in coagulation factors and fibrinogen associated with liver failure, thrombin generation in vitro is maintained or even increased in cirrhotic patients with platelet levels above 75,000/mm^3, due to the simultaneous decrease in coagulation inhibitors (protein C, protein S, antithrombin) and the increase in the procoagulant factor VIII. Elements of disseminated intravascular coagulation (DIC) and fibrinolysis (increase in D-dimer, thrombin-antithrombin complexes, fibrinopeptide A and soluble fibrin, decrease in clot lysis time) may also be observed, probably as a result of endotoxemia, which is common in cirrhosis, but the impact of these abnormalities is unknown [24].

Assessing haemostasis in cirrhosis is difficult. The usual tests do not correctly assess thrombin generation (prothrombin rate or INR). The INR was developed to monitor anti-vitamin K anticoagulation, not to assess thrombin time prolongation linked to liver disease. The thrombin generation test could be of interest, but its results are highly variable depending on the technique used, and it is not used routinely. Finally, platelet levels are not predictive of the risk of haemorrhage. Furthermore, digestive haemorrhage from ruptured oesophageal or gastric varices, the most frequent cause of bleeding in cirrhotic patients, is related to portal hypertension and not to haemostasis disorders.

Bacterial Infections

Cirrhosis significantly increases the risk of bacterial infection. It is estimated that the incidence of bacterial infections observed during hospitalisation in cirrhotic patients is in the region of 30–50%, compared with an average of 10% in non-cirrhotic patients [25]. The most frequent infections are urinary tract infections, pneumonia, bacteraemia and soft tissue infections. Bacterial infections are both a marker of the severity of cirrhosis and a factor often at the origin of cirrhosis decompensation. Overall mortality after an infectious episode is 30% at 1 month and over 60% at 1 year [26].

Among the mechanisms involved, bacterial translocation from the lumen of the digestive tract plays a key role. This is linked to a proliferation of digestive microbes, changes in the composition of the intestinal microbiota, an increase in intestinal permeability, and disturbances to the immune system (inhibition of Kupffer cells, other macrophagic cells in the body, and neutrophil polynuclear cells) [27]. Excessive alcohol consumption also promotes infection.

In addition to a particular sensitivity to bacterial infections, recent studies show that cirrhotic develop an inappropriate systemic inflammatory response in the event of sepsis. In these patients, sepsis induces abnormally high stimulation of monocytes, with blood concentrations of pro-inflammatory cytokines, including TNF-α and interleukin 6, higher than in non-cirrhotic patients [25]. This effect is more marked in patients with liver failure and decompensated cirrhosis than in patients with compensated cirrhosis, and contributes to the development of severe sepsis and multi-visceral failure. At the same time, secretion of interleukin 10, the main anti-inflammatory cytokine, is reduced in the monocytes. There are also quantitative and qualitative abnormalities in albumin during cirrhosis [28]. The antioxidant and anti-inflammatory properties of albumin are altered [28].

Conclusion

Pathophysiology of end-stage liver disease is complex and mechanisms are mainly due to systemic inflammation and hemodynamic changes. Most of complications are fully reversible after liver transplantation.

References

1. Huet PM, Pomier-Layrargues G, Villeneuve JP, et al. Intrahepatic circulation in liver disease. Semin Liver Dis. 1986;6:277–86.
2. Engelmann C, Claria J, Szabo G, et al. Pathophysiology of decompensated cirrhosis: portal hypertension, circulatory dysfunction, inflammation, metabolism and mitochondrial dysfunction. J Hepatol. 2021;75(Suppl 1):S49–66.
3. Wilde B, Katsounas A. Immune dysfunction and albumin-related immunity in liver cirrhosis. Mediat Inflamm. 2019;2019:7537649.
4. Durand F, Graupera I, Gines P, et al. Pathogenesis of Hepatorenal syndrome: implications for therapy. Am J Kidney Dis. 2016;67:318–28.
5. Gines P, Schrier RW. Renal failure in cirrhosis. N Engl J Med. 2009;361:1279–90.
6. Krag A, Bendtsen F, Henriksen JH, et al. Low cardiac output predicts development of hepatorenal syndrome and survival in patients with cirrhosis and ascites. Gut. 2010;59:105–10.
7. Stadlbauer V, Wright GA, Banaji M, et al. Relationship between activation of the sympathetic nervous system and renal blood flow autoregulation in cirrhosis. Gastroenterology. 2008;134:111–9.
8. Bernardi M, Moreau R, Angeli P, et al. Mechanisms of decompensation and organ failure in cirrhosis: from peripheral arterial vasodilation to systemic inflammation hypothesis. J Hepatol. 2015;63:1272–84.
9. Alobaidi R, Basu RK, Goldstein SL, et al. Sepsis-associated acute kidney injury. Semin Nephrol. 2015;35:2–11.
10. Langenberg C, Wan L, Egi M, et al. Renal blood flow in experimental septic acute renal failure. Kidney Int. 2006;69:1996–2002.
11. Langenberg C, Wan L, Egi M, et al. Renal blood flow and function during recovery from experimental septic acute kidney injury. Intensive Care Med. 2007;33:1614–8.
12. Prowle JR, Bellomo R. Sepsis-associated acute kidney injury: macrohemodynamic and microhemodynamic alterations in the renal circulation. Semin Nephrol. 2015;35:64–74.
13. Wiest R, Lawson M, Geuking M. Pathological bacterial translocation in liver cirrhosis. J Hepatol. 2014;60:197–209.
14. Albillos A, de la Hera A, Gonzalez M, et al. Increased lipopolysaccharide binding protein in cirrhotic patients with marked immune and hemodynamic derangement. Hepatology. 2003;37:208–17.

15. Thabut D, Massard J, Gangloff A, et al. Model for end-stage liver disease score and systemic inflammatory response are major prognostic factors in patients with cirrhosis and acute functional renal failure. Hepatology. 2007;46:1872–82.
16. Shah N, Dhar D, El Zahraa Mohammed F, et al. Prevention of acute kidney injury in a rodent model of cirrhosis following selective gut decontamination is associated with reduced renal TLR4 expression. J Hepatol. 2012;56:1047–53.
17. Shah N, Mohamed FE, Jover-Cobos M, et al. Increased renal expression and urinary excretion of TLR4 in acute kidney injury associated with cirrhosis. Liver Int. 2013;33:398–409.
18. Izzy M, VanWagner LB, Lin G, et al. Redefining cirrhotic cardiomyopathy for the modern era. Hepatology. 2020;71:334–45.
19. Moller S, Lee SS. Cirrhotic cardiomyopathy. J Hepatol. 2018;69:958–60.
20. Liu H, Naser JA, Lin G, et al. Cardiomyopathy in cirrhosis: from pathophysiology to clinical care. JHEP Rep. 2024;6:100911.
21. Rose CF, Amodio P, Bajaj JS, et al. Hepatic encephalopathy: novel insights into classification, pathophysiology and therapy. J Hepatol. 2020;73:1526–47.
22. Tripodi A, Mannucci PM. The coagulopathy of chronic liver disease. N Engl J Med. 2011;365:147–56.
23. Francoz C, Valla D, Durand F. Portal vein thrombosis, cirrhosis, and liver transplantation. J Hepatol. 2012;57:203–12.
24. O'Leary JG, Greenberg CS, Patton HM, et al. AGA clinical practice update: coagulation in cirrhosis. Gastroenterology. 2019;157(34–43):e31.
25. Gustot T, Durand F, Lebrec D, et al. Severe sepsis in cirrhosis. Hepatology. 2009;50:2022–33.
26. Dionigi E, Garcovich M, Borzio M, et al. Bacterial infections change natural history of cirrhosis irrespective of liver disease severity. Am J Gastroenterol. 2017;112:588–96.
27. Piano S, Fasolato S, Salinas F, et al. The empirical antibiotic treatment of nosocomial spontaneous bacterial peritonitis: results of a randomized, controlled clinical trial. Hepatology. 2016;63:1299–309.
28. Arroyo V, Garcia-Martinez R, Salvatella X. Human serum albumin, systemic inflammation, and cirrhosis. J Hepatol. 2014;61:396–407.

Candidate Evaluation for Liver Transplantation

3

Laia Aceituno Sierra, Vishan Seetahal, and Cynthia Tsien

Key Points

- Holistic Evaluation: Comprehensive assessment is essential to optimize outcomes for liver transplant candidates, addressing factors from liver anatomy to cardiovascular health, pulmonary function, renal status, nutritional status, infectious disease risks, and extra-hepatic malignancy screening.
- Cardiovascular Risk Management: Rigorous screening and management of cardiovascular risks are paramount due to their significant impact on post-transplant mortality, with strategies ranging from non-invasive stress tests to invasive coronary angiography for higher-risk patients.
- Nutritional and Frailty Assessment: Identification and management of sarcopenia, frailty, and nutritional deficiencies are crucial to reduce perioperative complications and improve overall survival post-transplant.

In this chapter, we are going to review the LT candidate evaluation.

Liver Anatomic Evaluation

All patients should undergo a contrast-enhanced computed tomography (CT) abdomen to determine the hepatic volume and size, assess the patency and anatomy of the vascular inflow and outflow of the liver for preoperative planning, and exclude conditions that could complicate the surgery, including large shunts [1].

L. Aceituno Sierra · V. Seetahal · C. Tsien (✉)
Multi-Organ Transplant, Toronto General Hospital, University Health Network, Toronto, ON, Canada

Department of Medicine (Gastroenterology and Hepatology), University of Toronto, Toronto, ON, Canada
e-mail: cynthia.tsien@uhn.ca

B. Eghtesad et al. (eds.), *Liver Transplantation*,
https://doi.org/10.1007/978-3-032-07072-2_3

It is also crucial for primary liver tumor staging and ruling out cholangiocarcinoma and metastatic lesions. If CT abdomen is unavailable or contraindicated in patients with a severe contrast allergy or renal impairment, ultrasonography (US) with doppler can be used, although it has limitations including poorer visibility, and requires patient cooperation and a trained sonographer. Magnetic Resonance Imaging (MRI) presents another option that can be safely used in candidates with renal dysfunction [2]. However, it also requires patient cooperation and is less cost-effective (Table 3.1).

Preoperative determination of the volume is critical to match the recipient and donor appropriately. In an ideal situation, the transplant organ should be similar in size to the native organ. Optimal results could be achieved with more technical difficulties if the donated liver is up to 20% larger than the ideal estimated volume [3].

Conversely, smaller grafts are better tolerated, and up to 50% smaller than the optimal volume is acceptable [4, 5]. Additionally, small livers could experience torsion, in which case the falciform ligament may need to be fixed.

Table 3.1 Pre-liver transplant work-up

Assessment	Test recommended
Blood work	Complete blood count with differential Complete biochemistry panel (including alanine aminotransferase, aspartate aminotransferase, total bilirubin and fractionated bilirubin, alkaline phosphatase, creatinine, eGFR, sodium, potassium, calcium, magnesium, and phosphate) Coagulation panel (PT/INR, APTT, serum fibrinogen levels) Blood group cross-match/typing Serum alpha-fetoprotein (AFP) Thyroid profile Lipid profile HbA1C, fasting, and post-prandial sugars
Endoscopic procedures	Gastroscopy Colonoscopy
Imaging	Abdomen-pelvis contrast-enhanced computed tomography (angio-CT) If any contraindication to CT: abdomen and pelvis Doppler US Mammography (for females in the age range)
Cardiovascular	ECG Transthoracic echocardiography (TTE) Stress test (when indicated) CT or conventional coronary angiography (when indicated)
Pulmonary	Chest X-ray Pulmonary function test Arterial blood gas analysis CT thorax (in select cases)
Kidney	If any alteration in the creatinine/eGFR: urine electrolytes, ultrasound with doppler of the kidneys
Sarcopenia, nutritional status and frailty	Liver frailty index Bone mineral density Nutritional assessment

(continued)

Table 3.1 (continued)

Assessment	Test recommended
Infectious diseases workup	HIV Hepatitis panel (HAV IgG, HBsAg, HBcore total, Anti-HCV) Rapid plasma reagin for syphilis Cytomegalovirus (CMV) IgG Epstein-Barr virus (EBV) IgG Herpes simplex virus serology Toxoplasmosis IgG SARS-CoV-2 (PCR test) Oral health
Special situations	CT or MRI of the brain for acute liver failure (ALF) and for individuals with a history of transient ischemic attack (TIA) or cerebrovascular accident (CVA) Electroencephalogram (EEG) for individuals with a history of seizure Females in the age range: pap smear + pregnancy test

Systematic evaluation of the hepatic artery, portal vein, and hepatic vein tracts is essential for identifying relevant vascular findings, such as vein thrombosis and anatomic variants of the hepatic artery (e.g., accessory or aberrant arterial origin). Portal vein thrombosis occurs in 5–12% of cirrhotic patients at the time of transplant evaluation. It is not considered a contraindication for liver transplantation with advances in surgical techniques and intravascular procedures allowing portal revascularization, although each case must be individually assessed [6].

Cardiovascular Evaluation

Cardiovascular complications are one of the leading earliest non-graft-related causes of death post-transplantation and the third most common cause of death overall [7]. The spectrum of cardiovascular events includes acute coronary syndromes (ACS), cardiac arrhythmias, right-heart failure, pulmonary edema, stroke, and pulmonary embolism [8]. Appropriate screening is essential for timely intervention to reduce these events.

Most ACS incidents after liver transplantation (LT) occur within the first month post-LT and are often due to preexisting coronary artery disease (CAD) [9]. Accurate pre-transplant CAD evaluation is crucial as the number and age of transplant candidates increase [10], and the epidemiology of liver disease changes. Metabolic dysfunction-associated steatosis liver diseases (MASLD) is an increasing indication for liver transplantation, but is also a CAD risk factor [11, 12]. These patients have a high prevalence of comorbid metabolic syndrome, diabetes, hypertension, and dyslipidemia. Screening for CAD in patients with end-stage liver disease (ESLD) is challenging because standard noninvasive tests have low sensitivity (13–32%) due to the cirrhotic hemodynamic changes: a hyperdynamic state with severe vasodilation; moreover, many patients are on beta-blockers [13, 15].

Cardiovascular Risk Stratification

The recommended approach for assessing cardiovascular risk (Fig. 3.1) starts with a comprehensive screening for cardiovascular comorbidities, including family history and physical examination. Baseline electrocardiogram and resting transthoracic echocardiogram (TTE) should be performed in all patients.

A risk-based approach is used, focusing on traditional cardiovascular risk factors (age, hypertension, smoking history, family or personal history of CAD, dyslipidemia, and diabetes) [16]. High-risk candidates should undergo invasive coronary angiography (ICA). Intermediate-risk patients should undergo noninvasive testing as outlined below, and if deemed to be high risk, an ICA should be performed. Low-risk patients do not require additional testing [17].

In order to risk-stratify patients into low or high cardiovascular risk, various scoring systems exist, with the CAD-LT score being the most commonly used [8]. It classifies patients with ESLD as low [2, 3], low-intermediate [4–6], high-intermediate [7, 8], or high risk [9–25] for CAD. Patients with risk factors, or intermediate CAD-LT risk score, should undergo non-invasive stress testing.

Functional stress tests are challenging in this population, especially for patients with decompensated ESLD due to ascites and some degree of hydrothorax, with limited exercise tolerance. Standard noninvasive testing includes dobutamine stress echocardiography (DSE) which in ESLD exhibits low sensitivity (13–32%) and a low negative predictive value (75%), and myocardial perfusion imaging (MPI)with low sensitivity (37%) for LT candidates who cannot exercise [13, 15].

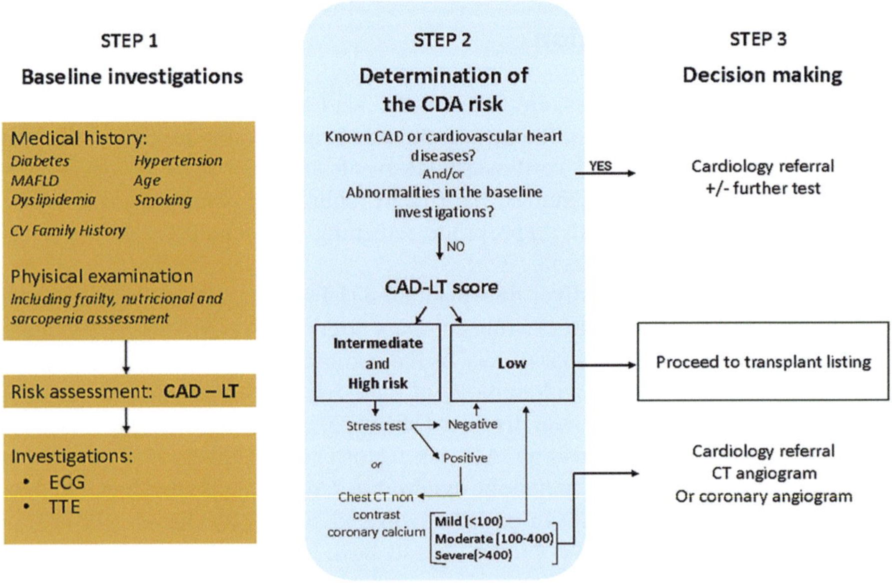

Fig. 3.1 Algorithm for screening for coronary artery diseases [8]

Coronary artery calcium (CAC) scoring has been shown to be predictive of cardiovascular events [18–20], although the optimum test and its exact role in conjunction with other risk stratification scores and noninvasive stress testing is still to be determined. Evaluating CAC on routine non-contrast chest CT is a cost-effective method of quantifying coronary calcium, with less radiation exposure compared with electrocardiogram-gated cardiac CT. In contrast, cardiac CT can identify subclinical CAD by calculating CAC scores and evaluating the degree of coronary calcium by the Agatston method [21] . In patients with high scores, ICA may be indicated even if LT candidates are asymptomatic, as the incidence of significant CAD requiring revascularization in this setting is as high as 24% [15, 22].

ICA remains the gold standard [8, 15] and it can be performed safely despite coagulopathy, thrombocytopenia and kidney impairment.

Management of Coronary Artery Disease

The management of CAD includes a Cardiology referral and, in many cases, a percutaneous coronary intervention (PCI) with drug-eluting stent (DES) insertion. This is usually followed by dual-antiplatelet therapy (DAPT), acknowledging the associated risk of hepatic decompensation and increased risk of upper gastrointestinal bleeding. The recommended duration is a short course of 3 months [23].

Coronary artery bypass alone is contraindicated in patients with a MELD score >13 or Child Pugh class B or C (score >7). In patients with diffuse cardiovascular disease or not amenable to revascularization, a simultaneous coronary bypass-LT with extreme caution could be considered at select transplant centers, due to the high risk of perioperative mortality and poor long-term outcomes [25].

Arrythmias

The primary screening for clinically significant arrhythmias (e.g., ventricular tachycardia, atrial fibrillation, and atrial flutter) is an electrocardiogram (ECG) [15]. Atrial fibrillation (AF) is the most common arrhythmia post-transplant; it has also been shown to be a marker of underlying hypertension and cirrhotic cardiomyopathy [25, 26]. It confers a higher risk of cardiovascular complications peri- and post-operatively. Any arrhythmias found during the evaluation should be accompanied by a referral to cardiology for further management.

Valvular Heart Disease

All LT candidates should undergo echocardiography. Any valvular disease should be referred to cardiology for further management. In severe valvular disease in LT candidates, pre-operative repair is recommended.

Aortic stenosis (AS) leads to pressure overload and left ventricular (LV) hypertrophy, along with reduced LV compliance. While asymptomatic mild to moderate AS is generally not considered a contraindication for liver transplantation (LT), severe or critical AS can cause hemodynamic instability during surgery and increase short and long-term mortality risk. Approximately 28% of LT candidates have mitral or tricuspid regurgitation, with tricuspid regurgitation (TR) being linked to poorer post-LT outcomes [27]. Transcatheter aortic valve replacement (TAVR) has become an important option for liver transplant candidates with severe aortic stenosis who face high surgical risks. The decision between TAVR and surgical aortic valve replacement requires careful evaluation of both technical and liver-specific factors, and is best made by a multidisciplinary team. Technical considerations include valve calcification patterns, particularly in bicuspid valves, along with access route feasibility and coronary obstruction risk based on coronary height and sinus of Valsalva dimensions. The liver disease itself introduces additional complexities, requiring careful coagulopathy management. Recent evidence shows that TAVR can be safely performed in selected end-stage liver disease patients, with post-procedure 1-year mortality and major adverse cardiac and cerebrovascular event (MACE) rate comparable to non-cirrhotic patients [28, 29].

Cardiomyopathy and Heart Failure

An ejection fraction (EF) below 40% is an absolute contraindication for LT, while an EF below 50% is considered as a relative contraindication [15]. An echocardiogram can detect heart failure with or without preserved ejection fraction. Cardiac magnetic resonance (CMR) can also be used to screen for structural or functional cardiac abnormalities.

Pulmonary Function Evaluation

Pulmonary complications can arise in patients with or without decompensation. Up to 70% of ESLD patients being evaluated for LT report dyspnea [30]. Additionally, around 45% of chronic liver disease patients in screening studies show abnormal arterial blood gas results [30].

Pulmonary disorders are commonly seen in patients with ESLD, either as a direct result of their liver condition or due to unrelated factors (e.g., smoking, asthma). To evaluate lung function (see Fig. 3.2), the assessment begins with a comprehensive screening for lung comorbidities (including a detailed smoking history if applicable) and a physical exam, chest X-ray, and pulmonary function testing with arterial blood gas. If any abnormalities are found, a high-resolution computed tomography (HRCT) scan of the chest should be performed before the transplant.

Chronic obstructive pulmonary disease (COPD) is a progressive condition marked by persistent airflow limitation due to inflammation and mucus hypersecretion. The epidemiology of ESLD remains unclear, but some studies suggest that

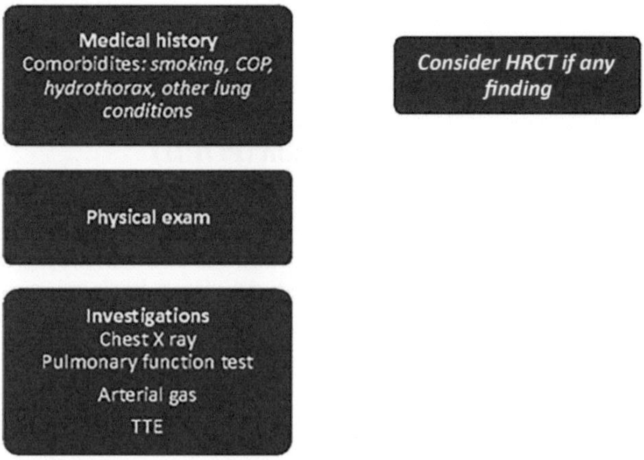

Fig. 3.2 Algorithm for lung function assessment prior to liver transplantation [27]

around 18% of liver transplant candidates are affected [31]. The forced expiratory volume in 1 s (FEV1) is commonly used to assess the severity of COPD, with lower FEV1 values indicating more severe obstruction. Active smoking and severe COPD are still considered contraindications for transplantation [32].

Special Situations

Hepatopulmonary Syndrome (HPS)

HPS is the most common pulmonary complication of portal hypertension, affecting 10–30% of patients undergoing LT evaluation [33]. It is characterized by intrapulmonary alveolar microvascular dilatation and arteriovenous shunts, leading to impaired gas exchange [34].

HPS can coexist with other pulmonary conditions, and its severity is determined by the degree of reduction in partial pressure of oxygen in arterial blood (PaO_2) levels [35].

Although pulse oximetry is suggested for screening significant hypoxemia, it lacks sensitivity and specificity.

The most effective screening method is contrast (bubbles) transthoracic echocardiography, normally, microbubbles (>10 mm in diameter) from agitated saline injected intravenously are only visible in the right heart and do not pass through the pulmonary vascular bed (8–15 mm in diameter). However, in the presence of extracardiac shunts (typically >15 mm), microbubbles can be seen in the left heart three or more cardiac cycles after appearing in the right heart.

A technetium-99 m labeled macroaggregated albumin lung perfusion scan can also detect and quantify shunts. Brain uptake >5–6% indicates an intracardiac or intrapulmonary shunt, as opposed to pulmonary parenchymal disease, which has uptake <5%.

HPS severity is categorized as follows: mild (PaO_2 > 80 mm Hg), moderate (PaO_2 60–80 mm Hg), severe (PaO_2 50–59 mm Hg), and very severe (PaO_2 < 50 mm

Hg). The only management includes oxygen and to prioritize patients with exceptions points on the wait list. While there is significant wait list mortality (20% 5-year survival), HPS usually will improve following LT.

Portopulmonary Hypertension (POPH)
POPH is characterized by the presence of pulmonary arterial hypertension (PAH) in the setting of portal HTN. In POPH, there is obstruction and remodeling of the pulmonary resistance arterial bed, which leads to pulmonary vasculature constriction and remodeling [36]. This leads to high pressure in the pulmonary artery, high right ventricular systolic pressure, and finally cardiac remodeling. POPH occurs in 5–10% of LT candidates. Autoimmune hepatitis and female sex are risk factors [37].

Routine screening echocardiogram will demonstrate right ventricular systolic pressure (RVSP), determined from peak tricuspid regurgitant velocity and estimated right atrial pressure. If RVSP is greater than 50 mm Hg, or in the presence of significant right ventricular hypertrophy or dysfunction, a right heart catheterization is indicated to distinguish from other causes of pulmonary hypertension, including volume overload and hyperdynamic circulation. Hemodynamic diagnostic criteria for PAH include mean pulmonary arterial pressure (mPAP) >20 mmHg, pulmonary vascular resistance (PVR) ≥2 Wood units, and pulmonary arterial wedge pressure ≤15 mmHg.

Elevated pulmonary artery systolic pressure (PASP) may indicate POPH, with a suggested threshold for further invasive testing being PASP >45 mm Hg. Mild POPH is defined by a mPAP of 25–34 mm Hg, while moderate to severe POPH is defined by mPAP ≥35 mm Hg. Patients with mPAP ≥35 mm Hg have a 50% mortality rate, increasing to 100% for those with mPAP ≥50 mm Hg [36, 38].

LT is feasible for patients with mild POPH. However, those with moderate to severe POPH should undergo a trial of vasodilator therapy (e.g., prostaglandins, phosphodiesterase inhibitors, or endothelin receptor antagonists) to reduce pulmonary pressures before LT can be considered [39].

Variceal Screening

All patients should have endoscopic screening for esophageal and gastric varices prior to transplantation. For patients with compensated cirrhosis undergoing transplantation for other indications (e.g., cholangitis, HCC), the Baveno VII criteria have established clear parameters for excluding high-risk varices in compensated cirrhotic patients. These criteria specifically identify patients at low risk when their liver stiffness measurement remains below 20 kPa and platelet count exceeds 150,000/μL, provided they have not experienced prior decompensation. For patients found to have high-risk varices, primary prophylaxis should be implemented using either non-selective beta-blockers or endoscopic band ligation based on patient-specific factors and preferences [40].

Hepatic Hydrothorax

Hepatic hydrothorax is a transudative pleural effusion in patients with portal hypertension, without primary cardiopulmonary abnormalities. It occurs in 4–12% of patients with decompensated cirrhosis and increases mortality risk [41]. Evaluation should include a chest X-ray and diagnostic thoracentesis to exclude other causes (e.g., infection, malignancy). Management before transplantation is conservative—the need for therapeutic thoracocentesis is guided mainly by patient symptoms such as shortness of breath or hypoxemia. The insertion of a chest tube is not recommended due to the risk of infection. For patients with refractory hepatic hydrothorax, transjugular intrahepatic portosystemic shunt (TIPS) placement can be carefully considered as a bridge to transplantation. The procedure can improve hydrothorax in 70–80% of cases [42]; however, precise stent placement is crucial as improper positioning may complicate or even preclude transplantation.

Renal Evaluation

Renal dysfunction before or after LT is usually multifactorial and critically impacts outcomes, including increased graft failure and decreased patient survival. Renal impairment is prevalent among cirrhosis patients due to functional kidney failure (hepato-renal syndrome), intrinsic kidney disease (like IgA nephropathy associated to alcohol consumption), or secondary to other comorbidities (diabetes or hypertensive nephropathy, for example), causing a multifactorial chronic kidney disease (CKD) [43–45].

Pre-LT kidney function is a crucial predictor of post-LT kidney outcomes [46, 47]. Acute kidney injury (AKI) post-transplant is very common, with a prevalence of 50%. This correlates with reduced long-term survival, increased acute graft rejection rates, infections, and longer ICU stays [46]. Pre-transplant factors linked to post-transplant renal dysfunction include diabetes and the presence of HRS [48].

Intraoperative factors like hypotension and acute blood loss, particularly in patients with decompensated cirrhosis, are risk factors for CKD development [49]. Terlipressin is recommended for patients with AKI-HRS, as response to terlipressin before LT can reduce the risk of CKD and the need for renal replacement therapy [50].

Patients with known CKD prior to LT may benefit from simultaneous liver-kidney transplantation (SLKT) [51]. However, predicting which patients will progress to kidney failure post-LT or who will recover remains challenging. If the patient has an Estimated Glomerular Filtration Rate (eGFR) $\leq$30 ml/min at the time of listing or has started regular dialysis, the patient should be evaluated by nephrology for SKLT [51]. Indications for SKLT are summarized in Table 3.2 [52].

Renal function evaluation includes creatinine level and eGFR. If the eGFR is below 60 ml/min, a comprehensive urinalysis, checking for red blood cells and proteinuria, urine protein-to-creatinine ratio, and a 24-h urinary estimation should be performed. In patients with kidney impairment, an abdominal US to measure

Table 3.2 UNOS/OPTN criteria for simultaneous liver-kidney transplantation [52]

CKD with a measured or calculated GFR ≤ 60 mL/min for > 90 consecutive days At least one of the following:	The candidate has started regular dialysis as a patient with ESRD in a hospital-based, independent non-hospital-based, or home setting At the time of registration on the kidney waiting list, the candidate's most recent measured or calculated CrCl or GFR is ≤30 mL/min
Sustained acute kidney injury At least one of the following, or a combination of both, for the last 6 weeks:	The candidate has been on dialysis at least once every 7 days The candidate has a measured or calculated CrCl or GFR ≤25 mL/min at least once every 7 days If the candidate's eligibility is not confirmed at least once every 7 days for the last 6 weeks, the candidate is not eligible to receive a liver and a kidney from the same donor
Diagnosis of at least one	Hyperoxaluria Atypical hemolytic uremic syndrome from mutations in factor H or factor I Familial nonneuropathic systemic amyloidosis Methylmalonic aciduria

kidney size, doppler studies, and prostate size assessment (in males) is recommended. In certain cases, a kidney biopsy may be necessary. All patients with an eGFR below 30 mL/min for more than 3 months must be assessed by a nephrologist as part of the evaluation.

Cystatin C has emerged as a potentially valuable biomarker for renal function assessment in liver transplant candidates, offering several advantages over traditional creatinine measurements. This protein's independence from muscle mass and bilirubin levels, coupled with its heightened sensitivity to early renal function changes, makes it particularly useful in the transplant population. However, accurate interpretation requires careful consideration of confounding factors, including inflammatory states, thyroid function, and steroid use, which can influence Cystatin C levels. Studies have demonstrated that Cystatin C-based equations provide more accurate GFR estimates in cirrhotic patients compared to creatinine-based formulas, though optimal assessment often combines both markers [53].

Special Situation

Hyponatremia

Dilutional hyponatremia predicts short-term mortality for LT candidates, independent of MELD score [54]. It has been shown that hyponatremia is associated with increased preoperative mortality [55]. Pretransplant hyponatremia also increases postoperative morbidity [56]. Any hyponatremia with sodium levels below 130 mEq/L should be investigated with serum and urine osmolality, and urine electrolytes. After ruling out other causes, it should be corrected with measures such as fluid restriction, cessation of diuretics, and albumin administration.

Sarcopenia, Nutritional Status, and Frailty

Patients with end-stage liver disease (ESLD) frequently develop sarcopenia, characterized by loss of muscle mass. This condition stems from multiple factors: altered taste sensation, dietary restrictions such as low-sodium diets, and the presence of ascites, all of which contribute to poor nutritional intake [57]. The challenge is compounded by patients' increased catabolic states, which demand higher protein requirements. Sarcopenia affects a significant portion of ESLD patients, ranging from 30% to 70%, and its implications are serious. Patients with sarcopenia face increased operative risks, higher mortality rates, more frequent hospital admissions, and poorer outcomes following transplantation [58].

Diagnosis of sarcopenia is made through various imaging techniques. Abdominal CT scans allow measurement of the skeletal muscle index (SMI), while alternatives include DEXA scans, muscle ultrasound, and bioimpedance analysis, depending on local resources. There are no standardized cut-offs that preclude LT [60]. For nutritional assessment, prealbumin has emerged as the preferred marker over albumin, owing to its shorter half-life of 2–3 days, making it more responsive to changes in metabolic status [45, 61–63]. During the pre-transplant period, patients are typically recommended to consume 1.2–1.5 g/kg/day of protein.

Frailty, which indicates increased vulnerability to health stressors, represents another crucial aspect of ESLD patient assessment [64, 65]. The 6-Minute Walk Test (6MWT) serves as a valuable tool for evaluating functional status. Research has shown that patients who can walk less than 250 meters during this test face a higher risk of post-transplant mortality. Conversely, each additional 100 meters achieved correlates significantly with improved survival prospects (hazard ratio 0.48, $p = 0.0001$) [59].

The liver-specific frailty index (FrAI LT) provides a comprehensive assessment framework specifically designed for ESLD patients [66]. This index evaluates three key components: grip strength measured with a hand-held dynamometer, the time required to complete five chair stands, and balance testing across various positions. Scores exceeding 4.5, typically seen in the 80th percentile of patients, indicate frailty. The FrAI LT has proven particularly valuable as it can enhance mortality risk predictions when used in conjunction with the MELD Na score. Importantly, the introduction of these frailty measurements into clinical practice has led to the development of pre-habilitation programs, which have shown promising results in improving patient outcomes [67–69].

Special Situations

Age

Currently, there is a demographic shift, whereby countries are moving to a more elderly population. While there is no absolute age limit for transplantation, post-operative complications are more prevalent and long-term outcomes may be suboptimal in elderly patients. Generally, the age threshold is 70 years old, although some studies showed that, instead of the age, it is more important to conduct a proper frailty evaluation [70]. Candidates in this age group are carefully screened for concomitant diseases, with some individuals deemed ineligible due to comorbid conditions or frailty that could negatively impact short-term outcomes.

Obesity

Obesity presents challenges in LT candidate selection and is increasingly prevalent due to the obesity epidemic. Pretransplant obesity, particularly class III (BMI >40), has been associated with higher waitlist mortality and increased risk of early posttransplant complications such as infection, respiratory failure, and wound dehiscence [71]. Some studies have shown reduced survival in patients with class I (BMI 30–34.9) and class II (BMI 35–39.9) obesity, although more recent studies have not demonstrated reduced survival in class III obesity patients (BMI >40); leading many centers to reconsider arbitrary BMI thresholds for candidacy [71–73].

Sleeve gastrectomy has shown promising results both before and during liver transplant. Elective bariatric surgery in patients with decompensated cirrhosis is generally approached with caution due to higher morbidity and mortality rates [74, 75].

Infectious Diseases Screening

A comprehensive evaluation from the infectious perspective is essential, as pretransplant infection increases the risk of post-transplant infection-related mortality. Screening includes a thorough medical history, with information on previous infections, vaccinations, travel, and occupational exposures to identify any increased risk for blood-borne or sexually transmitted pathogens. Physical examination should include skin and soft tissue assessment.

Standard screening laboratory tests should include serological testing for viral hepatitis (Hepatitis A, B, C), human immunodeficiency virus (HIV), Epstein-Barr virus (EBV), cytomegalovirus (CMV), herpes simplex virus (HSV), venereal disease research laboratory (VDRL) or rapid plasma reagin test (RPR), SARS-CoV-2 (PCR test), toxoplasma, and any testing as indicated by candidate's history. Tuberculosis testing using interferon-gamma release assay (QuantiFERON Test) is also tested at selected centers in high incidence areas.

Prior to transplant the patient's vaccination status should be updated, see Table 3.3 for the recommended vaccinations [71, 76] including the SARS CoV2 vaccine [78–80].

Special Situations: Oral Health

Poor oral health is linked to worse outcomes in patients with cirrhosis, prompting some centers to recommend dental evaluations [81, 82].

Table 3.3 Recommended immunization for adult patients prior to liver transplantation [76, 77, 80]

	Immunization schedule
Hepatitis B	2-dose Heplisav-B 4 weeks apart, or 3-dose Engerix-B, Recombivax-HB, or Twinrix at 0, 1, and 6 months
Hepatitis A	2 doses of Havrix 6–12 months apart, or Vaqta 6–18 months apart, or 3 doses of Twinrix at 0, 1, and 6 months
Pneumococcal	Dose of PCV13 followed by 3 doses of PPSV23 at: 8 weeks after PCV13 5 years after the previous dose When they turn 65 years (>5 years apart from the second PPSV23 dose)
Influenza (inactivated)	1 dose annually
Zoster	2 doses 4–8 weeks apart in seronegative candidates Zoster recombinant (Shingrix): **recommended pre-transplant** Zoster live attenuated (Zostavax): **not recommended**
Tetanus, diphtheria, and pertussis	1 dose of Tdap, then td or Tdap booster every 10 years
Measles, mumps, and rubella:	2 doses 4 weeks apart in seronegative LT candidates. Patients who have already received one injection must receive a second dose before LT
Human papillomavirus (HPV)	All patients should receive 3 doses through age 26
Meningococcal	**ACWY and B are r**ecommended for adults with additional risk factors/indications: Anatomical or functional asplenia Hematopoietic stem cell transplant Other additional factors
Hemophilus influenzae	Recommended for adults with additional risk factors/indications: Anatomical or functional asplenia Hematopoietic stem cell transplant Other additional factors
COVID-19	Options 3 doses of Pfizer-BioNTech mRNA, or 2 doses of Pfizer-BioNTech mRNA, or 3 doses of Moderna mRNA, or 2 doses of Moderna mRNA, or 2 doses of Novavax Adjuvanted, or 1 dose of Janssen adenoviral vector followed by mRNA vaccine Follow-up: all vaccination regimens should be followed by a booster dose of mRNA vaccines >2 months after the primary series

Extra-Hepatic Malignancy Screening

Pretransplant malignancy (PTM) in LT candidates increases the risk of cancer recurrence due to post-LT immunosuppression. The risk factors include the type of prior malignancy and the duration in remission. The decision regarding timing and candidacy for LT should involve a multidisciplinary team, assessing detailed staging, treatment history, cancer recurrence potential, treatment response, and disease stage. The specific waiting period between cancer diagnosis and LT listing varies based on the type of cancer and the effectiveness of treatment, as supported by evidence-based practices [83–86]. The recommendations made by international societies primarily reflect improved recurrence-free survival observed in the general population. Limited data are available specifically for LT or solid-organ transplant recipients, suggesting that modifications may be necessary.

Liver transplant candidates should undergo sex and age-appropriate screening for occult or underlying malignancy. Specifically, screening for colorectal cancer is required for individuals over 50 years old [87, 88]. If a colonoscopy is considered too risky, CT colonography may be an alternative option; however, it has not been validated in ESLD patients. The fecal immunochemical test (FIT) is a screening tool for individuals at average risk for colorectal cancer [89]. While several randomized trials are currently comparing FIT to colonoscopy for colorectal cancer screening, FIT has not yet been validated specifically for patients with end-stage liver disease (ESLD). In liver transplant candidates, colonoscopy remains the gold standard for colorectal cancer screening.

For patients with alcohol consumption and/or smoking history (current or past), it is essential to screen for pulmonary neoplasms [90], as well as oropharyngeal and esophageal malignancies [86]. It is recommended to include an ear, nose, and throat examination with nasofibroscopy, an oral cavity examination, and an upper gastrointestinal endoscopy.

Female patients should receive regular gynecological screening, including Pap smears and mammograms (starting at 40 if no risk factor) as needed [91]. Prostate disease screening should be conducted based on the urologist's recommendations.

The most common de novo cancer post-LT is skin cancer [92, 93]. LT candidates should undergo thorough skin examinations, noting that non-melanotic skin cancers typically do not contraindicate liver transplantation.

Psychosocial Considerations

Patients should have thorough evaluation by social work to ensure that they have adequate social support and no compliance issues prohibiting adherence to postoperative and follow-up care. This is outlined in more detail elsewhere in this book.

Conclusion

The evaluation of candidates for LT requires a comprehensive assessment to optimize outcomes in a challenging landscape of organ shortage and increasing patient complexity, underscoring the critical need for cautious patient selection to maximize survival benefits. Multidisciplinary collaboration remains essential, ensuring equitable allocation and optimal organ utilization.

Future research and clinical practice must continue to innovate strategies in candidate assessment and management to address ongoing challenges and enhance outcomes in LT recipients. By prioritizing meticulous evaluation and targeted intervention, we can improve both short-term outcomes and long-term survival rates.

References

1. Girometti R, Pancot M, Como G, Zuiani C. Imaging of liver transplantation. Eur J Radiol. 2017;93(2016):295–307. https://doi.org/10.1016/j.ejrad.2017.05.014.
2. Weinreb JC, Rodby RA, Yee J, Wang CL, Fine D, McDonald RJ, et al. Use of intravenous gadolinium-based contrast media in patients with kidney disease: Consensus Statements from the American College of Radiology and the National Kidney Foundation. Radiology. 2021;298(1):28–35. https://doi.org/10.1148/radiol.2020202903.
3. Addeo P, Noblet V, Naegel B, Bachellier P. Large-for-size Orthotopic liver transplantation: a systematic Review of definitions, outcomes, and solutions. J Gastrointest Surg. 2020;24(5):1192–200.
4. Hernandez-Alejandro R, Sharma H. Small-for-size syndrome in liver transplantation: new horizons to cover with a good launchpad. Liver Transpl. 2016;22:33–6.
5. Kow AWC, Liu J, Patel MS, De Martin E, Reddy MS, Soejima Y, et al. Post living donor liver transplantation small-for-size syndrome: definitions, timelines, biochemical, and clinical factors for diagnosis: guidelines from the ILTS-iLDLT-LTSI consensus conference. Transplantation. 2023;107(10):2226–37.
6. Fundora Y, Hessheimer AJ, Del Prete L, Maroni L, Lanari J, Barrios O, et al. Alternative forms of portal vein revascularization in liver transplant recipients with complex portal vein thrombosis. J Hepatol. 2023;78(4):794–804.
7. Altieri MH, Liu H, Lee SS. Cardiovascular events after liver transplantation: MACE hurts. Rev Cardiovasc Med. 2022;23, 91(3)
8. Martinez-Perez S, McCluskey SA, Davierwala PM, Kalra S, Nguyen E, Bhat M, et al. Perioperative cardiovascular risk assessment and management in liver transplant recipients: a review of the literature merging guidelines and interventions. J Cardiothorac Vasc Anesth. 2024;38(4):1015–30. https://doi.org/10.1053/j.jvca.2023.11.039.
9. Nicolau-Raducu R, Gitman M, Ganier D, Loss GE, Cohen AJ, Patel H, et al. Adverse cardiac events after Orthotopic liver transplantation: a cross-sectional study in 389 consecutive patients. Liver Transpl. 2015;21:13–21.
10. Durand F, Levitsky J, Cauchy F, Gilgenkrantz H, Soubrane O, Francoz C. Age and liver transplantation. J Hepatol. 2019;70(4):745–58. https://doi.org/10.1016/j.jhep.2018.12.009.
11. Wong RJ, Singal AK. Trends in liver disease etiology among adults awaiting liver transplantation in the United States, 2014–2019. JAMA Netw Open. 2020;3(2):3–7.
12. Huang DQ, Terrault NA, Tacke F, Gluud LL, Arrese M, Bugianesi E, et al. Global epidemiology of cirrhosis – aetiology, trends and predictions. Nat Rev Gastroenterol Hepatol. 2023;20(6):388–98.
13. Soldera J, Camazzola F, Rodríguez S, Brandão A. Dobutamine stress echocardiography, myocardial perfusion scintigraphy, invasive coronary angiography, and post-liver transplantation events: systematic review and meta-analysis. Clin Transpl. 2018;32(4):e13222.
14. Fede G, Privitera G, Tomaselli T, Spadaro L, Purrello F. Cardiovascular dysfunction in patients with liver cirrhosis. Ann Gastroenterol. 2015;28(1):31–40.
15. VanWagner LB, Harinstein ME, Runo JR, Darling C, Serper M, Hall S, et al. Multidisciplinary approach to cardiac and pulmonary vascular disease risk assessment in liver transplantation: an evaluation of the evidence and consensus recommendations. Am J Transplant. 2018;18(1):30–42.
16. Sampaio Rodrigues T, Narendren A, Cailes B, Lim RP, Weinberg L, Testro A, et al. Enhancing pre-transplant cardiac assessment: validation and utility of the CAD-LT score with CCTA in

liver transplant candidates. Int J Cardiol. 2024;403(2023):131895. https://doi.org/10.1016/j.ijcard.2024.131895.
17. Rachwan RJ, Kutkut I, Timsina LR, Bou Chaaya RG, El-Am EA, Sabra M, et al. CAD-LT score effectively predicts risk of significant coronary artery disease in liver transplant candidates. J Hepatol. 2021;75(1):142–9. https://doi.org/10.1016/j.jhep.2021.01.008.
18. Moss AJ, Williams MC, Newby DE, Nicol ED. The updated NICE guidelines: cardiac CT as the first-line test for coronary artery disease. Curr Cardiovasc Imaging Rep. 2017;10(5):15.
19. Budoff MJ, Nasir K, McClelland RL, Detrano R, Wong N, Blumenthal RS, et al. Coronary calcium predicts events better with absolute calcium scores than age-sex-race/ethnicity percentiles. MESA (multi-ethnic study of atherosclerosis). J Am Coll Cardiol. 2009;53(4):345–52. https://doi.org/10.1016/j.jacc.2008.07.072.
20. Detrano R, Guerci AD, Carr JJ, Bild DE, Burke G, Folsom AR, et al. Coronary calcium as a predictor of coronary events in four racial or ethnic groups. N Engl J Med. 2008;358(13):1336–45.
21. Raggi P, Callister TQ, Cooil B, He ZX, Lippolis NJ, Russo DJ, et al. Identification of patients at increased risk of first unheralded acute myocardial infarction by electron-beam computed tomography. Circulation. 2000;101(8):850–5.
22. Huded CP, Blair JE, Sweis RN, Flaherty JD. Transradial cardiac catheterization in liver transplant candidates. Am J Cardiol. 2014;113(10):1634–8. https://doi.org/10.1016/j.amjcard.2014.02.014.
23. Lu DY, Steitieh D, Feldman DN, Cheung JW, Wong SC, Halazun H, et al. Impact of cirrhosis on 90-day outcomes after percutaneous coronary intervention (from a Nationwide database). Am J Cardiol. 2020;125(9):1295–304. https://doi.org/10.1016/j.amjcard.2020.01.052.
24. Cheng XS, VanWagner LB, Costa SP, Axelrod DA, Bangalore S, Norman SP, et al. Emerging evidence on coronary heart disease screening in kidney and liver transplantation candidates: a scientific statement from the American Heart Association. Circulation. 2022;146(21):E299–324.
25. Bargehr J, Trejo-Gutierrez JF, Patel T, Rosser B, Aranda-Michel J, Yataco ML, et al. Preexisting atrial fibrillation and cardiac complications after liver transplantation. Liver Transpl. 2015;21:314–20.
26. Fleisher LA, Fleischmann KE, Auerbach AD, Barnason SA, Beckman JA, Bozkurt B, et al. ACC/AHA guideline on perioperative cardiovascular evaluation and management of patients undergoing noncardiac surgery A report of the American College of Cardiology/American Heart Association task force on practice guidelines. Circulation. 2014;130:278–333.
27. VanWagner LB, Harinstein ME, Runo JR, Darling C, Serper M, Hall S, et al. Multidisciplinary approach to cardiac and pulmonary vascular disease risk assessment in liver transplantation: an evaluation of the evidence and consensus recommendations. Am J Transplant. 2018;18(1):30–42. https://doi.org/10.1111/ajt.14531.
28. Ahmed T, Misumida N, Grigorian A, Tarantini G, Messerli AW. Transcatheter interventions for valvular heart diseases in liver cirrhosis patients. Trends Cardiovasc Med. 2023;33(4):242–9. https://doi.org/10.1016/j.tcm.2021.12.014.
29. Lak HM, Chawla S, Gajulapalli RD, Verma BR, Vural AF, Gad M, et al. Outcomes after Transfemoral Transcatheter aortic valve implantation with a SAPIEN 3 valve in patients with cirrhosis of the liver (a tertiary care center experience). Am J Cardiol. 2021;160:75–82. https://doi.org/10.1016/j.amjcard.2021.08.043.
30. Benz F, Mohr R, Tacke F, Roderburg C. Pulmonary complications in patients with liver cirrhosis. J Transl Intern Med. 2020;8(3):150–8.
31. Rybak D, Fallon MB, Krowka MJ Jr, RSB, Stadheim L, Faulk D, et al. Disease in candidates for. Liver Transpl. 2010;14(9):1357–65.
32. Kia L, Cuttica MJ, Yang A, Donnan EN, Whitsett M, Singhvi A, et al. The utility of pulmonary function testing in predicting outcomes following liver transplantation. Liver Transpl. 2016;22(6):805–11.
33. Raevens S, Boret M, Fallon MB. Hepatopulmonary syndrome. JHEP Rep. 2022;4(9):100527. https://doi.org/10.1016/j.jhepr.2022.100527.
34. Bommena S, Fallon MB. Pulmonary complications of portal hypertension. Clin Liver Dis. 2024;28(3):467–82. https://doi.org/10.1016/j.cld.2024.03.005.

35. Krowka MJ, Fallon MB, Kawut SM, Fuhrmann V, Heimbach JK, Ramsay MAE, et al. International liver transplant society practice guidelines: diagnosis and management of hepatopulmonary syndrome and portopulmonary hypertension. Transplantation. 2016;100(7):1440–52.
36. Jasso-Baltazar EA, Peña-Arellano GA, Aguirre-Valadez J, Ruiz I, Papacristofilou-Riebeling B, Jimenez JV, et al. Portopulmonary hypertension: an updated Review. Transplant Direct. 2023;9(8):E1517.
37. Kawut SM, Krowka MJ, Trotter JF, Roberts KE, Benza RL, Badesch DB, et al. Clinical risk factors for portopulmonary hypertension. Hepatology. 2008;48(1):196–203.
38. Aldenkortt F, Aldenkortt M, Caviezel L, Waeber JL, Weber A, Schiffer E. Portopulmonary hypertension and hepatopulmonary syndrome. World J Gastroenterol. 2014;20(25):8072–81.
39. Hemnes A, Robbins IM. Sildenafil monotherapy in Portopulmonary hypertension can facilitate liver transplantation. Liver Transpl. 2009;15:15–9.
40. de Franchis R, Bosch J, Garcia-Tsao G, Reiberger T, Ripoll C, Abraldes JG, et al. Baveno VII—renewing consensus in portal hypertension. J Hepatol. 2021; https://doi.org/10.1016/j.jhep.2021.12.022.
41. Raevens S, Boret M, De Pauw M, Fallon MB, Van Vlierberghe H. Pulmonary abnormalities in liver disease: relevance to transplantation and outcome. Hepatology. 2021;74(3):1674–86.
42. Lv Y, Han G, Fan D. Hepatic hydrothorax. Ann Hepatol. 2018;17(1):33–46. https://doi.org/10.5604/01.3001.0010.7533.
43. Raja K, Panackel C. Post liver transplant renal dysfunction—evaluation, management and immunosuppressive practice. J Clin Exp Hepatol. 2024;14(2):101306. https://doi.org/10.1016/j.jceh.2023.101306.
44. Lizaola-Mayo B, Vargas HE. Hepatorenal syndrome–acute kidney injury in liver transplantation. Clin Gastroenterol Hepatol. 2023;21(10):S20–6. https://doi.org/10.1016/j.cgh.2023.06.010.
45. Kulkarni AV, Rabiee A, Mohanty A. Management of portal hypertension. J Clin Exp Hepatol. 2022;12(4):1184–99. https://doi.org/10.1016/j.jceh.2022.03.002.
46. Dixon W, Fenton C, Feng S, Cullaro G. The type, duration, and severity of pretransplant kidney injury predict prolonged kidney dysfunction after liver transplantation. Liver Transpl. 2024; https://doi.org/10.1097/LVT.0000000000000386.
47. Chauhan K, Azzi Y, Faddoul G, Liriano-Ward L, Chang P, Nadkarni G, et al. Pre-liver transplant renal dysfunction and association with post-transplant end-stage renal disease: a single-center examination of updated UNOS recommendations. Clin Transpl. 2018;32(12):e13428.
48. Schlegel A, Linecker M, Kron P, Györi G, De Oliveira ML, Müllhaupt B, et al. Risk assessment in high- and low-MELD liver transplantation. Am J Transplant. 2017;17(4):1050–63.
49. Goren O, Matot I. Update on perioperative acute kidney injury. Curr Opin Crit Care. 2016;22(4):370–8.
50. Piano S, Gambino C, Vettore E, Calvino V, Tonon M, Boccagni P, et al. Response to Terlipressin and albumin is associated with improved liver transplant outcomes in patients with Hepatorenal syndrome. Hepatology. 2021;73(5):1909–19.
51. Singal AK, Kuo YF. Waitlist and post-transplant outcomes among candidates listed for liver transplant: liver alone versus simultaneous liver kidney listings. Aliment Pharmacol Ther. 2023;58(9):929–37.
52. Enestvedt CK. PRO: simultaneous liver-kidney transplantation in the current era: still the best option. Clin Liver Dis. 2020;16(6):266–71.
53. Singapura P, Ma T, Sarmast N, Gonzalez S, Durand F, Maiwall R, et al. Estimating glomerular filtration rate in cirrhosis using creatinine- and cystatin C- based equations: systematic review and meta-analysis. Liver Transpl. 2021;27(8):1538–52. https://doi.org/10.1002/lt.26216.
54. Gotthardt DN, Weiss KH, Rathenberg V, Schemmer P, Stremmel W, Sauer P. Persistent ascites after liver transplantation: etiology, treatment and impact on survival. Ann Transplant. 2013;18(1):378–83.
55. Ruf AE, Kremers WK, Chavez LL, Descalzi VI, Podesta LG, Villamil FG. Addition of serum sodium into the MELD score predicts waiting list mortality better than MELD alone. Liver Transpl. 2005;11(3):336–43.

56. Karapanagiotou A, Kydona C, Papadopoulos S, Dimitriadis C, Giasnetsova T, Rempelakos G, et al. The effect of hyponatremia on the outcome of patients after orthotopic liver transplantation. Transplant Proc. 2012;44(9):2724–6. https://doi.org/10.1016/j.transproceed.2012.09.095.
57. Warner ER, Satapathy SK. Sarcopenia in the cirrhotic patient: current knowledge and future directions. J Clin Exp Hepatol. 2023;13(1):162–77. https://doi.org/10.1016/j.jceh.2022.06.005.
58. Dasarathy S, Merli M. Sarcopenia from mechanism to diagnosis and treatment in liver disease. J Hepatol. 2016;65(6):1232–44. https://doi.org/10.1016/j.jhep.2016.07.040.
59. Carey EJ, Steidley DE, Aqel BA, Byrne TJ, Mekeel KL, Rakela J, et al. Six-minute walk distance predicts mortality in liver transplant candidates. Liver Transpl. 2010;16:1373.
60. Dhaliwal A, Armstrong MJ. Sarcopenia in cirrhosis: a practical overview. Clin Med (London). 2020;20(5):489–92. https://doi.org/10.7861/clinmed.2020-0089.
61. Caraceni P, O'Brien A, Gines P. Long-term albumin treatment in patients with cirrhosis and ascites. J Hepatol. 2022;76(6):1306–17. https://doi.org/10.1016/j.jhep.2022.03.005.
62. Devoto G, Gallo F, Marchello C, Racchi O, Garbarini R, Bonassi S, et al. Prealbumin serum concentrations as a useful tool in the assessment of malnutrition in hospitalized patients. Clin Chem. 2006;52(12):2281–5.
63. Carvalho JR, Machado MV. New insights about albumin and liver disease. Ann Hepatol. 2018;17(4):547–60. https://doi.org/10.5604/01.3001.0012.0916.
64. Fried LP, Tangen CM, Walston J, Newman AB, Hirsch C, Gottdiener J, et al. Frailty in older adults: evidence for a phenotype. J Gerontol Ser A Biol Sci Med Sci. 2001;56(3):146–57.
65. Guralnik JM, Ferrucci L, Simonsick EM, Salive ME, Wallace RB. Lower-extremity function in persons over the age of 70 years as a predictor of subsequent disability. N Engl J Med. 1995;332(9):556–62.
66. Lai JC, Covinsky KE, Dodge JL, Boscardin WJ, Segev DL, Roberts JP, et al. Development of a novel frailty index to predict mortality in patients with end-stage liver disease. Hepatology. 2017;66(2):564–74.
67. Bambha K. Implications of an aging liver transplant waiting list: survival benefit should be based upon "mile-age" and performance. Liver Transpl. 2015;21:1459–62.
68. Wang C, Covinsky K, Feng S, Hayssen H, Segev D, Lai JC. Functional impairment in older liver transplantation candidates: from the functional assessment in liver transplantation study. Liver Transpl. 2015;21:1465–70.
69. Morkane CM, Kearney O, Bruce DA, Melikian CN, Martin DS. An outpatient hospital-based exercise training program for patients with cirrhotic liver disease awaiting transplantation: a feasibility trial. Transplantation. 2020;104(1):97–103.
70. Gómez-Gavara C, Charco R, Tapiolas I, Ridaura N, Campos-Varela I, Dopazo C, et al. Recipient age for liver transplantation: should it be limited? A propensity score matching analysis of a large European series. Transplant Proc. 2020;52(5):1442–9. https://doi.org/10.1016/j.transproceed.2020.02.061.
71. Spengler EK, O'Leary JG, Te HS, Rogal S, Pillai AA, Al-Osaimi A, et al. Liver transplantation in the obese cirrhotic patient. Transplantation. 2017;101(10):2288–96.
72. Beckmann S, Drent G, Ruppar T, Nikolić N, de Geest S. Body weight parameters are related to morbidity and mortality after liver transplantation: a systematic review and meta-analysis. Transplantation. 2019;103(11):2287–303.
73. Schlansky B, Naugler WE, Orloff SL, Kristian Enestvedt C. Higher mortality and survival benefit in obese patients awaiting liver transplantation. Transplantation. 2016;100(12):2648–55.
74. Moctezuma-Velazquez C, Márquez-Guillén E, Torre A. Obesity in the liver transplant setting. Nutrients. 2019;11(11):1–19.
75. Iannelli A. Bariatric surgery and liver transplant. Liver Transpl. 2017;23(11):1369–70.
76. Valour F, Conrad A, Ader F, Launay O. Vaccination in adult liver transplantation candidates and recipients. Clin Res Hepatol Gastroenterol. 2020;44(2):126–34. https://doi.org/10.1016/j.clinre.2019.08.007.
77. Ballester MP, Jalan R, Mehta G. Vaccination in liver diseases and liver transplantation: recommendations, implications and opportunities in the post-COVID era. JHEP Rep. 2023;5(8):100776. https://doi.org/10.1016/j.jhepr.2023.100776.

78. Dufour JF, Marjot T, Becchetti C, Tilg H. COVID-19 and liver disease. Gut. 2022;71(11):2350–62.
79. Wu J, et al. Liver diseases in COVID-19: Etiology, treatment and prognosis. World J Gastroenterol. 2020;26(19):2286–93.
80. Cornberg M, Buti M, Eberhardt CS, Grossi PA, Shouval D. EASL position paper on the use of COVID-19 vaccines in patients with chronic liver diseases, hepatobiliary cancer and liver transplant recipients. J Hepatol. 2021;74(January):944–51.
81. Bajaj JS, Lai JC, Tandon P, Leary JGO, Garcia-tsao G, Vargas HE, et al. Insurance status but not race and ethnicity are associated with outcomes in a large hospitalized Cohort of Patients with Cirrhosis. Clin Gastroenterol Hepatol. 2024;21(7):1864–72.
82. Guggenheimer J, Eghtesad B, Close J, Shay C, Fung J. Dental health status of liver transplant candidates. Liver Transpl. 2007;13(5):767–8.
83. Al-Adra DP, Hammel L, Roberts J, Woodle ES, Levine D, Mandelbrot D, et al. Preexisting melanoma and hematological malignancies, prognosis, and timing to solid organ transplantation: a consensus expert opinion statement. Am J Transplant. 2021;21(2):475–83. https://doi.org/10.1111/ajt.16324.
84. Al-Adra DP, Hammel L, Roberts J, Woodle ES, Levine D, Mandelbrot D, et al. Pretransplant solid organ malignancy and organ transplant candidacy: a consensus expert opinion statement. Am J Transplant. 2021;21(2):460–74. https://doi.org/10.1111/ajt.16318.
85. Salcedo M, Vinaixa C, Javle M, Trapero-Marugán M, Bustamante J, Line PD. Evaluation and Management of Liver Transplant Candidates with prior nonhepatic cancer: guidelines from the ILTS/SETH consensus conference. Transplantation. 2022;106(1):E3–E11.
86. Burra P, Burroughs A, Graziadei I, Pirenne J, Valdecasas JC, Muiesan P, et al. EASL clinical practice guidelines: liver transplantation. J Hepatol. 2016;64(2):433–85. https://doi.org/10.1016/j.jhep.2015.10.006.
87. Argilés G, Tabernero J, Labianca R, Hochhauser D, Salazar R, Iveson T, et al. Localised colon cancer: ESMO clinical practice guidelines for diagnosis, treatment and follow-up†. Ann Oncol. 2020;31(10):1291–305. https://doi.org/10.1016/j.annonc.2020.06.022.
88. Lopes G, Stern MC, Temin S, Sharara AI, Cervantes A, Costas-Chavarri A, et al. Early detection for colorectal cancer: ASCO resource-stratified guideline. J Glob Oncol. 2019;2019(5):1–22.
89. Shaukat A, Levin TR. Current and future colorectal cancer screening strategies. Nat Rev Gastroenterol Hepatol. 2022;19(8):521–31.
90. Fu C, Li X, Chen Y, Long X, Liu K. Lung cancer incidences after liver transplantation: a systematic review and meta-analysis. Cancer Med. 2023;12(15):16119–28.
91. Ren W, Chen M, Qiao Y, Zhao F. Global guidelines for breast cancer screening: a systematic review. Breast. 2022;64(April):85–99. https://doi.org/10.1016/j.breast.2022.04.003.
92. Saglam K, Sahin TT, Ogut Z, Ince V, Usta S, Yilmaz S. De novo malignancies after liver transplantation: experience of a high-volume center. J Gastrointest Cancer. 2022;53(4):1020–7. https://doi.org/10.1007/s12029-021-00749-0.
93. Rodríguez-Perálvarez M, Colmenero J, González A, Gastaca M, Curell A, Caballero-Marcos A, et al. Cumulative exposure to tacrolimus and incidence of cancer after liver transplantation. Am J Transplant. 2022;22(6):1671–82.

Management of Portal Hypertension

4

Nicolas Chong Lugon and Guadalupe Garcia-Tsao

Portal Hypertension

Cirrhosis is the end-stage of any chronic liver disease. The main determinant of death in cirrhosis is the development of clinical decompensation, defined as the development/presence of complications of cirrhosis, specifically ascites, variceal hemorrhage and/or hepatic encephalopathy.

The main driver of decompensation is portal hypertension (PH) as determined by measurements of the hepatic venous pressure gradient (HVPG) [1]. While higher portal pressures increase the risk of complications, reductions in portal pressures are associated with improved outcomes [2]. HVPG is a measurement of hepatic sinusoidal pressure and, in cirrhosis, it is equivalent to direct measurements of portal pressure. HVPG is performed via catheterization of the hepatic vein through central venous access using a balloon catheter and obtaining a free pressure and an occluded pressure by inflating (occluded pressure) and deflating (free pressure) the balloon. The HVPG is obtained by subtracting the free from the occluded pressure and it correlates with direct measurement of portal pressure in most etiologies of cirrhosis. Normal HVPG is 3–5 mmHg, while, in cirrhosis, it is usually >5 mmHg. The development of clinical decompensation is associated with an HVPG ≥10 mmHg and this pressure defines clinically significant portal hypertension (CSPH) [1, 3, 4].

Measuring the HVPG remains the gold standard for the diagnosis of CSPH, but unfortunately, it is an invasive, nuanced test that can be cumbersome to perform and may not be readily available. Because of this, non-invasive methods of estimating CSPH have been developed. Liver stiffness measurements (LSM) measured by transient

N. C. Lugon · G. Garcia-Tsao (✉)
Yale University, Digestive Diseases Section, New Haven, CT, USA

Veterans Administration Healthcare System, Digestive Diseases Section, West Haven, CT, USA
e-mail: guadalupe.garcia-tsao@yale.edu

B. Eghtesad et al. (eds.), *Liver Transplantation*,
https://doi.org/10.1007/978-3-032-07072-2_4

elastography (TE), and platelet (PLT) count have been validated for the diagnosis of CSPH [5]. A LSM <10 kPa excludes the presence of cirrhosis, while a LSM >15 kPa indicates the presence of compensated advanced chronic liver disease (cACLD), the noninvasive term for advanced liver fibrosis/cirrhosis. A LSM >25 kPa or a LSM of 20–25 kPa in combination with a platelet count <150 predicts a greater than 60% risk of having CSPH [6]. While a higher portal pressure increases the risk of complications, reductions in portal pressure are associated with improved outcomes [2].

Therapeutic Strategies in the Management of Portal Hypertension

Non-Selective Beta-Blockers (NSBB)

The main pharmacological strategy to prevent/treat complications of cirrhosis is to lower portal pressure by using splanchnic vasoconstrictors and/or intrahepatic vasodilators. Non-selective beta-blockers (NSBBs) reduce portal pressure by splanchnic vasoconstriction via beta-1 and beta-2 adrenergic blockade, thereby reducing portal venous inflow.

Achieving a >20% reduction of HVPG or a HVPG of <12 mmHg after initiation of therapy has historically been used to determine if a patient is a responder to NSBB. While these goals apply to groups of patients in clinical trials, the role of routinely evaluating HVPG changes in individual patients has been questioned [7]. A meta-analysis evaluating HVPG changes in patients assigned to the placebo arm of 20 RCT found that while HVPG was unchanged on repeat measurements at a population level, there were significant changes at the individual level, with up to 25% of patients having a 10% improvement of HVPG despite not receiving a portal pressure-lowering drug [8]. Therefore, while assessing changes in HVPG is an important research endpoint for new portal-hypotensive drugs, it should not be used to guide portal hypertension therapy in individual patients [7].

Studies suggest that less than half of patients achieve a hemodynamic response with traditional NSBB, but the rate of response is significantly greater with carvedilol, with up to 75% of patients responding to this drug [9, 10]. Furthermore, carvedilol has a larger HVPG-lowering effect compared to traditional NSBB (propranolol, nadolol), and this effect is observed even in patient populations that had not responded initially to other NSBB [11, 12]. Given its better side-effect profile, and greater efficacy in reducing HVPG and improving clinical outcomes, the Baveno VII expert consensus recommends carvedilol as the preferred NSBB in patients with cirrhosis [6].

Observational studies have raised the concern that NSBB may have deleterious effects in patients with ascites, including increased incidence of acute kidney injury (AKI) and increased mortality [13, 14]. Subsequent studies have shown that the harmful effects of NSBBs occurred mostly in patients with refractory ascites and were caused by blunting the adaptive mechanisms that maintain renal perfusion in this group of patients [15, 16]. Despite this initial concern, recent studies have shown a survival benefit even in patients with refractory ascites and have helped determine parameters for a safer use of NSBBs in patients with decompensated cirrhosis and ascites [17]. NSBB can be used cautiously in patients with refractory ascites, maintaining adequate blood pressures (MAP >65 mmHg or systolic BP >90 mmHg), as these pressures help maintain renal perfusion and have been associated with increased survival [15]. NSBBs should be dose-reduced or discontinued in patients with persistent low blood pressures (MAP <60 mmHg or systolic blood pressures <90 mmHg) or with AKI [6].

Systemic Vasoconstrictors (Vasopressin, Terlipressin, Octreotide)

Systemic vasoconstrictors are used in the setting of acute variceal hemorrhage and include vasopressin, somatostatin, and its analogs terlipressin and octreotide, respectively. Vasopressin and terlipressin cause splanchnic vasoconstriction by directly stimulating arginine vasopressin (AVP) receptors, while somatostatin and octreotide decrease portal blood flow indirectly by inhibiting the release of vasodilator hormones. The use of systemic vasoconstrictors in patients with acute variceal hemorrhage have shown to decrease all-cause mortality, transfusion needs, and hospital stay, and improve rates of hemostasis [18]. Compared to vasopressin, octreotide has fewer side effects and is more effective in achieving hemostasis [19]. Meanwhile, octreotide, somatostatin and terlipressin have comparable efficacy in achieving hemostasis and reducing mortality [20] and the use of any of these vasoconstrictors is acceptable per recent guidelines [21].

Transjugular Intrahepatic Portosystemic Shunt (TIPS)

TIPS decrease portal hypertension by placing a stent that shunts flow from the high-pressure portal system to the low-pressure systemic circulation, bypassing the increased vascular resistance present in the cirrhotic liver. The main indications for TIPS are in the management of (1) refractory variceal bleeding, (2) recurrent variceal hemorrhage, and (3) refractory ascites [6, 21–23]. Most recently, preemptive placement of TIPS soon (within 72 hours and ideally 24 hours) after control of acute variceal bleeding has emerged as an additional indication in selected patients at high risk of rebleeding [21]. Common absolute contraindications for TIPS creation include heart failure with a reduced ejection fraction, severe pulmonary hypertension, sepsis, and severe hepatic encephalopathy, while relative contraindications include severe coagulopathy, unrelieved biliary obstruction, moderate pulmonary hypertension, and polycystic liver disease [22, 24].

Endoscopy/Endoscopic Ligation

In the era of non-invasive methods for diagnosing CSPH and pharmacological therapy to prevent complications of cirrhosis, the role of diagnostic and therapeutic endoscopy in patients without prior episodes of variceal hemorrhage has become less prominent.

Upper endoscopy continues to have an important role when TE is not available to diagnose CSPH (diagnostic role), and in patients already diagnosed with CSPH but unable to receive NSBB due to side effects or contraindications (therapeutic role). Combined therapy with serial endoscopies with endoscopic variceal ligation and NSBBs remains the standard of care for patients with a prior history of variceal hemorrhage (i.e., secondary prophylaxis of variceal hemorrhage, as outlined below).

Management of Portal Hypertension in Specific Patient Populations

Compensated Patient: NSBB in Prevention of First Decompensation

Given the marked difference in survival between compensated and decompensated cirrhosis (median survival >15 years vs. ~2 years once a decompensating event occurs), preventing decompensation is crucial in the management of patients with cirrhosis. While in the past emphasis had been placed on preventing variceal hemorrhage, emphasis is now on preventing any decompensating event, with ascites being the most common first decompensating event and the one associated with the highest mortality [25].

NSBB have been shown to decrease the first decompensation in patients with compensated cirrhosis and CSPH. The PREDESCI trial randomized 201 patients with compensated cirrhosis and CSPH and either no or small varices to receive either a NSBB (propranolol or carvedilol) or placebo. In a median follow-up of 37 months, an absolute risk reduction of 11% in the primary endpoint of decompensating event or death was observed in the NSBB group (16%) compared to the placebo group (27%), with a number needed to treat (NNT) of 9. The benefit observed in patients receiving NSBBs was due mostly to a decrease in the development of ascites, where the differences between those on NSBB and on placebo was significant (20% vs. 9% $p = 0.03$). Other complications were much less frequent and therefore were not significantly reduced, although the study did show a tendency for decreased progression of varices (which could indicate prevention of variceal hemorrhage) and decreased mortality [11].

In the past, guidelines recommended screening endoscopy for patients with compensated cirrhosis. For those with high-risk varices (large varices or varices with red wale marks), the standard approach was to initiate NSBB therapy or perform serial endoscopic variceal ligation (EVL) until variceal obliteration followed by serial endoscopies to assess for variceal recurrence. The primary goal was to prevent the first variceal hemorrhage.

However, the PREDESCI trial has shown that initiating NSBB therapy (preferably carvedilol) in patients with cirrhosis and CSPH (and this could include patients with no or small varices) not only prevents variceal hemorrhage but, by reducing portal/sinusoidal pressure, also prevents variceal growth and, perhaps more importantly, also reduces the risk of ascites [26–30]. Consequently, patients with compensated cirrhosis no longer require screening endoscopy unless they are intolerant or have contraindications to NSBB. A summary of the recommended doses of NSBB can be found in Table 4.1.

In patients with CSPH that are unable to receive NSBB due to side effects or contraindications, endoscopy is recommended with the goal of detecting high-risk varices and performing EVL, in order to prevent a first episode of variceal hemorrhage [6]; if no varices are identified, patients with CSPH should have endoscopic surveillance every 2–3 years, and if varices without high-risk features are detected, the surveillance interval is shortened to every 1–2 years [21]. If high-risk varices are detected during any endoscopy in these patients who are intolerant to NSBB, EVL is recommended, and serial endoscopies with EVL are then repeated every 2–4 weeks until complete eradication of varices is achieved [31, 32]. After complete eradication, endoscopies should be performed every 6–12 months with the goal of identifying recurring high-risk varices that would require repeat EVL [21].

While NSBBs in patients with CSPH decreases the risk of decompensation, starting beta-blockers in patients with cirrhosis without CSPH is unlikely to be beneficial and exposes patients to unnecessary side effects. Therefore, it is important to adequately select patients with compensated cirrhosis that will benefit from initiation of NSBBs. This was exemplified in a randomized clinical trial that included 213 patients with and without CSPH to receive timolol or placebo. There were no significant differences in rates of VH or other decompensating events between treatment groups, and patients who received beta-blockers had a significantly higher incidence of serious adverse events such as bradycardia, respiratory symptoms, and syncope [3]. An overview of the management of portal hypertension in patients with compensated cirrhosis/cACLD can be found in Figure 4.1.

Patient with Ascites and At-risk Varices: Prevention of Variceal Hemorrhage

In patients who have developed decompensated cirrhosis with ascites, the goal in management should shift towards preventing further decompensation by preventing

Table 4.1 Recommended doses of NSBB

Agent	Initial dose	Target or maximal dose	Comments
Carvedilol	6.25 mg daily[a]	12.5 mg[a]	Preferred NSBB. Dose can be increased up to 25 mg/day if well tolerated.
Propranolol	20–40 mg daily	320 mg/day (without ascites) 160 mg/day (with ascites)	
Nadolol	20–40 mg daily	160 mg/day (without ascites) 80 mg/day (with ascites)	

[a]Can be split to twice daily

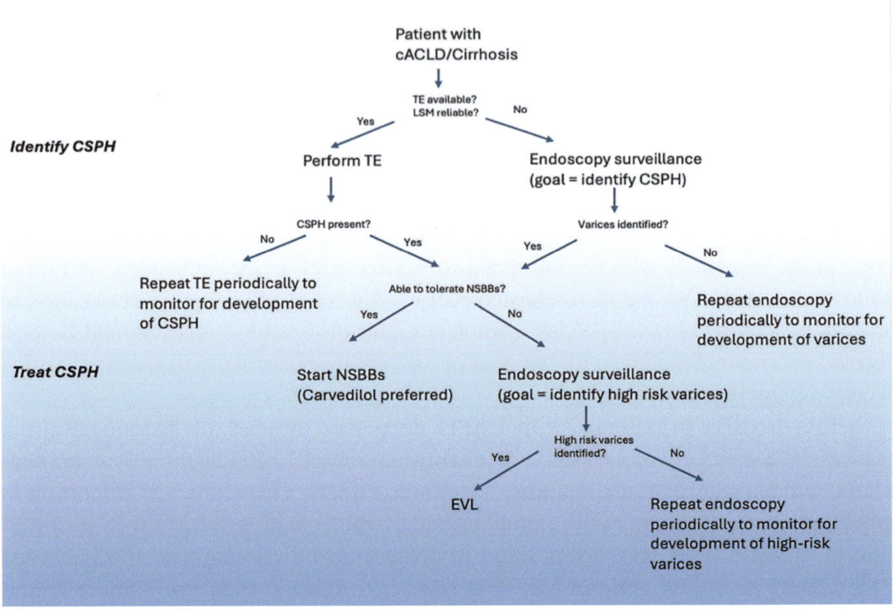

Fig. 4.1 Portal hypertension management in patients with cACLD/compensated cirrhosis. TE transient elastography, LSM liver stiffness measurement, CSPH clinically significant portal hypertension, NSBB non-selective beta-blockers, EVL endoscopic variceal ligation

a first episode of VH. NSBB in patients with ascites are effective in preventing VH and improving overall survival, and is recommended in this population [6]. Prior studies demonstrating the superiority of NSBB over EVL in preventing a first episode of VH included a majority of patients with ascites at baseline, demonstrating the effectiveness of NSBB in already decompensated patients [27]. Furthermore, subsequent subgroup analysis, including only patients with ascites continued to show the improved survival initially seen in populations including both compensated and decompensated patients receiving NSBB [28].

Patient Presenting with Variceal Hemorrhage (VH): Control of Hemorrhage

Standard of Care

In patients with acute variceal hemorrhage, the goals of therapy are to ensure hemodynamic stability and adequate oxygenation, achieve hemostasis, and prevent complications such as infections. Cardiovascular resuscitation and airway assessment should be performed, with consideration for endotracheal intubation in patients at risk of aspiration. A restrictive red blood cell transfusion goal is recommended with a target hemoglobin of 7 g/dL. Transfusion of platelets and fresh frozen plasma is not routinely recommended, as these blood products have not been shown to be beneficial, and additional intravascular volume can worsen portal pressures [21, 33, 34]. Intravenous systemic vasoactive agents (as discussed above) and antibiotics should be administered at the time of presentation, with upper endoscopy performed within 12 hours. EVL is the endoscopic therapy of choice for bleeding esophageal varices and type 1 gastro-esophageal varices (GOV-1; varices extending from the esophagus into the lesser curvature of the stomach) [21, 33]. Endoscopic interventions for the management of other less commonly encountered types of varices (e.g., isolated gastric varices, GOV-2) differ and are beyond the scope of this chapter.

Pre-emptive TIPS (pTIPS)

In patients with variceal hemorrhage, preemptive TIPS within 72 hours (and ideally within 24 hours) of initial endoscopy has demonstrated a mortality benefit in patients with a Child-Pugh class B score >7 with active bleeding seen on endoscopy and patients in Child-Pugh class C score 10–13, a population at higher risk of recurrent bleeding. Most studies have shown that pTIPS in this group is associated with increased transplant-free survival and decreased rate of recurrent bleeding. Exclusion criteria in these studies included advanced HCC, advanced acute or chronic kidney disease, age > 75 years, heart failure, and pregnancy [21, 35–37].

Refractory and Recurrent Variceal Bleeding

TIPS is recommended as a rescue intervention in patients with acute variceal bleeding who are unable to be adequately treated with endoscopic interventions. In the acute setting, TIPS should be considered in patients with active bleeding despite attempts to treat endoscopically (salvage TIPS), and in patients that develop recurrent bleeding shortly after the initial endoscopy achieves transient hemostasis (rescue TIPS). In the latter case, a second repeat endoscopy can be pursued before rescue TIPS is considered [21, 38, 39]. Patients requiring rescue TIPS are usually those who have met criteria for pTIPS and therefore identifying these patients at the time of initial endoscopy and placing a pTIPS within 72 hours of this initial endoscopy will prevent these patients from requiring a rescue TIPS which is associated with a very high mortality. An overview of the management of acute variceal bleeding can be found in Fig. 4.2.

Prevention of Recurrent Variceal Hemorrhage

Patients who recover from an initial episode of variceal hemorrhage without requiring TIPS should be started on secondary prophylaxis with serial endoscopies with EVL and NSBB. In this population, TIPS should be considered if a second episode of variceal hemorrhage occurs despite adherence to secondary prophylaxis [21, 22].

Multiple studies have shown that combining EVL and NSBBs is superior to either treatment alone in reducing the risk of recurrent VH [40, 41]. Furthermore, in patients with Child–Pugh class B or C cirrhosis, combination therapy also has a mortality benefit over EVL alone [42]. A meta-analysis including 955 patients found a 32% relative risk reduction with combination therapy compared to monotherapy, with a NNT of 8. Interestingly, the difference was only seen when comparing combined

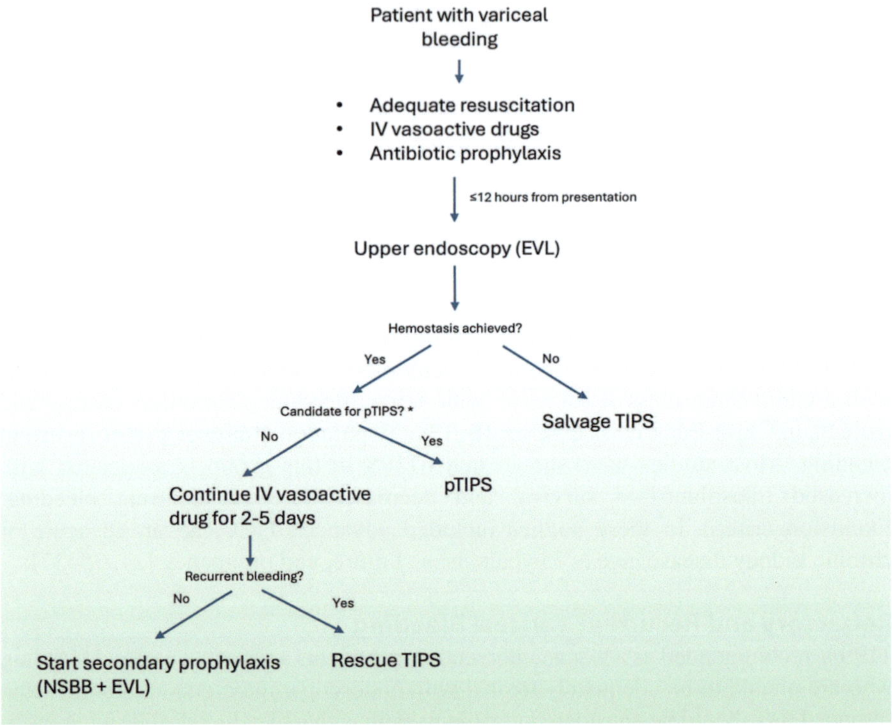

Fig. 4.2 Management of acute variceal bleeding. IV intravenous, EVL (endoscopic variceal ligation), TIPS transjugular intrahepatic portosystemic shunt, pTIPS pre-emptive TIPS, NSBB nonselective beta-blockers. *Indications for pTIPS: CTP B score >7 with active bleeding or CTP C score 10–13

therapy to EVL, and not to medical therapy alone, potentially signaling that most of the benefit obtained with combined therapy is driven by NSBBs [43].

In untreated patients, the risk of rebleeding is high and can be greater than 60% but varies significantly depending on factors such Child–Pugh class and size of esophageal varices [44]. Similarly, the reduction in rebleeding risk is not homogeneous in patients receiving appropriate therapy. Achieving a HVPG reduction of >20% reduces the risk of VH to less than 20%, while the risk of VH is less than 10% if HVPG decreases to <12 mmHg. On the other hand, the bleeding rate is as high as 40% in patients who receive appropriate therapy but do not achieve a significant HVPG reduction [45]. Nevertheless, measuring HVPG is not warranted outside of clinical trials to assess response to therapy.

Patient Presenting with Refractory Ascites

TIPS is more effective than serial large volume paracentesis (LVP) in patients with large ascites that is unable to be controlled adequately with diuretics [46]. TIPS is successful in controlling ascites in 80% of these patients by reducing hepatic sinusoidal pressure and increasing the effective circulation, thus blunting the renin-aldosterone-angiotensin system, and decreasing sodium retention [22, 23, 47]. In addition to its effectiveness in controlling ascites, a recent randomized controlled trial has also demonstrated a significant survival benefit in patients undergoing TIPS compared to serial LVPs [48].

References

1. Ripoll C, Groszmann R, Garcia-Tsao G, Grace N, Burroughs A, Planas R, et al. Hepatic venous pressure gradient predicts clinical decompensation in patients with compensated cirrhosis. Gastroenterology. 2007;133(2):481–8.
2. Turco L, Villanueva C, La Mura V, Garcia-Pagan JC, Reiberger T, Genesca J, et al. Lowering portal pressure improves outcomes of patients with cirrhosis, with or without ascites: a meta-analysis. Clin Gastroenterol Hepatol. 2020;18(2):313–27 e6.
3. Groszmann RJ, Garcia-Tsao G, Bosch J, Grace ND, Burroughs AK, Planas R, et al. Beta-blockers to prevent gastroesophageal varices in patients with cirrhosis. N Engl J Med. 2005;353(21):2254–61.
4. Sanyal AJ, Harrison SA, Ratziu V, Abdelmalek MF, Diehl AM, Caldwell S, et al. The natural history of advanced fibrosis due to nonalcoholic steatohepatitis: data from the simtuzumab trials. Hepatology. 2019;70(6):1913–27.
5. Abraldes JG, Bureau C, Stefanescu H, Augustin S, Ney M, Blasco H, et al. Noninvasive tools and risk of clinically significant portal hypertension and varices in compensated cirrhosis: the "Anticipate" study. Hepatology. 2016;64(6):2173–84.
6. de Franchis R, Bosch J, Garcia-Tsao G, Reiberger T, Ripoll C, Baveno VIIF. Baveno VII - renewing consensus in portal hypertension. J Hepatol. 2022;76(4):959–74.
7. Garcia-Tsao G. Can we rely on changes in HVPG in patients with cirrhosis? Hepatology. 2021;74(6):2945–7.
8. Bai W, Al-Karaghouli M, Stach J, Sung S, Matheson GJ, Abraldes JG. Test-retest reliability and consistency of HVPG and impact on trial design: a study in 289 patients from 20 randomized controlled trials. Hepatology. 2021;74(6):3301–15.
9. Albillos A, Banares R, Gonzalez M, Ripoll C, Gonzalez R, Catalina MV, et al. Value of the hepatic venous pressure gradient to monitor drug therapy for portal hypertension: a meta-analysis. Am J Gastroenterol. 2007;102(5):1116–26.
10. Reiberger T, Ulbrich G, Ferlitsch A, Payer BA, Schwabl P, Pinter M, et al. Carvedilol for primary prophylaxis of variceal bleeding in cirrhotic patients with haemodynamic non-response to propranolol. Gut. 2013;62(11):1634–41.
11. Villanueva C, Albillos A, Genesca J, Garcia-Pagan JC, Calleja JL, Aracil C, et al. beta blockers to prevent decompensation of cirrhosis in patients with clinically significant portal hypertension (PREDESCI): a randomised, double-blind, placebo-controlled, multicentre trial. Lancet. 2019;393(10181):1597–608.
12. Zacharias AP, Jeyaraj R, Hobolth L, Bendtsen F, Gluud LL, Morgan MY. Carvedilol versus traditional, non-selective beta-blockers for adults with cirrhosis and gastroesophageal varices. Cochrane Database Syst Rev. 2018;10(10):CD011510.
13. Serste T, Melot C, Francoz C, Durand F, Rautou PE, Valla D, et al. Deleterious effects of beta-blockers on survival in patients with cirrhosis and refractory ascites. Hepatology. 2010;52(3):1017–22.
14. Kim SG, Larson JJ, Lee JS, Therneau TM, Kim WR. Beneficial and harmful effects of non-selective beta blockade on acute kidney injury in liver transplant candidates. Liver Transpl. 2017;23(6):733–40.
15. Tergast TL, Kimmann M, Laser H, Gerbel S, Manns MP, Cornberg M, et al. Systemic arterial blood pressure determines the therapeutic window of non-selective beta blockers in decompensated cirrhosis. Aliment Pharmacol Ther. 2019;50(6):696–706.

16. Tellez L, Ibanez-Samaniego L, Perez Del Villar C, Yotti R, Martinez J, Carrion L, et al. Nonselective beta-blockers impair global circulatory homeostasis and renal function in cirrhotic patients with refractory ascites. J Hepatol. 2020;73(6):1404–14.
17. Chirapongsathorn S, Valentin N, Alahdab F, Krittanawong C, Erwin PJ, Murad MH, et al. Nonselective beta-blockers and survival in patients with cirrhosis and ascites: a systematic review and meta-analysis. Clin Gastroenterol Hepatol. 2016;14(8):1096–104 e9.
18. Wells M, Chande N, Adams P, Beaton M, Levstik M, Boyce E, et al. Meta-analysis: vasoactive medications for the management of acute variceal bleeds. Aliment Pharmacol Ther. 2012;35(11):1267–78.
19. Hwang SJ, Lin HC, Chang CF, Lee FY, Lu CW, Hsia HC, et al. A randomized controlled trial comparing octreotide and vasopressin in the control of acute esophageal variceal bleeding. J Hepatol. 1992;16(3):320–5.
20. Seo YS, Park SY, Kim MY, Kim JH, Park JY, Yim HJ, et al. Lack of difference among terlipressin, somatostatin, and octreotide in the control of acute gastroesophageal variceal hemorrhage. Hepatology. 2014;60(3):954–63.
21. Kaplan DE, Ripoll C, Thiele M, Fortune BE, Simonetto DA, Garcia-Tsao G, et al. AASLD Practice Guidance on risk stratification and management of portal hypertension and varices in cirrhosis. Hepatology. 2023;
22. Lee EW, Eghtesad B, Garcia-Tsao G, Haskal ZJ, Hernandez-Gea V, Jalaeian H, et al. AASLD Practice Guidance on the use of TIPS, variceal embolization, and retrograde transvenous obliteration in the management of variceal hemorrhage. Hepatology. 2024;79(1):224–50.
23. Biggins SW, Angeli P, Garcia-Tsao G, Gines P, Ling SC, Nadim MK, et al. Diagnosis, evaluation, and management of ascites, spontaneous bacterial peritonitis and hepatorenal syndrome: 2021 practice guidance by the American Association for the Study of Liver Diseases. Hepatology. 2021;74(2):1014–48.
24. Dariushnia SR, Haskal ZJ, Midia M, Martin LG, Walker TG, Kalva SP, et al. Quality improvement guidelines for transjugular intrahepatic portosystemic shunts. J Vasc Interv Radiol. 2016;27(1):1–7.
25. D'Amico G, Pasta L, Morabito A, D'Amico M, Caltagirone M, Malizia G, et al. Competing risks and prognostic stages of cirrhosis: a 25-year inception cohort study of 494 patients. Aliment Pharmacol Ther. 2014;39(10):1180–93.
26. Garcia-Tsao G, Abraldes JG, Berzigotti A, Bosch J. Portal hypertensive bleeding in cirrhosis: risk stratification, diagnosis, and management: 2016 practice guidance by the American Association for the study of liver diseases. Hepatology. 2017;65(1):310–35.
27. Tripathi D, Ferguson JW, Kochar N, Leithead JA, Therapondos G, McAvoy NC, et al. Randomized controlled trial of carvedilol versus variceal band ligation for the prevention of the first variceal bleed. Hepatology. 2009;50(3):825–33.
28. McDowell HR, Chuah CS, Tripathi D, Stanley AJ, Forrest EH, Hayes PC. Carvedilol is associated with improved survival in patients with cirrhosis: a long-term follow-up study. Aliment Pharmacol Ther. 2021;53(4):531–9.
29. Villanueva C, Torres F, Sarin SK, Shah HA, Tripathi D, Brujats A, et al. Carvedilol reduces the risk of decompensation and mortality in patients with compensated cirrhosis in a competing-risk meta-analysis. J Hepatol. 2022;77(4):1014–25.
30. Serper M, Kaplan DE, Taddei TH, Tapper EB, Cohen JB, Mahmud N. Nonselective beta blockers, hepatic decompensation, and mortality in cirrhosis: a national cohort study. Hepatology. 2023;77(2):489–500.
31. Sheibani S, Khemichian S, Kim JJ, Hou L, Yan AW, Buxbaum J, et al. Randomized trial of 1-week versus 2-week intervals for endoscopic ligation in the treatment of patients with esophageal variceal bleeding. Hepatology. 2016;64(2):549–55.
32. Yoshida H, Mamada Y, Taniai N, Yamamoto K, Kawano Y, Mizuguchi Y, et al. A randomized control trial of bi-monthly versus bi-weekly endoscopic variceal ligation of esophageal varices. Am J Gastroenterol. 2005;100(9):2005–9.
33. Gralnek IM, Camus Duboc M, Garcia-Pagan JC, Fuccio L, Karstensen JG, Hucl T, et al. Endoscopic diagnosis and management of esophagogastric variceal hemorrhage: European Society of Gastrointestinal Endoscopy (ESGE) guideline. Endoscopy. 2022;54(11):1094–120.

34. European Association for the Study of the L. EASL Clinical Practice Guidelines on prevention and management of bleeding and thrombosis in patients with cirrhosis. J Hepatol. 2022;76(5):1151–84.
35. Lv Y, Yang Z, Liu L, Li K, He C, Wang Z, et al. Early TIPS with covered stents versus standard treatment for acute variceal bleeding in patients with advanced cirrhosis: a randomised controlled trial. Lancet Gastroenterol Hepatol. 2019;4(8):587–98.
36. Garcia-Pagan JC, Di Pascoli M, Caca K, Laleman W, Bureau C, Appenrodt B, et al. Use of early-TIPS for high-risk variceal bleeding: results of a post-RCT surveillance study. J Hepatol. 2013;58(1):45–50.
37. Njei B, McCarty TR, Laine L. Early transjugular intrahepatic portosystemic shunt in US patients hospitalized with acute esophageal variceal bleeding. J Gastroenterol Hepatol. 2017;32(4):852–8.
38. Maimone S, Saffioti F, Filomia R, Alibrandi A, Isgro G, Calvaruso V, et al. Predictors of rebleeding and mortality among patients with refractory variceal bleeding undergoing salvage Transjugular Intrahepatic Portosystemic Shunt (TIPS). Dig Dis Sci. 2019;64(5):1335–45.
39. Azoulay D, Castaing D, Majno P, Saliba F, Ichai P, Smail A, et al. Salvage transjugular intrahepatic portosystemic shunt for uncontrolled variceal bleeding in patients with decompensated cirrhosis. J Hepatol. 2001;35(5):590–7.
40. Puente A, Hernandez-Gea V, Graupera I, Roque M, Colomo A, Poca M, et al. Drugs plus ligation to prevent rebleeding in cirrhosis: an updated systematic review. Liver Int. 2014;34(6):823–33.
41. Bosch J, Garcia-Pagan JC. Prevention of variceal rebleeding. Lancet. 2003;361(9361):952–4.
42. Albillos A, Zamora J, Martinez J, Arroyo D, Ahmad I, De-la-Pena J, et al. Stratifying risk in the prevention of recurrent variceal hemorrhage: results of an individual patient meta-analysis. Hepatology. 2017;66(4):1219–31.
43. Thiele M, Krag A, Rohde U, Gluud LL. Meta-analysis: banding ligation and medical interventions for the prevention of rebleeding from oesophageal varices. Aliment Pharmacol Ther. 2012;35(10):1155–65.
44. North Italian Endoscopic Club for the S, Treatment of Esophageal V. Prediction of the first variceal hemorrhage in patients with cirrhosis of the liver and esophageal varices. A prospective multicenter study. N Engl J Med. 1988;319(15):983–9.
45. D'Amico G, Garcia-Pagan JC, Luca A, Bosch J. Hepatic vein pressure gradient reduction and prevention of variceal bleeding in cirrhosis: a systematic review. Gastroenterology. 2006;131(5):1611–24.
46. Saab S, Nieto JM, Lewis SK, Runyon BA. TIPS versus paracentesis for cirrhotic patients with refractory ascites. Cochrane Database Syst Rev. 2006;2006(4):CD004889.
47. Tan HK, James PD, Sniderman KW, Wong F. Long-term clinical outcome of patients with cirrhosis and refractory ascites treated with transjugular intrahepatic portosystemic shunt insertion. J Gastroenterol Hepatol. 2015;30(2):389–95.
48. Bureau C, Thabut D, Oberti F, Dharancy S, Carbonell N, Bouvier A, et al. Transjugular intrahepatic portosystemic shunts with covered stents increase transplant-free survival of patients with cirrhosis and recurrent ascites. Gastroenterology. 2017;152(1):157–63.

Management of Critically Sick Patient with End-Stage Liver Disease (Acute Liver Failure and Acute-on-Chronic Liver Failure)

5

Julie Gorham and Thierry Gustot

Acute Liver Failure

Definition

The clinical course of acute liver failure (ALF) is initiated by a severe acute liver injury (ALI) defined by an acute deterioration of liver blood tests and an impaired liver function such as coagulopathy (International Normalized Ratio (INR) >1.5 or prolongation of prothrombin time (PT)) and potentially jaundice without underlying chronic liver disease. The following development of hepatic encephalopathy (HE), which can be subtle, is required for the diagnosis of ALF [1]. There are some exceptions to this definition: even if there is an underlying chronic liver disease, patients with an acute de novo presentation of autoimmune hepatitis, Budd-Chiari syndrome or Wilson disease are considered as having ALF if they develop HE. Depending on the delay between the presentation of jaundice and the onset of

J. Gorham
Intensive Care Unit, H.U.B. Hôpital Erasme, Brussels, Belgium

T. Gustot (✉)
Department of Transplantation, H.U.B. Hôpital Erasme, Brussels, Belgium

Liver Transplant Unit, Department of Gastroenterology, Hepato-Pancreatology and Digestive Oncology, H.U.B. Hôpital Erasme, Brussels, Belgium

Laboratory of Experimental Gastroenterology, Université Libre de Bruxelles, Brussels, Belgium

Inserm Unité 1149, Centre de Recherche sur l'inflammation (CRI), Paris, France

UMR S_1149, Université Paris Diderot, Paris, France

EASL CLIF Consortium, European Foundation of Chronic Liver Failure (EF-Clif), Barcelona, Spain
e-mail: thierry.gustot@hubruxelles.be

B. Eghtesad et al. (eds.), *Liver Transplantation*,
https://doi.org/10.1007/978-3-032-07072-2_5

HE, several classifications of ALF have been described including O'Grady's and Bernau's classifications. The O'Grady's classification has a prognostic value and divided patients into three categories: hyperacute, acute and subacute if patients develop HE within 7 days, 8 to 28 days or 4 to 12 weeks of onset of jaundice [1]. Concerning the Bernau's classification, a delay between jaundice and HE less than 2 weeks is categorized as fulminant and subfulminant when there is a delay between 2 and 12 weeks [2].

Criteria for Liver Transplant Center and ICU Admission

The diagnosis of severe ALI and particularly ALF justifies an admission to a liver transplant center due to unpredictable outcome. The presence or probability of a hyperacute form (acetaminophen intoxication and mushrooms ingestion), an extra-hepatic organ failure such as renal failure (oliguria and/or elevated creatinine), elevated lactate and/or hypotension unresponsive to fluid resuscitation, metabolic acidosis (arterial pH < 7.30 or $HCO3 < 18$), altered level of consciousness (grade II EH) and hypoglycemia are criteria for admitting patients in intensive care unit (ICU). This admission is justified by the required intense monitoring.

Prognostication

There has been an improvement in the prognosis of ALF patients due to transplantation and improvement in intensive care management [3]. The prognosis depends on the etiology of ALF and the rapidity of onset of HE. In patients with subacute ALF, usually caused by idiosyncratic drug liver injury (DILI), hepatitis B (HBV) infection or autoimmune hepatitis, the prognosis is poor. Conversely, hyperacute presentations have greater chance of spontaneous recovery, even if there are more at risk of cerebral edema [4]. Indeed, even if acetaminophen-induced ALF is often associated with a progressive multi-organ failure (MOF) and HE, patients who do not have criteria for emergency liver transplantation (LT) have a good prognosis (<10% mortality) compared to patients with DILI where mortality without LT is 80% [5]. Concerning viral etiologies, which remains a major cause of ALF worldwide, hepatitis A (HAV)-related ALF has a good prognosis (70% of spontaneous survival rate) compared to HBV-related ALF (25% of spontaneous survival rate) [6]. ALF in the setting of a HBV reactivation, that can occur during or after treatment-induced immunosuppression for cancer, has a worse prognosis than de novo infections [7].

Management

General Management A complete history, a physical examination, extensive laboratory tests with viral, autoimmune and toxicology screening, an arterial blood gas as well as a baseline echocardiography and a liver ultrasound need to be done at admission in every patient. Axial computed tomography (CT) imaging should be considered to identify patients with underlying chronic liver disease.

Etiological Management N-acetyl cysteine (NAC) therapy has shown a benefit on survival in case of acetaminophen-induced ALF and therefore should be given in this case. In addition, to protect the liver by restoring glutathione levels, beneficial effects of NAC may be mediated by its antioxidant and vasodilatory effects. Concerning the use of NAC in non-acetaminophen-related ALF, although its use is increased in clinical practice probably due to its safety and tolerability profile, there is no evidence of benefit on survival [8]. There are other specific therapies for certain etiologies (Table 5.1).

Neurological Management ALF can lead to neurological dysfunction varying from HE to brain oedema and intracranial hypertension (ICH). Even if the pathogenesis is complex and multifactorial, there is evidence that ammonia plays a central role [9]. To reduce the level of ammonia, continuous renal replacement therapy (CRRT) has been shown to be effective in patients with ALF [10]. The use of lactulose or rifaximin cannot be recommended in this setting due to the fact that their efficacy and safety have not been assessed. A neurological examination should be performed every 2 hours. Endotracheal intubation is required for patients with grade III/IV EH to ensure airway protection Placement of intracranial pressure (ICP) devices is not recommended due to the high rate of bleeding and infectious complications and the fact that there is limited evidence on survival benefit. Several indirect non-invasive monitoring ICP tool have been proposed, with transcranial Doppler ultrasonography likely the most useful [11]. Therapeutic options for the management of brain oedema consist of general measures such as elevation of the head of the bed to 30-degree and avoidance of fever, hypo- or hyperglycemia and hyponatremia. Development of clinical signs (i.e., fixed dilated pupils) of ICH

Table 5.1 Etiology and specific therapies

Etiology	Treatment	RCT
Auto-immune hepatitis	Immunosuppression (corticosteroids)	No
Hepatitis B virus	Nucleos(t)ide analogs	No
Acetaminophen	N-acetylcysteine	Yes
Wilson	D-penicillamine	No
Herpes virus	Acyclovir/foscarnet	No
Budd-Chiari	Anticoagulation/TIPS	No
Amantia phalloides	Penicillin G/Silymarin	No
Ischemic injury	Cardiovascular support	No
Malignancy	Anti-neoplastic	No
Other DILI	Drug withdrawal	No

RCT randomized controlled trial, *TIPS* transjugular intrahepatic porto-systemic shunt, *DILI* drug-induced liver injury should be treated by a bolus of hypertonic saline to target sodium levels between 145 and 155 mEq/L or intravenous mannitol (0.5 g/kg 4–6 times per day). Sedation with propofol should be used in patients for whom osmotic therapy is not sufficient to reduce ICH [12]. In case of refractory ICH, reducing arterial $PaCO_2$ to 25–30 mmHg with a short period of hyperventilation, may be required but with the risk of cerebral ischemia due to the resultant vasoconstriction induced by hypocapnia. Even if barbiturates are effective in lowering ICP, they are not recommended due to their major side effects. Concerning hypothermia, clinical studies have shown that moderate hypothermia (34°) may be effective in controlling refractory ICH but without impact on survival. Nevertheless, the use of prophylactic hypothermia in patient with high-grade EH does not prevent ICH [13]. Hepatectomy is a theoretical possibility as a bridging procedure to LT for patients with refractory ICH, with no chance of spontaneous survival [14]. Seizures are commonly expected to occur in patients with ALF having cerebral edema; therefore, a continuous electroencephalography (EEG) monitoring should be done and antiepileptic drugs administered in case of seizure, with levetiracetam being the most frequently used. The prophylactic use of antiepileptic drugs is not recommended [15].

Cardiovascular Management Most patients with ALF are hypovolemic on admission due to multifactorial factors (i.e., poor oral intake, fluid losses through vomiting) and require initial fluid resuscitation. Concerning the type of fluid, crystalloid fluid is preferred over colloid [14]. Balanced solutions can be used to avoid hyperchloremia and acute kidney injury. However, Ringer's lactate is not recommended in ICH due to hypotonicity and balanced solutions buffered with acetate should not be used in ALF due to the risk of a decreased metabolic capacity. Intravenous albumin is not recommended. Excessive fluid overload is independently associated with poor outcomes and should be avoided [16]. Persistent hypotension despite adequate volume loading requires invasive monitoring and vasopressor administration. It is important to note that ALF is characterized by a hyperdynamic state with a low systemic vascular resistance. The vasopressor of choice is norepinephrine, with a mean arterial pressure (MAP) target of 65 mmHg. The role of vasopressin and analogs is controversial. Relative adrenal insufficiency is observed in nearly 50% but the administration of hydrocortisone is not routinely recommended due to the additive infectious risk.

Renal Management Acute renal injury (AKI) is common in patients with ALF [17]. Nephrotoxics should be minimized (drugs or contrast). As well as classic indications (i.e., uremia, fluid overload, hyperkalemia, acidosis), RRT may be used in ALF patients also to manage metabolic disturbances such as hyperammonemia and dysnatremia, and brain edema [10]. Continuous modes of RRT are preferred to intermittent dialysis, providing more hemodynamic stability and less metabolic fluctuations [18]. Concerning the choice of anticoagulation, an alternative to systemic anticoagulation with heparin in patients with high risk of bleeding is the use of anticoagulation free CRRT circuits with predilutional fluid replacement, but with the risk of clotting. Studies have shown that regional anticoagulation with citrate is another alternative, improving circuit patency and reducing bleeding complications [19, 20]. If citrate is used as an anticoagulant, close monitoring of the total calcium/ionized calcium ratio is required, knowing that in case of severe liver failure, citrate metabolism is impaired with a risk of citrate accumulation [21].

Respiratory Management The management of patients with ALF who require ventilatory support for hypoxemia and acute respiratory distress syndrome (ARDS) consists of standard sedation with propofol, avoidance of fluid overload and lung protective ventilator techniques with low tidal volume (6 ml/kg/ideal body weight), plateau pressure limited to 30 cm H2O, high frequency rate to ensure adequate minute ventilation and appropriate level of positive end-expiratory pressure (PEEP) [22]. However, some adaptations need to be done in case of cerebral edema, such as the regulation of the respiratory rate, avoiding hyper- and hypocapnia and maintaining the lowest PEEP that achieves adequate oxygenation. Once the patient is hemodynamically stable, a neutral or a negative fluid balance must be achieved.

Coagulation Management Prophylactic administration of coagulation factors should be avoided because it will influence artificial coagulation tests, and should be limited to specific situations, such as invasive procedures or active bleeding. It should be noted that although laboratory tests indicate a bleeding diathesis in ALF patients (i.e., prolonged INR, thrombocytopenia), thrombotic complications can be more frequent than bleeding complications because of a loss of synthesis in both pro- and anticoagulant factors in these patients [23].

Infectious Management Sepsis, as well as multi-organ failure, is a common cause of death in patients with ALF [24]. Therefore, we should have a low threshold for microbiological (mainly bacteria and fungi) assessment, for starting antibiotics (rapid unexplained progression of HE to grade III/IV, multiple organ failure, invasive mechanical ventilation), and line changes. However, we cannot recommend routine antibiotic prophylaxis or bowel decontamination [25].

Metabolic Management Hypoglycemia, common in patients with ALF, is associated with increased mortality and needs to be corrected. Hyperglycemia should also be avoided because of the risk of increased ICP. Enteral or parenteral nutrition, if enteral nutrition is contraindicated, should be initiated early because patients with ALF have a 30% increase in metabolic needs [26].

Extracorporeal Liver Support High-volume plasma exchange (8–12 L exchanged per session) for 3 consecutive days to remove damage-associated molecular patterns and cytokines is the only efficient treatment in terms of transplant-free survival compared to standard of care (SOC) in a randomized trial [27]. Another open-label RCT confirmed these results even if the exchanged volume was lower (1.5 to 2 plasma volumes per session) [28]. Other devices, such as albumin dialysis, MARS, failed to show a survival benefit in RCT [29]. Bioartificial liver supports, such as hepatassist containing porcine hepatocytes and ELAD containing C3A human-derived hepatoblastoma cells, were not able to improve the survival of patients with ALF compared to SOC [30, 31].

Indication for Liver Transplantation

An "As soon as possible" recognition of ALF patients who will die without LT is the main step in clinical management. Different prognostic tools have been developed. The most studied one is the King's College criteria (Table 5.2) which is characterized by acceptable specificity but relatively low sensitivity in acetaminophen (APAP) and non-APAP induced ALF [32]. Recent studies have unraveled that a substantial number of patients fulfilling transplant criteria will experience spontaneous recovery due to the progress of critical care management. Young patients with less severe HE or multiorgan failure and with APAP-induced ALF have a higher transplant-free survival rate [33]. By studying non-transplanted patients with APAP-induced ALF, it has been shown that improvements of INR and arterial lactate within 24 hours are associated with transplant-free survival underlining the importance of the early dynamic profile in the outcome prediction [34].

Table 5.2 Criteria for liver transplantation in acute liver failure (ALF)

King's College criteria
ALF due to paracetamol
Arterial pH < 7.3 after resuscitation and >24 hours since ingestion
Lactate > 3 mmol/L or
The 3 following criteria:
HE ≥ Stage III
Serum creatinine > 3.4 mg/dL (300 μmol/L)
INR > 6.5
ALF not due to paracetamol
INR > 6.5 (irrespective of grade of encephalopathy) or
3 out of 5 following criteria:
Indetermined etiology, non-A non-B viral hepatitis, drug-induced hepatitis
Age < 10 years or > 40 years
Interval jaundice encephalopathy > 7 days
Total bilirubin > 17 mg/dL (300 μmol/L)
INR > 3.5

HE hepatic encephalopathy, *INR* international normalized ratio

Currently, post-LT survival for patients with ALF is particularly good (~90% at 3 years) [35]. Different predictors of post-LT poor outcomes have been identified: increased age, multiorgan failure (high dose of vasopressors and high-grade HE) and APAP etiology. Currently, criteria to define inappropriate LT for ALF patients are lacking and decisions are made on a case-by-case basis considering the predicting factors of poor outcomes. An irreversible brain injury, extrahepatic malignancy and psychiatric disorders are criteria contraindicating LT. A controlled bacteremia is not a contraindication. Progressive vasoplegic shock with rapidly rising vasopressor requirement is considered a relative contraindication, as is severe hemorrhagic pancreatitis, extensive small bowel ischemia and uncontrolled ARDS [14].

Acute-on-Chronic Liver Failure

Definitions

Different definitions of Acute-on-Chronic Liver Failure have been proposed from different consortia (Asia Pacific Association for the Study of the Liver [APASL], European Association for the Study of the Liver-Chronic Liver Failure [EASL-CLIF] Consortium and North American Consortium for the Study of End-Stage Liver Disease [NACSELD]) [36]. The EASL-CLIF definition has been externally validated in different continents [37, 38]. The EASL-CLIF-defined ACLF is characterized by an acute decompensation of cirrhosis, occurrence of organ failures and a high risk of short-term mortality (>15%), due to an acute precipitating event (i.e., intrahepatic or extrahepatic insults) clinically apparent or not [36]. Organ failures are identified with the use of the CLIF-C organ failure (OF) score (Table 5.3) [39]. Based on the presence of organ failure(s) and renal and/or cerebral dysfunction, patients with acutely decompensated cirrhosis were divided into four prognostic grades (ACLF grades 1,2 and 3) (Table 5.4) [36].

Criteria for ICU Admission

Patients with ACLF have organ failure(s) and often life-threatening complications requiring management in ICU [40]. In recent years, there has been an improvement in the prognosis of these critically ill ACLF patients [41] and their outcomes are not significantly different from patients (matched for comorbidities and severity of critical illness) admitted to ICU for sepsis or medical reasons [42]. Therefore, criteria for deciding ICU admission among patients with ACLF should not be different to those applied in the general population. Need for close monitoring or organ support such as vasopressors, mechanical ventilation, or renal replacement therapy, massive bleeding or grade 3–4 encephalopathy (West-Haven) without airway protection are indications for ICU admissions; in contrast, severe frailty, advanced neoplasm and comorbidities associated with poor short-term prognosis are contra-indications to ICU admission [43].

Table 5.3 The CLIF-OF system

Organ/system	1 point	2 points	3 points
Liver	Bilirubin < 6mg/dl	Bilirubin ≥ 6mg/dl and < 12 mg/dl	Bilirubin ≥ 12mg/dl
Kidney	Creatinine < 2mg/dl	Creatinine ≥ 2mg/dl and < 3.5mg/dl	Creatinine ≥ 3.5mg/dl or RRT
Brain (West-Haven grade for HE)	Grade 0	Grade 1-2	Grade 3-4
Coagulation	INR < 2	INR ≥ 2 and < 2.5	INR ≥ 2.5
Circulatory	MAP ≥ 70mmHg	MAP < 70mmHg	Vasopressor requirement
Respiratory	PaO2/FiO2 > 300 Or SpO2/FiO2 > 357	PaO2/FiO2 > 201 and ≤ 300 or SpO2/FiO2 > 214 and ≤ 357	PaO2/FiO2 ≤ 200 or SpO2/FiO2 ≤ 214

Each organ system function receives a score ranging from 1 point (close to normal) to 3 points (abnormal). The dark-gray cells indicate the definition of each organ failure, and the light-gray cells the definition of each organ dysfunction. Patients treated with MV received a respiratory score of 3 points. Patients submitted to MV because of HE and not due to respiratory failure were considered as presenting a cerebral score of 3 points.

Table 5.4 ACLF grades and 28-day free-transplantation mortality

Grade	Definition	28-day mortality without LT (%)
Absence of ACLF	No OF	4.4
Absence of ACLF	A single non-renal OF without KD and BD	6.3
ACLF-1a	Single KF	18.6
ACLF-1b	Single non-renal OF with KD or/and BD	27.8
ACLF-2	Two OFs	32
ACLF-3a	Three OFs	68
ACLF-3b	Four to six OFs	88.9

BD brain dysfunction, *KD* kidney dysfunction, *OF* organ failure, *KF* kidney failure

Supportive Management

General Management Infections, most often bacterial, are frequent precipitating factors in patients with ACLF [44, 45]. It is important to identify and treat them as soon as possible, as well as the other commonest precipitants such as alcohol-related hepatitis, gastrointestinal hemorrhage, and hepatitis virus infection (Table 5.5).

Circulatory Management Circulatory failure in ACLF patients should be managed like in patients without cirrhosis. There is no evidence of advantage of colloid solutions, in particular albumin, against crystalloids despite a quicker resolution of hypotension but a higher rate of pulmonary edema [46]. Thus, crystalloids should be used as initial fluid and human albumin is suggested if patients with ACLF require substantial amounts of fluids and vasopressors [43]. Patients not responding to fluid therapy require the rapid initiation of vasopressors to preserve organ perfusion and prevent organ damage [47]. Norepinephrine (NE) is considered the first-line vasopressor in patients and continuous administration of terlipressin or vasopressin as second-line [48, 49]. A small open-label RCT comparing terlipressin to NE suggested that terlipressin administration was associated with more rapid hemodynamic stabilization, lower risk of variceal bleeding and improved survival at 48 hours but similar hospital survival and higher rate of adverse events (peripheral ischemia and lactic acidosis) [50]. Relative adrenal insufficiency is highly prevalent in patients with ACLF and refractory septic shock, and is associated with poor outcome [51]. Stress dose steroids (hydrocortisone 200 mg/day) may be used in patients with ACLF who require moderate or high doses of norepinephrine (>0.25 μg/kg/min) for hypotension [43].

Renal Management More than half of ACLF patients have AKI [36] which can be due to intrinsic renal causes, post renal obstruction, hypoperfusion due to hypovolemia and hepatorenal syndrome (HRS) [52]. The first-line therapy for HRS-AKI, is volume expansion with albumin (20–40 g/ day) and in case of non-response, the use of vasoconstrictors (NE or bolus or continuous terlipressin). RRT should be initiated in patients whose renal function fails to respond to medical treatment.

Table 5.5 Treatments for most common precipitating events

Precipitating events	Validated treatments
Bacterial infection	Prompt and adequate antibiotics for 5–7 days + albumin 1.5 g/kg day 0, 1 g/kg day 3 for spontaneous bacterial peritonitis[a]
Severe alcohol-related hepatitis	Prednisone 40 mg for 28 days ± NAC for 5 days[b]
Variceal bleeding	Vasoactive drugs[c] for 5 days + endoscopic treatment + appropriate antibiotics for 7 days
Flare-up or exacerbation of HBV	Nucleot(s)ide analogs
Paracetamol-induced liver injury	NAC[b]
Flare-up of autoimmune hepatitis	Prednisone 1 mg/kg ± azathioprine 1–2 mg/kg

[a]in absence of septic shock
[b]N-acetylcysteine (NAC) dosage: On day 1, 150 mg/kg over a period of 30 minutes, 50 mg/kg over 4 hours, and 100 mg/kg over 16 hours
[c]Terlipressin (bolus of 2 mg followed by 1 mg every 6 hours), somatostatin (bolus of 250 μg followed by 250 μg/hour continuous infusion) or octreotide (bolus of 50 μg followed by 25 μg/hour continuous infusion)

Continuous modes of RRT are preferred, and the use of citrate as anticoagulation seems to be safe [53].

Neurological Management HE is the most common neurological complication in ACLF patients [54]. Precipitating factors need to be identified and managed [55, 56]. Lactulose and possibly rifaximin are currently the main specific therapies for HE in cirrhotic patients, although their efficacy in ACLF is unknown. In refractory encephalopathy, RRT and extracorporeal liver support have some efficacy [55, 56]. Endotracheal intubation is required if the airway cannot be protected. Due to altered pharmacokinetics, benzodiazepines should be avoided for sedation [57].

Coagulation Management Conventional coagulation tests such as PT, INR, and activated partial thromboplastin time (APTT), do not accurately reflect the hemostatic status of ACLF patients [58]. Thromboelastography and rotational thromboelastometry (ROTEM) provide superior insights into hemostatic balance, particularly guiding transfusion in patients who are actively bleeding [59]. Systematic correction of coagulopathy with fresh frozen plasma is not recommended. While thrombocytopenia is common in cirrhosis, VWF elevation preserves platelet adhesion in vitro [60]. Maintaining a platelet count $>50 \times 10^9$/L is the practical clinical target in cases of active bleeding or as prophylaxis before procedures. Critically ill ACLF patients are at high risk of developing deep vein thrombosis and/or pulmonary embolism (PE), warranting thromboprophylaxis unless contraindications such as recent or active bleeding and significant thrombocytopenia are present.

Respiratory Management Currently, the impact of different respiratory supports (non-invasive or mechanical ventilation) has not been studied in ACLF patients. Standard protective lung ventilation strategy should be applied in patients with ACLF with low tidal volume (6 ml/kg/ideal body weight), plateau pressure limited to 30 cm H2O, high frequency rate to ensure adequate minute ventilation, and appropriate level of positive end-expiratory pressure (PEEP) [22].

Nutrition Management The screening of malnutrition using validated tools is indicated for all patients with ACLF [43]. The energy target is 30–35 kcal/kg/day with a protein target of 1.2–1.5 g/kg/day [43]. Protein intake restriction should be avoided. Oral intake should be encouraged; if not possible, enteral nutrition is recommended. If enteral nutrition is not tolerated, parenteral nutrition can be considered, like in other critically ill patients.

Extracorporeal Liver Support Extra-corporeal albumin dialysis systems have shown promise in clearing accumulated toxic metabolites. However, while MARS®

and Prometheus® improve serum bilirubin levels and HE, they have not demonstrated a significant impact on survival [61, 62]. A post-hoc analysis indicates that patients with ACLF-2 or 3 who undergo more than 4 albumin dialysis sessions may experience short-term survival benefits (2–3 weeks), suggesting albumin dialysis as a potential bridge to LT. Recently, a new liver dialysis device, DIALIVE, which combines a filter (Septex, Baxter, USA) for albumin and cytokine ultrafiltration and a second (Oxiris, Baxter, USA) for pathogen and damage-associated molecular pattern adsorption, was assessed in a pilot RCT involving 32 patients [63]. DIALIVE appears to be safe and permits a faster resolution of ACLF, without a 28-day survival benefit compared to standard medical care. A larger study is planned to evaluate the efficacy endpoint. Plasma exchange (PE) is commonly used in Asia, particularly for HBV-related ACLF, with some retrospective reports suggesting a survival benefit. An ongoing large RCT ($n = 380$, APACHE Trial: NCT03702920) aims to assess its impact on transplant-free survival.

Prognostication

The CLIF-C ACLF score predicted more accurately the 28-day and 90-day transplant-free mortality than MELD, MELD-Na and Child-Pugh scores [39]. However, this prognostic score was more accurate when assessed 3 to 7 days after full organ support than at ICU admission, understanding that ACLF patients may have a steady or a dynamic course with the possibility of resolution, improvement, or worsening within a few days [64]. A CLIF-C ACLF score > 64–70 points or the presence of ≥4 organ failures 3 to 7 days after initiation of intensive care support, without LT option, are criteria indicating potential futility of ongoing ICU support, and palliative care needs to be discussed [64, 65].

Indication for Liver Transplantation

LT is the only life-saving treatment for patients with severe ACLF with adequate post-transplant outcomes for highly selected patients, even in those with ACLF-3 [64, 66, 67]. Then, after early intensive management of ACLF patients, a transfer to a liver transplant center should be evaluated. Currently, the selection of patients for LT is based on a case-by-case approach and proven predictors of poor post-LT outcomes (advanced age, portal vein thrombosis, extra-hepatic comorbidities). A consensus of experts suggested some relative contraindications: severe frailty (defined by a clinical frailty scale ≥7), ongoing sepsis except for urinary tract infections, appropriate antimicrobial treatment of spontaneous bacterial peritonitis or pneumonia <72 hours, previous infection with pan-drug resistant bacteria, lung failure with PaO_2/FiO_2 ratio <150, hemodynamic instability requiring dose of norepinephrine >1 μg/kg/min, arterial lactate >9 mmol/L and worsening of the clinical course at the time of graft proposal [68]. Two scores have been developed to define if a patient is too sick to be transplanted (TAM score, SALT-M) but these scores have been designed on retrospective studies and were not externally validated [69, 70]. Every patient with severe ACLF (ACLF-2 or 3) should be assessed for LT, in particular those with a worse clinical course.

References

1. Williams R, Schalm SW, O'Grady JG. Acute liver failure: redefining the syndromes. Lancet. 1993;342(8866):273–5.
2. Bernuau J, Benhamou JP. Classifying acute liver failure. Lancet. 1993;342(8866):252–3.
3. Donnelly MC, Davidson JS, Martin K, Baird A, Hayes PC, Simpson KJ. Acute liver failure in Scotland: changes in aetiology and outcomes over time (the Scottish Look-Back Study). Aliment Pharmacol Ther. 2017;45(6):833–43.
4. Arshad MA, Murphy N, Bangash MN. Acute liver failure. Clin Med. 2020;20(5):505–8.
5. Stravitz RT, Lee WM. Acute liver failure. Lancet. 2019;394(10201):869–81.
6. Manka P, Verheyen J, Gerken G, Canbay A. Liver failure due to acute viral hepatitis (A-E). Visc Med. 2016;32(2):80–5.
7. Mindikoglu AL, Regev A, Schiff ER. Hepatitis B virus reactivation after cytotoxic chemotherapy: the disease and its prevention. Clin Gastroenterol Hepatol. 2006;4(9):1076–81.
8. Siu JT, Nguyen T, Turgeon RD. N-acetylcysteine for non-paracetamol (acetaminophen)-related acute liver failure. Cochrane Hepato-Biliary Group, éditeur. Cochrane Database of Systematic Reviews [Internet]. 9 déc 2020 [cité 29 mars 2024];2020(12). Disponible sur: http://doi.wiley.com/10.1002/14651858.CD012123.pub2.
9. Butterworth RF. Pathogenesis of hepatic encephalopathy and brain edema in acute liver failure. J Clin Exp Hepatol. 2015;5:S96–103.
10. Slack AJ, Auzinger G, Willars C, Dew T, Musto R, Corsilli D, et al. Ammonia clearance with haemofiltration in adults with liver disease. Liver Int. 2014;34(1):42–8.
11. Aggarwal S, Brooks DM, Kang Y, Linden PK, Patzer JF. Noninvasive monitoring of cerebral perfusion pressure in patients with acute liver failure using transcranial doppler ultrasonography. Liver Transpl. 2008;14(7):1048–57.
12. Wijdicks EFM, Nyberg SL. Propofol to control intracranial pressure in fulminant hepatic failure. Transplant Proc. 2002;34(4):1220–2.
13. Ribaud J, McLernon S, Auzinger G. Targeted temperature management in acute liver failure: a systematic review. Nurs Crit Care. 2022;27(6):784–95.
14. Wendon J, Cordoba J, Dhawan A, Larsen FS, Manns M, Nevens F, et al. EASL clinical practical guidelines on the management of acute (fulminant) liver failure. J Hepatol. 2017;66(5):1047–81.
15. Bhatia V, Batra Y, Acharya SK. Prophylactic phenytoin does not improve cerebral edema or survival in acute liver failure—a controlled clinical trial. J Hepatol. 2004;41(1):89–96.
16. Mitchell KH, Carlbom D, Caldwell E, Leary PJ, Himmelfarb J, Hough CL. Volume overload: prevalence, risk factors, and functional outcome in survivors of septic shock. Annals ATS. 2015;12(12):1837–44.
17. Tujios SR, Hynan LS, Vazquez MA, Larson AM, Seremba E, Sanders CM, et al. Risk factors and outcomes of acute kidney injury in patients with acute liver failure. Clin Gastroenterol Hepatol. 2015;13(2):352–9.
18. Davenport A. The clinical application of CRRT—current status: continuous renal replacement therapies in patients with liver disease. Semin Dial. 2009;22(2):169–72.
19. Schultheiß C, Saugel B, Phillip V, Thies P, Noe S, Mayr U, et al. Continuous venovenous hemodialysis with regional citrate anticoagulation in patients with liver failure: a prospective observational study. Crit Care. 2012;16(4):R162.
20. Agarwal B, Shaw S, Hari MS, Burroughs AK, Davenport A. Continuous renal replacement therapy (CRRT) in patients with liver disease: is circuit life different? J Hepatol. 2009;51(3):504–9.

21. Oudemans-van Straaten HM, Ostermann M. Bench-to-bedside review: citrate for continuous renal replacement therapy, from science to practice. Crit Care. 2012;16(6):249.
22. Fan E, Del Sorbo L, Goligher EC, Hodgson CL, Munshi L, Walkey AJ, et al. An Official American Thoracic Society/European Society of Intensive Care Medicine/Society of Critical Care Medicine clinical practice guideline: mechanical ventilation in adult patients with acute respiratory distress syndrome. Am J Respir Crit Care Med. 2017;195(9):1253–63.
23. Lisman T, Bakhtiari K, Adelmeijer J, Meijers JCM, Porte RJ, Stravitz RT. Intact thrombin generation and decreased fibrinolytic capacity in patients with acute liver injury or acute liver failure. J Thromb Haemost. 2012;10(7):1312–9.
24. Maiwall R, Kulkarni AV, Arab JP, Piano S. Acute liver failure. Lancet. 2024;404(10454):789–802.
25. Karvellas CJ, Cavazos J, Battenhouse H, Durkalski V, Balko J, Sanders C, et al. Effects of antimicrobial prophylaxis and blood stream infections in patients with acute liver Failure: a retrospective cohort study. Clin Gastroenterol Hepatol. 2014;12(11):1942–1949.e1.
26. Abenavoli L, Maurizi V, Boccuto L, Di Berardino A, Giostra N, Santori P, et al. Nutritional support in acute liver failure. Diseases. 2022;10(4):108.
27. Larsen FS, Schmidt LE, Bernsmeier C, Rasmussen A, Isoniemi H, Patel VC, et al. High-volume plasma exchange in patients with acute liver failure: an open randomised controlled trial. J Hepatol. 2016;64(1):69–78.
28. Maiwall R, Bajpai M, Singh A, Agarwal T, Kumar G, Bharadwaj A, et al. Standard-volume plasma exchange improves outcomes in patients with acute liver failure: a randomized controlled trial. Clin Gastroenterol Hepatol. 2022;20(4):e831–54.
29. Saliba F, Camus C, Durand F, Mathurin P, Letierce A, Delafosse B, et al. Albumin dialysis with a noncell artificial liver support device in patients with acute liver failure: a randomized, controlled trial. Ann Intern Med. 2013;159(8):522.
30. Demetriou AA, Brown RS, Busuttil RW, Fair J, McGuire BM, Rosenthal P, et al. Prospective, randomized, multicenter, controlled trial of a bioartificial liver in treating acute liver failure. Ann Surg. 2004;239(5):660–70.
31. Ellis AJ, Hughes RD, Wendon JA, Dunne J, Langley PG, Kelly JH, et al. Pilot–controlled trial of the extracorporeal liver assist device in acute liver failure. Hepatology. 1996;24(6):1446–51.
32. McPhail MJW, Farne H, Senvar N, Wendon JA, Bernal W. Ability of King's college criteria and model for end-stage liver disease scores to predict mortality of patients with acute liver failure: a meta-analysis. Clin Gastroenterol Hepatol. 2016;14(4):516–525.e5.
33. Bernal W, Hyyrylainen A, Gera A, Audimoolam VK, McPhail MJW, Auzinger G, et al. Lessons from look-back in acute liver failure? A single centre experience of 3300 patients. J Hepatol. 2013;59(1):74–80.
34. Bernal W, Wang Y, Maggs J, Willars C, Sizer E, Auzinger G, et al. Development and validation of a dynamic outcome prediction model for paracetamol-induced acute liver failure: a cohort study. Lancet Gastroenterol Hepatol. 2016;1(3):217–25.
35. Karvellas CJ, Leventhal TM, Rakela JL, Zhang J, Durkalski V, Reddy KR, et al. Outcomes of patients with acute liver failure listed for liver transplantation: a multicenter prospective cohort analysis. Liver Transplant. 2023;29(3):318–30.
36. Moreau R, Jalan R, Gines P, Pavesi M, Angeli P, Cordoba J, et al. Acute-on-chronic liver failure is a distinct syndrome that develops in patients with acute decompensation of cirrhosis. Gastroenterology. 2013;144(7):1426–1437.e9.
37. Hernaez R, Kramer JR, Liu Y, Tansel A, Natarajan Y, Hussain KB, et al. Prevalence and short-term mortality of acute-on-chronic liver failure: a national cohort study from the USA. J Hepatol. 2019;70(4):639–47.
38. Farias AQ, Curto Vilalta A, Momoyo Zitelli P, Pereira G, Goncalves LL, Torre A, et al. Genetic ancestry, race, and severity of acutely decompensated cirrhosis in Latin America. Gastroenterology. 2023;165(3):696–716.
39. Jalan R, Saliba F, Pavesi M, Amoros A, Moreau R, Ginès P, et al. Development and validation of a prognostic score to predict mortality in patients with acute-on-chronic liver failure. J Hepatol. 2014;61(5):1038–47.

40. Arroyo V, Moreau R, Jalan R. Acute-on-chronic liver failure. Longo DL, éditeur. N Engl J Med. 2020;382(22):2137–45.
41. McPhail MJW, Parrott F, Wendon JA, Harrison DA, Rowan KA, Bernal W. Incidence and outcomes for patients with cirrhosis admitted to the United Kingdom critical care units*. Crit Care Med. 2018;46(5):705–12.
42. Meersseman P, Langouche L, Du Plessis J, Korf H, Mekeirele M, Laleman W, et al. The intensive care unit course and outcome in acute-on-chronic liver failure are comparable to other populations. J Hepatol. 2018;69(4):803–9.
43. Moreau R, Tonon M, Krag A, Angeli P, Berenguer M, Berzigotti A, et al. EASL clinical practice guidelines on acute-on-chronic liver failure. J Hepatol. 2023;79(2):461–91.
44. Xu Z, Zhang X, Chen J, Shi Y, Ji S. Bacterial infections in acute-on-chronic liver Failure: epidemiology, diagnosis, pathogenesis, and management. J Clin Transl Hepatol. 2024;12(7):667.
45. Fernández J, Acevedo J, Wiest R, Gustot T, Amoros A, Deulofeu C, et al. Bacterial and fungal infections in acute-on-chronic liver failure: prevalence, characteristics and impact on prognosis. Gut. 2018;67(10):1870–80.
46. Maiwall R, Kumar A, Pasupuleti SSR, Hidam AK, Tevethia H, Kumar G, et al. A randomized-controlled trial comparing 20% albumin to plasmalyte in patients with cirrhosis and sepsis-induced hypotension [ALPS trial]. J Hepatol. 2022;77(3):670–82.
47. Russell JA, Gordon AC, Williams MD, Boyd JH, Walley KR, Kissoon N. Vasopressor therapy in the intensive care unit. Semin Respir Crit Care Med. 2021;42(01):059–77.
48. Backer DD, Chochrad D, Gottignies P. Comparison of dopamine and norepinephrine in the treatment of shock. N Engl J Med. 2010.
49. Delmas A, Leone M, Rousseau S, Albanèse J, Martin C. Clinical review: vasopressin and terlipressin in septic shock patients. Crit Care. 2004;9(2):212.
50. Choudhury A, Kedarisetty CK, Vashishtha C, Saini D, Kumar S, Maiwall R, et al. A randomized trial comparing terlipressin and noradrenaline in patients with cirrhosis and septic shock. Liver Int. 2017;37(4):552–61.
51. Fernández J, Escorsell A, Zabalza M, Felipe V, Navasa M, Mas A, et al. Adrenal insufficiency in patients with cirrhosis and septic shock: effect of treatment with hydrocortisone on survival. Hepatology. 2006;44(5):1288–95.
52. Velez JCQ, Therapondos G, Juncos LA. Reappraising the spectrum of AKI and hepatorenal syndrome in patients with cirrhosis. Nat Rev Nephrol. 2020;16(3):137–55.
53. Peng B, Lu J, Guo H, Liu J, Li A. Regional citrate anticoagulation for replacement therapy in patients with liver failure: a systematic review and meta-analysis. Front Nutr. 2023;10:1031796.
54. Córdoba J, Mínguez B. Hepatic encephalopathy. Semin Liver Dis. 2008;28(1):070–80.
55. Vilstrup H, Amodio P, Bajaj J, Cordoba J, Ferenci P, Mullen KD, et al. Hepatic encephalopathy in chronic liver disease: 2014 practice guideline by the American Association for the Study of Liver Diseases and the European Association for the Study of the Liver: Vilstrup et al. Hepatology. 2014;60(2):715–35.
56. Acharya C, Bajaj JS. Current Management of Hepatic Encephalopathy. Am J Gastroenterol. 2018;113(11):1600–12.
57. Bakti G, Fisch HU, Karlaganis G, Minder C, Bircher J. Mechanism of the excessive sedative response of cirrhotics to benzodiazepines: model experiments with triazolam. Hepatology. 1987;7(4):629–38.
58. Tripodi A, Caldwell SH, Hoffman M, Trotter JF, Sanyal AJ. Review article: the prothrombin time test as a measure of bleeding risk and prognosis in liver disease. Aliment Pharmacol Ther. 2007;26(2):141–8.
59. Kumar M, Ahmad J, Maiwall R, Choudhury A, Bajpai M, Mitra LG, et al. Thromboelastography-guided blood component use in patients with cirrhosis with nonvariceal bleeding: a randomized controlled trial. Hepatology. 2020;71(1):235–46.
60. De Oliveira SE, D'Amico ÉA, Flores Da Rocha TR, Marcondes Ferreira C, Medeiros Batista J, Carneiro D'Albuquerque LA, et al. Preservation of platelet function in patients with cirrhosis and thrombocytopenia undergoing esophageal variceal ligation. Hepatobiliary Pancreat Dis Int. 2020;19(6):555–60.

61. Bañares R, Nevens F, Larsen FS, Jalan R, Albillos A, Dollinger M, et al. Extracorporeal albumin dialysis with the molecular adsorbent recirculating system in acute-on-chronic liver failure: the RELIEF trial. Hepatology. 2013;57(3):1153–62.
62. Kribben A, Gerken G, Haag S, Herget–Rosenthal S, Treichel U, Betz C, et al. Effects of fractionated plasma separation and adsorption on survival in patients with acute-on-chronic liver failure. Gastroenterology. 2012;142(4):782–789.e3.
63. Agarwal B, Cañizares RB, Saliba F, Ballester MP, Tomescu DR, Martin D, et al. Randomized, controlled clinical trial of the DIALIVE liver dialysis device versus standard of care in patients with acute-on-chronic liver failure. J Hepatol. 2023;79(1):79–92.
64. Gustot T, Fernandez J, Garcia E, Morando F, Caraceni P, Alessandria C, et al. Clinical course of acute-on-chronic liver failure syndrome and effects on prognosis. Hepatology. 2015;62(1):243–52.
65. Engelmann C, Thomsen KL, Zakeri N, Sheikh M, Agarwal B, Jalan R, et al. Validation of CLIF-C ACLF score to define a threshold for futility of intensive care support for patients with acute-on-chronic liver failure. Crit Care. 2018;22(1):254.
66. Artru F, Goldberg D, Kamath PS. Should patients with acute-on-chronic liver failure grade 3 receive higher priority for liver transplantation? J Hepatol. 2023;78(6):1118–23.
67. Sundaram V, Kogachi S, Wong RJ, Karvellas CJ, Fortune BE, Mahmud N, et al. Effect of the clinical course of acute-on-chronic liver failure prior to liver transplantation on post-transplant survival. J Hepatol. 2020;72(3):481–8.
68. Weiss E, Saner F, Asrani SK, Biancofiore G, Blasi A, Lerut J, et al. When is a critically ill cirrhotic patient too sick to transplant? Development of consensus criteria by a multidisciplinary panel of 35 international experts. Transplantation. 2021;105(3):561–8.
69. Artzner T, Michard B, Weiss E, Barbier L, Noorah Z, Merle JC, et al. Liver transplantation for critically ill cirrhotic patients: stratifying utility based on pretransplant factors. Am J Transplant. 2020;20(9):2437–48.
70. Hernaez R, Karvellas CJ, Liu Y, Sacleux SC, Khemichian S, Stein LL, et al. The novel SALT-M score predicts 1-year post-transplant mortality in patients with severe acute-on-chronic liver failure. J Hepatol. 2023;79(3):717–27.

Kidney in Liver Transplant Candidates (Pre-transplant Evaluation)

6

Sapna V. Shah, Fadi A. Tohme, and Mitra K. Nadim

AKI has an estimated prevalence of over 50% in hospitalized patients with end-stage liver disease at the time of transplantation; however, the incidence varies based on the heterogeneity in severity of illness, the etiology of AKI, the presence of underlying co-morbidities (e.g., chronic kidney disease (CKD), diabetes) and the diversity of clinical settings. AKI occurs most often in the presence of sepsis, spontaneous bacterial peritonitis (SBP), and ascites and is associated with an increase in in-hospital morbidity and mortality as well as an increased risk of progression to CKD, especially in patients requiring renal replacement therapy (RRT) [1–6]. A diagnosis of AKI (even stage 1 AKI) is associated with an increased risk of mortality at 30 days, 90 days and 1 year, compared to those patients without AKI, even in the presence of renal recovery [3, 6].

Assessment of Kidney Function

Precise assessment of renal function in patients with cirrhosis facilitates accurate diagnosis and staging of kidney injury, appropriate drug dosing, and defines the need for simultaneous liver-kidney transplantation (SLK) [7]. Serum creatinine (sCr), the most widely used marker for kidney function, is affected by decrease in

S. V. Shah (✉) · M. K. Nadim
Division of Nephrology and Hypertension, Keck School of Medicine, University of Southern California, Los Angeles, CA, USA
e-mail: sapna.shah@med.usc.edu

F. A. Tohme
Division of Nephrology and Hypertension, Keck School of Medicine, University of Southern California, Los Angeles, CA, USA

Division of Pulmonary and Critical Care, Keck School of Medicine, University of Southern California, Los Angeles, CA, USA

B. Eghtesad et al. (eds.), *Liver Transplantation*,
https://doi.org/10.1007/978-3-032-07072-2_6

creatine production by the liver, malnutrition, sarcopenia, fluid overload, [8] bilirubin interference [9], large volume blood transfusions and significant portion of GFR must be lost before changes in sCr are detected. A SCr within the normal range, therefore, does not exclude kidney impairment in patients with cirrhosis.

Serum cystatin C (CysC), is unaffected by sarcopenia, sex, and hepatic function and has been shown to have better diagnostic accuracy and to be a useful prognostic marker for kidney outcomes and mortality in patients with decompensated cirrhosis, with rising levels often preceding changes in SCr by 48 h [10–12]. CysC use has not yet been widely adopted due to higher cost, and levels are affected by inflammation, infections, and use of steroids.

Estimated GFR (eGFR), which is used to determine candidacy for SLKT, overestimates the true GFR by 10–20 ml/min/1.73 m^2, especially in patients with a GFR <40 ml/min/1.73 m^2 and/or ascites [13, 14]. In a meta-analysis of 25 studies ($n = 4565$), the least bias was demonstrated with the use of CysC-based eGFR equation (10.3 mL/min/1.73 m^2) [13]. In 2021, a new eGFR equation (CKD-EPI), which included the removal of race as a variable, was introduced and widely implemented as an effort to eliminate disparities in the care of patients with kidney disease [15, 16]. Preliminary data in patients with cirrhosis indicate acceptable performance [17].

Diagnostic Criteria for AKI and HRS

Over the last 15 years, the diagnostic criteria for AKI and HRS have undergone several revisions by the Acute Disease Quality Initiative (ADQI) and International Club of Ascites (ICA) [18–20]. In 2023, In a Joint Multidisciplinary Consensus Meeting between ADQI and ICA, significant updates were made to the definition of AKI and HRS (Table 6.1) [20, 21]. As such, patients could either fulfill AKI criteria through a change in SCr, a change in urine output or both. Transient oliguria has been shown to identify AKI in patients, including those with cirrhosis, without any elevation of SCr levels, reclassify AKI cases to higher stages, and be associated with a higher risk of mortality in critically ill patients [6, 22]. Volume resuscitation (preferentially crystalloids) is recommended only when indicated, with the time window for assessing response to be completed within 24 h, to ensure early diagnosis and initiation of treatment for HRS-AKI [20, 21, 23, 24]. In patients with clinical and imaging evidence of intravascular volume overload, albumin infusion for the diagnosis of HRS-AKI will risk further worsening of the volume overload state and therefore is no longer recommended by the expert panel. It is important to recognize that HRS-AKI can co-exist with other causes of AKI and/or with pre-existing CKD.

The diagnosis of AKI and staging of AKI depends on the identification of a prior sCr value. If no previous sCr value is available, ADQI/ICA recommends following recommendation proposed by KDIGO, i.e., the use of the lower value of the admission SCr or SCr derived from eGFR equation assuming a baseline GFR of 75 ml/min/1.73 m^2, to decide the reference SCr [20]. It should be noted that this method may still underestimate the incidence and severity of AKI; however, it has been

Table 6.1 Diagnostic criteria for AKI and HRS [20]

Variable	Definition
Baseline sCr	Lowest stable SCr value obtained in the previous 3 months
	If no values are available in previous 3 months, most recent value up to 12 months prior may be used.
	If more than one SCr value is available, median SCr may be used. However, if significant fluctuations exist in the multiple SCr values, clinical judgement is crucial to determine the SCr that best reflects the most appropriate baseline value.
	In the absence of a known prior SCr, the lower value of the following should be considered as reference SCr: SCr on admission or SCr value back calculated from an estimated GFR of 75 ml/min/1.73 m^2.
AKI	Increase in sCr >0.3 mg/dL within 48 h or
	Increase in sCr >1.5 times baseline levels over 7 days or
	Urine output <0.5 ml/kg/h in 6 h
AKI Stage	*Stage 1*: increase in sCr ≥0.3 mg/dl or ≥1.5–2 times baseline level
	Stage 2: increase in sCr >2–3 times baseline level *Stage 3*: increase in sCr >3 times baseline level or ≥4.0 mg/dl with an acute increase ≥0.5 mg/dl or initiation of renal-replacement therapy
HRS—AKI	Cirrhosis with ascites
	Increase sCr ≥0.3 mg/dl or ≥50% baseline level within the prior 7 days or urinary output <0.5 ml/kg/h for ≥6 h
	Absence of improvement in sCr and/or urine output within 12–24 h following adequate volume resuscitation (when clinically indicated)
	Absence of strong evidence for an alternative explanation as the primary cause of AKI

**AKD* Acute Kidney Disease

shown to correlate more accurately with rates of AKI, even in patients with cirrhosis [4, 6, 25–27].

Just as the incidence of metabolic dysfunction-associated liver disease is increasing, so is the incidence of CKD due to diabetes and hypertension [28]. As such, the diagnostic criteria for HRS-AKI were recently revised by ADQI/ICA (Table 6.1) [20]. The presence of isolated proteinuria related to comorbidities (e.g., diabetes) and/or pre-existing CKD should not rule out the presence of HRS-AKI. Depending on the timing and duration of impaired kidney function, the historical terminologies for HRS (HRS type-1 and HRS type-2) have been replaced by HRS-AKI, HRS-AKD and HRS-CKD [20, 29].

Pathophysiology of HRS-AKI

The pathophysiology involves complex physiological processes, including circulatory dysfunction, systemic inflammation, and impaired renal microcirculation and inflammation [20, 30]. Advanced hepatic fibrosis causes increased intravascular resistance and increased shear stress in the splanchnic vascular beds and is associated with the production of several vasodilators, including nitric oxide and prostacyclins. The resulting splanchnic dilation and decrease in effective arterial circulating blood volume initially results in increased cardiac output. With time, however, even increased cardiac output cannot maintain effective circulating volume [20, 30]. Due to the hyperdynamic circulatory state of cirrhosis, renal blood flow is extremely susceptible to events associated with a decrease in effective arterial blood volume. Activation of neurohormonal systems, specifically the renin-angiotensin-aldosterone system, results in sodium and water retention to restore the effective circulating volume through vasoconstriction of the renal afferent artery. In response to reduced renal blood flow, there is increased secretion of renal prostaglandins that serve to maintain glomerular pressure. Over time, these compensatory mechanisms are insufficient, and reduced renal blood flow results in decrease in GFR and a pre-renal injury that fails to correct with volume expansion. Progression of cirrhosis and portal hypertension leads to further vasodilatation and consequent increased activation of these neurohumoral systems, leading to ascites, extreme renal vasoconstriction, and ultimately, HRS-AKI. Cardiac dysfunction may also contribute to the development of AKI; however, the mechanisms remain controversial. During the early phase of decompensated cirrhosis, the cardiac output increases; however, the release of cardio-depressive substances leads to subclinical changes in the myocardium, which, coupled with cardio-depression and diastolic dysfunction, result in what is referred to as "cirrhotic cardiomyopathy" [31]. Finally, systemic inflammation is common in patients with decompensated cirrhosis, and the presence of bacterial/ bacterial products translocation and/or overt infection is fundamental in the development of HRS-AKI [32, 33].

Prevention of AKI

Prevention of AKI, especially HRS-AKI, is important in order to improve patient outcomes and reduce liver-related mortality [34–36]. Volume depletion should be prevented, and volume status should be optimized with careful use of diuretics. The use of IV albumin following large volume paracentesis (>5 L) and in patients with SBP have been shown to decrease the incidence of AKI, specifically HRS-AKI [20, 37, 38]. However, however, the optimal dose and timing of IV albumin remains to be determined.

Administration of albumin in patients with infections other than SBP does not improve mortality and has been associated with increased risk of pulmonary edema [39]. Continuous infusions of albumin, both in the inpatient and outpatient setting, to maintain serum albumin >3 g/dL are not beneficial in randomized controlled studies and may be associated with an increased risk of pulmonary edema [40, 41]. In those patients with ascites refractory to medical management, transjugular intrahepatic portosystemic shunt placement controls ascites, and thus, may play a role in the prevention of AKI / HRS-AKI in patients with refractory ascites.

Workup and Management of AKI/HRS-AKI

Successful treatment of AKI depends on identifying and addressing the underlying causes contributing to renal dysfunction. Etiology of AKI is obtained by careful review of the patient's history and physical examination, urine studies (e.g., urine sediment), and response to volume challenge and diuretic withdrawal when indicated.

Nearly half of all cases of AKI in hospitalized patients with cirrhosis is related to renal hypoperfusion, most often from hypovolemia [30, 42, 43]. Intrinsic causes, most often ATN, account for approximately 30% while post-obstructive causes of AKI are seen in <1% of hospitalized patients with AKI [43]. Glomerular diseases may occur in patients with viral hepatitis due to the formation of immune complexes, antibody production against altered hepatocytes, or direct virus cytopathic effects [44].

Fractional excretion of sodium (FENa) has been shown to be unhelpful to differentiate ATN from HRS-AKI, since FENa <1% is common in patients with cirrhosis, even in the absence of AKI [45, 46]. Lower threshold of FENa <0.2% in combination with other urinary biomarkers such as neutrophil gelatinase-associated lipocalin (uNGAL), along with clinical judgement improves specificity in identifying HRS-AKI; however, many laboratories do not report urine sodium values <20 mEq/L [45, 47]. uNGAL value of ~220–250 μg/g may help distinguish patients with ATN from other phenotypes, in addition to determining response to terlipressin; however, overlap between different phenotypes has been shown in various studies [47, 48]. The combination use of various functional (e.g., sCr, CysC) and stress-and injury-related (e.g., albuminuria, uNGAL) potentially may allow the clinicians to detect those at risk of AKI, allow earlier detection of AKI, and allow the identification of AKI sub-phenotypes suitable for precise therapeutic interventions [49, 50].

Pharmacologic Therapy

IV Fluids

When indicated, volume resuscitation (preferentially with crystalloids) and assessment of response to IV fluids should be completed within 24 h, to ensure early diagnosis and initiation of treatment for HRS-AKI [20, 23]. Failure to respond to 48 h of volume resuscitation is no longer recommended by the ADQI / ICA consensus meeting as a pre-requisite for the definition of HRS-AKI, as this may lead to fluid accumulation and delay in the initiation of vasopressor therapy in those who are euvolemic or hypervolemic [51]. When volume status is equivocal, a fluid challenge of 250–500 ml of crystalloid or 1–1.5 g/kg of 20–25% albumin may be considered [20].

Assessment of intravascular volume can be difficult in patients with cirrhosis, and most hemodynamic monitoring tools have not been well-studied in patients with advanced liver disease [20, 23, 24]. The choice of tool depends on the patient's location (ICU vs general ward) and clinical discretion, as no study has demonstrated superiority of a particular method. It is important to assess volume status repeatedly and to monitor UO closely in order to prevent complications of iatrogenic volume overload. Bedside point-of-care ultrasonography may help guide volume resuscitation in patients with cirrhosis; however, its use is challenging in the presence of significant ascites and is prone to inter-observer variability [52–54].

Vasoconstrictors

The cornerstone of therapy for HRS-AKI involves the use of vasoactive drugs combined with albumin to counter the systemic vasodilation that occurs with cirrhosis; however, its use has not been shown to improve transplant-free survival. The consequent improvement in mean arterial pressure improves renal blood flow and may decrease kidney injury [55, 56]. However, a higher risk of pulmonary edema, respiratory failure, mainly due to pulmonary edema, is seen in those treated with terlipressin [57]. Norepinephrine may have comparable effects to terlipressin for reversal of HRS-AKI, and can be used if terlipressin is not available; however, it requires admission to the ICU and placement of central access. Reversal of HRS-AKI with pharmacologic treatment may result in lowering the MELD score and potentially affect the wait time for those listed for liver transplantation, resulting in higher waitlist mortality, especially in regions with high MELD scores at the time of transplant [58–60].

Trans-Jugular Intrahepatic Portosystemic Shunt (TIPS)

TIPS may improve kidney function in those with refractory ascites by decreasing portal pressures and redistributing blood volume, but it is not well studied as a treatment for HRS-AKI [61, 62]. The Liver-HERO Trial is currently ongoing to assess how terlipressin and albumin vs TIPS placement affects outcomes in those with HRS-AKI [63].

Renal Replacement Therapy

There is currently no consensus on the timing, dose, or duration of RRT in patients with cirrhosis and AKI [30, 64]. The decision regarding when to initiate RRT should be individualized, with consideration of the trajectory of both kidney and liver health and, before the occurrence of overt complications [65, 66]. Early initiation of RRT should be considered in those with intravascular volume overload without adequate response to diuretics (even in the absence of AKI). Uremic symptoms can often overlap with hepatic encephalopathy; as such, initiation of RRT should be considered earlier, especially if encephalopathy persists despite appropriate treatment [64]. Initiation of RRT in patients who are listed or undergoing evaluation for LT, should be viewed as a condition optimization and a bridge to LT. Multidisciplinary discussions with the patient and/or caretakers should be held for those who are not candidates for LT regarding goals of therapy and the overall prognosis, as transplant-free survival is extremely low, especially in patients with high MELD scores [20, 58, 64, 67].

Liver Transplantation

LT is the definitive treatment for patients with HRS-AKI. SLKT should be considered in patients with prolonged kidney dysfunction; however, predicting the level and duration of renal dysfunction (including RRT) after which renal recovery is unlikely following LT remains a challenge [68, 69]. In the USA, listing criteria for SLKT include duration of AKI and RRT, and presence of CKD [68, 70]. A safety net policy has also been established to prioritize those patients who develop severe kidney dysfunction (eGFR < 20 ml/min/1.73 m^2 or dialysis dependency) between 60 to 365 days following LT to receive a kidney transplant. The role of biomarkers to predict reversibility of AKI after LT in recent studies has been promising and may allow more accurate allocation of kidney grafts [71, 72].

References

1. Patidar KR, Belcher JM, Regner KR, St Hillien SA, Simonetto DA, Asrani SK, et al. Incidence and outcomes of acute kidney injury including hepatorenal syndrome in hospitalized patients with cirrhosis in the US. J Hepatol. 2023;79:1408.
2. Tariq R, Hadi Y, Chahal K, Reddy S, Salameh H, Singal AK. Incidence, mortality and predictors of acute kidney injury in patients with cirrhosis: a systematic review and meta-analysis. J Clin Transl Hepatol. 2020;8(2):135–42.
3. Tandon P, James MT, Abraldes JG, Karvellas CJ, Ye F, Pannu N. Relevance of new definitions to incidence and prognosis of acute kidney injury in hospitalized patients with cirrhosis: a retrospective population-based cohort study. PLoS One. 2016;11(8):e0160394.
4. Patidar KR, Naved MA, Grama A, Adibuzzaman M, Aziz Ali A, Slaven JE, et al. Acute kidney disease is common and associated with poor outcomes in patients with cirrhosis and acute kidney injury. J Hepatol. 2022;77(1):108–15.
5. Cullaro G, Rubin JB, Fortune BE, Crawford CV, Verna EC, Hsu C-Y, et al. Association between kidney dysfunction types and mortality among hospitalized patients with cirrhosis. Dig Dis Sci. 2022;67(7):3426–35.
6. Amathieu R, Al-Khafaji A, Sileanu FE, Foldes E, DeSensi R, Hilmi I, et al. Significance of oliguria in critically ill patients with chronic liver disease. Hepatology. 2017;66(5):1592–600.
7. Piano S, Romano A, Di Pascoli M, Angeli P. Why and how to measure renal function in patients with liver disease. Liver Int. 2017;37(S1):116–22.
8. Macedo E, Bouchard J, Soroko SH, Chertow GM, Himmelfarb J, Ikizler TA, et al. Fluid accumulation, recognition and staging of acute kidney injury in critically-ill patients. Crit Care. 2010;14(3):R82.
9. Verna EC, Connelly C, Dove LM, Adem P, Babic N, Corsetti J, et al. Center-related bias in MELD scores within a liver transplant UNOS region: a call for standardization. Transplantation. 2020;104(7):1396–402.
10. Markwardt D, Holdt L, Steib C, Benesic A, Bendtsen F, Bernardi M, et al. Plasma cystatin C is a predictor of renal dysfunction, acute-on-chronic liver failure, and mortality in patients with acutely decompensated liver cirrhosis. Hepatology. 2017;66(4):1232–41.
11. Slack AJ, McPhail MJ, Ostermann M, Bruce M, Sherwood R, Musto R, et al. Predicting the development of acute kidney injury in liver cirrhosis – an analysis of glomerular filtration rate, proteinuria and kidney injury biomarkers. Aliment Pharmacol Ther. 2013;37(10):989–97.
12. Maiwall R, Kumar A, Bhardwaj A, Kumar G, Bhadoria AS, Sarin SK. Cystatin C predicts acute kidney injury and mortality in cirrhotics: a prospective cohort study. Liver Int. 2018;38(4):654–64.

13. Singapura P, Ma TW, Sarmast N, Gonzalez SA, Durand F, Maiwall R, et al. Estimating glomerular filtration rate in cirrhosis using creatinine-based and cystatin C-based equations: systematic review and meta-analysis. Liver Transpl. 2021;27(11):1538–52.
14. Francoz C, Nadim MK, Baron A, Prie D, Antoine C, Belghiti J, et al. Glomerular filtration rate equations for liver-kidney transplantation in patients with cirrhosis: validation of current recommendations. Hepatology. 2014;59(4):1514–21.
15. Inker LA, Eneanya ND, Coresh J, Tighiouart H, Wang D, Sang Y, et al. New creatinine- and cystatin C-based equations to estimate GFR without race. N Engl J Med. 2021;385(19):1737–49.
16. Delgado C, Baweja M, Crews DC, Eneanya ND, Gadegbeku CA, Inker LA, et al. A unifying approach for GFR estimation: recommendations of the NKF-ASN task force on reassessing the inclusion of race in diagnosing kidney disease. J Am Soc Nephrol. 2021;32(12):2994–3015.
17. Panchal S, Serper M, Bittermann T, Asrani SK, Goldberg DS, Mahmud N. Impact of race-adjusted glomerular filtration rate estimation on eligibility for simultaneous liver-kidney transplantation. Liver Transpl. 2022;28(6):959–68.
18. Nadim MK, Kellum JA, Davenport A, Wong F, Davis C, Pannu N, et al. Hepatorenal syndrome: the 8th international consensus conference of the acute dialysis quality initiative (ADQI) group. Crit Care. 2012;16(1):R23.
19. Angeli P, Gines P, Wong F, Bernardi M, Boyer TD, Gerbes A, et al. Diagnosis and management of acute kidney injury in patients with cirrhosis: revised consensus recommendations of the International Club of Ascites. J Hepatol. 2015;62(4):968–74.
20. Nadim MK, Kellum JA, Forni L, Francoz C, Asrani SK, Ostermann M, et al. Acute kidney injury in patients with cirrhosis: acute disease quality initiative (ADQI) and international Club of ascites (ICA) joint multidisciplinary consensus meeting. J Hepatol. 2024;81:163.
21. Nadim MK, Forni LG, Ostermann M, Panel AIE. Hepatorenal syndrome in the intensive care unit. Intensive Care Med. 2024;50(6):978–81.
22. Bianchi NA, Stavart LL, Altarelli M, Kelevina T, Faouzi M, Schneider AG. Association of Oliguria with acute kidney injury diagnosis, severity assessment, and mortality among patients with critical illness. JAMA Netw Open. 2021;4(11):e2133094.
23. Durand F, Kellum JA, Nadim MK. Fluid resuscitation in patients with cirrhosis and sepsis: a multidisciplinary perspective. J Hepatol. 2023;79:240.
24. Nadim MK, Durand F, Kellum JA, Levitsky J, O'Leary JG, Karvellas CJ, et al. Management of the critically ill patient with cirrhosis: a multidisciplinary perspective. J Hepatol. 2016;64(3):717–35.
25. Rosi S, Piano S, Frigo AC, Morando F, Fasolato S, Cavallin M, et al. New ICA criteria for the diagnosis of acute kidney injury in cirrhotic patients: can we use an imputed value of serum creatinine? Liver Int. 2015;35(9):2108–14.
26. Kidney Disease: Improving Global Outcomes (KDIGO) Acute Kidney Injury Work Group. KDIGO clinical practice guideline for acute kidney injury. Kidney Inter Suppl. 2012;2:1–138.
27. Tonon M, Rosi S, Gambino CG, Piano S, Calvino V, Romano A, et al. Natural history of acute kidney disease in patients with cirrhosis. J Hepatol. 2021;74(3):578–83.
28. Cullaro G, Verna EC, Lee BP, Lai JC. Chronic kidney disease in liver transplant candidates: a rising burden impacting post–liver transplant outcomes. Liver Transpl. 2020;26(4):498–506.
29. Angeli P, Garcia-Tsao G, Nadim MK, Parikh CR. News in pathophysiology, definition and classification of hepatorenal syndrome: a step beyond the International Club of Ascites (ICA) consensus document. J Hepatol. 2019;71(4):811–22.
30. Nadim MK, Garcia-Tsao G. Acute kidney injury in patients with cirrhosis. N Engl J Med. 2023;388(8):733–45.
31. Izzy M, VanWagner LB, Lin G, Altieri M, Findlay JY, Oh JK, et al. Redefining cirrhotic cardiomyopathy for the modern era. Hepatology. 2020;71(1):334–45.
32. Arroyo V, Angeli P, Moreau R, Jalan R, Clària J, Trebicka J, et al. The systemic inflammation hypothesis: towards a new paradigm of acute decompensation and multiorgan failure in cirrhosis. J Hepatol. 2021;74(3):670–85.

33. Trebicka J, Amoros A, Pitarch C, Titos E, Alcaraz-Quiles J, Schierwagen R, et al. Addressing profiles of systemic inflammation across the different clinical phenotypes of acutely decompensated cirrhosis. Front Immunol. 2019;10:476.
34. O'Leary JG, Levitsky J, Wong F, Nadim MK, Charlton M, Kim WR. Protecting the kidney in liver transplant candidates: practice-based recommendations from the American Society of Transplantation Liver and Intestine community of practice. Am J Transplant. 2016;16(9):2516–31.
35. Fede G, D'Amico G, Arvaniti V, Tsochatzis E, Germani G, Georgiadis D, et al. Renal failure and cirrhosis: a systematic review of mortality and prognosis. J Hepatol. 2012;56(4):810–8.
36. Belcher JM, Garcia-Tsao G, Sanyal AJ, Bhogal H, Lim JK, Ansari N, et al. Association of AKI with mortality and complications in hospitalized patients with cirrhosis. Hepatology. 2013;57(2):753–62.
37. Biggins SW, Angeli P, Garcia-Tsao G, Gines P, Ling SC, Nadim MK, et al. Diagnosis, evaluation, and management of ascites, spontaneous bacterial peritonitis and hepatorenal syndrome: 2021 practice guidance by the American Association for the Study of Liver Diseases. Hepatology. 2021;74(2):1014–48.
38. European Association for the Study of the Liver. Electronic address eee, European Association for the Study of the L. EASL clinical practice guidelines for the management of patients with decompensated cirrhosis. J Hepatol. 2018;69(2):406–60.
39. Fernández J, Angeli P, Trebicka J, Merli M, Gustot T, Alessandria C, et al. Efficacy of albumin treatment for patients with cirrhosis and infections unrelated to spontaneous bacterial peritonitis. Clin Gastroenterol Hepatol. 2020;18(4):963–73.e14.
40. China L, Freemantle N, Forrest E, Kallis Y, Ryder SD, Wright G, et al. A randomized trial of albumin infusions in hospitalized patients with cirrhosis. N Engl J Med. 2021;384(9):808–17.
41. Caraceni P, Riggio O, Angeli P, Alessandria C, Neri S, Foschi FG, et al. Long-term albumin administration in decompensated cirrhosis (ANSWER): an open-label randomised trial. Lancet. 2018;391(10138):2417–29.
42. Garcia-Tsao G, Parikh CR, Viola A. Acute kidney injury in cirrhosis. Hepatology. 2008;48(6):2064–77.
43. Patidar KR, Belcher JM, Regner KR, St. Hillien SA, Simonetto DA, Asrani SK, et al. Incidence and outcomes of acute kidney injury including hepatorenal syndrome in hospitalized patients with cirrhosis in the US. J Hepatol. 2023;79(6):1408–17.
44. Muciño-Bermejo M-J. Mechanisms of kidney dysfunction in the cirrhotic patient: non-hepatorenal acute-on-chronic kidney damage considerations. Ann Hepatol. 2020;19(2):145–52.
45. Belcher JM, Garcia-Tsao G, Sanyal AJ, Thiessen-Philbrook H, Peixoto AJ, Perazella MA, et al. Urinary biomarkers and progression of AKI in patients with cirrhosis. Clin J Am Soc Nephrol. 2014;9(11):1857–67.
46. Belcher JM, Sanyal AJ, Peixoto AJ, Perazella MA, Lim J, Thiessen-Philbrook H, et al. Kidney biomarkers and differential diagnosis of patients with cirrhosis and acute kidney injury. Hepatology. 2014;60(2):622–32.
47. Huelin P, Sola E, Elia C, Sole C, Risso A, Moreira R, et al. Neutrophil gelatinase-associated lipocalin for assessment of acute kidney injury in cirrhosis: a prospective study. Hepatology. 2019;70(1):319–33.
48. Gambino C, Piano S, Stenico M, Tonon M, Brocca A, Calvino V, et al. Diagnostic and prognostic performance of urinary neutrophil gelatinase-associated lipocalin in patients with cirrhosis and acute kidney injury. Hepatology. 2023;77(5):1630–8.
49. Francoz C, Nadim MK, Durand F. Kidney biomarkers in cirrhosis. J Hepatol. 2016;65(4):809–24.
50. Asrani SK, Shankar N, da Graca B, Nadim MK, Cardenas A. Role of novel kidney biomarkers in patients with cirrhosis and after liver transplantation. Liver Transpl. 2022;28(3):466–82.
51. Nadim MK, Kellum JA, Forni L, Francoz C, Asrani SK, Ostermann M, et al. Acute kidney injury in patients with cirrhosis: Acute Disease Quality Initiative (ADQI) and International Club of Ascites (ICA) joint multidisciplinary consensus meeting. J Hepatol. 2024;81:163.

52. Díaz-Gómez JL, Mayo PH, Koenig SJ. Point-of-care ultrasonography. N Engl J Med. 2021;385(17):1593–602.
53. Kaptein EM, Oo Z, Kaptein MJ. Hepatorenal syndrome misdiagnosis may be reduced using inferior vena cava ultrasound to assess intravascular volume and guide management. Ren Fail. 2023;45(1):2185468.
54. Velez JCQ, Petkovich B, Karakala N, Huggins JT. Point-of-care echocardiography unveils misclassification of acute kidney injury as hepatorenal syndrome. Am J Nephrol. 2019;50(3):204–11.
55. Stadlbauer VP, Wright GAK, Banaji M, Mukhopadhya A, Mookerjee R, Moore K, et al. Relationship between activation of the sympathetic nervous system and renal blood flow autoregulation in cirrhosis. Gastroenterology. 2008;134(1):111–9.e2.
56. Velez JCQ, Nietert PJ. Therapeutic response to vasoconstrictors in hepatorenal syndrome parallels increase in mean arterial pressure: a pooled analysis of clinical trials. Am J Kidney Dis. 2011;58(6):928–38.
57. Wong F, Pappas SC, Curry MP, Reddy KR, Rubin RA, Porayko MK, et al. Terlipressin plus albumin for the treatment of type 1 hepatorenal syndrome. N Engl J Med. 2021;384(9):818–28.
58. Nadim MK, DiNorcia J, Ji L, Groshen S, Levitsky J, Sung RS, et al. Inequity in organ allocation for patients awaiting liver transplantation: rationale for uncapping the model for end-stage liver disease. J Hepatol. 2017;67(3):517–25.
59. Przybyszewski EM, Wilechansky RM, McLean Diaz P, Allegretti AS, Vanwagner LB, Cullaro G, et al. Controversies in terlipressin and transplantation in the United States: how do we MELD the two? Liver Transpl. 2024;30:753.
60. Angeli P, Gines P. Hepatorenal syndrome, MELD score and liver transplantation: an evolving issue with relevant implications for clinical practice. J Hepatol. 2012;57(5):1135–40.
61. Charilaou P, Devani K, Petrosyan R, Reddy C, Pyrsopoulos N. Inpatient mortality benefit with transjugular intrahepatic portosystemic shunt for hospitalized hepatorenal syndrome patients. Dig Dis Sci. 2020;65(11):3378–88.
62. Gonzalez-Garay AG, Serralde-Zúñiga AE, Velasco Hidalgo L, Flores García NC, Aguirre-Salgado MI. Transjugular intrahepatic portosystemic shunts for adults with hepatorenal syndrome. Cochrane Database Syst Rev. 2024;1(1):CD011039.
63. Ripoll C, Platzer S, Franken P, Aschenbach R, Wienke A, Schuhmacher U, et al. Liver-HERO: hepatorenal syndrome-acute kidney injury (HRS-AKI) treatment with transjugular intrahepatic portosystemic shunt in patients with cirrhosis-a randomized controlled trial. Trials. 2023;24(1):258.
64. Shah SV, Nadim MK. KRT in patients with AKI and cirrhosis. Clin J Am Soc Nephrol. 2024;19:914.
65. Rosner MH, Ostermann M, Murugan R, Prowle JR, Ronco C, Kellum JA, et al. Indications and management of mechanical fluid removal in critical illness. Br J Anaesth. 2014;113(5):764–71.
66. Ostermann M, Zarbock A, Goldstein S, Kashani K, Macedo E, Murugan R, et al. Recommendations on acute kidney injury biomarkers from the acute disease quality initiative consensus conference: a consensus statement. JAMA Netw Open. 2020;3(10):e2019209.
67. Scherer JS, Holley JL. The role of time–limited trials in dialysis decision making in critically ill patients. Clin J Am Soc Nephrol. 2016;11(2):344–53.
68. Nadim MK, Sung RS, Davis CL, Andreoni KA, Biggins SW, Danovitch GM, et al. Simultaneous liver-kidney transplantation summit: current state and future directions. Am J Transplant. 2012;12(11):2901–8.
69. Levitsky J, Baker T, Ahya SN, Levin ML, Friedewald J, Gallon L, et al. Outcomes and native renal recovery following simultaneous liver-kidney transplantation. Am J Transplant. 2012;12(11):2949–57.
70. Formica RN, Aeder M, Boyle G, Kucheryavaya A, Stewart D, Hirose R, et al. Simultaneous liver-kidney allocation policy: a proposal to optimize appropriate utilization of scarce resources. Am J Transplant. 2016;16(3):758–66.

71. Levitsky J, Asrani SK, Abecassis M, Ruiz R, Jennings LW, Klintmalm G. External validation of a pretransplant biomarker model (REVERSE) predictive of renal recovery after liver transplantation. Hepatology. 2019;70(4):1349–59.
72. Levitsky J, Asrani SK, Klintmalm G, Schiano T, Moss A, Chavin K, et al. Discovery and validation of a biomarker model (PRESERVE) predictive of renal outcomes after liver transplantation. Hepatology. 2020;71(5):1775–86.

Cardiopulmonary Issues in Patients with End-Stage Liver Disease

7

Elena Gavrila, Lisa B. VanWagner, and Dempsey L. Hughes

Abbreviations

AF	Atrial fibrillation
ALD	Alcohol-associated liver disease
AS	Aortic stenosis
CABG	Coronary artery bypass graft
CAD	Coronary artery disease
CCM	Cirrhotic cardiomyopathy
CCTA	Coronary ct angiography
CNI	Calcineurin inhibitors
CVD	Cardiovascular disease
DAPT	Dual anti-platelet therapy
ESLD	End-stage liver disease
FFR	Fractional flow reserve
HH	Hepatic hydrothorax
HF	Heart failure
HFrEF	Heart failure with reduced ejection fraction
HPS	Hepatopulmonary syndrome

E. Gavrila
Department of Internal Medicine, University of Texas Southwestern Medical Center, Dallas, TX, USA

L. B. VanWagner (✉)
Department of Internal Medicine, Division of Digestive and Liver Diseases, University of Texas Southwestern Medical Center, Dallas, TX, USA
e-mail: lisa.vanwagner@utsouthwestern.edu

D. L. Hughes
Department of Medicine, Division of Gastroenterology and Hepatology, Northwestern University Feinberg School of Medicine, Chicago, IL, USA

B. Eghtesad et al. (eds.), *Liver Transplantation*,
https://doi.org/10.1007/978-3-032-07072-2_7

LT	Liver transplant
ICA	Invasive coronary angiography
IPVD	Intrapulmonary vascular dilatations
LV	Left ventricle
LVEF	Left ventricular ejection fraction
MACE	Major adverse cardiovascular event
MASH	Metabolic-dysfunction associated steatohepatitis
MELD	Model for end-stage liver disease
MS	Mitral stenosis
mTOR	Mammalian target of rapamycin
PAH	Pulmonary arterial hypertension
PCI	Percutaneous coronary intervention
POPH	Portopulmonary hypertension
RHC	Right heart catheterization
SAVR	Surgical aortic valve replacement
SVR	Systemic vascular resistance
TAVR	Transcatheter aortic valve replacement
TIPS	Transjugular intrahepatic portosystemic shunt
TTE	Transthoracic echocardiography
TR	Tricuspid regurgitation
VHD	Valvular heart disease

Introduction

Cardiopulmonary conditions present with distinct physical features and clinical significance among patients with end-stage liver disease (ESLD). Many of these conditions result from the pathophysiology of decompensated cirrhosis, characterized by progressive hyperdynamic circulation and decreased peripheral vascular resistance. This results in decreased effective arterial blood volume and mean arterial pressure and increased cardiac output and heart rate [1]. Hyperdynamic circulation leads to myocardial stress through the renin-angiotensin-aldosterone system (RAAS) activation and increased sympathetic nervous system activity. Physical manifestations of this complex pathophysiology can ultimately lead to cardiac dysfunction and pulmonary vascular disease. Cardiopulmonary conditions in ESLD include heart failure (HF) and cirrhotic cardiomyopathy (CCM), coronary artery disease (CAD), arrhythmias, valvular heart disease (VHD), portopulmonary hypertension (POPH), hepatopulmonary syndrome (HPS), and hepatic hydrothorax (HH). These conditions portend prognostic significance and, in severe forms, may serve as a contraindication to liver transplantation (LT). In the following chapter, we present the spectrum of cardiopulmonary conditions with special attention to implementing evidence-based screening methods and effective management strategies.

Cardiac Complications

Heart Failure and Cirrhotic Cardiomyopathy

The presentation of HF among patients with ESLD can range from subclinical cardiac dysfunction to overt structural heart disease. Subclinical cardiac dysfunction is highly prevalent, occurring in 20–47% of LT candidates depending on the underlying etiology of cirrhosis (e.g., metabolic-dysfunction associated steatohepatitis (MASH) [2] 47%, alcohol-associated liver disease (ALD) 33%, other etiologies 20%) [3]. In ESLD, the cardiac response to physiologic and pathophysiologic stimuli such as exercise, infection, and surgery is abnormal, a condition termed "cirrhotic cardiomyopathy" (CCM). CCM is estimated to affect about one-third of patients with ESLD, though the true prevalence is unknown given evolving diagnostic criteria [3]. The pathophysiology of CCM is complex but is largely driven by oxidative stress, inflammation, and fibrosis, resulting in systolic and/or diastolic dysfunction (Fig. 7.1). Additionally, CCM is characterized by impaired β-adrenergic receptor function and increased cardiac output [4]. Of note, the severity of subclinical dysfunction appears to worsen with progressive hepatic decompensation. CCM is usually asymptomatic (latent) cardiac dysfunction (both systolic and diastolic), but can become unmasked under stress, such as an acute change in hemodynamic loading conditions during transjugular intrahepatic portosystemic shunt (TIPS) creation or LT surgery, progressing to symptomatic, overt HF [5, 6]. CCM diagnostic criteria (Fig. 7.1) have been revised in line with contemporary echocardiography guidelines [7].

Apart from CCM, several etiologies of liver disease can also be associated with cardiomyopathy, including hemochromatosis, alcohol, or infiltrative diseases (sarcoidosis, amyloidosis). In alcohol-related cardiomyopathy, LV systolic function is

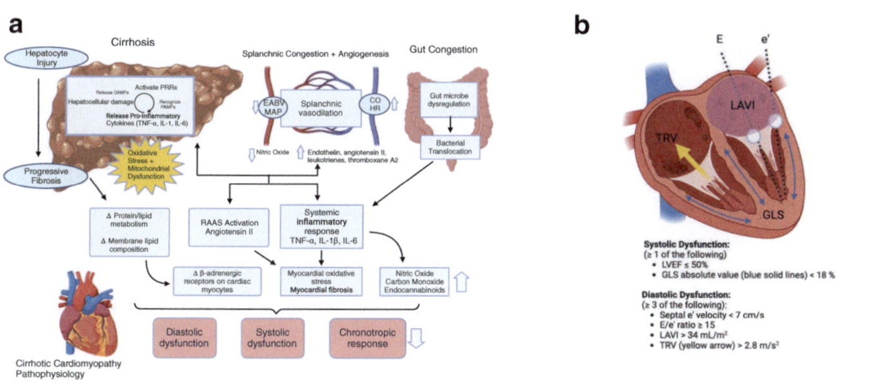

Fig. 7.1 Pathophysiology (**a**) and diagnostic criteria (**b**) for cirrhotic cardiomyopathy. Abbreviations: CO cardiac output, DAMPs damage-associated molecular pattern molecules, EABV estimated arterial blood volume, HR heart rate, MAP mean arterial pressure, PAMPs pathogen-associated molecular patterns, PRRs pattern recognition receptors, RAAS renin-angiotensin-aldosterone system

reduced due to impaired contractile protein synthesis and immunogenic cardiac protein acetaldehyde adducts [4]. Patients may have asymptomatic myocardial dysfunction with myocardial fibrosis, impaired systolic function, and LV dilation [8]. For patients with sarcoidosis, the presence of high-grade AV block is the most common initial sign of cardiac involvement [9]. Hemochromatosis may be associated with concomitant cardiac disease due to iron deposition in the myocardium and conduction system. This can result in rhythm disturbances (tachyarrhythmias, premature ventricular beats, nodal block) and, less commonly, overt HF or pulmonary hypertension. The cardiomyopathy may be restrictive or dilated. TTE may show increased atrial and ventricular mass, and diastolic dysfunction with or without systolic dysfunction [10]. Obesity, hypertension, hyperlipidemia, diabetes, and CAD are highly prevalent in LT candidates, particularly in those with MASH [11], and contribute to risk for ischemic cardiomyopathy [12, 13]. Finally, unrelated to the etiology of cirrhosis is hypertrophic cardiomyopathy (HCM), an autosomal dominant disorder with an estimated prevalence of 0.5% in LT candidates [14].

TTE should be pursued for any patients meeting clinical suspicion for cardiomyopathy. However, due to the low SVR (afterload) associated with ESLD, left ventricular ejection fraction (LVEF) is frequently inflated and may not capture cardiac dysfunction that can manifest once a normal afterload is restored. Other TTE metrics including assessment of diastolic function, myocardial strain, left atrial, and right ventricular function are of particular importance to risk-stratify patients for unmasked myocardial dysfunction in the periprocedural period [3, 15]. The absence of contractile or diastolic reserve on stress imaging may be a useful marker of subclinical LV dysfunction [16–19]. Cardiopulmonary exercise testing may be used to identify patients with cardiovascular limitation and to differentiate patients with advanced liver disease who may have severe exercise limitation and low pVO2 due to other mechanisms [7]. Other investigations to be considered when assessing TIPS or LT candidates with cardiomyopathy include cardiac magnetic resonance imaging, which enables accurate assessment of wall thickness, detection of HCM phenotype and apical aneurysms, and can help differentiate HCM from other thick-walled heart conditions such as amyloidosis or hypertensive cardiomyopathy [20]. In the general population, biomarkers like B-type natriuretic peptide (BNP), NT-proBNP and cardiac troponins (cTn) have prognostic impact and can help identify subjects at high-risk of HF [21]. In LT candidates, preoperative levels of cTn and BNP have been shown to predict early post-LT mortality and may be used to improve prognostication [22–24].

When detected, the severity of HF can have direct impact on ESLD management. Per consensus guidelines, severe HF with reduced ejection fraction (HFrEF, LVEF $< 40\%$) and moderate to severe right HF are considered absolute contraindications to LT alone, and in these cases, combined heart-liver transplantation must be considered [7, 25]. Relative contraindications to LT alone are LVEF $< 50\%$ and HCM with resting left ventricular outflow tract obstruction [12, 26]. Management of HF requires a multidisciplinary approach including careful consideration for RAAS inhibition, β-blockers, and mineralocorticoid receptor antagonists. In patients with ESLD, use of RAAS inhibitors is limited due to renal insufficiency and hypotension

[27]. LT candidates with identified subclinical cardiomyopathy should undergo surveillance TTE every 6 months prior to LT, and at 6–12 month intervals post-LT to monitor for progressive cardiac dysfunction [7].

Coronary Artery Disease

CAD is the formation of atherosclerotic plaques within the lumen of the coronary arteries supplying blood to the myocardium. In addition to traditional epicardial disease, CAD also includes microvascular disease of the myocardium, which may be driven by inflammatory processes [28]. In the current age of steatotic-predominant cirrhosis, LT candidates increasingly present with older age and higher CVD burden. Because of these evolving patient demographics, prevalence of both traditional risk factors for CAD and CAD itself have increased [29]. CAD prevalence is as high as 36.8% in patients with ESLD, with the highest prevalence (52.8%) among patients with MASH [30]. CAD is a major contributor to post-LT major adverse cardiovascular events (MACE), which include myocardial infarction, coronary revascularization, HF, sustained ventricular tachycardia, atrial fibrillation, cardiac arrest, and stroke [13]. Notably, 1 in 3 LT recipients experience a MACE event within a year of transplant, and associated cardiac death accounts for 40% of all LT recipient deaths within 30 days post-LT [31–33].

Accordingly, it is imperative to screen LT candidates for CAD to inform LT recipient selection and to institute interventions to mitigate cardiac risk. Although there are currently many screening methods for significant CAD, there is wide variation in practice across centers [34]. Contemporary AHA guidelines recommend stratifying patients by pretest probability for significant CAD, rather than a universal CAD testing protocol, to promote effective clinical resource utilization and timeliness to complete LT evaluation [27].

Predictors of significant CAD in LT candidates include male sex, hypertension, hyperlipidemia, active smoking, age > 60 years, LV hypertrophy, prior CVD, chronic kidney disease, diabetes, and MASH [11, 35, 36]. LT candidates are most likely to have obstructive CAD if they have ≥3 risk factors [37]. MASH and diabetes should be considered as CAD equivalents in LT candidates given the increased risks of MACE and mortality in these conditions [38].

One approach to establishing pretest probability for significant CAD and MACE is to use clinical risk scores. A variety of clinical risk scores are available to risk-stratify patients before major noncardiac surgery, but their discrimination and calibration in LT candidates are suboptimal (C statistic, 0.66–0.73) [39–41]. Three LT-specific clinical risk scores, CAR-OLT, CAD-LT, and CARI scores, have recently been published for risk prediction in LT candidates, which predict global CV event risk, CAD-specific risk and cardiac arrest-specific risk, respectively, with good discrimination (bias-corrected C-statistics 0.76–0.77) and may be calculated in LT candidates to inform CV risk discussions.

All LT candidates should be evaluated with a cardiac physical exam, electrocardiogram (ECG), and TTE [27]. Additional testing for CAD should be pursued based on risk stratification. In patients with low to intermediate risk, myocardial stress testing can be considered, whereas in high-risk patients (≥2 traditional risk factors, diabetes, or MASH) anatomic coronary imaging is recommended [12, 27]. Table 7.1 outlines risk stratification methods and available testing to assess for CAD.

Dobutamine stress echocardiography (DSE) was previously recommended in all LT candidates as an initial CAD screening test [42]. However, DSE has poor sensitivity (13–37%) for significant CAD or MACE and a high rate of non-diagnostic testing due to the inability of patients with ESLD to achieve the target rate because of blunted chronotropy and reduced cardiopulmonary fitness, leading to increased rates of subsequent invasive testing [27, 43]. Other non-invasive modalities for assessment of CAD in asymptomatic LT candidates, including nuclear stress testing, have limited accuracy in the ESLD population, with a sensitivity of 62.5% and specificity of 66.7% for post-LT CAD events [43, 44]. However, a strength of nuclear imaging is the ability to assess for both epicardial CAD and myocardial perfusion at the microvascular level. A recent study examining use of MPI PET-CT in LT candidates found reduced global myocardial flow reserve (MFR) ≤ 1.38 was associated with a higher risk of MACE [HR = 3.42 (1.23–9.47), $p = 0.019$]. This is particularly important because in patients with MASH, microvascular dysfunction is highly prevalent and predictive of MACE [45]. Further data is needed to confirm diagnostic and prognostic utility of PET MPI in ESLD and LT candidates [46]. Finally, the coronary artery calcium score (CACS), measured using noncontrast CT imaging, has a strong negative predictive value (95–100%) for significant CAD and therefore may be incorporated into algorithms to risk stratify LT candidates [47].

Coronary angiography, noninvasive or invasive, has emerged as the most accurate test for excluding obstructive CAD in patients with ESLD [48]. Coronary CT angiography (CCTA) has a negative predictive value of 99% in the general population for excluding significant stenosis (≥50% obstruction) [49]. However, the positive predictive value of CCTA for ischemia-causing lesions ranges from 76% to 88%. The diagnostic utility of CCTA can be increased with the addition of CT-derived fractional flow reserve (FFR). FFR can help determine the functional significance of epicardial stenosis; however, its use in patients with ESLD can be limited due to chronic vasodilation [50]. More data is needed on the utility of FFR, whether CT-derived or invasive, in ESLD.

Invasive coronary angiography (ICA) should be reserved for patients with evidence of high-risk features on noninvasive testing, known obstructive CAD, or history of revascularization [51]. In preparation for ICA, providers should perform a risk-benefit analysis pertaining to potential for revascularization and associated need for dual antiplatelet (DAPT) and statin therapy to prevent delays in coronary intervention and the need for repeat ICA. The risks of ICA include contrast-induced nephropathy and bleeding [52]. Management of thrombocytopenia and coagulopathies, as well as minimizing sheath size, may reduce vascular and bleeding complications related to angiography in patients with ESLD [53].

Coronary revascularization is indicated in patients with obstructive CAD, and revascularization has been demonstrated to have post-LT survival benefit [54]. Percutaneous coronary intervention (PCI) with newer generation drug-eluting stents

Table 7.1 Summary of evaluation and considerations in patients with end stage liver disease

Test for CAD	Test component and performance characteristics	Positive Test characteristic	Positive test implication	Considerations in patients with ESLD
Risk factor stratification, ECG, TTE	Presence of risk factors can be used to calculate risk scores such as CAD-LT and CAR-OLT	Signs of ischemia (Q-waves on ECG, inverted T-waves) Wall region abnormalities and reduced EF on echo	Proceed to further testing with a non-invasive or invasive screening method	Guidelines recommended as universal testing in every liver transplant candidate
Cardiopulmonary exercise resting	Sensitivity: 86% Specificity: 98%	No specific cutoff for obstructive CAD has been published	VO_2 peak <15 mL/min/kg predicts poor prognosis after LT Reduction in AT predicts poor outcomes in LT candidates and at 90 & 100 days post-LT AT <0.9 mL/min/kg associated with reduced 90-day survival	VO_2 max is achieved in <35% of patients with ESLD Testing requires specific equipment and expertise
Dobutamine stress echo	Sensitivity: 13–32% Specificity: 78%	New or worsening wall motion abnormalities	Low sensitivity to predict both peri-operative (9%) and postoperative (5.6%) cardiovascular events	Patients with ESLD may not achieve maximal chronotropy
Stress CMR	Sensitivity: 50% Specificity: 98%	Perfusion defect	No current studies	May be limited by ability to lie flat for extended period of time

(continued)

Table 7.1 (continued)

Test for CAD	Test component and performance characteristics	Positive Test characteristic	Positive test implication	Considerations in patients with ESLD
CCTA	Sensitivity: 93% Specificity: 63%	Identifying a segment with a diameter >2 mm and >50% reduction in luminal diameter (>70% stenosis)	Early progression of atherosclerosis is seen in LT	IV contrast can worsen kidney function Patient needs to be able to lie still Target HR < 60 bpm needs to be achieved Patient has to tolerate breath holding technique
CAC scoring	Sensitivity: 100% Specificity: 31%	CAC > 400 = high risk CAC > 234 = significant obstructive CAD	CAC score > 400 predicts: Significant CAD requiring revascularization 1 month post LT complications	Ability to tolerate CT
Invasive coronary angiography	Gold standard for diagnosing CAD	Significant CAD: ≥70% stenosis in a major vessel FFR < 0.8 (if measured)	Pretransplant ASCVD associated with MACE within 1 year of transplant	Transradial approach is preferred to minimize bleeding risks, use of smallest sheath possible

Abbreviations: ASCVD atherosclerotic cardiovascular disease, *AT* aerobic threshold, *CAC* coronary artery calcification, *CAD* coronary artery disease, *CAD-LT* coronary artery disease in liver transplantation score, *CAR-OLT* coronary artery risk in orthotopic liver transplantation score, *CCTA* coronary computed tomography angiography, *CMR* cardia magnetic resonance, *ECG* electrocardiogram, *EF* ejection fraction, *ESLD* end-stage liver disease, *FFR* fractional flow reserve, *HR* heart rate, *IV* intravenous, *LT* liver transplantation, *MACE* major adverse cardiovascular event (MACE), *TTE* transthoracic echocardiogram, VO_2 maximal rate of oxygen consumption during physical exertion can be performed with a DAPT duration of 3–6 months and PPI use to minimize risk for gastrointestinal bleeding [27]. The duration of DAPT can be shortened to as little as 1 month based on stent choice to minimize bleeding risks [27]. Patients with multivessel CAD can be considered for combined coronary artery bypass graft (CABG) either in advance or at the time of LT, depending on the severity of ESLD, though this requires multidisciplinary review and collaboration at highly experienced centers [27]. CAD not amenable to revascularization is a contraindication to LT [12, 27].

Statin therapy should be based on cardiovascular disease (CVD) benefit and not lipid level, particularly since lipid production is decreased in ESLD and serum lipids do not reflect total body lipid burden in this population [27]. Although patients with ESLD have a higher risk of muscle-related side effects, statin use is safe and beneficial in Child class A compensated cirrhosis. Statins should not be initiated in Child class C decompensated cirrhosis and should be used with caution in Child class B decompensated cirrhosis [55, 56]. Aspirin use for secondary prevention should be considered on a case-by-case basis, as patients with ESLD have an increased bleeding risk [27]. Non-selective β-blockers are used for primary and secondary prevention of variceal bleeding. Carvedilol has been shown to have the greatest effect on reducing portal pressure and can have anti-anginal effects in patients with symptomatic CAD [27]. Further management with RAAS inhibition (ACE-inhibitors, angiotensin receptor blockers) is limited due to hypotension and renal insufficiency in patients with decompensated cirrhosis [27].

In the post-LT setting, atherosclerotic CVD has additional clinical significance. Within the first 12 months of LT, CAD requiring revascularization compromises 12% of cardiovascular complications [57]. Incidence of CVD is as high as 30% in LT recipients by 8 years post-LT, and CVD-related death is a leading cause of mortality after LT [58]. Both pre-LT CAD plus substantial risk of new onset or worsening cardiometabolic comorbidities, including hypertension, hyperlipidemia, diabetes, chronic kidney disease, and obesity, contribute to this observation [59, 60]. Chronic immunosuppression with calcineurin inhibitors (CNI) carry the highest risk of metabolic side effects as well as nephrotoxicity. Diabetes and hypertension are the most common side effects seen with CNIs, while dyslipidemia is seen more often with mammalian target of rapamycin (mTOR) inhibitors [61]. In general, steroids should be tapered quickly post-LT as able, and used sparingly given the risk of inciting hyperglycemia and associated risk of de novo or exacerbation of diabetes [62]. However, decisions regarding immunosuppression focused on cardiovascular outcomes are of little impact if they are not accompanied by a multidisciplinary, protocolized and targeted management of cardiovascular risk factors after LT [63]. Blood pressure and weight monitoring, smoking cessation counseling, and annual biochemical disease screening (lipid panel, hemoglobin A1c) are strongly recommended [64].

Arrhythmias

The most common ECG abnormality in patients with ESLD is QT-interval prolongation [65]. A prolonged corrected QT-interval (QTc) is defined as >0.45 milliseconds for males and >0.47 milliseconds for females. There is an increased risk of sudden cardiac death with a prolonged QTc >500 milliseconds due to ventricular arrhythmias [65, 66]. For patients with prolonged QTc, it is important to obtain a family history of hereditary prolonged QTc syndromes, careful medication review to eliminate any QT-prolonging agents, and correct any electrolyte abnormalities as they arise.

Atrial fibrillation (AF) is the most common arrhythmia in adults and is associated with increased morbidity and all-cause mortality in LT candidates [31, 67]. AF is prevalent in 7.5% of hospitalized patients with ESLD and pre-existing AF is associated with an increased risk of 90-day post-LT MACE [31, 68]. Patients with ESLD have been excluded from most cardiovascular drug trials, so there is limited data on AF medical management in ESLD [69]. Generally, AF management centers on rate control strategies. In patients with early cirrhosis, β-blockers are indicated if the patient has a concurrent CVD, such as HF or CAD and can reduce risk of portal hypertensive bleeding [70]. However, β-blockers may be contraindicated in more advanced disease due to hypotension, decreased cardiac output, and renal failure [70]. In LT recipients, rate control should be primarily obtained with β-blockers, but not non-dihydropyridine calcium channel blockers as these inhibit CYP450 and can interact with CNI [71]. Rhythm control with amiodarone is an alternative both pre- and post-LT. Amiodarone can pose a risk of hepatotoxicity, so use should be considered with caution and close monitoring [72]. In general, amiodarone should be avoided in patients with ALT levels two times greater than the upper limit of normal [72]. In lower-risk patients, the lowest dose of amiodarone should be used, and liver function tests monitored regularly.

Anticoagulation is recommended in AF to reduce risk of arterial thromboembolic events. Choice of anticoagulation agent, if any, in ESLD requires a careful risk-benefit analysis. The CHA_2DS_2VASc score [73] has proven useful in LT recipients to predict the risk of stroke [74]. The HAS-BLED score, which accounts for liver disease, can be used to estimate the 1-year risk of a major bleeding event in patients with AF [75]. The use of oral anticoagulants, such as warfarin, has better risk reduction of ischemic stroke and similar risk of intracranial hemorrhage compared to antiplatelet therapies such as aspirin [76]. Early data on the use of direct-acting oral anticoagulants in patients with cirrhosis and non-valvular AF has suggested comparable efficacy with warfarin, but prospective studies and longitudinal data on both efficacy and safety are needed [77].

Valvular Heart Disease

LT candidates should be evaluated for significant VHD, which, if uncorrected, may represent an absolute contraindication to LT. The most common VHD is aortic stenosis (AS), which is present in an estimated 2–7% of the general population [78, 79]. Given the multiple shared cardiometabolic risk factors between AS and MASH (e.g., diabetes, hypertension), AS is increasingly common among patients with MASH [12, 35]. Severe AS can lead to systemic hypoperfusion and LV hypertrophy, which can progress to LV failure and ventricular arrhythmias, including ventricular tachycardia. Severe AS is associated with high mortality (50% at 1 year). Thus, severe AS not amenable to therapeutic intervention is a medical contraindication to LT [80].

Methods of AS repair include transcatheter aortic valve replacement (TAVR) and surgical aortic valve replacement (SAVR). In patients with ESLD and severe AS, TAVR may be preferable to SAVR since it is minimally invasive and avoids general anesthesia or the use of a cardiopulmonary bypass pump [81]. For LT candidates, balloon valvuloplasty or TAVR can be considered as bridge therapy to LT with the intent to later pursue SAVR for definitive management once stable post-LT [82]. In rare cases, SAVR may be performed at the time of LT. Given the limited data to guide treatment strategies, a multidisciplinary case review is imperative to determining the appropriate course of action for AS management.

Significant tricuspid regurgitation (TR) and mitral stenosis (MS) also require careful consideration in LT candidates. TR can be present as either structural VHD or functional regurgitation, the latter secondary to asymmetric dilation of the tricuspid valve annulus [83]. This annular dilation is usually in the setting of right ventricular enlargement due to left heart dysfunction. TR can cause congestive hepatopathy in patients with ESLD pre-LT and lead to graft hypoperfusion post-LT [84]. In patients with clinically significant TR, multidisciplinary management is warranted to optimize any right heart function with consideration for valve replacement if severe. Right-sided HF secondary to MS can have similar effects. There is less evidence regarding the repair of MS in the LT population, although minimally invasive repair with a MitralClip procedure can be performed when MS is moderate to severe [85].

Given the associated morbidity and mortality posed by VHD, all LT candidates should undergo TTE as routine screening for valvular dysfunction. Presence of moderate to severe VHD warrants multidisciplinary case review and management (Table 7.2) to optimize valve function and prevent associated poor clinical outcomes.

Table 7.2 Summary of valvular heart disease recommendations and management in patients with cirrhosis

	Valvular heart disease	Management
Aortic stenosis	Severe: Mean gradient > 40 mmHg Peak aortic velocity (Vmax) ≥ 4 m/s Moderate—Severe: Mean gradient 30–40 mmHg Peak aortic velocity ≥ 3 m/s Moderate: Mean gradient 20–30 mmHg Peak aortic velocity ≥ 3 m/s	Severe: TAVR SAVR (if age < 65) Moderate—Severe: TTE monitoring SAVR v. TAVR Moderate: TTE monitoring
Aortic regurgitation	Moderate—Severe: Jet width > 25% of LVOT Regurgitant volume > 30 Regurgitant fraction > 30%	Moderate—Severe: TTE monitoring Consider replacement
Mitral regurgitation	Moderate—Severe: Central jet MR > 40% LA (or holosystolic eccentric jet MR) Regurgitant volume ≥ 60 mL Regurgitant fraction ≥40% ERO ≥ 0.40 cm^2	Moderate—Severe: TTE monitoring 6–12 months Mitral valve replacement or repair
Mitral stenosis	Moderate—Severe: MV area ≤ 1.5 cm^2 Diastolic pressure half-time ≥ 150 ms Any LA enlargement +/− elevated PASP	Moderate—Severe: TTE monitoring yearly Mitral valve replacement or repair Management of comorbidities such as atrial fibrillation
Tricuspid regurgitation	Moderate—Severe: Central jet ≥ 50% RA ERO ≥ 0.40 cm^2 Regurgitant volume ≥ 45 m Left Hepatic vein systolic flow reversal	Moderate—Severe: TTE monitoring yearly Tricuspid valve replacement or repair PAH management if present Atrial fibrillation management if present

Abbreviations: *ERO* effective regurgitant orifice area, *LA* left atrium, *LVOT* left ventricular outflow tract obstruction, *MV* mitral valve, *PAH* pulmonary arterial hypertension, *PASP* pulmonary artery systolic pressure, *RA* right atrium, *TAVR* transcatheter aortic valve replacement, *TTE* transthoracic echocardiogram, *SAVR* surgical aortic valve replacement

Pulmonary Complications

Portopulmonary Hypertension

POPH is defined as pulmonary arterial hypertension (PAH) that develops specifically in the setting of portal hypertension, even in the absence of cirrhosis. POPH belongs to the Group 1 PAH clinical classification, and accounts for approximately 5–15% of all PAH cases [86]. POPH is estimated to affect 5–6% of patients with ESLD, though interestingly severity of POPH does not appear to correlate with either the severity of portal HTN or liver disease [87, 88]. POPH is associated with

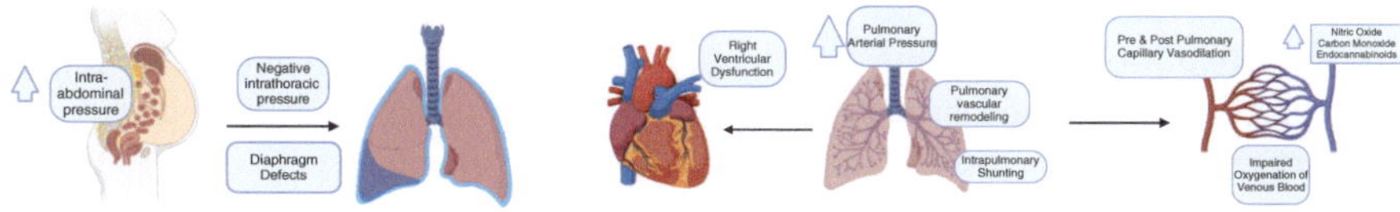

	HH	POPH	HPS

Definition	Transudative pleural effusion in setting of cirrhosis with ascites
	• PF/serum protein ratio < 0.5
	• PF/serum LDH ratio < 0.6
	• Low protein (< 2.5 g/dL)
	• **Serum to pleural fluid** albumin gradient > 1.1 g/dL
		• mPAP > 20mmHg
		• Group 1: Pre-Capillary PH (includes porto-pulmonary hypertension)
		  • PAWP ≤ 15mmHg
		  • PVR ≥ 2 WU
			• Alveolar-arterial oxygen gradient (AaPO2) >15
			• Evidence of shunting on echo

Pathophysiology	Due to increased intra-abdominal pressure and defects in the diaphragm, **ascites fluid moves into the** pleural space due to negative intrathoracic pressure	Increased pulmonary vascular remodeling and pulmonary arterial pressure cause right ventricular dysfunction	Intrapulmonary vascular dilatations result in ventilation-perfusion mismatch, diffusion restriction and arteriovenous shunts thereby causing gas exchange impairment
Management	• AVOID Chest Tube • Diuretics • Low- salt diet • Thoracentesis • TIPS consideration	• Caution in use of beta-blockers due to worsening exercise capacity and right ventricular impairment • Diuretics • Oxygen if hypoxemia is present • Consideration of prostacyclin derivatives, endothelin receptor blockers, and phosphodiesterase-5 inhibitors	Oxygen supplementation especially if PaO2 < 60 mmHg
LT Consideration	**LT is definitive** treatment and provides **survival benefit.**	• mPAP > 45-50 mmHg is an absolute contraindication • LT should be considered in patients with mPAP ≤ 35 mmHg who are responding to medical therapy for PH	Indication for LT if severe HPS (PaO2 < 60 mmHg). MELD exception points may be granted

Fig. 7.2 Pulmonary considerations in ESLD. Abbreviations: HH hepatic hydrothorax, HPS hepatopulmonary syndrome, LT liver transplant, MELD model for end-stage liver disease, mPAP mean pulmonary arterial pressure, PAWP pulmonary arterial wedge pressure, PH pulmonary hypertension, POPH portopulmonary hypertension, PVR pulmonary vascular resistance, TIPS transjugular intrahepatic portosystemic shunt

high rates of hospital admissions, reduced survival even compared to idiopathic PAH, and higher perioperative risk among LT candidates [89].

Screening for POPH via TTE is indicated for all LT candidates and any patients with portal hypertension meeting clinical suspicion for POPH by cardiac physical exam [90]. TTE findings suggestive of POPH include right ventricular systolic pressure (RVSP) > 38 mmHg, RV dilation or dysfunction, flattening of the interventricular septum, or a pulmonary artery diameter > 25 mm [91]. Patients should undergo diagnostic right heart catheterization (RHC) for definitive diagnosis (see Fig. 7.2 for diagnostic criteria) [92, 93]. POPH is diagnosed by the following on RHC: (i) mean pulmonary arterial pressure (mPAP) > 20 mmHg, (ii) pulmonary arterial wedge pressure ≤ 15 mmHg, and (iii) pulmonary vascular resistance ≥240 dynes*sec/cm^5 [86].

While the exact pathophysiology of POPH remains unknown, the most widely accepted mechanism is an imbalance of vasoconstrictive and vasodilatory mediators, wherein humoral substances such as endothelin-1 bypass hepatic metabolism and reach the pulmonary circulation through portosystemic shunts, leading to PAH [94]. Patients with POPH often respond to standard PAH therapeutics (Fig. 7.2). Patients with POPH who receive PAH therapies as a bridge to LT have improved perioperative cardiopulmonary outcomes and reduced risk of right HF [95]. Effective POPH management requires a multidisciplinary team as some portal hypertension therapeutics may conflict with management of PAH. For example, non-selective β-blockers, while effectively providing variceal hemorrhage prophylaxis, should be avoided in patients with POPH given risk of exacerbating mPAP and worsening right heart function [96].

Prognosis in POPH is primarily impacted by LT. LT is not curative of POPH, but nearly 50% of patients with POPH have improvement or resolution of POPH after LT [95]. Thus, patients with POPH are awarded model for end-stage liver disease (MELD) exception points to improve waitlist prioritization. Criteria for appropriate LT recipient selection and MELD exception points include mPAP < 35 mmHg and PVR < 400 dynes*sec/cm^5 on surveillance RHC [95, 97]. However, patients with POPH carry an increased in 1-year mortality and graft loss after LT compared to patients without POPH [98]. Pre-transplant PVR is a predictor of post-LT survival; thus, optimizing treatment with PAH therapeutics is important in patients with POPH [99]. Severe POPH (mPAP > 45–50 mmHg) refractory to PAH therapy is associated with LT perioperative mortality of nearly 100% due to inciting right HF and cardiac arrest; it is therefore considered an absolute contraindication to LT [100]. Given the survival b,enefit of patients who are treated for POPH it is imperative to screen for, treat, and consider LT in eligible patients.

Hepato-Pulmonary Syndrome

HPS is the most common cause of respiratory insufficiency in patients with ESLD, affecting 10–30% of patients [101]. HPS consists of intrapulmonary vascular dilatations (IPVD), resulting in ventilation-perfusion mismatch, diffusion restriction, and arteriovenous shunts, causing hypoxemia [102]. Like CCM and POPH, the pro-inflammatory pathway seen in progressive cirrhotic portal hypertension is thought to be a significant mediator of HPS. The prolonged stimulation of inflammatory and vasoactive mediators ultimately leads to progressive vasodilation in the pulmonary capillary network (IPVD formation) [103]. Macrophages are recruited and release vasodilatory molecules, leading to progressive capillary vasodilation and impaired gas exchange.

Most patients with HPS are asymptomatic, but symptoms and signs including dyspnea, platypnea, and clubbing develop with progressive hypoxemia. Patients with HPS develop substantially reduced functional capacity and have two-fold increased mortality compared to patients without HPS [104]. Beyond supplemental oxygen, medical therapy for HPS is limited. Only LT is considered potentially curative and severe HPS (PaO2 < 60 mmHg on room air) is an indication for LT [105].

All LT candidates and any patient with ESLD exhibiting respiratory insufficiency should be screened for HPS with pulse oximetry. Patients with room air oxygen saturation < 96% should undergo further diagnostic testing. HPS diagnosis is based on the presence of (i) ESLD, (ii) hypoxemia per arterial blood gas, and (iii) shunt pathology, which can be identified by late passage of microbubbles into the left heart on contrast-enhanced TTE [106]. Stages of HPS are based on the degree of arterial hypoxemia. Severe hypoxemia pre-LT, specifically PaO2 < 44 mmHg, is associated with higher post-LT mortality [105]. Early post-LT interventions for HPS are largely center-dependent and variable, including use of extracorporeal membrane oxygenation and high-flow nasal cannulation. Clinical outcomes data in post-HPS management remain limited, hence coordinated multidisciplinary care is needed to develop successful perioperative ventilation strategies.

Hepatic Hydrothorax

A HH is a transudative pleural effusion, typically right-sided and occurring in patients with cirrhosis and ascites [107]. HH develops due to fluid shifts through small defects in the diaphragm, driven by a pressure gradient from higher intra-abdominal pressure to a negative intra-thoracic pressure. HH is present in 5–10% of patients with ESLD and is associated with reduced survival compared to those without HH [108]. Refractory HH, occurring in 20–25% of cases, is an established independent predictor of mortality in ESLD and an indication for LT [109]. Diagnosis is made by chest imaging and confirmed by fluid analysis per thoracentesis.

Management of HH is similar to ascites: dietary sodium restriction, diuretics, and thoracentesis. It is important to avoid chest tubes in patients with HH due to the risk of high volume and protein loss that could incite renal dysfunction and increased risk for infection [107]. TIPS is effective in treating refractory HH, especially for patients awaiting LT [110]. LT is the definitive management of HH and post-LT outcomes for HH are similar for patients with non-HH indications for LT [111].

Conclusion

There is a broad array of cardiac and pulmonary conditions among patients with ESLD, and each harbors distinct clinical significance, including higher morbidity and mortality compared to patients without these complications. Thus, while cardiopulmonary conditions may not always be anticipated in patients with ESLD, their clinical impact should never be underestimated. Providers should be aware of these conditions, and their respective diagnostic and therapeutic strategies, given the associated impact on patient prognosis, including consideration for LT. Lastly, these cardiopulmonary conditions reflect the marked importance of multidisciplinary management required to attain optimal patient outcomes in ESLD.

References

1. Dourakis SP, Geladari E, Geladari C, Vallianou N. Cirrhotic cardiomyopathy: the interplay between liver and cardiac muscle. How does the cardiovascular system react when the liver is diseased? Curr Cardiol Rev. 2021;17(1):78–84.
2. Rinella ME, Lazarus JV, Ratziu V, Francque SM, Sanyal AJ, Kanwal F, et al. A multisociety Delphi consensus statement on new fatty liver disease nomenclature. Hepatology. 2023;78(6):1966–86.

3. Izzy M, Soldatova A, Sun X, Angirekula M, Mara K, Lin G, et al. Cirrhotic cardiomyopathy predicts posttransplant cardiovascular disease: revelations of the new diagnostic criteria. Liver Transpl. 2021;27(6):876–86.
4. Moller S, Henriksen JH. Cirrhotic cardiomyopathy: a pathophysiological review of circulatory dysfunction in liver disease. Heart. 2002;87(1):9–15.
5. Izzy M, Oh J, Watt KD. Cirrhotic cardiomyopathy after transplantation: neither the transient nor innocent bystander. Hepatology. 2018;68(5):2008–15.
6. Izzy MJ, VanWagner LB. Current concepts of cirrhotic cardiomyopathy. Clin Liver Dis. 2021;25(2):471–81.
7. Izzy M, VanWagner LB, Lin G, Altieri M, Findlay JY, Oh JK, et al. Redefining cirrhotic cardiomyopathy for the modern era. Hepatology. 2020;71(1):334–45.
8. Lazarevic AM, Nakatani S, Neskovic AN, Marinkovic J, Yasumura Y, Stojicic D, et al. Early changes in left ventricular function in chronic asymptomatic alcoholics: relation to the duration of heavy drinking. J Am Coll Cardiol. 2000;35(6):1599–606.
9. Lehtonen J, Uusitalo V, Poyhonen P, Mayranpaa MI, Kupari M. Cardiac sarcoidosis: phenotypes, diagnosis, treatment, and prognosis. Eur Heart J. 2023;44(17):1495–510.
10. Joshi PK, Patel SC, Shreya D, Zamora DI, Patel GS, Grossmann I, et al. Hereditary hemochromatosis: a cardiac perspective cureus. 2021;13(11):e20009.
11. Vanwagner LB, Bhave M, Te HS, Feinglass J, Alvarez L, Rinella ME. Patients transplanted for nonalcoholic steatohepatitis are at increased risk for postoperative cardiovascular events. Hepatology. 2012;56(5):1741–50.
12. Tsochatzis EA, Watt KD, VanWagner LB, Verna EC, Berzigotti A. Evaluation of recipients with significant comorbidity – patients with cardiovascular disease. J Hepatol. 2023;78(6):1089–104.
13. Barman PM, VanWagner LB. Cardiac risk assessment in liver transplant candidates: current controversies and future directions. Hepatology. 2021;73(6):2564–76.
14. Maraj S, Jacobs LE, Maraj R, Contreras R, Rerkpattanapipat P, Malik TA, et al. Inducible left ventricular outflow tract gradient during dobutamine stress echocardiography: an association with intraoperative hypotension but not a contraindication to liver transplantation. Echocardiography. 2004;21(8):681–5.
15. Meucci MC, Hoogerduijn Strating MM, Butcher SC, van Rijswijk CSP, Van Hoek B, Delgado V, et al. Left atrial dysfunction is an independent predictor of mortality in patients with cirrhosis treated by transjugular intrahepatic portosystemic shunt. Hepatol Commun. 2022;6:3163.
16. Koshy AN, Farouque O, Cailes B, Testro A, Ramchand J, Sajeev JK, et al. Impaired cardiac reserve on dobutamine stress echocardiography predicts the development of hepatorenal syndrome. Am J Gastroenterol. 2020;115(3):388–97.
17. Nasis A, Moir S, Meredith IT, Barton TL, Nerlekar N, Wong DT, et al. Abnormal left ventricular contractile response to exercise in the absence of obstructive coronary artery disease is associated with resting left ventricular long-axis dysfunction. J Am Soc Echocardiogr. 2015;28(1):95–105.
18. Kim SA, Shim CY, Kim JM, Lee HJ, Choi DH, Choi EY, et al. Impact of left ventricular longitudinal diastolic functional reserve on clinical outcome in patients with type 2 diabetes mellitus. Heart. 2011;97(15):1233–8.
19. Rustad LA, Amundsen BH, Slørdahl SA, Støylen A. Upright bicycle exercise echocardiography in patients with myocardial infarction shows lack of diastolic, but not systolic, reserve: a tissue Doppler study. Eur J Echocardiogr. 2009;10(4):503–8.
20. Dungu JN, Hardy-Wallace A, Dimarco AD, Savage HO. Hypertrophic cardiomyopathy. Curr Heart Fail Rep. 2024;21:428.
21. Upadhya B, Hegde S, Tannu M, Stacey RB, Kalogeropoulos A, Schocken DD. Preventing new-onset heart failure: intervening at stage a. Am J Prev Cardiol. 2023;16:100609.
22. Moon YJ, Kwon HM, Jung KW, Kim KS, Shin WJ, Jun IG, et al. Preoperative high-sensitivity troponin I and B-type natriuretic peptide, alone and in combination, for risk stratification of mortality after liver transplantation. Korean J Anesthesiol. 2021;74(3):242–53.

23. Park J, Lee SH, Han S, Jee HS, Lee SK, Choi GS, et al. Preoperative cardiac troponin level is associated with all-cause mortality of liver transplantation recipients. PLoS One. 2017;12(5):e0177838.
24. Watt KD, Coss E, Pedersen RA, Dierkhising R, Heimbach JK, Charlton MR. Pretransplant serum troponin levels are highly predictive of patient and graft survival following liver transplantation. Liver Transpl. 2010;16(8):990–8.
25. VanWagner LB, Harinstein ME, Runo JR, Darling C, Serper M, Hall S, et al. Multidisciplinary approach to cardiac and pulmonary vascular disease risk assessment in liver transplantation: an evaluation of the evidence and consensus recommendations. Am J Transplant. 2018;18(1):30–42.
26. Pai SL, Aniskevich S 3rd, Logvinov II, Matcha GV, Palmer WC, Blackshear JL. Hypertrophic cardiomyopathy in liver transplantation patients. Transplant Proc. 2018;50(5):1466–9.
27. Cheng XS, VanWagner LB, Costa SP, Axelrod DA, Bangalore S, Norman SP, et al. Emerging evidence on coronary heart disease screening in kidney and liver transplantation candidates: a scientific statement from the American Heart Association: endorsed by the American Society of Transplantation. Circulation. 2022;146(21):e299–324.
28. Stark K, Massberg S. Interplay between inflammation and thrombosis in cardiovascular pathology. Nat Rev Cardiol. 2021;18(9):666–82.
29. Martinez-Perez S, McCluskey SA, Davierwala PM, Kalra S, Nguyen E, Bhat M, et al. Perioperative cardiovascular risk assessment and management in liver transplant recipients: a review of the literature merging guidelines and interventions. J Cardiothorac Vasc Anesth. 2024;38(4):1015–30.
30. Patel SS, Nabi E, Guzman L, Abbate A, Bhati C, Stravitz RT, et al. Coronary artery disease in decompensated patients undergoing liver transplantation evaluation. Liver Transpl. 2018;24(3):333–42.
31. VanWagner LB, Serper M, Kang R, Levitsky J, Hohmann S, Abecassis M, et al. Factors associated with major adverse cardiovascular events after liver transplantation among a national sample. Am J Transplant. 2016;16(9):2684–94.
32. Albeldawi M, Aggarwal A, Madhwal S, Cywinski J, Lopez R, Eghtesad B, et al. Cumulative risk of cardiovascular events after orthotopic liver transplantation. Liver Transpl. 2012;18(3):370–5.
33. VanWagner LB, Lapin B, Levitsky J, Wilkins JT, Abecassis MM, Skaro AI, et al. High early cardiovascular mortality after liver transplantation. Liver Transpl. 2014;20(11):1306–16.
34. Barman PM, Chadha RM, VanWagner LB. Cardiac risk assessment in liver transplant candidates: a survey of National Practice Patterns. Liver Transpl. 2022;28(3):501–4.
35. Safadi A, Homsi M, Maskoun W, Lane KA, Singh I, Sawada SG, et al. Perioperative risk predictors of cardiac outcomes in patients undergoing liver transplantation surgery. Circulation. 2009;120(13):1189–94.
36. Rachwan RJ, Kutkut I, Timsina LR, Bou Chaaya RG, El-Am EA, Sabra M, et al. CAD-LT score effectively predicts risk of significant coronary artery disease in liver transplant candidates. J Hepatol. 2021;75(1):142–9.
37. Skaro AI, Gallon LG, Lyuksemburg V, Jay CL, Zhao L, Ladner DP, et al. The impact of coronary artery disease on outcomes after liver transplantation. J Cardiovasc Med (Hagerstown). 2016;17(12):875–85.
38. Kim D, Konyn P, Sandhu KK, Dennis BB, Cheung AC, Ahmed A. Metabolic dysfunction-associated fatty liver disease is associated with increased all-cause mortality in the United States. J Hepatol. 2021;75(6):1284–91.
39. Josefsson A, Fu M, Bjornsson E, Kalaitzakis E. Prevalence of pre-transplant electrocardiographic abnormalities and post-transplant cardiac events in patients with liver cirrhosis. BMC Gastroenterol. 2014;14:65.
40. Di Maira T, Rubin A, Puchades L, Aguilera V, Vinaixa C, Garcia M, et al. Framingham score, renal dysfunction, and cardiovascular risk in liver transplant patients. Liver Transpl. 2015;21(6):812–22.

41. Park YS, Moon YJ, Jun IG, Song JG, Hwang GS. Application of the revised cardiac risk index to the model for end-stage liver disease score improves the prediction of cardiac events in patients undergoing liver transplantation. Transplant Proc. 2018;50(4):1108–13.
42. Martin P, DiMartini A, Feng S, Brown R Jr, Fallon M. Evaluation for liver transplantation in adults: 2013 practice guideline by the American Association for the Study of Liver Diseases and the American Society of Transplantation. Hepatology. 2014;59(3):1144–65.
43. Tiwari N, Margapuri J, Katamreddy A, Jubbal S, Madan N. Diagnostic accuracy of cardiac testing for coronary artery disease in potential liver transplant recipients: a systematic review and meta-analysis. Int J Cardiol Heart Vasc. 2021;32:100714.
44. Malik MU, Russell SD, Pustavoitau A, Chacko M, Cosar AM, Thompson CB, et al. The predictors of post-transplant coronary events among liver transplant recipients. Hepatol Int. 2016;10(6):974–82.
45. Vita T, Murphy DJ, Osborne MT, Bajaj NS, Keraliya A, Jacob S, et al. Association between nonalcoholic fatty liver disease at CT and coronary microvascular dysfunction at myocardial perfusion PET/CT. Radiology. 2019;291(2):330–7.
46. Hughes DL, Pan J, Answine AR, Sonnenday CJ, Waits SA, Kumar SS, et al. Positron emission tomography myocardial perfusion imaging (PET MPI) findings predictive of post-liver transplant major adverse cardiac events. Liver Transpl. 2023;29(9):970–8.
47. West BH, Low CG, Bista BB, Yang EH, Vorobiof G, Busuttil RW, et al. Significance of coronary artery calcium found on non-electrocardiogram-gated computed tomography during preoperative evaluation for liver transplant. Am J Cardiol. 2019;124(2):278–84.
48. McCarthy KJ, Motta-Calderon D, Estrada-Roman A, Cajiao KM, Curry MP, Bonder A, et al. Introduction of a standardized protocol for cardiac risk assessment in candidates for liver transplant – a retrospective cohort analysis. Ann Hepatol. 2022;27(2):100582.
49. Dangl M, Eisenberg T, Grant JK, Vincent L, Colombo R, Sancassani R, et al. A comprehensive review of coronary artery disease in patients with end-stage liver disease. Transplant Rev (Orlando). 2022;36(3):100709.
50. Kumar P, Kim JS, Gordin J, Honda HM, Suh W, Lee MS, et al. Fractional flow reserve in end-stage liver disease. Am J Cardiol. 2022;166:122–6.
51. Lee MS, Wadia S, Yeghiazarians Y, Matthews R, White CJ, Herrmann HC, et al. Cardiology assessment of patients undergoing evaluation for orthotopic liver transplantation. J Soc Cardiovasc Angiogr Interv. 2023;2(1):100528.
52. Rear R, Bell RM, Hausenloy DJ. Contrast-induced nephropathy following angiography and cardiac interventions. Heart. 2016;102(8):638–48.
53. Pillarisetti J, Patel P, Duthuluru S, Roberts J, Chen W, Genton R, et al. Cardiac catheterization in patients with end-stage liver disease: safety and outcomes. Catheter Cardiovasc Interv. 2011;77(1):45–8.
54. Satapathy SK, Vanatta JM, Helmick RA, Flowers A, Kedia SK, Jiang Y, et al. Outcome of liver transplant recipients with revascularized coronary artery disease: a comparative analysis with and without cardiovascular risk factors. Transplantation. 2017;101(4):793–803.
55. Abraldes JG, Villanueva C, Aracil C, Turnes J, Hernandez-Guerra M, Genesca J, et al. Addition of simvastatin to standard therapy for the prevention of variceal rebleeding does not reduce rebleeding but increases survival in patients with cirrhosis. Gastroenterology. 2016;150(5):1160–70 e3.
56. Francis P, Forman L. Use of statins in patients with and without liver disease. Clin Liver Dis (Hoboken). 2020;15(1):40–5.
57. VanWagner LB, Ning H, Whitsett M, Levitsky J, Uttal S, Wilkins JT, et al. A point-based prediction model for cardiovascular risk in orthotopic liver transplantation: the CAR-OLT score. Hepatology. 2017;66(6):1968–79.
58. Konerman MA, Fritze D, Weinberg RL, Sonnenday CJ, Sharma P. Incidence of and risk assessment for adverse cardiovascular outcomes after liver transplantation: a systematic review. Transplantation. 2017;101(7):1645–57.

59. Madhwal S, Atreja A, Albeldawi M, Lopez R, Post A, Costa MA. Is liver transplantation a risk factor for cardiovascular disease? A meta-analysis of observational studies. Liver Transpl. 2012;18(10):1140–6.
60. Izzy M, VanWagner LB, Lee SS, Altieri M, Angirekula M, Watt KD. Understanding and managing cardiovascular outcomes in liver transplant recipients. Curr Opin Organ Transplant. 2019;24(2):148–55.
61. Dadlani A, Lee TH. Management of metabolic syndrome after liver transplant. Clin Liver Dis (Hoboken). 2023;21(6):155–9.
62. Gu J, Wu X, Lu L, Zhang S, Bai J, Wang J, et al. Role of steroid minimization in the tacrolimus-based immunosuppressive regimen for liver transplant recipients: a systematic review and meta-analysis of prospective randomized controlled trials. Hepatol Int. 2014;8(2):198–215.
63. Sastre L, García R, Viñals C, Amor AJ, Yago G, Hervás A, et al. Results of a multidisciplinary strategy to improve the management of cardiovascular risk factors after liver transplantation. Liver Transpl. 2022;28(8):1332–44.
64. Izzy M, Fortune BE, Serper M, Bhave N, deLemos A, Gallegos-Orozco JF, et al. Management of cardiac diseases in liver transplant recipients: comprehensive review and multidisciplinary practice-based recommendations. Am J Transplant. 2022;22(12):2740–58.
65. Kim KS, Kwon HM, Jung KW, Sang BH, Moon YJ, Kim B, et al. Markedly prolonged QTc interval in end-stage liver disease and risk of 30-day cardiovascular event after liver transplant. J Gastroenterol Hepatol. 2021;36(3):758–66.
66. Gibbs C, Thalamus J, Heldal K, Holla OL, Haugaa KH, Hysing J. Predictors of mortality in high-risk patients with QT prolongation in a community hospital. Europace. 2018;20(FI1):f99–f107.
67. Bargehr J, Trejo-Gutierrez JF, Patel T, Rosser B, Aranda-Michel J, Yataco ML, et al. Preexisting atrial fibrillation and cardiac complications after liver transplantation. Liver Transpl. 2015;21(3):314–20.
68. Han H, Qin Y, Yu Y, Wei X, Guo H, Ruan Y, et al. Atrial fibrillation in hospitalized patients with end-stage liver disease: temporal trends in prevalence and outcomes. Liver Int. 2020;40(3):674–84.
69. Vandenberk B, Altieri MH, Liu H, Raj SR, Lee SS. Review article: diagnosis, pathophysiology and management of atrial fibrillation in cirrhosis and portal hypertension. Aliment Pharmacol Ther. 2023;57(3):290–303.
70. Ge PS, Runyon BA. The changing role of beta-blocker therapy in patients with cirrhosis. J Hepatol. 2014;60(3):643–53.
71. Zhou SF, Xue CC, Yu XQ, Li C, Wang G. Clinically important drug interactions potentially involving mechanism-based inhibition of cytochrome P450 3A4 and the role of therapeutic drug monitoring. Ther Drug Monit. 2007;29(6):687–710.
72. Sileno S, Chirila RM, Harris DM. Use of statins, amiodarone, direct oral anticoagulants and NSAIDs in chronic liver disease: a guide for general clinicians. Rom J Intern Med. 2020;58(4):181–7.
73. Lip GY, Nieuwlaat R, Pisters R, Lane DA, Crijns HJ. Refining clinical risk stratification for predicting stroke and thromboembolism in atrial fibrillation using a novel risk factor-based approach: the euro heart survey on atrial fibrillation. Chest. 2010;137(2):263–72.
74. Koshy AN, Enyati A, Weinberg L, Han HC, Horrigan M, Gow PJ, et al. Postoperative atrial fibrillation and long-term risk of stroke in patients undergoing liver transplantation. Stroke. 2021;52(1):111–20.
75. Lip GY, Frison L, Halperin JL, Lane DA. Comparative validation of a novel risk score for predicting bleeding risk in anticoagulated patients with atrial fibrillation: the HAS-BLED (hypertension, abnormal renal/liver function, stroke, bleeding history or predisposition, labile INR, elderly, drugs/alcohol concomitantly) score. J Am Coll Cardiol. 2011;57(2):173–80.
76. Kuo L, Chao TF, Liu CJ, Lin YJ, Chang SL, Lo LW, et al. Liver cirrhosis in patients with atrial fibrillation: would oral anticoagulation have a net clinical benefit for stroke prevention? J Am Heart Assoc. 2017;6(6).

77. Karapedi E, Papadopoulos N, Trifylli EM, Koustas E, Deutsch M, Aloizos G. Anticoagulation in patients with atrial fibrillation and liver cirrhosis. Ann Gastroenterol. 2022;35(6):557–67.
78. Coffey S, Cairns BJ, Iung B. The modern epidemiology of heart valve disease. Heart. 2016;102(1):75–85.
79. Osnabrugge RL, Mylotte D, Head SJ, Van Mieghem NM, Nkomo VT, LeReun CM, et al. Aortic stenosis in the elderly: disease prevalence and number of candidates for transcatheter aortic valve replacement: a meta-analysis and modeling study. J Am Coll Cardiol. 2013;62(11):1002–12.
80. Leon MB, Smith CR, Mack M, Miller DC, Moses JW, Svensson LG, et al. Transcatheter aortic-valve implantation for aortic stenosis in patients who cannot undergo surgery. N Engl J Med. 2010;363(17):1597–607.
81. Ahmed T, Misumida N, Grigorian A, Tarantini G, Messerli AW. Transcatheter interventions for valvular heart diseases in liver cirrhosis patients. Trends Cardiovasc Med. 2023;33(4):242–9.
82. Giménez-Milà M, Blasi A, Sabaté M, Regueiro A. Crossing the boundaries of treatment of valvular heart disease in patients with liver cirrhosis. J Cardiothorac Vasc Anesth. 2022;36(12):4237–40.
83. Watt TMF, Brescia AA, Williams AM, Bolling SF. Functional tricuspid regurgitation: indications, techniques, and outcomes. Indian J Thorac Cardiovasc Surg. 2020;36(Suppl 1):131–9.
84. Aghaulor B, VanWagner LB. Cardiac and pulmonary vascular risk stratification in liver transplantation. Clin Liver Dis. 2021;25(1):157–77.
85. Lozano M, Molina M, Zarauza J, Castillo F, Fernández-Santiago R, Anderson EJ, et al. Cardiovascular assessment of candidates for liver transplant. J Liver Transpl. 2023;10:10.
86. Humbert M, Kovacs G, Hoeper MM, Badagliacca R, Berger RMF, Brida M, et al. 2022 ESC/ERS guidelines for the diagnosis and treatment of pulmonary hypertension. Eur Heart J. 2022;43(38):3618–731.
87. Jasso-Baltazar EA, Pena-Arellano GA, Aguirre-Valadez J, Ruiz I, Papacristofilou-Riebeling B, Jimenez JV, et al. Portopulmonary hypertension: an updated review. Transplant Direct. 2023;9(8):e1517.
88. Shao Y, Yin X, Qin T, Zhang R, Zhang Y, Wen X. Prevalence and associated factors of portopulmonary hypertension in patients with portal hypertension: a case-control study. Biomed Res Int. 2021;2021:5595614.
89. Lazaro Salvador M, Quezada Loaiza CA, Rodriguez Padial L, Barbera JA, Lopez-Meseguer M, Lopez-Reyes R, et al. Portopulmonary hypertension: prognosis and management in the current treatment era – results from the REHAP registry. Intern Med J. 2021;51(3):355–65.
90. Porres-Aguilar M, Altamirano JT, Torre-Delgadillo A, Charlton MR, Duarte-Rojo A. Portopulmonary hypertension and hepatopulmonary syndrome: a clinician-oriented overview. Eur Respir Rev. 2012;21(125):223–33.
91. Augustine DX, Coates-Bradshaw LD, Willis J, Harkness A, Ring L, Grapsa J, et al. Echocardiographic assessment of pulmonary hypertension: a guideline protocol from the British Society of Echocardiography. Echo Res Pract. 2018;5(3):G11–24.
92. Frost A, Badesch D, Gibbs JSR, Gopalan D, Khanna D, Manes A, et al. Diagnosis of pulmonary hypertension. Eur Respir J. 2019;53(1):1801904.
93. Savale L, Guimas M, Ebstein N, Fertin M, Jevnikar M, Renard S, et al. Portopulmonary hypertension in the current era of pulmonary hypertension management. J Hepatol. 2020;73(1):130–9.
94. Huertas A, Guignabert C, Barberà JA, Bärtsch P, Bhattacharya J, Bhattacharya S, et al. Pulmonary vascular endothelium: the orchestra conductor in respiratory diseases: highlights from basic research to therapy. Eur Respir J. 2018;51(4):1700745.
95. Cartin-Ceba R, Burger C, Swanson K, Vargas H, Aqel B, Keaveny AP, et al. Clinical outcomes after liver transplantation in patients with portopulmonary hypertension. Transplantation. 2021;105(10):2283–90.
96. Provencher S, Herve P, Jais X, Lebrec D, Humbert M, Simonneau G, et al. Deleterious effects of beta-blockers on exercise capacity and hemodynamics in patients with portopulmonary hypertension. Gastroenterology. 2006;130(1):120–6.

97. Porres-Aguilar M, Bartolome SD, Duarte-Rojo A. MELD exception for liver transplantation in portopulmonary hypertension: current implementation and future considerations. Ann Hepatol. 2014;13(6):719–21.
98. Huang B, Shi Y, Liu J, Schroder PM, Deng S, Chen M, et al. The early outcomes of candidates with portopulmonary hypertension after liver transplantation. BMC Gastroenterol. 2018;18(1):79.
99. Guglin M, Mehra S, Mason TJ. Comparison of drugs for pulmonary hypertension reversibility testing: a meta-analysis. Pulm Circ. 2013;3(2):406–13.
100. Colle IO, Moreau R, Godinho E, Belghiti J, Ettori F, Cohen-Solal A, et al. Diagnosis of portopulmonary hypertension in candidates for liver transplantation: a prospective study. Hepatology. 2003;37(2):401–9.
101. Fallon MB, Krowka MJ, Brown RS, Trotter JF, Zacks S, Roberts KE, et al. Impact of hepatopulmonary syndrome on quality of life and survival in liver transplant candidates. Gastroenterology. 2008;135(4):1168–75.
102. Raevens S, Boret M, Fallon MB. Hepatopulmonary syndrome. JHEP Rep. 2022;4(9):100527.
103. Thenappan T, Goel A, Marsboom G, Fang YH, Toth PT, Zhang HJ, et al. A central role for CD68(+) macrophages in hepatopulmonary syndrome. Reversal by macrophage depletion. Am J Respir Crit Care Med. 2011;183(8):1080–91.
104. Krowka MJ. Hepatopulmonary syndrome and Portopulmonary hypertension: the pulmonary vascular enigmas of liver disease. Clin Liver Dis (Hoboken). 2020;15(Suppl 1):S13–24.
105. Goldberg DS, Krok K, Batra S, Trotter JF, Kawut SM, Fallon MB. Impact of the hepatopulmonary syndrome MELD exception policy on outcomes of patients after liver transplantation: an analysis of the UNOS database. Gastroenterology. 2014;146(5):1256–65 e1.
106. Fuhrmann V, Krowka M. Hepatopulmonary syndrome. J Hepatol. 2018;69(3):744–5.
107. Garbuzenko DV, Arefyev NO. Hepatic hydrothorax: an update and review of the literature. World J Hepatol. 2017;9(31):1197–204.
108. Matei D, Craciun R, Crisan D, Procopet B, Mocan T, Pasca S, et al. Hepatic hydrothorax-an independent decompensating event associated with long-term mortality in patients with cirrhosis. J Clin Med. 2021;10(16):3688.
109. Panackel C, Fawaz M, Jacob M, Raja K. Pulmonary assessment of the liver transplant recipient. J Clin Exp Hepatol. 2023;13(5):895–911.
110. Ditah IC, Al Bawardy BF, Saberi B, Ditah C, Kamath PS. Transjugular intrahepatic portosystemic stent shunt for medically refractory hepatic hydrothorax: a systematic review and cumulative meta-analysis. World J Hepatol. 2015;7(13):1797–806.
111. Osman KT, Naritsin A, Amuchi B, Qamar AA. Liver transplantation for refractory hepatic hydrothorax is associated with a greater survival benefit compared to other complications of cirrhosis. Liver Transpl. 2024;30(2):142–50.

Pre-transplant Infectious Problems

8

Carmen Vinaixa Aunés and Rosa Blanes-Hernández

Introduction

Several infectious-related problems must be addressed before LT: (a) chronic HBV and HCV infections, (b) evaluation of HIV-infected LT candidates, (c) management of infections by pathogenic bacteria and colonizations, (d) management of fungal infections, (e) management of latent tuberculosis, and (f) serological infectious testing to screen for infections that can reactivate in the post-LT setting and indicate pre-LT vaccination when necessary.

Management of Chronic Viral Hepatitis Pre-LT

Chronic HBV and HCV infections are one of the leading indications of liver transplantation worldwide, along with alcohol liver-related disease (ALD) and metabolic-associated steatotic liver disease (MASLD) [1].

Hepatitis B viral (HBV) infection can be an indication for LT in two different scenarios: cirrhotic stage, or non-cirrhotic chronic hepatitis with hepatocellular carcinoma meeting transplant criteria. In either case, viral suppression with nucleos(t)ide analogues (entecavir, tenofovir, or tenofovir alafenamide) is indicated before LT and must be continued in the post-LT setting. Screening for hepatitis delta (HDV) coinfection is also mandatory in patients infected with HBV. Active HDV

C. V. Aunés (✉)
Hepatology Unit, Digestive Diseases Department, Hospital Universitario y Politécnico La Fe, Valencia, Spain

CIBERehd, Instituto de Salud Carlos III, Madrid, Spain

R. Blanes-Hernández
Infectious Diseases Unit, Internal Medicine Department, Hospital Universitario y Politécnico La Fe, Valencia, Spain

B. Eghtesad et al. (eds.), *Liver Transplantation*,
https://doi.org/10.1007/978-3-032-07072-2_8

replication is not a contraindication for LT, but it can be the cause of pre-LT deterioration in an HBV infected patient [2–4].

Hepatitis C-related cirrhosis has been the leading indication for LT in the Western world for decades, but its incidence is declining since the advent of direct-acting antiviral (DAA) agents in 2015. Currently, most patients listed with HCV cirrhosis have already achieved sustained virological response (SVR) and their indication for LT is hepatocellular carcinoma [5]. However, if active HCV infection is present, it can be easily treated with DAA either pre- or post-LT. Pre-LT antiviral treatment is preferred whenever possible, as it prevents the universal reinfection of the graft [6]. In addition, antiviral treatment of patients listed for decompensated cirrhosis can significantly improve their liver function and thus may avoid the need for LT [7].

Selection of HIV Infected Candidates for LT

Liver disease is responsible for significant comorbidity in people living with human immunodeficiency virus (PLWH), due to viral coinfections with HBV or HCV, and also increasingly ALD and MASLD, leading to end-stage liver disease (ESLD) and hepatocellular carcinoma, which may necessitate a LT. Currently, a controlled HIV infection is not a contraindication for LT, as multiple series have shown favorable post-LT outcomes, comparable to non-HIV-infected patients [8–11]. Current eligibility criteria for LT in PLWH include: CD4 cell count >100 cells/mm^3, stable antiretroviral regimen, suppressed viral replication (or expected suppression with treatment), no active opportunistic infection or cancer, and no history of chronic cryptosporidiosis, visceral Kaposi's sarcoma, primary central nervous system lymphoma, progressive multifocal leukoencephalopathy, or drug-resistant fungal infection [12, 13].

In the post-LT setting, the incidence of bacterial infections in PLWH undergoing LT is variable across series but generally not increased as compared to non-HIV-infected patients [14, 15]. Similarly, the occurrence of opportunistic infections and HIV-related malignancies is uncommon [16].

Infectious Diseases Screening Pre-LT and Vaccinations

Screening for bacterial and viral latent infections before LT is required in order to prevent reactivation or exacerbation in the post-LT setting, as it may lead to significant morbidity. See Table 8.1.

Tuberculosis (discussed separately, see below) and syphilis, if detected, must be treated pre-LT.

Regarding vaccination, vaccination response is decreased in ESLD and even more in the first 6 months post-LT. Therefore, ideally, pre-LT vaccinations must be performed as early as possible. In addition, live attenuated vaccines (as measles, rubella, mumps, varicella) are contraindicated post-LT, so these particular vaccinations must be considered pre-LT. Live vaccines must be administered at least

Table 8.1 Infectious screening testing pre-LT

All LT candidates	HIV 1 and 2 antibodies
	HBV serology If HBsAg positive: HBeAg/HBe Ab; HBV-DNA, Hepatitis D virus (HDV) IgG If HBcAb positive: HBV-DNA
	HCV antibodies → if positive: HCV RNA and genotype
	HAV and HEV serology
	CMV serology
	Mycobacterium tuberculosis: PPD-Mantoux & IFN-gamma release assays (IGRA)
	HSV 1 and 2 serology
	EBV serology
	VZV serology
	Treponema pallidum serology (rpr)
	Toxoplasma gondii IgG antibodies
	Measles, mumps, rubella (MMR) serology
	Dentist review
Depending on endemic diseases, local epidemiology and comorbidities	Drug exposure → Aspergillosis monitoring
	MDRO gram negative and/or Vancomicin-resistant Enterococcus (VRE) rectal swab
	Malaria blood test
	Southern and Central America, Southeastern United States → Trypanosome serology
	Mediterranean, Eastern Europe, Africa, Southern and Central America, Southeastern Asia → Leishmania serology
	Southern and Central America, Southeastern United States → Human T cell lymphotropic viruses (HTLV) 1 and 2 serologies
	West Nile Virus (WNV) endemic areas → WNV serology and PCR
	Histoplasma, coccidiomycosis, schistosoma serologies

4 weeks pre-LT. Even if administration of inactivated vaccines is allowed in the post-LT period, the immune response is decreased, and therefore, vaccination before LT is also preferred, if possible. LT candidates must be tested to determine the presence of antibodies before vaccination against hepatitis A virus (HAV), HBV, varicella, measles, mumps, and rubella. If negative, they must be vaccinated against HAV, HBV, varicella (live attenuated), and/or zoster (inactive, if previously immune to varicella). In addition, LT candidates must also be vaccinated against tetanus, diphtheria, *Streptococcus pneumoniae* (conjugated or polysaccharide inactive vaccine), influenza, SARS-CoV-2, and Human Papilloma Virus (HPV) when indicated (young female recipients under 26 years old), with no previous determination of antibodies required [3, 17].

Active Pathogenic Infections

Infections are responsible for significant comorbidity and short-term mortality in ESLD patients, as they can trigger acute hepatic decompensations and acute-on-chronic liver failure (ACLF) [18, 19]. ESLD is characterized by impaired liver function, immune paralysis, intestinal microbiome imbalance, liver microcirculation, and local and systemic inflammatory responses disturbances, all of which can favor infections. The classical example is bacterial translocation from the gut to the peritoneal space with ascitic fluid, the underlying mechanism causing spontaneous bacterial peritonitis (SBP). Patients with acute decompensations or ACLF with concomitant infections, and those who are decompensated triggered by an infection, have been reported to have worse outcomes than patients without infections [20, 21]. Therefore, adequate management and treatment of infections improves outcomes in ESLD patients, decreasing the dropout risk from the transplant waiting list and improving the post-LT outcome [22, 23].

Up to 40–50% of infections in cirrhotic patients are nosocomial or health-care related [24, 25]. Infections and colonization with multi-drug resistant organisms (MDRO) have the highest mortality rates [19, 25, 26]. MDRO infections have increased in frequency in the last two decades, and account for one-third of all infections in hospitalized cirrhotic patients [27]. Risk factors for MDRO colonization and infections include recent antibiotic therapy, recent hospitalization or ICU admission, nosocomial or health care-associated infections [28], and even non-antibiotic drugs [29] as metformin (effect on gut microbiota composition), proton-pump inhibitors (increase in small intestinal bacterial overgrowth), or laxatives. In a recent study, terlipressin administration was found to be associated with a significantly increased risk for MDRO colonization, although this finding requires further validation. The proposed mechanism was an increase in inaction genes for antibiotics in the microbiome of these patients [30].

Any clinical sign of infection in an LT candidate must be investigated to give the most appropriate treatment. It is paramount to perform systematic culturing to guide antimicrobial therapy. Local epidemiology of bacterial resistance must also be considered to guide the choice of empirical antibiotic treatment. The most frequent infection in cirrhotic patients, and also in those awaiting LT, is SBP in 20–35% of cases, followed by urinary tract infections, pneumonia, cellulitis, and catheter-associated bloodstream infections [28, 31]. Serum albumin increases the survival of patients with SBP and is therefore an essential part of the treatment of SBP [32]. However, concomitant use of albumin is not currently recommended for other infection sites. The proposed empirical treatment for the most common bacterial and fungal infections in cirrhosis is presented in Table 8.2. Local epidemiology and antimicrobial resistance should be considered over these general recommendations.

The performance of acute-phase serum proteins as C-reactive protein (CRP) and procalcitonin (PCT) for bacterial infection detection is generally similar in patients with and without cirrhosis, but the production of these acute-phase proteins could be reduced in patients with advanced liver failure and therefore should be

Table 8.2 Proposed empirical antimicrobial therapy in cirrhosis

	Community-adquired	Nosocomial or health-care related
SBP and spontaneous bacteriemia	Cefotaxime 2 g/12 h IV or Amoxicillin-Clavulanic acid 1–0.2 g/6–8 h IV or Piperacillin/tazobactam 4 g/8 h IV	Meropenem (1 g/8 h IV) or Piperacillin/tazobactam (4 g/8 h IV) + Vancomycin (15–20 mg/kg/12 h)/Daptomycin (8–10 mg/kg/24 h)/Linezolid (600 mg/12 h) if suspected or confirmed *Enteroccoccae*
Pneumonia	Ceftriaxone 1 g/12–24 h IV or amoxicillin-clavulanic acid 1–0.2 g/6–8 h IV and a macrolide or levofloxacin (500 mg/24 h IV or PO) Ceftarollin if risk of MRSA	Meropenem (1 g/8 h IV) or Ceftazidime (2 g/8 h IV) + Levofloxacin (500 mg IV). IV Vancomycin or Linezolid should be added in patients with risk of MRSA
Urinary tract Infection	Cefotaxime 2 g/12 h IV or Ceftriaxone 1 g/12–24 h IV or Amoxicillin-Clavulanic acid 1–0.2 g/6–8 h IV in patients with sepsis. In uncomplicated infections: Cotrimoxazole (160–800 mg/12 h PO) or Nitrofurantoin (50 mg/6 h PO) if ESBL-producing Enterobacteriaceae	Fosfomycin (2 g/6 h IV) if uncomplicated or Meropenem (1 g/8 h IV) or Ceftazidime (2 g/8 h IV) + IV Vancomycin or Daptomycin
Soft tissue infections	Amoxicillin-clavulanic acid 1–0.2 g/6–8 h IV or Ceftriaxone 1 g/12–24 h IV + Clindamycin 600 mg/6 h (if toxic signs)	Meropenem (1 g/8 h IV) or Ceftazidime (2 g/8 h IV) or Piperacillin/tazobactam (4 g/8 h IV) + Daptomycin (8–10 mg/kg/24 h) or Vancomycin (15–20 mg/kg/12 h) or Linezolid (600 mg/12 h)
Catheter-associated bloodstream infections	Piperacillin/tazobactam (4 g/8 h IV) or Meropenem 1 g/8 h IV + Daptomycin (8–10 mg/kg/24 h) or Vancomycin (15–20 mg/kg/12 h) or Linezolid (600 mg/12 h)	
Candidemia	Anidulafungin (200 mg/24 h 24 h → 100 mg/24 h) or Micafungin (100 mg/24 h)	
Aspergillosis	Voriconazole (400 mg/12 h 24 h → 200 mg/12 h) or Isavuconazole (200 mg/8 h 48 h → 200 mg/24 h)	

interpreted with caution in patients with Child–Pugh C cirrhosis [33, 34]. Elevated levels of CRP and PCT are correlated with the presence and prognosis of sepsis [28].

The LT team must be notified of any infectious event occurring in a patient in the LT waiting list, as the patient must be temporarily inactivated from the waiting list (WL), until the infection is controlled. Active ongoing sepsis is a contraindication for LT. Therefore, identification, decolonization, and eradication of infections is mandatory [3]. The time period during which the patient is temporarily inactivated from the WL is not defined, as it will depend on the type of infection and the clinical evolution of the patient. In general, if infection signs are improving or resolving, LT should not be delayed [35]. Patients should undergo active surveillance for post-LT infections and be treated promptly when needed.

Regarding specific antibiotic families in cirrhotic patients, the risk of drug-induced liver injury (DILI) and hepatic metabolism must be considered. Most beta-lactams and partial quinolones (ciprofloxacin and levofloxacin) are safe and effective in ESLD patients. Amoxicillin/Clavulanic acid and penicillinase-resistant penicillines may cause elevation of liver enzymes. Most cephalosporins and carbapenems may be used at conventional dosage in ESLD patients. Some quinolones as moxifloxacin or gatifloxacin, also exhibit risk of DILI. Aminoglycosides must be avoided due to renal toxicity, particularly in patients with refractory ascites and/or hepatorenal syndrome. Most macrolides are metabolized by the liver and should therefore be avoided, but the use of azithromycin and clarithromycin is safe. Tetracyclines should generally also be avoided as they may cause steatosis and cholestatic DILI, though doxycycline and minocycline can be safely used. The dosage of tigecycline must be reduced in Child–Pugh C patients. Clindamycin and metronidazole may have some risk of DILI as they are metabolized by the liver. Sulfonamides are also contraindicated in ESLD patients. Linezolid can cause pancytopenia and lactic acidosis, and is a bacteriostatic agent with limited efficacy on bacteriemia and endocarditis.

Fungal Infections

Fungal infections are less frequent than bacterial infections in cirrhosis, representing up to 7% of culture-positive infections and being mainly nosocomial [27, 36]. Fungal infections can present as colonization or invasive infection (IFI), particularly in patients with multiple risk factors, as broad-spectrum antibiotherapy, invasive procedures, and parenteral nutrition. In general, IFI are associated with an extremely poor short-term prognosis in ESLD patients, despite adequate antifungal treatment.

Candidemia or invasive candidiasis is the most frequent IFI (70–90%) followed by invasive aspergillosis. In particular, in patients with Primary Sclerosing Cholangitis (PSC) and dominant strictures, *Candida* species may be identified in up to 44% of bile samples [37]. Candidemia should be treated with equinocandins and not with fluconazole due to the emergence of non-albicans *Candida* species resistant to fluconazole. Anidulafungine and Micafungine are preferred over Caspofungine as they do not require dose adjustments due to impaired liver function [38].

The presence of an IFI is a contraindication to LT. For example, in the case of an invasive aspergillosis, the LT candidate must be treated until there is clinical, radiographic, and microbiological resolution. However, in cirrhotic patients, classical radiographic signs of pulmonary aspergillosis such as cavitated nodules are not always present, but rather show only non-specific pulmonary infiltrates.

Antifungal prophylaxis in high-risk patients or in those who are colonized by *Candida* or *Aspergillus* is still a matter of debate. Dose and treatment duration have not been established.

Latent Tuberculosis

Latent tuberculosis is not a contraindication to LT, but requires treatment, either pre- or post-LT [3, 39]. The gold standard test for tuberculosis diagnosis in cirrhotic patients is interferon-gamma release assays (IGRA), as there is a high proportion of false-negative PPD tests (Mantoux) in immunodeficient patients. Prophylactic treatment of tuberculosis must be considered in all candidates to LT with a positive test or recent close exposure to a person with active tuberculosis, given the high rate of active tuberculosis infection with a high case fatality rate in LT recipients as compared to the general population [40]. Consultation with an Infectious Diseases specialist is recommended. Ideally, antimicrobial therapy should be started prior to LT, if preserved liver function (Child–Pugh score < 10), but it may also be delayed to the first weeks post-LT period when liver function tests are normalized. The first-line recommended treatment schedule is Isoniazid 300 mg plus pyridoxine (vitamin B6) 50 mg daily for 6 months. Treatment extension to 9 months may be considered if advanced cirrhosis and/or more severely immunodepressed patients. Isoniazide may be hepatotoxic and thus monitoring of liver enzymes and liver function tests is mandatory. Other treatment regimens are weekly isoniazid and rifapentine for 3 months, or rifampicin 600 mg daily for 4 months. In case of isoniazid resistance or intolerance, rifampicin 10 mg/kg/day for 4 months or ethambutol plus levofloxacin can be used as alternative regimens [41, 42]. Rifampicin interacts with calcineurin inhibitors and should be avoided in settings with short waiting times to LT.

References

1. Hill AL, Khan M, Kiani AZ, et al. Global liver transplantation: emerging trends and ethical challenges. Langenbeck's Arch Surg. 2023;408(1):418. https://doi.org/10.1007/s00423-023-03144-4.
2. European Association For The Study Of The Liver. EASL clinical practice guidelines: management of chronic hepatitis B virus infection. J Hepatol. 2012;57(1):167–85. https://doi.org/10.1016/j.jhep.2012.02.010.
3. EASL Clinical Practice Guidelines. Liver transplantation. J Hepatol. 2016;64(2):433–85. https://doi.org/10.1016/j.jhep.2015.10.006.
4. Terrault NA, Lok ASF, McMahon BJ, et al. Update on prevention, diagnosis, and treatment of chronic hepatitis B: AASLD 2018 hepatitis B guidance. Hepatol Baltim Md. 2018;67(4):1560–99. https://doi.org/10.1002/hep.29800.
5. Crespo G, Trota N, Londoño MC, et al. The efficacy of direct anti-HCV drugs improves early post-liver transplant survival and induces significant changes in waiting list composition. J Hepatol. 2018;69(1):11–7. https://doi.org/10.1016/j.jhep.2018.02.012.
6. Belli LS, Duvoux C, Berenguer M, et al. ELITA consensus statements on the use of DAAs in liver transplant candidates and recipients. J Hepatol. 2017;67(3):585–602. https://doi.org/10.1016/j.jhep.2017.03.006.
7. Belli LS, Berenguer M, Cortesi PA, et al. Delisting of liver transplant candidates with chronic hepatitis C after viral eradication: a European study. J Hepatol. 2016;65(3):524–31. https://doi.org/10.1016/j.jhep.2016.05.010.

8. Mindikoglu AL, Regev A, Magder LS. Impact of human immunodeficiency virus on survival after liver transplantation: analysis of United Network for Organ Sharing database. Transplantation. 2008;85(3):359–68. https://doi.org/10.1097/TP.0b013e3181605fda.
9. Miro JM, Montejo M, Castells L, et al. Outcome of HCV/HIV-coinfected liver transplant recipients: a prospective and multicenter cohort study. Am J Transplant. 2012;12(7):1866–76. https://doi.org/10.1111/j.1600-6143.2012.04028.x.
10. Terrault NA, Roland ME, Schiano T, et al. Outcomes of liver transplant recipients with hepatitis C and human immunodeficiency virus coinfection. Liver Transplant. 2012;18(6):716–26. https://doi.org/10.1002/lt.23411.
11. Campos-Varela I, Dodge JL, Berenguer M, et al. Temporal trends and outcomes in liver transplantation for recipients with HIV infection in Europe and United States. Transplantation. 2020;104(10):2078–86. https://doi.org/10.1097/TP.0000000000003107.
12. Roland ME, Barin B, Huprikar S, et al. Survival in HIV-positive transplant recipients compared with transplant candidates and with HIV-negative controls. AIDS Lond Engl. 2016;30(3):435–44. https://doi.org/10.1097/QAD.0000000000000934.
13. Lynch EN, Russo FP. Liver transplantation in people living with HIV: still an experimental procedure or standard of care? Life. 2023;13(10):1975. https://doi.org/10.3390/life13101975.
14. Moreno A, Cervera C, Fortún J, et al. Epidemiology and outcome of infections in human immunodeficiency virus/hepatitis C virus-coinfected liver transplant recipients: a FIPSE/GESIDA prospective cohort study. Liver Transplant. 2012;18(1):70–81. https://doi.org/10.1002/lt.22431.
15. Teicher E, Boufassa F, Vittecoq D, et al. Infectious complications after liver transplantation in human immunodeficiency virus-infected recipients. Transpl Infect Dis. 2015;17(5):662–70. https://doi.org/10.1111/tid.12422.
16. Santos ME, Protopopescu C, Sogni P, et al. HCV-related mortality among HIV/HCV coinfected patients: the importance of behaviors in the HCV cure era (ANRS CO13 HEPAVIH Cohort). AIDS Behav. 2020;24(4):1069–84. https://doi.org/10.1007/s10461-019-02585-7.
17. Danziger-Isakov L, Kumar D, AST Infectious Diseases Community of Practice. Vaccination in solid organ transplantation. Am J Transplant. 2013;13(Suppl 4):311–7. https://doi.org/10.1111/ajt.12122.
18. Moreau R, Jalan R, Gines P, et al. Acute-on-chronic liver failure is a distinct syndrome that develops in patients with acute decompensation of cirrhosis. Gastroenterology. 2013;144(7):1426–37, 1437.e1–9. https://doi.org/10.1053/j.gastro.2013.02.042.
19. Fernández J, Prado V, Trebicka J, et al. Multidrug-resistant bacterial infections in patients with decompensated cirrhosis and with acute-on-chronic liver failure in Europe. J Hepatol. 2019;70(3):398–411. https://doi.org/10.1016/j.jhep.2018.10.027.
20. Fernández J, Acevedo J, Wiest R, et al. Bacterial and fungal infections in acute-on-chronic liver failure: prevalence, characteristics and impact on prognosis. Gut. 2018;67(10):1870–80. https://doi.org/10.1136/gutjnl-2017-314240.
21. Mücke MM, Rumyantseva T, Mücke VT, et al. Bacterial infection-triggered acute-on-chronic liver failure is associated with increased mortality. Liver Int. 2018;38(4):645–53. https://doi.org/10.1111/liv.13568.
22. Reddy KR, O'Leary JG, Kamath PS, et al. High risk of delisting or death in liver transplant candidates following infections: results from the North American consortium for the study of end-stage liver disease. Liver Transplant. 2015;21(7):881–8. https://doi.org/10.1002/lt.24139.
23. Martin-Mateos R, Martínez-Arenas L, Carvalho-Gomes Á, et al. Multidrug-resistant bacterial infections after liver transplantation: prevalence, impact, and risk factors. J Hepatol. 2024:S0168827824001284. https://doi.org/10.1016/j.jhep.2024.02.023.
24. Merli M, Lucidi C, Giannelli V, et al. Cirrhotic patients are at risk for health care-associated bacterial infections. Clin Gastroenterol Hepatol. 2010;8(11):979–85. https://doi.org/10.1016/j.cgh.2010.06.024.
25. Waidmann O, Kempf VA, Brandt C, Zeuzem S, Piiper A, Kronenberger B. Colonisation with multidrug-resistant bacteria is associated with increased mortality in patients with cirrhosis. Gut. 2015;64(7):1183–4. https://doi.org/10.1136/gutjnl-2014-309104.

26. Trebicka J, Fernandez J, Papp M, et al. PREDICT identifies precipitating events associated with the clinical course of acutely decompensated cirrhosis. J Hepatol. 2021;74(5):1097–108. https://doi.org/10.1016/j.jhep.2020.11.019.
27. Piano S, Singh V, Caraceni P, et al. Epidemiology and effects of bacterial infections in patients with cirrhosis worldwide. Gastroenterology. 2019;156(5):1368–1380.e10. https://doi.org/10.1053/j.gastro.2018.12.005.
28. Jalan R, Fernandez J, Wiest R, et al. Bacterial infections in cirrhosis: a position statement based on the EASL Special Conference 2013. J Hepatol. 2014;60(6):1310–24. https://doi.org/10.1016/j.jhep.2014.01.024.
29. Maier L, Pruteanu M, Kuhn M, et al. Extensive impact of non-antibiotic drugs on human gut bacteria. Nature. 2018;555(7698):623–8. https://doi.org/10.1038/nature25979.
30. Mücke MM, Hernández-Tejero M, Gu W, et al. Terlipressin therapy is associated with increased risk of colonisation with multidrug-resistant bacteria in patients with decompensated cirrhosis. Aliment Pharmacol Ther. 2024;59(7):877–88. https://doi.org/10.1111/apt.17899.
31. Fischer SA, Lu K, AST Infectious Diseases Community of Practice. Screening of donor and recipient in solid organ transplantation. Am J Transplant. 2013;13(Suppl 4):9–21. https://doi.org/10.1111/ajt.12094.
32. Sort P, Navasa M, Arroyo V, et al. Effect of intravenous albumin on renal impairment and mortality in patients with cirrhosis and spontaneous bacterial peritonitis. N Engl J Med. 1999;341(6):403–9. https://doi.org/10.1056/NEJM199908053410603.
33. Mackenzie I, Woodhouse J. C-reactive protein concentrations during bacteraemia: a comparison between patients with and without liver dysfunction. Intensive Care Med. 2006;32(9):1344–51. https://doi.org/10.1007/s00134-006-0251-1.
34. Tsiakalos A, Karatzaferis A, Ziakas P, Hatzis G. Acute-phase proteins as indicators of bacterial infection in patients with cirrhosis. Liver Int. 2009;29(10):1538–42. https://doi.org/10.1111/j.1478-3231.2009.02088.x.
35. Incicco S, Tonon M, Zeni N, et al. Impact of bacterial infections prior to liver transplantation on post-transplant outcomes in patients with cirrhosis. JHEP Rep. 2023;5(9):100808. https://doi.org/10.1016/j.jhepr.2023.100808.
36. Bajaj JS, O'Leary JG, Reddy KR, et al. Second infections independently increase mortality in hospitalized patients with cirrhosis: the north american consortium for the study of end-stage liver disease (NACSELD) experience: Hepatology. Hepatology. 2012;56(6):2328–35. https://doi.org/10.1002/hep.25947.
37. Kulaksiz H, Rudolph G, Kloeters-Plachky P, Sauer P, Geiss H, Stiehl A. Biliary candida infections in primary sclerosing cholangitis. J Hepatol. 2006;45(5):711–6. https://doi.org/10.1016/j.jhep.2006.07.022.
38. Pappas PG, Kauffman CA, Andes DR, et al. Clinical Practice Guideline for the Management of Candidiasis: 2016 update by the Infectious Diseases Society of America. Clin Infect Dis. 2016;62(4):e1–e50. https://doi.org/10.1093/cid/civ933.
39. Fagiuoli S, Colli A, Bruno R, et al. Management of infections pre- and post-liver transplantation: report of an AISF consensus conference. J Hepatol. 2014;60(5):1075–89. https://doi.org/10.1016/j.jhep.2013.12.021.
40. Torre-Cisneros J, Doblas A, Aguado JM, et al. Tuberculosis after solid-organ transplant: incidence, risk factors, and clinical characteristics in the RESITRA (Spanish Network of Infection in Transplantation) Cohort. Clin Infect Dis. 2009;48(12):1657–65. https://doi.org/10.1086/599035.
41. Aguado JM, Torre-Cisneros J, Fortún J, et al. Tuberculosis in solid-organ transplant recipients: consensus statement of the Group for the Study of Infection in Transplant Recipients (GESITRA) of the Spanish Society of Infectious Diseases and Clinical Microbiology. Clin Infect Dis. 2009;48(9):1276–84. https://doi.org/10.1086/597590.
42. Subramanian A, Dorman S. Mycobacterium tuberculosis in solid organ transplant recipients. Am J Transplant. 2009;9:S57–62. https://doi.org/10.1111/j.1600-6143.2009.02894.x.

Liver Transplantation for Malignancies

9

Christian T. J. Magyar, Luckshi Rajendran, Laia Aceituno, Owen Jones, Anudari Zorigtbaatar, and Gonzalo Sapisochin

C. T. J. Magyar
Department of Surgery, University of Toronto, Toronto, ON, Canada

HPB Surgical Oncology, University Health Network, Toronto, ON, Canada

Multi-Organ Transplant Program, University Health Network, Toronto, Canada

Department of Visceral Surgery and Medicine, Inselspital, Bern University Hospital, University of Bern, Bern, Switzerland

L. Rajendran · O. Jones · A. Zorigtbaatar
Department of Surgery, University of Toronto, Toronto, ON, Canada

HPB Surgical Oncology, University Health Network, Toronto, ON, Canada

Multi-Organ Transplant Program, University Health Network, Toronto, Canada
e-mail: lrajend1@hfhs.org; Owen.Jones@uhn.ca; anudari.zorigtbaatar@mail.utoronto.ca

L. Aceituno
Multi-Organ Transplant Program, University Health Network, Toronto, Canada

Department of Medicine, Faculty of Medicine, Universitat Autònoma de Barcelona, Barcelona, Spain
e-mail: Laia.Aceitunosierra@uhn.ca

G. Sapisochin (✉)
Department of Surgery, University of Toronto, Toronto, ON, Canada

HPB Surgical Oncology, University Health Network, Toronto, ON, Canada

Multi-Organ Transplant Program, University Health Network, Toronto, Canada

Department of Medicine, Faculty of Medicine, Universitat Autònoma de Barcelona, Barcelona, Spain
e-mail: Gonzalo.sapisochin@uhn.ca

B. Eghtesad et al. (eds.), *Liver Transplantation*,
https://doi.org/10.1007/978-3-032-07072-2_9

Transplant Oncology

The term *transplant oncology* is defined as the treatment of cancer through transplant medicine and surgery, and comprises four conceptual pillars, which are summarized in Fig. 9.1a [1–6].

To achieve these pillars, four patient- and tumour-related conceptual termini need to be accurately used: *resectability*, *operability*, *transplantability*, and *curability*. The definition of *resectability* is assigned to liver tumors based on assessment of tumor and surgery-related factors. Its definition remains ambiguous, poorly objectivized, and confined to surgical expertise and judgment. Within the field of transplant oncology, *resectability* is mainly applicable to other curative-intent interventions, i.e. bridging or downstaging procedures. *Operability* refers to the relative risk of an intervention, as determined by the physiologic state and perioperative anaesthesiologic risk (patient-related factors). The term *transplantability* refers to the national or institutional criteria for listing for transplantation, which considers post-transplant mortality and waitlist dropout due to death or disease progression. Epidemiologically, *curability* is when the patient's mortality risk returns to the same level as that observed in the general population, which can be quantified with 'cure fractions' and 'time to cure' (population-level), or overall survival (OS), recurrence, and disease-free survival (patient-level).

These four concepts allow for a detailed balance of expectations from a patient-centered and public-health perspective (Fig. 9.1b). A hallmark work in transplant

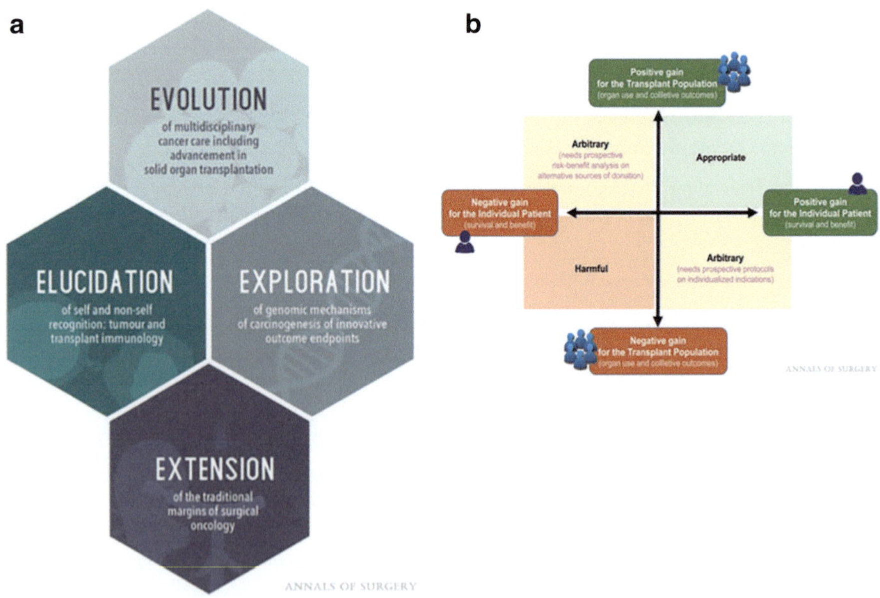

Fig. 9.1 (**a**) The pillars of transplant oncology. (**b**) Balance of individual versus population-based perspective in transplantation applied to hepato-biliary cancer. (Reprints with permission from Sapisochin et al. [1])

oncology is the Milan criteria (MC) from 1996 [7], showing the contingency of oncological transplant criteria.

Hepatocellular Carcinoma

Primary liver tumour is the sixth most common tumour type worldwide (906,000 new diagnoses per annum), and is the third leading cause of carcinoma-related deaths (830,000 deaths per annum) [8]. Hepatocellular carcinoma (HCC) accounts for 80–90% of all primary liver tumours.

HCC is considered a prototypical inflammation-associated cancer, and develops in approximately 90% of cases of chronic liver disease [9, 10]. Hepatitis B virus (HBV) and hepatitis C virus (HCV) are the most common risk factors for HCC and chronic liver disease worldwide [11, 12]. In Western countries, non-alcoholic fatty liver disease (NAFLD; now referred to as Metabolic Dysfunction-Associated Steatotic Liver Disease [MASLD]), and alcohol abuse have become the most common risk factors [12]. HCC-related guidelines include the European Association for the Study of the Liver (EASL) [13], American Association for the Study of Liver Diseases (AASLD) [14], Japan Society of Hepatology [15], and the Korean Liver Cancer Study Group [16] guidelines. Among the plethora of guidelines, the most commonly recommended staging system is the Barcelona Clinic Liver Cancer (BCLC) classification [17].

Transplantability

Sixty years ago, when liver transplantation (LT) was a novel therapy, the prognosis for patients with HCC was poor, with OS rates of 18–40%, and very high rates of tumour recurrence [18–22]. This led the transplant community to abandon LT for primary liver tumors, as concluded in 1989, when the US Department of Health declared HCC a relative contraindication to LT. The patient selection was the primary barrier for the success of LT, and was revolutionised by the MC in 1996 (Table 9.1) [7]. LT is now the standard treatment option for early to intermediate staged HCC, with patient selection remaining critical [33]. As outcomes after LT improve, scientific effort is given to extend the transplant indications [33, 34], with various existing criteria (Table 9.1). The International Liver Transplantation Society (ILTS) 2020 consensus recommends that tumour biology, tumour size and number, transplant benefit, including quality of life and probability of survival, waitlist composition, and organ availability, all be included when defining local transplant criteria [4].

Downstaging

In patients who have tumour burden beyond conventional criteria, "*downstaging*" is the process of reducing the tumour burden in order to achieve eligibility. Since

Table 9.1 Different liver transplantation criteria for hepatocellular carcinoma

Name	Criteria	References	Prognoses
Milan criteria	Singular ≤5 cm Multiple (≤ 3) ≤3 cm No vascular invasion No nodal involvement No extrahepatic spread	Mazzaferro et al. [23]	4-year OS: 75% 4-year RFS: 83%
UCSF criteria	Singular ≤6.5 cm Multiple (≤ 3) ≤4.5 cm Total tumor diameter ≤ 8 cm	Yao et al. [24]	5-year OS: 75.2% 5-year RFS: 80.7%
UNOS criteria	AFP ≤1000 ng/mL Singular 2–5 cm Multiple (≤ 3) <3 cm No macrovascular involvement No extrahepatic disease	Lucey et al. [25]	
Up to 7 criteria	Sum of the size of the largest tumor (in cm) and number of tumors <7 No microvascular invasion	Mazzaferro et al. [26]	5-year OS: 71.2%
TTV/AFP	TTV ≤115 cm^3 AFP ≤400 ng/mL In centers with at least 8-mo waiting time	Toso et al. [27]	4-year OS: 74.6% 4-year RFS: 68%
AFP French model	Point system based on tumor size, number, AFP levels	Duvoux et al. [28]	5-year OS: 68% low risk (0–2) 5-year RFS: 66.6%
Hangzhou criteria	Total tumor diameter ≤ 8 cm Total tumor diameter > 8 cm with histopathologic grade I or II and preoperative AFP level ≤ 400 ng/mL	Zheng et al. [29]	5-year OS: 70.7% 5-year RFS: 62.4%
(Extended) Toronto criteria	No tumor size or number restrictions No systemic symptoms Not poorly differentiated (beyond Milan tumors only)	DuBay et al. [30, 31]	5-year OS: 68% (beyond Milan within ETC) 5-year recurrence rate: 30% (beyond Milan within ETC)
Ontario criteria	TTV ≤145cm^3 AFP ≤1000ug/L LI-RADS 5 or otherwise biopsy proven HCC nodule No evidence of macrovascular invasion No evidence of extrahepatic spread No mixed types with predominance of cholangiocarcinoma	Trillium Gift of Life Network [32]	

Abbreviations: *AFP* alpha fetoprotein, *ETC* extended Toronto criteria, *HCC* hepatocellular carcinoma, *LI-RADS* Liver Imaging Reporting and Data System, *RFS* recurrence free survival, *OS* overall survival, *TTV* total tumor volume, *UCSF* University of California San Francisco, *UNOS* United Network for Organ Sharing many policies are based on the MC [7], this process is often reported as downstaging from "beyond" MC to "within" MC. A shift towards including biological/biochemical consideration has resulted in "downstaging" being required in patients otherwise considered within radiologic criteria [35]. A meta-analysis yielded a successful downstaging rate of 55.2% with a low risk of hepatic decompensation reported as low (3.6%; 95%CI: 2.0, 6.3%) [36]. In the subgroup receiving LT, the cumulative incidence of HCC recurrence LT was 16.0% [36, 37]. The open-label phase IIb/III randomized control 'XXL' trial has shown that in successfully downstaged patients, a subsequent LT to attribute to an improved OS (HR 0.32; 95%CI: 0.11, 0.92; p-value = 0.035), and recurrence-free survival (HR 0.20; 95%CI: 0.07, 0.57; p-value = 0.003) when compared to observation alone [38]. Patients with successful downstaging require defined transplant protocols [4].

Bridging

In waitlisted patients fulfilling LT criteria, the process of "*bridging*" intends to prevent or minimize waitlist dropout due to disease progression [35]. In a cohort of patients with bridging therapy (BT) the dropout rate at 6 months from listing was demonstrated to be 2.8% [39], compared to 23% in those without BT [40]. The European Society of Medical Oncology (ESMO) guidelines recommend offering bridging if a waitlist time of >3 months is anticipated [41]. One meta-analysis demonstrated that locoregional BT improves OS at one-year (HR 0.54; 95%CI: 0.35, 0.86; p-value = 0.009; $I^2 = 0\%$), with no significance at 3 years (p-value = 0.73), or 5 years (p-value = 0.74) [42].

A consensus report on *bridging* and *downstaging* by the European Society of Organ Transplantation (ESOT) was published in 2023 [43]. The recommendation for up to three lesions each ≤3 cm is to receive radiofrequency ablation (RFA) or microwave ablation (MWA), and for one lesion >3 cm is to undergo liver resection or transarterial chemoembolization (TACE) ± RFA/MWA [43]. Due to the recent rapid advances of immunotherapy options for patients with HCC, trials for its use in the neoadjuvant setting are being evaluated [44].

Future Directions

Salvage transplantation encompasses patients with recurrent disease who have undergone prior intention-to-cure resection. Salvage LT for HCC appears to have equivalent oncological outcome as primary LT (moderate quality of evidence) [4].

Immunotherapy (including programmed death 1 inhibitors, programmed death ligand 1 inhibitors, and anti-cytotoxic T-lymphocyte-associated protein 4 agents) has emerged as the first line treatment option for advanced HCC. However, concerns remain regarding the risk of rejection post-transplant. Case series, case reports, and a prospective study have shown the safety of immune checkpoint inhibitors (ICIs), reporting rejection rates comparable to those observed in non-ICI populations when used in selected patients [45]. The optimal washout period between the last dose of ICIs and transplantation remains a challenge. Current recommendations suggest a washout period of at least 2–3 half-lives of the specific agent to minimize risks [45–47]. Despite growing evidence, a consensus for the recommended wash-out period, preferred ICI agent, and induction therapy in these patients awaiting LT to minimize the risk of rejection is still warranted [48]. Ongoing clinical trials aim to provide clearer guidance on the use of ICIs in the context of LT.

Another emerging tool in the pre- and post-transplant period is liquid biopsy (e.g., circulating tumor DNA (ctDNA), circulating tumour cells (CTC), and circulating mRNA/miRNA) [49]. By detecting and dynamically assessing somatic mutations, this tool is thought to be able to transform risk prognosis and help in informing transplant eligibility criteria as well as guiding post-transplant management [50, 51]. In 50 patients, CTC at pre-transplant outperformed all other relevant factors for recurrence in a multivariable model with a risk ratio of 5.4 [52].

Cholangiocarcinoma

Cholangiocarcinoma (CCA) is the second most common primary liver cancer [53]. CCA is defined by the on location within the biliary tree into intrahepatic cholangiocarcinoma (iCCA), perihilar cholangiocarcinoma (pCCA), and distal/extrahepatic cholangiocarcinoma (dCCA or eCCA) [54]. Differentiation of these types might be challenging and requiring specific biliary imaging, and molecular characterization. For iCCA and pCCA, LT is an option in selected cases, and is part of a multimodal protocol [55]. For dCCA, LT is not an available treatment option, as the removal of the pancreatic head is required. Available guidelines include ESMO [56], EASL-ILCA [57], AASLD [58], Pan-Asian [59] and ILTS [60].

Intrahepatic Cholangiocarinoma

iCCA accounts for less than 10% of primary liver cancers, with an incidence of 1.3/100000/year in Western countries [61]. In Europe, 56% of all cholangiocarcinoma are iCCA [62]. Across all-comers with iCCA the 5-year OS is 14%, with a median OS (mOS) of 13 months (95%CI: 12, 14) [63].

The cellular origins of iCCA are a matter of ongoing debate [64, 65], with different molecular classifications of subtypes continuously being evaluated [66]. The 2019 World Health Organization (WHO) classified iCCA into small-duct type and large-duct type [67]. iCCA can arise in both cirrhotic and non-cirrhotic diseased livers and may occur as singular or multicentric lesions. The pattern of growth is mass-forming in 93%, with positive regional lymph nodes in 50%, and distant metastasis (predominantly lung, peritoneum, or distant lymph nodes) in 24% of patients at the time of diagnosis [62]. Surgical *resectability* concepts have been discussed elsewhere [68].

For iCCA, LT may be an option when the tumour is confined to the liver [60]. The two main indications for LT are:

1. Very early (≤2 cm) iCCA in patients who are not resection candidates (i.e., underlying liver dysfunction) [57, 58].
2. Locally advanced iCCA that renders the disease not-resectable or inoperable [60, 69].

Other treatment options include: resection, locoregional therapies, and systemic treatment [66, 70]. In non-cirrhotic patients with advanced iCCA, neoadjuvant treatment with observed disease stability is recommended to serve as a selection process [60].

Perihilar Cholangiocarcinoma

Perihilar CCA compromise about 27% of all cholangiocarcinoma [62]. It is classified according to the Bismuth–Corlette classification (I-IV) [71]. The pattern of growth is periductal-infiltrating (57%), and mass-forming (27%) [62]. 45% of patients will have regional lymph node invasion and 27% will have distant metastasis (predominantly to liver, peritoneum, or lung) at the time of diagnosis [62]. pCCA can occur in association with primary sclerosing cholangitis or other types of chronic bile duct inflammation [62]. ESMO guideline treatment recommendations are available [56], with in-depth surgical resectability considerations elsewhere [72].

In patients with early-stage unresectable pCCA, LT may be considered. The ESMO guidelines state that LT can be offered through participation in clinical trials [56], whereas in the USA, patients with pCCA are eligible for LT-waitlisting exception points since 2009 [73]. The ILTS recommends considering LT for selected patients with unresectable pCCA [60]: neoadjuvant therapy, no evidence of intra- or extrahepatic metastasis, size <3 cm, localised above the cystic duct, and where the tumour is unresectable or poor hepatic functional reserve co-exists. The Mayo Clinic protocol (Table 9.2) was introduced for this population, consisting of neoadjuvant chemoradiation, followed by LT [76]. Percutaneous biopsy is considered a contraindication due to needle-track seeding. A modified neoadjuvant chemoradiation protocol has been published by a group in Toronto [77].

In a meta-analysis including 13 studies, the 1-year, 3-year, and 5-year OS after LT were reported to range from 85.8–86.8%, 40.3–70.7%, to 38–60.1%, respectively [78]. Cumulative recurrence rates range from 28.7% to 36.3% [78].

Table 9.2 Eligibility criteria for patients with perihilar cholangiocarcinoma to the Mayo protocol [74, 75]

Inclusion criteria	Exclusion criteria
Diagnosis: Intraluminal brush cytology or Intraluminal biopsy or Carcinoma antigen 19.9 > 100 ng/ml with radiographic malignant stricture or Biliary ploidy by FISH with a malignant with radiographic malignant stricture	Intrahepatic cholangiocarcinoma
Unresectable Experienced hepatobiliary surgeon	Gallbladder involvement
Complete clinical staging Chest and abdomen computed tomography Liver ultrasound Bone scan Endoscopic ultrasound with fine needle aspiration of suspicious lymph nodes	Presence of extrahepatic disease (including regional lymph node involvement)
No restrictions of vascular encasement	Previous chemotherapy or radiotherapy
Radial diameter (from bile duct) < 3 cm No longitudinal limits for bile duct involvement	Previous malignancy other than skin or cervical cancer within 5 years
Candidate for liver transplantation	Operative/transperitoneal biopsy
	Attempted resection of the tumor
	Uncontrolled infection

Abbreviation: *FISH* Fluorescence in situ hybridization

Colorectal Liver Metastasis

Patients with unresectable colorectal liver metastasis (CRLM) receiving palliative systemic therapy have a 5-year OS of 5–8%, with a mOS of 11.7–24.3 months [79]. In patients with unresectable CRLM LT may be an option [80–82], with recently emerged high-quality evidence (TransMet trial [83]). In 2006, a pilot study highlighted four important predictive post-transplant outcome factors [84]:

- Tumour diameter > 5.5 cm
- Carcinoembryonic antigen (CEA) >80 µg/L
- Time interval from resection of the primary to LT < 2 years
- Progression of the metastatic disease while on chemotherapy

The presence of each factor comprise the 'Oslo score' (range 0–4) [84]. A management algorithm for the evaluation and workup processes of patients with CRLM being considered for LT has been proposed by the International Hepato-Pancreato-Biliary Association (Fig. 9.2) [85]. An algorithm leveraging living donor LT (LDLT) is ongoing being evaluated (NCT02864485) [86]. The open-label

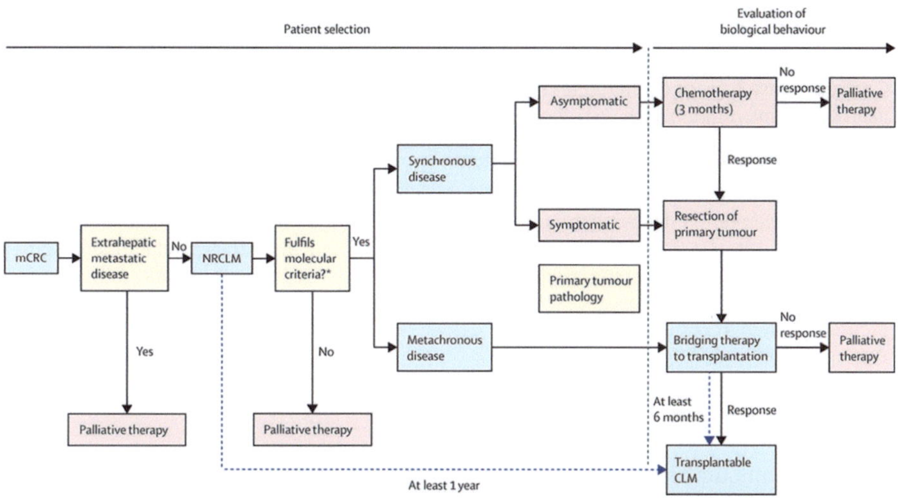

Fig. 9.2 Management algorithm as proposed by the International Hepato-Pancreato-Biliary Association. Abbreviations: CLM colorectal liver metastases, mCRC metastatic colorectal cancer, NRCLM non-resectable CLM. (Reprints with permission from Bonney et al. [85])

randomized-control trial 'TransMet' demonstrated in unresectable CRLM the superiority of chemotherapy followed by LT, compared to chemotherapy alone, in an intention-to-treat (HR 0.37; 95%CI: 0.21, 0.65; $p < 0.003$), as well as per-protocol arms (HR 0.16; 95%CI: 0.07, 0.33; $p < 0.001$) [83]. The 5-year OS was 56.6% (95%CI: 43.2, 74.1) in the chemotherapy+LT arm, with a median gain of mean survival time of 12.6 months (95%CI: 4.9, 20.4) [83]. The initial cohort encompassed 157 screened patients, of which 60% were randomised. Of these included patients in the interventional arm 19% have failed to reach LT due to disease progression [87].

In patients with synchronous CRLM with asymptomatic colorectal carcinoma the sequence of (1) neoadjuvant chemoradiation, (2) resection of primary, (3) bridging with observation of stable disease for ≥6 months, and (4) LT [85]. The selection of potential trial candidates involves an extensive multidisciplinary team with involvement of radiologists, medical oncologists, colorectal surgeons, transplant hepatologists, and hepatobiliary-liver transplantation surgeons. The oncological outcome after LT for unresectable CRLM is excellent, reaching in patients with Oslo score of 0 points a mOS of 12.6 years, and a 5-year OS of 89% [88]. Currently, there is little evidence on the utility of LT for resectable CRLM.

Others

Other cancer-related indications for LT include neuroendocrine tumour liver metastasis (NETLM) [80], hepatoblastoma [80], hepatic epithelioid hemangioendothelioma (HEHE) [2], mixed HCC-CCA [60], fibrolamellar HCC [89] and undifferentiated embryonal cell sarcoma [90].

Table 9.3 Milan criteria for neuroendocrine tumor liver metastasis [92]

Inclusion criteria	Exclusion criteria
Confirmed histology of carcinoid tumor (low-grade neuroendocrine tumors) with or without syndrome Primary tumor drained by the portal system (pancreas and intermediate gut: from distal stomach to sigmoid colon) removed with a curative resection (pre-transplant removal of all extra-hepatic tumor deposits) through surgical procedures different and separate from transplantation Metastatic diffusion to liver parenchyma 6 50% 4. Good response or stable disease for at least 6 months during the pre-transplantation period Age ≤ 55 years	Small-cell carcinoma and high-grade neuroendocrine carcinomas (non-carcinoid tumors) Other medical/surgical conditions contraindicating liver transplantation, including previous tumors Non-gastrointestinal carcinoids or tumors not-drained by the portal system

For patients undergoing LT for unresectable NETLM, a 5-year OS of 63% was observed [91], with distinct Milan criteria developed for NETLM [92] (Table 9.3). Using these Milan criteria for NETLM, excellent 5-year OS of 97% and 10-year OS of 89% was seen. In their multivariable model, no transplantation compared to LT was associated with a seven-fold increased hazard rate of mortality (HR 7.4, p-value = 0.001) [93].

Outlook and Future Directions

Amongst the challenges of transplantation disparities, the organ shortage remains the bottleneck to expand the application of LT. The demand for solutions with an increasing patient population may be reduced by LDLT programs, methods of donor organ preservation and optimization (i.e., machine perfusion), transplant eligibility criteria, donor evaluation criteria, as well as further advances in xenotransplantation and organoid transplantation. Intertwined with this aspect, is the complexity of competing organ allocation equity between patients with end-stage liver disease and patients with oncological disease. There have been adaptations through the integration of exception points for patients with oncological disease.

Recently, multiple exciting trials of potential neoadjuvant treatment options (tyrosine-kinase inhibitors or immunotherapy, vaccines, and chimeric antigen receptors-T cells) have been initiated [94–96]. These options might be implemented as future adjuncts in *bridging* and *downstaging* protocols. Currently, many trials are ongoing and have shown very promising results in improving outcomes within the field of transplant oncology [34]. In contrast to the organ shortage, these therapeutic options will hopefully allow us to continue to push the limits of transplant oncology.

Summary

LT is a multidisciplinary treatment option for HCC, iCCA, pCCA, CRLM, NETLM and other rare diseases affecting the liver. We highlighted the different precision medicine aspects in transplant oncology—specifically for the aspects of *transplantability* and *curability*. The *transplantability* criteria are continuously being explored and evolve. Challenges of identifying and selecting patients and a lack of multidisciplinary centre experience remain.

Disclosure Reuse of figures had been approved and issued by Wolters Kluwer Health, Inc. (License Number 5742080007214) and Elsevier (License Number 5742080499024).

Conflict of Interest Discloses consultancy for Astra-Zeneca, Roche, Natera, Novartis, Integra and HepaRegeniX. Gonzalo Sapisochin has received financial compensation for talks for Roche, Astra-Zeneca, Eisai, Chiesi, and Integra. Gonzalo Sapisochin has received a grant from Roche. Gonzalo Sapisochin has research collaborations with AstraZeneca, Natera, Roche, Stryker and HeparegeniX.

References

1. Sapisochin G, Hibi T, Toso C, et al. Transplant oncology in primary and metastatic liver tumors: principles, evidence, and opportunities. Ann Surg. 2021;273(3):483–93. https://doi.org/10.1097/SLA.0000000000004071.
2. Krendl FJ, Bellotti R, Sapisochin G, et al. Transplant oncology—Current indications and strategies to advance the field. JHEP Reports. Published online November 2023:100965. https://doi.org/10.1016/j.jhepr.2023.100965.
3. Hibi T, Sapisochin G. What is transplant oncology? Surgery. 2019;165(2):281–5. https://doi.org/10.1016/j.surg.2018.10.024.
4. Mehta N, Bhangui P, Yao FY, et al. Liver transplantation for hepatocellular carcinoma. Working group report from the ILTS transplant oncology consensus conference. Transplantation. 2020;104(6):1136–42. https://doi.org/10.1097/TP.0000000000003174.
5. Sapisochin G, Hibi T, Ghobrial M, Man K. The ILTS consensus conference on transplant oncology: setting the stage. Transplantation. 2020;104(6):1119–20. https://doi.org/10.1097/TP.0000000000003175.
6. Ciria R, Ivanics T, Aliseda D, et al. Liver transplantation for primary and secondary liver tumours. Patient-level meta-analyses compared to unos conventional indications. Hepatology. 2024; Online; https://doi.org/10.1097/HEP.0000000000001129.
7. Mazzaferro V, Regalia E, Doci R, et al. Liver transplantation for the treatment of small hepatocellular carcinomas in patients with cirrhosis. N Engl J Med. 1996;334(11):693–9. https://doi.org/10.1056/NEJM199603143341104.
8. Sung H, Ferlay J, Siegel RL, et al. Global cancer statistics 2020: GLOBOCAN estimates of incidence and mortality worldwide for 36 cancers in 185 countries. CA Cancer J Clin. 2021;71(3):209–49. https://doi.org/10.3322/caac.21660.
9. Brown ZJ, Tsilimigras DI, Ruff SM, et al. Management of hepatocellular carcinoma: a review. JAMA Surg Published online February 15, 2023. https://doi.org/10.1001/JAMASURG.2022.7989.

10. Llovet JM, Kelley RK, Villanueva A, et al. Hepatocellular carcinoma. Nat Rev Dis Primers. 2021;7(1) https://doi.org/10.1038/S41572-020-00240-3.
11. Kulik L, El-Serag HB. Epidemiology and management of hepatocellular carcinoma. Gastroenterology. 2019;156(2):477–491.e1. https://doi.org/10.1053/j.gastro.2018.08.065.
12. Yang JD, Hainaut P, Gores GJ, Amadou A, Plymoth A, Roberts LR. A global view of hepatocellular carcinoma: trends, risk, prevention and management. Nat Rev Gastroenterol Hepatol. 2019;16(10):589–604. https://doi.org/10.1038/S41575-019-0186-Y.
13. Galle PR, Forner A, Llovet JM, et al. EASL clinical practice guidelines: management of hepatocellular carcinoma. J Hepatol. 2018;69(1):182–236. https://doi.org/10.1016/j.jhep.2018.03.019.
14. Marrero JA, Kulik LM, Sirlin CB, et al. Diagnosis, staging, and Management of Hepatocellular Carcinoma: 2018 practice guidance by the American Association for the Study of Liver Diseases. Hepatology. 2018;68(2):723–50. https://doi.org/10.1002/hep.29913.
15. Hasegawa K, Takemura N, Yamashita T, et al. Clinical practice guidelines for hepatocellular carcinoma: the Japan Society of Hepatology 2021 version (5th JSH-HCC guidelines). Hepatol Res. 2023;53(5):383–90. https://doi.org/10.1111/hepr.13892.
16. Park JW. 2022 KLCA-NCC Korea practice guidelines for the management of hepatocellular carcinoma. Korean J Radiol. 2022;23(12):1126. https://doi.org/10.3348/kjr.2022.0822.
17. Reig M, Forner A, Rimola J, et al. BCLC strategy for prognosis prediction and treatment recommendation: the 2022 update. J Hepatol. 2022;76(3):681–93. https://doi.org/10.1016/j.jhep.2021.11.018.
18. Ismail T, Angrisani L, Gunson BK, et al. Primary hepatic malignancy: the role of liver transplantation. Br J Surg. 1990;77(9):983–7. https://doi.org/10.1002/bjs.1800770908.
19. Haug CE, Jenkins RL, Rohrer RJ, et al. Liver transplantation for primary hepatic cancer. Transplantation. 1992;53(2):376–82. https://doi.org/10.1097/00007890-199202010-00021.
20. Iwatsuki S, Gordon RD, Shaw BW, Starzl TE. Role of liver transplantation in cancer therapy. Ann Surg. 1985;202(4):401–7. https://doi.org/10.1097/00000658-198510000-00001.
21. Olthoff KM, Millis JM, Rosove MH, Goldstein LI, Ramming KP, Busuttil RW. Is liver transplantation justified for the treatment of hepatic malignancies? Arch Surg. 1990;125(10):1261–6; discussion 1266–8. https://doi.org/10.1001/archsurg.1990.01410220045007.
22. Ringe B, Wittekind C, Bechstein WO, Bunzendahl H, Pichlmayr R. The role of liver transplantation in hepatobiliary malignancy. A retrospective analysis of 95 patients with particular regard to tumor stage and recurrence. Ann Surg. 1989;209(1):88–98. https://doi.org/10.1097/00000658-198901000-00013.
23. Mazzaferro V, Regalia E, Doci R, et al. Liver transplantation for the treatment of small hepatocellular carcinomas in patients with cirrhosis. N Engl J Med. 1996;334(11):693–700. https://doi.org/10.1056/NEJM199603143341104.
24. Yao F, Ferrell L, Bass N, et al. Liver transplantation for hepatocellular carcinoma: expansion of the tumor size limits does not adversely impact survival. Hepatology. 2001;33(6):1394–403. https://doi.org/10.1053/jhep.2001.24563.
25. Lucey MR, Brown KA, Everson GT, et al. Minimal criteria for placement of adults on the liver transplant waiting list: a report of a national conference organized by the American Society of Transplant Physicians and the American Association for the Study of Liver Diseases. Liver Transpl Surg. 1997;3(6):628–37. https://doi.org/10.1002/lt.500030613.
26. Mazzaferro V, Llovet JM, Miceli R, et al. Predicting survival after liver transplantation in patients with hepatocellular carcinoma beyond the Milan criteria: a retrospective, exploratory analysis. Lancet Oncol. 2009;10(1):35–43. https://doi.org/10.1016/S1470-2045(08)70284-5.
27. Toso C, Asthana S, Bigam DL, Shapiro AMJ, Kneteman NM. Reassessing selection criteria prior to liver transplantation for hepatocellular carcinoma utilizing the scientific registry of transplant recipients database. Hepatology. 2009;49(3):832–8. https://doi.org/10.1002/hep.22693.
28. Duvoux C, Roudot–Thoraval F, Decaens T, et al. Liver transplantation for hepatocellular carcinoma: a model including α-fetoprotein improves the performance of Milan criteria. Gastroenterology. 2012;143(4):986–994.e3. https://doi.org/10.1053/j.gastro.2012.05.052.

29. Sen ZS, Xu X, Wu J, et al. Liver transplantation for hepatocellular carcinoma: Hangzhou experiences. Transplantation. 2008;85(12):1726–32. https://doi.org/10.1097/TP.0b013e31816b67e4.
30. DuBay D, Sandroussi C, Sandhu L, et al. Liver transplantation for advanced hepatocellular carcinoma using poor tumor differentiation on biopsy as an exclusion criterion. Ann Surg. 2011;253(1):166–72. https://doi.org/10.1097/SLA.0b013e31820508f1.
31. Sapisochin G, Goldaracena N, Laurence JM, et al. The extended Toronto criteria for liver transplantation in patients with hepatocellular carcinoma: a prospective validation study. Hepatology. 2016;64(6):2077–88. https://doi.org/10.1002/hep.28643.
32. Trillium Gift of Life Network. Ontario's adult referral and listing criteria for liver/liver-bowel transplantation. 2021. Accessed 19 Nov 2024. https://www.giftoflife.on.ca/en/professionals.htm.
33. Sapisochin G, Bruix J. Liver transplantation for hepatocellular carcinoma: outcomes and novel surgical approaches. Nat Rev Gastroenterol Hepatol. 2017;14(4):203–17. https://doi.org/10.1038/nrgastro.2016.193.
34. Magyar CTJ, O'Kane GM, Aceituno L, et al. Liver transplantation for hepatocellular carcinoma: an expanding cornerstone of Care in the era of immunotherapy. J Clin Oncol. 2024; Online; https://doi.org/10.1200/JCO.24.00857.
35. Ogawa K, Takada Y. Role of Pretransplant treatments for patients with hepatocellular carcinoma waiting for liver transplantation. Cancers (Basel). 2022;14(2):396. https://doi.org/10.3390/cancers14020396.
36. Tan DJH, Lim WH, Yong JN, et al. UNOS Down-staging criteria for liver transplantation of hepatocellular carcinoma: systematic review and meta-analysis of 25 studies. Clin Gastroenterol Hepatol. 2023;21(6):1475–84. https://doi.org/10.1016/j.cgh.2022.02.018.
37. Parikh ND, Waljee AK, Singal AG. Downstaging hepatocellular carcinoma: a systematic review and pooled analysis. Liver Transpl. 2015;21(9):1142–52. https://doi.org/10.1002/lt.24169.
38. Mazzaferro V, Citterio D, Bhoori S, et al. Liver transplantation in hepatocellular carcinoma after tumour downstaging (XXL): a randomised, controlled, phase 2b/3 trial. Lancet Oncol. 2020;21(7):947–56. https://doi.org/10.1016/S1470-2045(20)30224-2.
39. Ashoori N, Bamberg F, Paprottka P, et al. Multimodality treatment for early-stage hepatocellular carcinoma: a bridging therapy for liver transplantation. Digestion. 2012;86(4):338–48. https://doi.org/10.1159/000342813.
40. Llovet JM, Fuster J, Bruix J. Intention-to-treat analysis of surgical treatment for early hepatocellular carcinoma: resection versus transplantation. Hepatology. 1999;30(6):1434–40. https://doi.org/10.1002/hep.510300629.
41. Vogel A, Cervantes A, Chau I, et al. Hepatocellular carcinoma: ESMO clinical practice guidelines for diagnosis, treatment and follow-up. Ann Oncol. 2018;29(Supplement 4):iv238–55. https://doi.org/10.1093/annonc/mdy308.
42. Kostakis ID, Dimitrokallis N, Iype S. Bridging locoregional treatment prior to liver transplantation for cirrhotic patients with hepatocellular carcinoma within the Milan criteria: a systematic review and meta-analysis. Ann Gastroenterol. 2023;36(4):449–58. https://doi.org/10.20524/aog.2023.0812.
43. Claasen MPAW, Sneiders D, Rakké YS, et al. European Society of Organ Transplantation (ESOT) consensus report on Downstaging, bridging and immunotherapy in liver transplantation for hepatocellular carcinoma. Transpl Int. 2023;36(September):11648. https://doi.org/10.3389/ti.2023.11648.
44. Lindemann J, Yu J, Doyle MBM. Downstaging hepatocellular carcinoma before transplantation. Surg Oncol Clin N Am. Published online September 2023:1–16. https://doi.org/10.1016/j.soc.2023.07.001.
45. Rezaee-zavareh MS, Yeo YH, Wang T, et al. Impact of pre-transplant immune checkpoint inhibitor use on post-transplant outcomes in HCC: a systematic review and individual patient data meta-analysis. J Hepatol. Published online 2024. https://doi.org/10.1016/j.jhep.2024.06.042.

46. Tabrizian P, Holzner M, Ajmera V, et al. Intention-to-treat outcomes of patients with hepatocellular carcinoma receiving immunotherapy before liver transplant: the multicenter VITALITY study. J Hepatol. Published online 2024. https://doi.org/10.1016/j.jhep.2024.09.003.
47. Tabrizian P, Marino R, Bhoori S, et al. Neoadjuvant atezolizumab plus bevacizumab prior liver transplantation for hepatocellular carcinoma. J Hepatol Rep. 2024:101246. https://doi.org/10.1016/j.jhepr.2024.101246.
48. European Association for the Study of the Liver. Electronic address: easloffice@easloffice.eu, Clinical Practice Guideline Panel: Chair, Samuel D, et al. EASL clinical practice guidelines on liver transplantation. J Hepatol. 2024;81:1–47. https://doi.org/10.1016/j.jhep.2024.07.032.
49. Gonvers S, Tabrizian P, Melloul E, et al. Is liquid biopsy the future commutator of decision-making in liver transplantation for hepatocellular carcinoma? Front Oncol. 2022;12(August):1–12. https://doi.org/10.3389/fonc.2022.940473.
50. Terrault NA, Francoz C, Berenguer M, Charlton M, Heimbach J. Liver transplantation 2023: status report, current and future challenges. Clin Gastroenterol Hepatol. 2023;21(8):2150–66. https://doi.org/10.1016/j.cgh.2023.04.005.
51. Lindemann J, Doyle MBM. Expanding the boundaries for liver transplantation for hepatocellular carcinoma. Surg Clin N Am. Published online September 2023. https://doi.org/10.1016/j.suc.2023.08.006.
52. Chen Z, Lin X, Chen C, et al. Analysis of preoperative circulating tumor cells for recurrence in patients with hepatocellular carcinoma after liver transplantation. Ann Transl Med. 2020;8(17):1067. https://doi.org/10.21037/atm-20-2751.
53. Arnold M, Abnet CC, Neale RE, et al. Global burden of 5 major types of gastrointestinal cancer. Gastroenterology. 2020;159(1):335–349.e15. https://doi.org/10.1053/J.GASTRO.2020.02.068.
54. Blechacz B, Komuta M, Roskams T, Gores GJ. Clinical diagnosis and staging of cholangiocarcinoma. Nat Rev Gastroenterol Hepatol. 2011;8(9):512–22. https://doi.org/10.1038/nrgastro.2011.131.
55. Gorji L, Brown ZJ, Limkemann A, Schenk AD, Pawlik TM. Liver transplant as a treatment of primary and secondary liver neoplasms. JAMA Surg. Published online December 6, 2023:1–8. https://doi.org/10.1001/jamasurg.2023.6083.
56. Vogel A, Bridgewater J, Edeline J, et al. Biliary tract cancer: ESMO clinical practice guideline for diagnosis, treatment and follow-up. Ann Oncol. 2023;34(2):127–40. https://doi.org/10.1016/j.annonc.2022.10.506.
57. Alvaro D, Gores GJ, Walicki J, et al. EASL-ILCA clinical practice guidelines on the management of intrahepatic cholangiocarcinoma. J Hepatol. 2023;79(1):181–208. https://doi.org/10.1016/j.jhep.2023.03.010.
58. Bowlus CL, Arrivé L, Bergquist A, et al. AASLD practice guidance on primary sclerosing cholangitis and cholangiocarcinoma. Hepatology. 2023;77(2):659–702. https://doi.org/10.1002/hep.32771.
59. Chen LT, Vogel A, Hsu C, et al. Pan-Asian adapted ESMO clinical practice guidelines for the diagnosis, treatment and follow-up of patients with biliary tract cancer. ESMO Open. 2024;9(8):103647. https://doi.org/10.1016/j.esmoop.2024.103647.
60. Sapisochin G, Javle M, Lerut J, et al. Liver transplantation for Cholangiocarcinoma and mixed hepatocellular Cholangiocarcinoma: working group report from the ILTS transplant oncology consensus conference. Transplantation. 2020;104(6):1125–30. https://doi.org/10.1097/TP.0000000000003212.
61. Vithayathil M, Khan SA. Current epidemiology of cholangiocarcinoma in Western countries. J Hepatol. 2022;77(6):1690–8. https://doi.org/10.1016/j.jhep.2022.07.022.
62. Izquierdo-Sanchez L, Lamarca A, La Casta A, et al. Cholangiocarcinoma landscape in Europe: diagnostic, prognostic and therapeutic insights from the ENSCCA registry. J Hepatol. 2022;76(5):1109–21. https://doi.org/10.1016/j.jhep.2021.12.010.
63. Xing H, Tan B, Yang C, Zhang M. Incidence trend and competing risk analysis of patients with intrahepatic Cholangiocarcinoma: a population-based study. Front Med (Lausanne). 2022;9(March):1–16. https://doi.org/10.3389/fmed.2022.846276.

64. Banales JM, Marin JJG, Lamarca A, et al. Cholangiocarcinoma 2020: the next horizon in mechanisms and management. Nat Rev Gastroenterol Hepatol. 2020;17(9):557–88. https://doi.org/10.1038/s41575-020-0310-z.
65. Calvisi DF, Boulter L, Vaquero J, et al. Criteria for preclinical models of cholangiocarcinoma: scientific and medical relevance. Nat Rev Gastroenterol Hepatol. 2023;20 https://doi.org/10.1038/s41575-022-00739-y.
66. Ilyas SI, Affo S, Goyal L, et al. Cholangiocarcinoma — novel biological insights and therapeutic strategies. Nat Rev Clin Oncol. 2023;20(July):470–86. https://doi.org/10.1038/s41571-023-00770-1.
67. Nagtegaal ID, Odze RD, Klimstra D, et al. The 2019 WHO classification of tumours of the digestive system. Histopathology. 2020;76(2):182–8. https://doi.org/10.1111/his.13975.
68. Machairas N, Lang H, Jayant K, Raptis DA, Sotiropoulos GC. Intrahepatic cholangiocarcinoma: limitations for resectability, current surgical concepts and future perspectives. Eur J Surg Oncol. 2020;46(5):740–6. https://doi.org/10.1016/j.ejso.2020.01.028.
69. Sapisochin G, Ivanics T, Heimbach J. Liver transplantation for intrahepatic Cholangiocarcinoma: ready for prime time? Hepatology. 2022;75(2):455–72. https://doi.org/10.1002/hep.32258.
70. Rizvi S, Khan SA, Hallemeier CL, Kelley RK, Gores GJ. Cholangiocarcinoma — evolving concepts and therapeutic strategies. Nat Rev Clin Oncol. 2018;15(2):95–111. https://doi.org/10.1038/nrclinonc.2017.157.
71. Bismuth H, Corlette MB. Intrahepatic cholangioenteric anastomosis in carcinoma of the hilus of the liver. Surg Gynecol Obstet. 1975;140(2):170–8.
72. Pratt CG, Whitrock JN, Shah SA, Fong ZV. How to determine unresectability in hilar Cholangiocarcinoma. Surg Clin N Am. 2023;73:1–18. https://doi.org/10.1016/j.suc.2023.09.001.
73. United Network for Organ Sharing. Submitting standardized MELD/PELD exception scores - change 2009. 2010. Accessed 20 Nov 2024. https://unos.org/news/submitting-standardized-meldpeld-exception-scores/
74. Rea DJ, Heimbach JK, Rosen CB, et al. Liver transplantation with Neoadjuvant Chemoradiation is more effective than resection for hilar Cholangiocarcinoma. Ann Surg. 2005;242(3):451–61. https://doi.org/10.1097/01.sla.0000179678.13285.fa.
75. Acher AW, Weber SM, Pawlik TM. Liver transplantation for perihilar cholangiocarcinoma: patient selection and outcomes. Expert Rev Gastroenterol Hepatol. 2021;15(5):555–66. https://doi.org/10.1080/17474124.2021.1890584.
76. Heimbach JK, Gores GJ, Haddock MG, et al. Liver transplantation for unresectable perihilar cholangiocarcinoma. Semin Liver Dis. 2004;24(2):201–7. https://doi.org/10.1055/s-2004-828896.
77. Loveday BPT, Knox JJ, Dawson LA, et al. Neoadjuvant hyperfractionated chemoradiation and liver transplantation for unresectable perihilar cholangiocarcinoma in Canada. J Surg Oncol. 2018;117(2):213–9. https://doi.org/10.1002/jso.24833.
78. Machairas N, Kostakis ID, Tsilimigras DI, Prodromidou A, Moris D. Liver transplantation for hilar cholangiocarcinoma: a systematic review. Transplant Rev. 2020;34(1):100516. https://doi.org/10.1016/j.trre.2019.100516.
79. Masi G, Vasile E, Loupakis F, et al. Randomized trial of two induction chemotherapy regimens in metastatic colorectal cancer: an updated analysis. J Natl Cancer Inst. 2011;103(1):21–30. https://doi.org/10.1093/jnci/djq456.
80. Hibi T, Rela M, Eason JD, et al. Liver transplantation for colorectal and neuroendocrine liver metastases and Hepatoblastoma. Working group report from the ILTS transplant oncology consensus conference. Transplantation. 2020;104(6):1131–5. https://doi.org/10.1097/TP.0000000000003118.
81. Line PD, Dueland S. Transplantation for colorectal liver metastasis. Curr Opin Organ Transplant. 2023;7(4):311–6. https://doi.org/10.1097/MOT.0000000000001126.
82. Schepers EJ, Hartman SJ, Whitrock JN, Quillin RC. Liver transplantation for colorectal liver metastases. Surg Clin N Am. 2024;104(1):227–42. https://doi.org/10.1016/j.suc.2023.08.003.

83. Adam R, Piedvache C, Chiche L, et al. Liver transplantation plus chemotherapy versus chemotherapy alone in patients with permanently unresectable colorectal liver metastases (TransMet): results from a multicentre, open-label, prospective, randomised controlled trial. Lancet. 2024;404(10458):1107–18. https://doi.org/10.1016/S0140-6736(24)01595-2.
84. Hagness M, Foss A, Line PD, et al. Liver transplantation for nonresectable liver metastases from colorectal cancer. Ann Surg. 2013;257(5):800–6. https://doi.org/10.1097/SLA.0b013e3182823957.
85. Bonney GK, Chew CA, Lodge P, et al. Liver transplantation for non-resectable colorectal liver metastases: the international Hepato-Pancreato-biliary association consensus guidelines. Lancet Gastroenterol Hepatol. 2021;6(11):933–46. https://doi.org/10.1016/S2468-1253(21)00219-3.
86. Rajendran L, Claasen MP, McGilvray ID, et al. Toronto management of initially unresectable liver metastasis from colorectal cancer in a living donor liver transplant program. J Am Coll Surg. 2023;237(2) https://doi.org/10.1097/XCS.0000000000000734.
87. Adam R, Badrudin D, Chiche L, et al. Safety and feasibility of chemotherapy followed by liver transplantation for patients with definitely unresectable colorectal liver metastases: insights from the TransMet randomised clinical trial. EClinicalMedicine. 2024;72:102608. https://doi.org/10.1016/j.eclinm.2024.102608.
88. Dueland S, Smedman TM, Syversveen T, Grut H, Hagness M, Line PD. Long-term survival, prognostic factors, and selection of patients with colorectal cancer for liver transplant. JAMA Surg. 2023;158(9):e232932. https://doi.org/10.1001/jamasurg.2023.2932.
89. Atienza LG, Berger J, Mei X, et al. Liver transplantation for fibrolamellar hepatocellular carcinoma: a national perspective. J Surg Oncol. 2017;115(3):319–23. https://doi.org/10.1002/jso.24515.
90. Babu BI, Bigam DL, Gilmour SM, Dajani KZ, Shapiro AMJ, Kneteman NM. Liver transplantation in locally Unresectable, undifferentiated embryonal cell sarcoma. Transplant Direct. 2021;7(2):e654. https://doi.org/10.1097/TXD.0000000000001106.
91. Moris D, Tsilimigras DI, Ntanasis-Stathopoulos I, et al. Liver transplantation in patients with liver metastases from neuroendocrine tumors: a systematic review. Surgery (United States). 2017;162(3):525–36. https://doi.org/10.1016/j.surg.2017.05.006.
92. Mazzaferro V, Pulvirenti A, Coppa J. Neuroendocrine tumors metastatic to the liver: how to select patients for liver transplantation? J Hepatol. 2007;47(4):460–6. https://doi.org/10.1016/j.jhep.2007.07.004.
93. Mazzaferro V, Sposito C, Coppa J, et al. The long-term benefit of liver transplantation for hepatic metastases from neuroendocrine tumors. Am J Transplant. 2016;16(10):2892–902. https://doi.org/10.1111/ajt.13831.
94. Zhou M, Liu B, Shen J. Immunotherapy for hepatocellular carcinoma. Clin Exp Med. 2022;23(3):569–77. https://doi.org/10.1007/s10238-022-00874-5.
95. Tabrizian P, Yu A, Debnath N, Myers B, Marron T. Immunotherapy and liver transplantation. Surg Clin N Am. 2024;104(1):163–82. https://doi.org/10.1016/j.suc.2023.07.009.
96. Adjei M, Kim IK. Current use of immunosuppression in liver transplantation. Surg Clin N Am. 2024;104(1):11–25. https://doi.org/10.1016/j.suc.2023.08.004.

Metabolic Liver Diseases and Their Management

10

Lindsey Creech and Manhal Izzy

MASLD

In 2023, a global Delphi consensus process recommended a nomenclature change of nonalcoholic fatty liver disease (NAFLD) to metabolic dysfunction–associated steatotic liver disease (MASLD) due to its potential stigmatizing nature and the lack of root cause recognition of the condition [12]. With this change, the overarching concept of steatotic liver disease (SLD) was chosen to better classify individuals with hepatic steatosis. SLD can be divided into MASLD, metabolic dysfunction with alcohol-associated steatotic liver disease (MetALD), and alcohol-associated liver disease (ALD) [12]. This new definition allows for coexistence of more than one disease driver with MASLD creating a more personalized care approach for patients. Further differentiation is made in the case of alcohol with the terms MetALD or ALD, which are dependent on the extent of alcohol intake [12]. As the prevalence of obesity and other metabolic comorbid diseases (insulin resistance, dyslipidemia, and hypertension) increase, liver disease continues to rise in parallel necessitating providers to increase vigilance for early detection, as well as knowledge of disease management and time for referral for liver transplantation, when applicable [14, 17, 23].

Due to its variability with clinical setting, geographic distribution, and race/ethnicity, the prevalence of MASLD is difficult to ascertain but is estimated to be 25–30% of the general population [15, 30]. The prevalence of MASLD increases

L. Creech
The University of Florida, Department of Internal Medicine, Gainesville, FL, USA
e-mail: Lindsey.creech@ufl.edu

M. Izzy (✉)
Vanderbilt University Medical Center, Division of Gastroenterology, Hepatology, and Nutrition, Nashville, TN, USA
e-mail: manhal.izzy@vumc.org

B. Eghtesad et al. (eds.), *Liver Transplantation*,
https://doi.org/10.1007/978-3-032-07072-2_10

depending on the comorbidities, rising to 80–90% in adults with obesity, 30–50% in patients with diabetes mellitus, and greater than 90% in those with hyperlipidemia [14]. Overall, studies project that 33.5% of the general population will be affected by MASLD by 2030 [4]. With this rise, the incidence of hepatic decompensation, hepatocellular carcinoma (HCC), and death related to MASH (metabolic-dysfunction associated steatohepatitis)-related cirrhosis is expected to increase two- to threefold by 2030 [4]. Likewise, the need for liver transplantation (LT) will increase to become not only the leading cause of LT in women and those greater than 65, as it already is, but the leading cause of LT overall by 2030 [14, 23].

Figure 10.1 outlines the proposed management approach for MASLD. Per the American Association of Clinical Endocrinology Clinical Practice and AASLD (American Association for the Study of Liver Diseases) Guidelines, initial evaluation of a person with hepatic steatosis on imaging should include investigations into

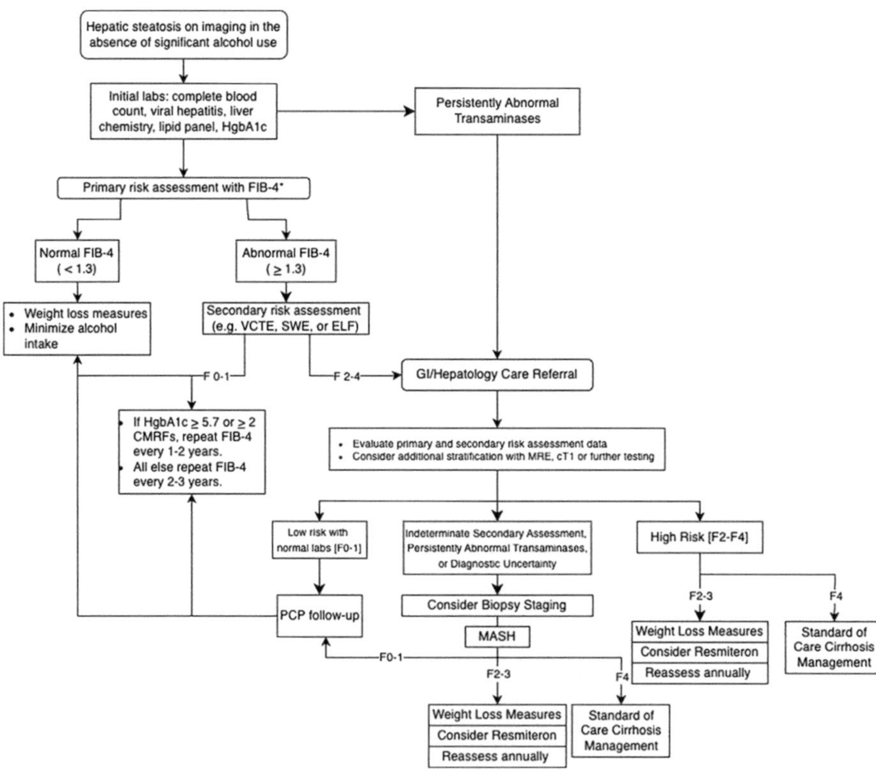

Fig. 10.1 Algorithm for hepatic steatosis and MASLD diagnosis and treatment. *In patients older than age 65, a FIB-4 cutoff of greater than 2.0 should be used for abnormal FIB-4. Additionally, in patients less than 35 years old with two or more cardiometabolic risk factors, patients should proceed directly to secondary risk assessment. Abbreviations: F fibrosis, CMRFs cardiometabolic risk factors, PCP primary care provider, HgbA1c Hemoglobin A1c, MASLD metabolic-associated steatotic liver disease, SWE, Ultrasound Shear Wave Elastography, VCTE vibration-controlled elastography, ELF Enhanced Liver Fibrosis, MRE magnetic resonance elastography [23]

other competing causes of hepatic steatosis with viral hepatitis serology, as well as serum testing that includes hepatic chemistry panel, lipid panel, and glycated hemoglobin (HgbA1c) [3, 23]. If elevated liver chemistries are present, further workup to assess for concurrent hepatic pathologies should include serum ferritin (SF), transferrin saturation (TS), ceruloplasmin, antimitochondrial antibodies, antinuclear antibodies, anti-smooth muscle antibodies, immunoglobulin G level, and alpha-1 antitrypsin (A1AT) genotype [3, 23].

When assessing for MASLD, the presence of hepatic steatosis with findings of any cardiometabolic risk factors (CMRFs) would confer a diagnosis if there are no other causes of hepatic steatosis [12]. These CMRFs include body mass index greater than 25, waist circumference greater than 94 centimeters for a male or greater than 80 centimeters for a female, elevated fasting blood glucose, prediabetes, treatment for Type II diabetes, blood pressure greater than 130 over 85, treatment for hypertension, triglycerides greater than 150 milligrams per deciliter (mg/dL), lipid-lowering treatment, or high density lipoprotein less than 40 mg/dL for a male or less than 50 mg/dL for a female [12]. Per the 2023 AASLD Practice Guidance, individuals with hepatic steatosis on imaging or a clinical suspicion of MASLD, such as those with CMRFs or unexplained elevation in liver chemistries, should undergo further evaluation [23]. For patients who do not have a diagnosis of diabetes or have less than two CMRFs, this evaluation should include a Fibrosis-4 (FIB-4) Index for Liver Fibrosis every 2 to 3 years followed by appropriate non-invasive testing (NIT) if the FIB-4 score is at an elevated risk [23]. Individuals with elevated risk, such as those with Type II diabetes, greater than two CMRFs, family history of cirrhosis, or increased alcohol consumption, should be screened for advanced fibrosis with FIB-4 reassessed every 1 to 2 years [23]. Per AASLD Practice Guidelines of 2023, general population-based screening for MASLD is not advised [23].

As seen in Fig. 10.1, initial primary risk assessment, per AASLD 2023 Practice Guidance, should be done with a FIB-4 [23]. FIB-4 is a calculation based on age, aspartate transaminase (AST), alanine aminotransferase (ALT), and platelet count, which can categorize individuals into low risk (< 1.3), intermediate risk (1.3–2.67), and high risk (> 2.67) for advanced hepatic fibrosis (i.e., stage 3 or 4 fibrosis [F3-F4]) [23]. In patients older than age 65, a FIB-4 cutoff of >2.0 should be used for intermediate risk [23]. Patients who are determined to have an intermediate or high risk of advanced liver disease (FIB-4 >1.3) should undergo further assessment with NIT, such as vibration-controlled elastography (VCTE), ultrasound-based shear wave elastography (SWE), or enhanced liver fibrosis (ELF). VCTE or SWE can be favored over magnetic resonance elastography (MRE) in outpatient setting as initial NITs due to financial considerations though MRE provides more precise assessment of hepatic fibrosis especially in obese patients [23, 26]. If imaging is unavailable for further risk assessment, the Enhanced Liver Fibrosis (ELF) test, a serum test consisting of three elements involved in matrix turnover: hyaluronic acid, tissue inhibitor of metalloproteinase-1, and N-terminal procollagen III peptide, can be utilized [23, 29]. ELF has breakthrough device designation per the Food and Drug Administration (FDA) for the diagnosis and prognostication of liver disease when advanced fibrosis is suspected. Note that in patients with confirmed or suspected advanced fibrosis, an ELF ≥11.3 is a predictor of future liver-related events [23]. As referenced in Fig. 10.1, if the patient continues to have a secondary risk assessment that is intermediate or high, then the individual should be referred to hepatology for further evaluation. If hepatology is not available, a gastroenterology referral is acceptable [23].

Once diagnosed with MASLD, individuals should be screened for modifiable comorbidities, such as dyslipidemia, diabetes, obstructive sleep apnea (OSA), and alcohol intake. Patients with MASLD are twice as likely to have lipid abnormalities compared to those without MASLD leading to an increased risk for coronary artery disease. Management of this dyslipidemia includes moderate to high-intensity statins based on atherosclerotic cardiovascular risk scores [23]. Of note, elevated liver enzymes due to MASLD/MASH should not prohibit or limit the initiation of statins. Importantly, the presence of MASLD is associated with a two to five-fold risk of diabetes, underlining that all patients affected by MASLD should have Hgb A1c testing [23]. Overweight or obese patients with MASLD should also be screened for OSA with polysomnography, if appropriate [23]. Next, alcohol intake should be addressed on a regular basis due to the synergistic effects of alcohol intake and insulin resistance on liver disease progression, leading to increased risk of cirrhosis, liver injury and death from liver disease [23]. It is suggested that individuals with MASLD partake in alcohol to keep consumption to mild alcohol intake, defined as up to 20 grams (women) and 30 grams (men) per day [23]. A safe amount of alcohol consumption in patients with MASLD is unknown; therefore, it is reasonable to avoid alcohol in patients with MASLD.

The mainstay of treatment for MASLD is weight loss. Notably, weight loss of 10% or greater can improve MASH and cause regression of fibrosis [23]. Individuals who are obese or overweight are recommended to follow a diet with a caloric deficit. According to the 2023 AASLD Practice Guidelines, excessive fructose consumption, such as sugar-sweetened beverages, is associated with an increased risk of MASLD, MASH, and advanced fibrosis independent of calorie intake [16]. Thus, regardless of weight, patients with MASLD are encouraged to not only decrease fructose intake but also to maintain a diet with limited carbohydrates and saturated fats with an increased fiber and unsaturated fat intake [23]. Most uniquely in epidemiological studies and meta-analyses drinking three or more cups of coffee per day, independent of caffeine content, has been shown to reduce risk for MASLD and liver fibrosis [23]. Patients are also recommended to increase their activity level to improve insulin resistance, aid in weight loss, and improve functional status. Finally, regarding pharmacotherapy, there are FDA-approved weight loss medications, Tirzepatide and Semaglutide, that show benefits in patients with MASH [18, 21]. Notably, these medications are anti-diabetic, cardioprotective and nephroprotective, which is an important consideration in this patient population with increased prevalence of cardiac and renal disease. Recently, the FDA approved the first medication for treatment of MASH (with stage 2 or 3 fibrosis) in early 2024 called Resmetirom. Resmetirom is an oral, liver-directed, thyroid hormone receptor beta–selective agonist which has been shown to be superior to placebo in MASH resolution and improvement in liver fibrosis by at least one stage [11]. Ultimately, the only cure for patients with end-stage liver disease (or decompensated cirrhosis) due to MASH or non-resectable early HCC in the setting of MASLD is LT [2].

Hereditary Hemochromatosis

The prevalence of HFE-related Hereditary Hemochromatosis (HH) has been observed to be similar in the United States, Europe, and Australia, with approximately 1 case in every 200 to 400 persons [13]. The highest prevalence exists among those of Northern European descent and is least prevalent in those of African descent [1]. A European meta-analysis, which used a pooled cohort of 127,613 individuals, calculated that the allelic frequency of C282Y in the general population approaches 6.2% [5]. However, the penetrance of the disease is variable across studies, with data supporting variability across genders with more males having both biochemical and clinical prevalence of HH [13]. Due to this variability, universal screening for HH is not recommended [13].

According to the American College of Gastroenterology (ACG) guidelines, any patient with elevated liver enzymes or suspicion for HH based on symptoms or family history of HH should be screened with SF and TS [13]. If TS is less than 45% and SF is normal, further evaluation is not required, as this criterion has a negative predictive value of 97% for excluding iron overload as the cause of hepatic steatosis [13]. If TS is greater than or equal to 45% and/or SF is elevated (defined as greater than 300 nanograms per milliliter (ng/mL) in men and greater than 200 nanograms per milliliter (ng/mL) in women), HFE gene testing should be performed [13]. According to EASL (European Association for the Study of the Liver) 2022 Hemochromatosis Guidelines, males should be advised to get HFE genotype testing when the TS is greater than 50% and SF greater than 300 ng/mL [7]. HFE gene testing assesses common variants within the HFE gene, such as C282Y homozygotes, which can implicate a diagnosis of HH [7]. All patients who are C282Y homozygotes should proceed directly to phlebotomy unless their SF is greater than 1000 ng/mL or the liver enzymes are elevated as more investigation should be pursued [7, 13]. If the patient meets either of the earlier criteria, a liver biopsy is suggested to rule out concurrent liver disease and fibrosis staging. Utilizing MRI for fibrosis assessment via elastography and iron quantification via specialized imaging techniques (e.g., T2 or R2 mapping) can be a reliable alternative to biopsy. Per the 2019 ACG Guidelines, in the patient who is not a C282Y homozygote, evaluation for other causes of elevated iron indices should be performed, including liver and hematologic disorders [13]. It is notable that chronic, non-HH, liver disease (viral liver disease, MASH, ALD) is a common cause of secondary hyperferritinemia. Therefore, before committing patients with C282Y heterozygosity to phlebotomy, Hepatology consultation (or Gastroenterology if hepatology is not available) may be warranted.

In HH, the goal of phlebotomy is to reduce the SF to 50–100 ng/mL to reduce the risk of developing complications related to liver disease or liver cancer [13].

Phlebotomy initially occurs weekly, with 500 milliliters removed with each session. Once the goal SF has been reached, maintenance phlebotomy typically occurs three to four times a year. The patients' dietary iron intake does not need to be restricted when undergoing serial phlebotomy, but the patient should continue to avoid iron and vitamin C supplements [13]. Certain clinical manifestations of HH do not improve with frequent phlebotomy, including cirrhosis, arthropathy, diabetes, and hypogonadism. However, there have been reports of improvements in mild to moderate liver fibrosis after the removal of excess iron [8]. Additionally, patients with advanced fibrosis (greater than or equal to F3) should be screened with liver ultrasound and AFP every 6 months to assess for HCC [13]. If a patient with HH decompensated cirrhosis or HCC, they should continue to receive serial phlebotomies barring intolerance to medical therapy [13]. Also, a referral for liver transplantation should be considered as it is curative and normalizes hepcidin levels and iron metabolism.

Alpha 1 Antitrypsin Deficiency

Alpha 1 Antitrypsin (A1AT) deficiency is a genetic condition with variable penetrance that affects approximately 1 in 2000 to 6000 individuals, which can predispose patients to liver disease and/or early-onset emphysema [20]. A1AT is an enzyme inhibitor synthesized in the liver whose primary function is to protect lung tissue against the enzyme neutrophil elastase [27]. Point mutations in the A1AT genotype can lead to retention of enzyme inhibitor within the liver, precipitating liver disease, whereas a loss-of-function mutation causes a lack of circulating A1AT which predisposes homozygotes with severe deficiency to early-onset emphysema [27]. Thus, if an individual has elevated liver chemistries, then an A1AT genotype should be pursued. The A1AT genotype can assess if a patient has a normal proteinase inhibitor (PI) genotype (MM), PI MZ genotype (heterozygous Z carrier), a PI ZZ genotype (homozygous Z allele), or other less common A1AT genotypes [27]. Heterozygotes with Z gene are at risk for cirrhosis when there are other risk factors such as excessive alcohol use, MASLD or hepatitis C [28]. Thus, in individuals with Z gene heterozygosity with normal synthetic liver function and no liver fibrosis, it is recommended to avoid being overweight/obesity and significant alcohol drinking [27]. If a patient has PI ZZ or has Z heterozygosity with hepatic fibrosis, abstinence from alcohol is recommended [27].

To risk-stratify and assess for potential complications, A1AT deficiency patients should be offered liver biochemistry, non-invasive fibrosis assessment (i.e., elastography), and liver ultrasound at the time of diagnosis [10]. Due to the poor correlation between liver chemistry and underlying liver disease, all individuals with at least one Z-allele, despite normal biomarkers, should be screened with elastography [22]. In non-cirrhotic individuals, liver enzymes should be obtained at least every 6–12 months and an assessment of liver fibrosis every 1–2 years. A liver ultrasound can be considered once a year [10]. In patients with cirrhosis, it is recommended to monitor liver disease with liver ultrasound with alpha fetoprotein testing every

6 months to screen for HCC [9, 27]. Notably, all PI ZZ carriers should be monitored with a hepatologist due to their high propensity for progression to end-stage liver disease and high risk for HCC [27, 28]. Ultimately, there is no FDA-approved therapy for liver disease associated with A1AT deficiency other than LT in advanced disease (i.e., decompensated cirrhosis or early HCC), which is curative [27, 28].

Wilson's Disease

An additional cause of hepatic steatosis that should be considered in individuals with liver abnormalities of uncertain cause is Wilson's Disease (WD). Wilson's disease is an autosomal recessive disorder of copper (Cu) metabolism caused by a mutation in the ATPase copper-transporting beta (ATP7B) gene [24]. The estimated prevalence of WD is about 1 in 30,000 to 50,000 in the United States, Europe, and Asia [24]. Due to higher mutation rates or consanguinity, the genetic prevalence was found to be 3–4 times higher in Middle Eastern countries, Pakistan, and India, as well as Croatia and Sardinia [24].

WD should be considered in patients with elevated liver enzymes or unexplained liver disease with neurological or psychiatric disorders. Age alone should not be the sole basis for excluding this diagnosis [25]. Initial assessment should include serum ceruloplasmin (CPN), 24-hour urine copper, and ophthalmologic examination to assess for Keyser-Flescher (KF) rings [25]. In patients without KF rings, if the CPN is equal or less than 10 milligrams per deciliter (mg/dL) and the basal 24-hour urinary Cu is greater than two times the upper limit of normal or 80 micrograms per 24 hour (mcg/24 hour), then a diagnosis of WD is established [25]. Due to the increased likelihood of a WD diagnosis being found with the presence of KF rings, diagnosis is secured with a CPN less than 20 mg/dL with a urinary copper greater than 40 mcg/24 hour or urinary copper level greater than 80 mcg/24 hour with CPN greater than 20 mg/dL [25]. A liver biopsy is typically pursued to quantify the copper deposits in the liver under three circumstances: an individual with KF rings who has CPN greater than 20 mg/dL with a 24-urine Cu less than 80 mcg/24 hour, individual without KF rings has CPN less then 10 mg/dL with urine Cu less than 40 mcg/24 hour or individual with CPN greater than 10 mg/dL with urine Cu greater than 40 mcg/24 hour [25]. A diagnosis of WD is established by liver biopsy if the liver copper is greater than 250 nanograms per gram dry weight (ng/g dry wgt) liver. If the quantified copper in the liver is inconclusive, between 50 and 250 ng/g dry wgt liver, a genotype analysis assessing disease-specific ATP7B mutations can provide diagnostic confirmation of WD when biochemical testing is not definitive [25]. Additionally, first-degree relatives of patients newly diagnosed with WD must be screened for WD.

After a diagnosis of WD is determined, a liver ultrasound evaluation should be pursued. If the patient is diagnosed with cirrhosis, the individual should have HCC screening with liver ultrasound and AFP every 6 months [9]. The treatment of WD is based on patient symptoms, such as jaundice and ascites, or biochemical markers (i.e. elevated AST/ALT). For symptomatic patients, chelating agents, such as penicillamine or trientine, are first-line medications [25]. According to AASLD and EASL Wilson's Disease Guidelines, in asymptomatic individuals, initial therapy can be zinc or a chelating agent [6, 25]. Titration of medication to maintenance therapy is based on favorable clinical and biochemical responses by measuring 24-hour urinary copper excretion, serum copper, and non-ceruloplasmin-bound copper of X (CuEXC), as well as time on therapy. The urinary Cu excretion is highest after starting treatment with penicillamine or trientine but averages 200–500 mcg/24 hour on maintenance therapy [25]. Low serum copper or CuEXC can indicate adequate treatment or overtreatment if very low. Additionally, AASLD 2022 Practice Guidelines on WD recommends that patients maintain copper intake to less than the recommended dietary allowance of 0.9 milligrams per day [25]. Counseling patients on low-copper diet includes assessing the copper content of drinking water and emphasizing the avoidance of foods high in copper content. Most non-dairy milks, nuts, chocolate, shellfish, soy-based products, mushrooms, and organ meats should be avoided in at least the first year of treatment [25]. Failure of dietary changes and chelation therapy is determined by monitoring biochemical and clinical response with lab work and physical exam, and hepatic fibrosis progression with elastography. Persons with WD and end-stage liver disease who fail to respond to or tolerate therapy should be considered for LT, which is curative and does not require post-transplant chelation treatment [25].

Table 10.1 summarizes the prevalence and needed testing for evaluation of the metabolic diseases discussed in this chapter.

When to Refer for Liver Transplant Evaluation

Liver transplantation is the only curative intervention for patients with end-stage liver disease, including those with metabolic liver diseases. Referral to a transplant center for evaluation of the candidacy for liver transplantation should be considered when patients have decompensated cirrhosis (i.e., cirrhosis complicated by variceal bleeding, ascites, hepatic hydrothorax, or hepatic encephalopathy), liver disease with a Model for End-stage Liver Disease (MELD) score $\geq$ 15, early hepatocellular carcinoma (i.e., non-metastatic disease, without vascular invasion), hepatopulmonary syndrome, or portopulmonary hypertension, irrespective of the liver disease pathology [19]. Notably, even when the decompensated component of cirrhosis (e.g., ascites) is medically controlled, LT evaluation should not be deferred, and the patient should still be referred to a transplant center [19]. LT evaluation in the aforementioned conditions should not be delayed, as patients may decompensate further unpredictably and become too sick to transplant. Ultimately, the evaluation process is multidisciplinary, involving cardiac, pulmonary, surgical, psychosocial, and financial assessments.

Appendix

Table 10.1 Prevalence of types of metabolic liver disease in the general population and the diagnostic testing needed

Type of liver disease	Prevalence	Diagnostic testing
Metabolic associated steatotic liver disease	1 in 4 [15]	Any cardiometabolic risk factors without any other causes of hepatic steatosis
Hereditary hemochromatosis	1 in 200 to 400 [13]	Transferrin saturation, Serum ferritin, and HFE gene testing
Alpha-1 antitrypsin deficiency	1 in 2000 to 6000 [20]	A1AT genotype
Wilson's disease	1 in 30,000 to 50,000 [24]	Ceruloplasmin, urinary copper, quantitative copper in liver biopsy, and ATP7B gene testing

References

1. Adams PC. Epidemiology and diagnostic testing for hemochromatosis and iron overload. Int J Lab Hematol. 2015;37:25–30.
2. Battistella S, D'Arcangelo F, Grasso M, et al. Liver transplantation for non-alcoholic fatty liver disease: indications and post-transplant management. Clin Mol Hepatol. 2023;29(Suppl):S286–301. https://doi.org/10.3350/cmh.2022.0392.
3. Cusi K, Isaacs S, Barb D, Basu R, Caprio S, Garvey WT, Kashyap S, Mechanick JI, Mouzaki M, Nadolsky K, Rinella ME, Vos MB, Younossi Z. American Association of Clinical Endocrinology Clinical Practice Guideline for the Diagnosis and Management of Nonalcoholic Fatty Liver Disease in Primary Care and Endocrinology Clinical Settings: co-sponsored by the American Association for the Study of Liver Diseases (AASLD). Endocr Pract. 2022;28(5):528–62. https://doi.org/10.1016/j.eprac.2022.03.010.
4. Estes C, Razavi H, Loomba R, Younossi Z, Sanyal AJ. Modeling the epidemic of nonalcoholic fatty liver disease demonstrates an exponential increase in burden of disease. Hepatology. 2018;67(1):123–33.
5. European Association For the Study of the Liver (EASL). EASL clinical practice guidelines for HFE hemochromatosis. J Hepatol. 2010;53(1):3–22.
6. European Association for the Study of the Liver. EASL clinical practice guidelines: Wilson's disease. J Hepatol. 2012;56(3):671–85. https://doi.org/10.1016/j.jhep.2011.11.007.
7. European Association for the Study of the Liver. EASL clinical practice guidelines on haemochromatosis. J Hepatol. 2022;77(2):479–502. https://doi.org/10.1016/j.jhep.2022.03.033.
8. Falize L, Guillygomarc'h A, Perrin M, Lainé F, Guyader D, Brissot P, et al. Reversibility of hepatic fibrosis in treated genetic hemochromatosis: a study of 36 cases. Hepatology. 2006;44(2):472–7.
9. Guillaud O, Dumortier J, Couchonnal-Bedoya E, Ruiz M. Wilson disease and Alpha1-antitrypsin deficiency: a review of non-invasive diagnostic tests. Diagnostics (Basel, Switzerland). 2023;13(2):256. https://doi.org/10.3390/diagnostics13020256.
10. Hamesch K, Strnad P. Non-invasive assessment and management of liver involvement in adults with Alpha-1 antitrypsin deficiency. Chronic Obstr Pulm Dis (Miami, Fla.). 2020;7(3):260–71. https://doi.org/10.15326/jcopdf.7.3.2019.0161.

11. Harrison SA, Bedossa P, Guy CD, Schattenberg JM, Loomba R, Taub R, et al. A phase 3, randomized, controlled trial of resmetirom in NASH with liver fibrosis. N Engl J Med. 2024;390(6):497–509.
12. Kanwal F, Neuschwander-Tetri BA, Loomba R, Rinella ME. Metabolic dysfunction–associated steatotic liver disease: update and impact of new nomenclature on the American Association for the Study of Liver Diseases practice guidance on nonalcoholic fatty liver disease. Hepatology. 2023. Advance online publication. https://doi.org/10.1097/HEP.0000000000000670.
13. Kowdley KV, Brown KE, Ahn J, Sundaram V. ACG clinical guideline: hereditary hemochromatosis. Am J Gastroenterol. 2019;114(8):1202–18. https://doi.org/10.14309/ajg.0000000000000315.
14. Kudaravalli P, John S. Nonalcoholic fatty liver. In: StatPearls. Springer Basic Publishing; 2023.
15. Le MH, Yeo YH, Li X, Li J, Zou B, Wu Y, et al. 2019 Global NAFLD prevalence: a systematic review and meta-analysis. Clin Gastroenterol Hepatol. 2022;20(12):2809–17.
16. Lee D, Chiavaroli L, Ayoub-Charette S, et al. Important food sources of fructose-containing sugars and non-alcoholic fatty liver disease: a systematic review and meta-analysis of controlled trials. Nutrients. 2022;14(14):2846. https://doi.org/10.3390/nu14142846.
17. Lim Y, Boster J. Obesity and comorbid conditions. In: StatPearls [Internet]. Treasure Island: Springer Basic Publishing; 2024. Available from: https://www.ncbi.nlm.nih.gov/books/NBK574535/.
18. Loomba R, Hartman ML, Lawitz EJ, Vuppalanchi R, Boursier J, Bugianesi E, et al. Tirzepatide for metabolic dysfunction–associated steatohepatitis with liver fibrosis. N Engl J Med. 2024;391:299.
19. Martin P, DiMartini A, Feng S, Brown R Jr, Fallon M. Evaluation for liver transplantation in adults: 2013 practice guideline by the American Association for the Study of Liver Diseases and the American Society of Transplantation. Hepatology. 2014;59(3):1144–65. https://doi.org/10.1002/hep.26972.
20. Meseeha M, Sankari A, Attia M. Alpha-1 antitrypsin deficiency. In: StatPearls [Internet]. Treasure Island: Springer Basic Publishing; 2024. Available from: https://www.ncbi.nlm.nih.gov/books/NBK442030/.
21. Newsome PN, Buchholtz K, Cusi K, Linder M, Okanoue T, Ratziu V, et al. A placebo-controlled trial of subcutaneous semaglutide in nonalcoholic steatohepatitis. N Engl J Med. 2021;384(12):1113–24.
22. Pons M, Núñez A, Esquinas C, Torres-Durán M, Rodríguez-Hermosa JL, Calle M, Tubio-Pérez R, Belmonte I, Rodríguez-Frías F, Rodríguez E, Genescà J, Miravitlles M, Barrecheguren M. Utility of transient elastography for the screening of liver disease in patients with Alpha1-antitrypsin deficiency. J Clin Med. 2021;10(8):1724. https://doi.org/10.3390/jcm10081724.
23. Rinella ME, Neuschwander-Tetri BA, Siddiqui MS, Abdelmalek MF, Caldwell S, Barb D, Kleiner DE, Loomba R. AASLD Practice Guidance on the clinical assessment and management of nonalcoholic fatty liver disease. Hepatology. 2023;77(5):1797–835. https://doi.org/10.1097/HEP.0000000000000323.
24. Sandahl TD, Laursen TL, Munk DE, Vilstrup H, Weiss KH, Ott P. The prevalence of Wilson's disease: an update. Hepatology (Baltimore, Md.). 2020;71(2):722–32. https://doi.org/10.1002/hep.30911.
25. Schilsky ML, Roberts EA, Bronstein JM, Dhawan A, Hamilton JP, Rivard AM, Washington MK, Weiss KH, Zimbrean PC. A multidisciplinary approach to the diagnosis and management of Wilson disease: 2022 practice guidance on Wilson disease from the American Association for the Study of Liver Diseases. Hepatology. 2022. Advance online publication. https://doi.org/10.1002/hep.32801.
26. Singh S, Venkatesh SK, Loomba R, Wang Z, Sirlin C, Chen J, Yin M, Miller FH, Low RN, Hassanein T, Godfrey EM, Asbach P, Murad MH, Lomas DJ, Talwalkar JA, Ehman RL. Magnetic resonance elastography for staging liver fibrosis in non-alcoholic fatty liver disease: a diagnostic accuracy systematic review and individual participant data pooled analysis. Eur Radiol. 2016;26(5):1431–40. https://doi.org/10.1007/s00330-015-3949-z.

27. Strnad P, McElvaney NG, Lomas DA. Alpha1-antitrypsin deficiency. N Engl J Med. 2020;382(15):1443–55. https://doi.org/10.1056/NEJMra1910234.
28. Suri AM, Patel D, Teckman J. Alpha-1-antitrypsin deficiency. Clin Liver Disease. 2022;19(3):89–92. https://doi.org/10.1002/cld.1147.
29. Vali Y, Lee J, Boursier J, Spijker R, Löffler J, Verheij J, Brosnan MJ, Böcskei Z, Anstee QM, Bossuyt PM, Zafarmand MH, LITMUS systematic review team. Enhanced liver fibrosis test for the non-invasive diagnosis of fibrosis in patients with NAFLD: a systematic review and meta-analysis. J Hepatol. 2020;73(2):252–62. https://doi.org/10.1016/j.jhep.2020.03.036.
30. Younossi ZM, Koenig AB, Abdelatif D, Fazel Y, Henry L, Wymer M. Global epidemiology of nonalcoholic fatty liver disease—meta-analytic assessment of prevalence, incidence, and outcomes. Hepatology. 2016;64(1):73–84. https://doi.org/10.1002/hep.28431.

11 Role of Social Workers in the Evaluation of Candidates for Liver Transplantation

Sonali Pendharkar

Introduction

Social workers are an integral part of the multidisciplinary team [1], and are tasked with providing an opinion to the transplant team regarding a patient's suitability and readiness for liver transplantation [2]. In the evaluation of liver transplant candidates, the social worker's primary role is to conduct thorough psychosocial assessments [1, 2], present their findings at multidisciplinary case conferences [3], and provide ongoing supportive counseling, psychoeducation, and resource navigation to patients and caregivers for the duration of their transplant journey.

It is critical to note that the transplant social worker has a dual role. On one hand, their role is to support patients being considered for transplantation and provide the necessary information and interventions to help meet transplant suitability criteria. On the other hand, as stewards of a scarce resource [1, 3–5], social workers are tasked with determining whether an individual has the capacity to manage the demands of receiving a new organ [1, 4, 5].

Psychosocial Assessment

The psychosocial assessment is a necessary component of the evaluation of transplant candidates and is mandated by organ procurement agencies around the world [2, 6–9]. The purpose of the psychosocial assessment is to develop a holistic picture of a transplant candidate [7], including their own perception of strengths and challenges [5]. The information gathered in the psychosocial assessment, as well as corroborative information from family and other health care providers [1], is used to

S. Pendharkar (✉)
University Health Network, Toronto, Canada
e-mail: sonali.pendharkar@uhn.ca

B. Eghtesad et al. (eds.), *Liver Transplantation*,
https://doi.org/10.1007/978-3-032-07072-2_11

determine transplant suitability and to help predict transplant outcomes [10]. It also gives clinicians an opportunity to evaluate behaviors, identify interventions [11, 12], and facilitate community referrals, as available and appropriate.

At the Ajmera Transplant Centre in Toronto, Canada, all patients must undergo a thorough psychosocial assessment conducted by a social worker with a Master of Social Work degree. These psychosocial assessments are initially scheduled as a comprehensive single-session interview. In the interview, the patient's understanding of their current health issues and transplant processes, their personal history (including biological family and current family/social networks), their employment and financial situation (including medication coverage), their substance use and mental health histories, their patterns of adherence, and their motivation to proceed with transplant are explored.

Assessment Considerations

Psychosocial assessments should be conducted with interpretation support, when needed. When English is not a patient's primary language, third-party interpreters, rather than family, ensure patients and their caregivers are able to have a fulsome discussion with their social worker, and fully understand the expectations and requirements of proceeding with liver transplantation. Interpreters also help to ensure that the thoughts and values of the patient are being documented rather than solely the family's wishes for the patient [1, 13].

Given the lifesaving nature of transplantation, many individuals are conditioned to understand that without a transplant, their loved one will die; therefore, the patient and family's reluctance to identify or admit to psychosocial barriers to transplant [14], including existing caregiver burden [15], is high. For this reason, the assessment should start with a clear explanation of the social worker's dual role. Additionally, ongoing rapport building is instrumental in ensuring patients and families feel safe to be truthful in their assessment.

In Ontario, the Trillium Gift of Life Network (TGLN) governs liver transplantation. TGLN psychosocial contraindications guide the focus of the liver transplant social work assessment and related interventions. These contraindications include poor social support, recent illicit drug misuse, unstable mental health issues, and documented and ongoing nonadherence [9]. For individuals being considered for liver transplantation secondary to alcohol-related liver disease, additional criteria regarding stable housing, abstinence, and relapse prevention therapy are also included [9].

The elements of the psychosocial assessment are discussed in detail below and referenced in Table 11.1.

Table 11.1 Elements of the Psychosocial Assessment and Considerations

Elements of Psychosocial Assessment	Discussion, Questions, and Considerations
Health history and transplant knowledge	Review patients' health history, including diagnosis of liver disease and transplant discussions. Does the patient understand the cause of their liver disease? Does the patient understand current treatments and medications (including names and purpose)? Does the patient understand transplant processes and requirements?
Social support	Discuss current social network (including family, friends, and community). Who will provide practical and instrumental support to patients for the entire transplant trajectory? Are these identified caregivers aware of the patient's health status? Are they willing and able to commit to this process?
Finances (including medication coverage)	Discuss the source of household income, medication coverage, and extended health/disability benefits. Does the patient have medication coverage? Does the patient have the necessary financial resources to manage the out-of-pocket costs associated with transplant? Does the patient have the means to continue to manage these costs posttransplant while also maintaining day-to-day expenses?
Substance use/misuse	Discuss substance use/misuse history (past and present). Are there any active substance use/misuse concerns? Are these absolute contraindications to transplant? If not an absolute contraindication, how will their substance use influence transplant adherence?
Mental health	Discuss adjustment to illness and functional decline. Are there any new or worsening mental health concerns? Is there a history of documented mental health concerns? Are there any undiagnosed or unstable major mental health concerns? What mental health interventions have been previously explored, and what may currently be indicated?
Adherence to transplantation expectations and requirements	Discuss the history of adherence/nonadherence. Does the patient have a history of nonadherence to medications, follow-up appointments, or recommendations for care? Is the patient committed to lifelong management of a new organ (including medication adherence, attendance at follow-up appointments, responding to adverse medical events, and a collaborative partnership with the transplant team)?
Motivation to pursue transplantation	Does the patient want to pursue transplantation? Are there any concerns with transplant motivation that will prevent the patient from responding to an organ offer or following through with transplant requirements?

Health History and Transplant Knowledge

In the psychosocial assessment, social workers can facilitate knowledge development of a patient's understanding of their health history and transplant processes by asking them to share their liver disease "story." Research shows that patients who demonstrate understanding of their illness have greater engagement in their health care management, a better sense of control and patient satisfaction, and adherence [16]. Conversely, patients who lack understanding have demonstrated higher rates of ambivalence and nonadherence [16]. In telling their story, patients can share what led to their diagnosis, when transplant discussions started, and what information they have retained about transplantation. This often provides insight into their initial thoughts and feelings about transplant, as well as any knowledge gaps that need to be explored and addressed by the medical team.

Social Support

Caregivers play a significant role in positive transplant outcomes [13, 17, 18], and many transplant programs across North America require a dedicated caregiver to participate in the transplant journey [2, 19, 20]. Cognitive impairment caused by hepatic encephalopathy is common in the pretransplant period [15, 21] and can impact an individual's ability to actively participate in the psychosocial assessment and transplant planning. For this reason, the caregiver's responsibilities often begin before the transplant evaluation even starts [22].

Social support is typically provided by informal networks, including a spouse or partner, immediate and/or extended family, and friends [10, 23]. The primary responsibilities of caregivers include acting as a substitute decision-maker/health care proxy, participating in evaluation appointments [22, 24], supporting recipients in completing documentation (financial assistance application, medication coverage enrolment, etc.), providing caregiving and supervision [19], providing practical support at home (cooking, cleaning, laundry, etc.), and providing transportation and accompaniment to medical appointments [25]. They are also responsible for liaising with medical teams if/when recipients are unable [19], supporting discharge planning while in hospital after transplant [2], supporting new medication regimes after transplant [15], and supporting patient motivation [15]. As part of this caregiving, individuals may require time away from paid employment or other household responsibilities [19, 20, 22], relocation to the patient's residence, or relocation with the patient to a transplant center [20, 26].

Most of the caregiving responsibilities outlined above require overlap from pre- to posttransplant [18]; therefore, long-term commitment is required, with the duration varying based on the length of waiting time for transplant. Assessment of a caregiver's suitability - as well as their willingness and readiness to provide long-term support - must be completed, given the significant responsibility placed on them throughout the transplant journey.

Caregiver burden and burnout is also common in this population [15, 16], manifesting as depression and anxiety [15, 18]. Identified risk factors are multifactorial [15, 24, 27] and should not be ignored by the medical team [15, 18].

Finances and Medication Coverage

Transplant expenses vary by province, state, and country. Proceeding with transplant requires patients and families to make a significant financial commitment to carry transplant-related costs for the rest of their lives [5, 15, 20]. Given the functional decompensation related to chronic liver disease, patients often become too burdened by medical appointments or too unwell to maintain regular gainful employment while waiting for transplant [24]. As a result, many experience work loss or absenteeism [22, 24]. In the case of patients with hepatic encephalopathy, caregivers are also required to miss or give up work to address their caregiving responsibilities [2, 20]. Understandably, this fiscal loss adds an additional layer of financial uncertainty, anxiety, and caregiver distress [22, 28] and can lead to financial, food, and transportation insecurity, as well as housing instability throughout the transplant journey [24, 29]. These stressors may not improve after transplant, as the cumulative effect of pretransplant financial losses continues to exist after transplant surgery and recovery [20, 22, 24].

The psychosocial assessment aims to assess a patient's income source, insurance coverage, disability benefits, and medication coverage [10]. In addition to acknowledging and supporting the distress that financial insecurity causes, the social worker's role is to educate patients about potential out-of-pocket costs and to ensure they have the resources to manage these expenses. These expenditures include both direct (health care costs) and indirect (travel, food, and accommodation) expenses [20, 26], as well as day-to-day costs (rent/mortgage, utilities, food, childcare, etc.) [20, 24].

When faced with a fiscal crisis, patients are left with complex decision-making between day-to-day factors (e.g., food, housing, schooling, and childcare) or taking medications as prescribed [22, 30] and seeking medical care [22]. For some, their decision-making favors the former, and their health care needs are neglected. Unfortunately, as is well documented, treatment nonadherence is a significant cause of graft loss [18, 21], increased hospitalizations [22], poor prognosis [18, 31], and patient morbidity [21].

Transplant assessment and financial planning must therefore take into consideration whether a patient and/or caregiver will return to gainful employment, if they will return to their pretransplant level of employment, and whether a dependence on disability health insurance benefits will be a deterrent for seeking paid work [21].

Substance Use/Misuse

Substance use/misuse includes smoking, alcohol, illicit drug use, and prescription drugs. While many transplant centers do not view smoking as an absolute contraindication despite clear documentation of the negative effects of tobacco on transplant outcomes [21], program requirements about drug and alcohol misuse tend to be much more stringent. Maldonado (2019) states, "a history of substance use disorder has been found to be both highly predictive of post-transplant substance use and of post-transplant treatment nonadherence" [13].

For all substances, the psychosocial assessment collects information about the substance use history—including amount used, duration of use, and time and circumstance around abstinence [13]—any underlying mental health challenges that contributed to the substance misuse (more pertinent in illicit and prescription drug and/or alcohol misuse), potential triggers, and coping strategies to mitigate relapse. Corroborative information about substance use/misuse should also be gathered from a support person. The assessment guides the transplant team in their discussions around risk of relapse, the need for more in-depth addiction assessment [25], and for preventative interventions.

Mental Health

As part of the psychosocial assessment, a robust discussion around past and current mental health challenges, both formally diagnosed and those perceived by the patient and/or caregiver, is required, including discussion around suicidal ideation and attempts. This is also an ideal time to discuss a patient's adjustment to diagnosis, illness, and functional decline.

The purpose of this discussion is to ensure psychiatric stability [9, 14], optimize patient and caregiver well-being while waiting for transplant, and to provide information to the medical team to help predict any concerns for posttransplant challenges secondary to physical and medical changes related to immunosuppression medications [21]. Where appropriate, referrals to mental health services can supplement transplant social work interventions. From a transplant suitability perspective, major mental health challenges can have a significant impact on posttransplant outcomes [1] and have been shown to demonstrate an increased risk of posttransplant graft-loss, treatment nonadherence [18], and mortality [10, 21].

Adherence

Adherence relates to a patient's ability to work with their transplant team, take medications, attend appointments [18, 23], medical procedures, and laboratory tests [18], respond to adverse health events requiring medical intervention [23], and participate in general self-care regimes (exercise and diet) [16, 21]. There are several contributing factors to pre- and posttransplant nonadherence, including mental health (depression, anxiety, and uncontrolled major mental health illnesses) [18], finances [22, 24], health literacy, social support, and treatment complexity [18, 21, 32]. Psychosocial assessments can preemptively identify some of these risk factors and work toward mitigating posttransplant nonadherence by providing appropriate referrals and interventions in the pre- and peri-transplant period.

Motivation

Patient motivation to proceed with liver transplantation must be explored in the psychosocial assessment [13] to ensure that individuals are prepared to assume the lifelong responsibilities associated with liver transplantation [1, 13]. Pretransplant, patients may not feel ready for transplant. They may be in denial about the severity of illness or have not yet experienced a justifiable change in their quality of life to warrant proceeding with such a major surgery. Often, patients proceed with evaluation at the insistence of family members or to "see what happens" in the assessment phase before making a final decision. In this period, if a patient has not overtly acknowledged low motivation, it can manifest as nonadherence with medical follow-up, failure to complete laboratory testing and/or medical procedures, and an unwillingness to respond to organ offers. Posttransplant motivation can be impacted by mental health challenges and significant changes to the patient's physical and emotional health. Low motivation after transplant is most often expressed as treatment nonadherence.

Discussions around transplant motivation should also include hopes for the future (e.g., after liver transplantation), as well as a patient or caregiver's worries about the future. Discussing a patient's worries in this space and providing supportive counseling around these concerns allows for increased rapport building, open communication between the team and patient/caregiver, and improved patient and caregiver well-being.

Interventions

Embedded throughout the psychosocial assessment and evaluation period are supportive counseling, psychoeducation, and resource navigation.

Supportive Counseling

The morbidity and mortality for patients with chronic liver disease and/or cirrhosis have been well documented [15, 24]. The physical changes and life-limiting implications of this disease are felt in all aspects of an individual's life—financial [2, 22, 24], social (e.g., change in family structure [19] and/or family dynamics), and psychological (new or worsening mental health challenges) [10, 21], as well as in caregiver burden and burnout [15, 16, 24, 27]. These stressors are often brought to the surface during psychosocial assessments and create an opportunity to acknowledge feelings associated with these significant changes. Opportunities are also presented to discuss coping strategies, find community resources and support, and to look for hope in the face of adversity.

In the psychosocial assessment, many patients and caregivers discuss their distress about the wait for a new organ [10, 25]. They worry they will not qualify for transplant or will become ineligible for transplant due to a change in their health status and/or medical complications [10, 25]. Others fear they will not live long enough to receive a new liver. While the wait for transplant is uncertain, social workers have a unique opportunity to encourage patients and caregivers to be hopeful about transplant, while remaining aware of the realities of organ scarcity [25].

Psychoeducation

Transplant social workers have an ongoing responsibility to ensure patients and caregivers understand the transplant process and expectations, and how they can maintain transplant readiness while waiting for a new organ. Coupling transplant education with transplant planning gives social workers an opportunity to explain to patients and caregivers what to expect while waiting for an organ, during recovery, and beyond, while also assessing their transplant plans for attendance at follow-up appointments, management of lifelong medication requirements, and return to work, etc.

Resource Navigation

Inherent in the social work role is knowledge of government and community resources. The social worker can provide education to patients and families about general and transplant-specific resources related to their liver disease, caregiving support and benefits, mentorship programs, income support programs, medication coverage, medical travel, and relocation funding, as well as relapse prevention therapy, smoking cessation, and mental health services, to name only a few.

Standardized Assessment Tools

Transplant programs around the world utilize standardized assessment tools in the evaluation of solid organ transplant candidates [13]. The Stanford Integrated Psychosocial Assessment for Transplant (SIPAT) [7, 13, 16, 33] and the Psychosocial Assessment of Candidates for Transplantation (PACT) [8, 13] are two examples. These tools ensure equity and fairness in determining suitability for transplant [33] but should not be used in isolation and must be accompanied by a thorough psychosocial evaluation conducted by a qualified clinician [7].

Further Considerations

While not addressed in this chapter, it is important to note that the role of social workers on the transplant team, and the interventions they provide, are not limited to pretransplant psychosocial assessment and intervention. In addition to the initial assessment, transplant social workers follow patients (as needed) while waiting for transplant, during their posttransplant admission to the hospital (including discharge planning), and lifelong after transplant [9].

Conclusion

The role of the social worker on the transplant team is essential to ensuring that those who have the capacity to care for organs are moved forward in the process. The multifaceted interventions provided by social workers, including psychosocial assessments, supportive counseling, psychoeducation, and resource navigation, are complex and nuanced and require unique expertise. While the focus of this chapter has been the role of the social worker in the evaluation of liver transplant candidates specifically, it is important to note that the assessment of, and support with, many psychosocial issues (e.g., medication coverage, finances, adherence, and substance use) are lifelong factors that must continue to be considered once an individual has received a lifesaving liver transplant. To ensure ongoing stewardship of these scarce resources, transplant social workers are often called upon to support patients with challenges in these areas long after surgical recovery.

References

1. Bramstedt K, Chalfant A, Wright C. Emergency consults in the setting of transplant medicine: dilemmas for social workers and bioethicists. Prog Transplant. 2007;17(1):36–9.
2. West CJ, Winnike K. Social work interventions in end-stage organ disease and transplant patients. In: Sher Y, Maldonado J, editors. Psychosocial care of end-stage organ disease and transplant patients. Cham: Springer; 2019. https://doi.org/10.1007/978-3-319-94914-7_44.
3. Volk ML, Biggins SW, Huang MA, Argo CK, Fontana RJ, Anspach RR. Decision making in liver transplant selection committees. Ann Intern Med. 2011;155(8):503–8. https://doi.org/10.1059/0003-4819-155-8-201110180-00006.
4. Sas C. The psychosocial evaluation is an essential part of the pretransplant workup for patients with end-stage renal disease: a social worker's perspective [Viewpoint]. Health Soc Work. 2019;44:208–11. https://doi.org/10.1093/hsw/hlz012.
5. Olbrisch ME, Levenson JL. Psychosocial assessment of organ transplant candidates: current status of methodological and philosophical issues. Psychosomatics. 1995;36:236–43.
6. Deutsch-Link S, Weinberg EM, Bittermann T, McDougal M, Dhariwal A, Jones LS, Weinrieb RM, Banerjee AG, Addis S, Serper M. The Stanford integrated psychosocial assessment for transplant is associated with outcomes before and after liver transplantation. Liver Transp. 2021;27(5):652–67. https://doi.org/10.1002/lt.25975.
7. Weinrieb RM, DiMartini AF. The role of psychosocial screening tools in the evaluation of transplantation patients with alcohol-related liver disease. Liver Transpl. 2022;28(6):915–7. https://doi.org/10.1002/lt.26449.

8. Schneekloth TD, Hitschfeld MJ, Petterson TM, Narayanan P, Niazi SK, Jowsey-Gregoire SG, Thusius NJ, Vasquez AR, Kremers WK, Watt KD, Rummans TA. Psychosocial risk impacts mortality in women after liver transplantation. Psychosomatics. 2019;60(1):56–65.
9. Trillium Gift of Life Network. Ontario's adult referral and listing criteria for liver transplantation. Government of Ontario; 2018.
10. Rivera MN, Jowsey S, Alsina AE, Torres EA. Factors contributing to health disparities in liver transplantation in a hispanic population. P R Health Sci J. 2012;31(4):199–204.
11. Becker JH, Shemesh E, Shenoy A, Posillico A, Knight CS, Kim S-K, Florman SS, Schiano T. The utility of a pre-transplant psychosocial evaluation in predicting post-liver transplant outcomes. Prog Transplant. 2021;31(1):4–12. https://doi.org/10.1177/1526924820978605.
12. Weiss E, Kabacam G, Gorvin L, Spiro M, Raptis DA, Keskin O, Orloff S, Belghiti J. The role of preoperative psychosocial counselling on the improvement of the recipient compliance and speed of recovery after liver transplantation—A systemic review of the literature and expert panel recommendations. Clin Transpl. 2022;36:e14632. https://doi.org/10.1111/ctr.14632.
13. Maldonado JR. The psychosocial evaluation of transplant candidates. In: Sher Y, Maldonado J, editors. Psychosocial care of end-stage organ disease and transplant patients. Cham: Springer; 2019. https://doi.org/10.1007/978-3-319-94914-7_3.
14. Carlson J, Potter L, Pennington S, Nour B, Sebatian A, Paris W. Liver transplantation in a patient at psychosocial risk. Prog Transplant. 2000;10(4):209–14.
15. Shrestha D, Rathi S, Grover S, Taneja S, Duseja A, Chawla YK, Dhiman RK. Factors affecting psychological burden on the informal caregiver of patients with cirrhosis: looking beyond the patient. J Clin Exp Hepatol. 2020;10(1):9–16. https://doi.org/10.1016/j.jceh.2019.06.002.
16. Maldonado JR. Why it is important to consider social support when assessing organ transplant candidates? Am J Bioeth. 2019;19(11):1–8. https://doi.org/10.1080/15265161.2019.1671689.
17. Verma M, Horrow J, Carmody S, Navarro V. Unmet needs and burden of caregivers of patients being evaluated for a liver transplant are similar to those of cancer caregivers. Am J Hospice Palliat Med. 2024;41(4):391–7. https://doi.org/10.1177/10499091231176297.
18. Schmajuk M, DeGuzman E, Allen N. Psychotherapy in transplant patients. In: Sher Y, Maldonado J, editors. Psychosocial care of end-stage organ disease and transplant patients. Cham: Springer; 2010. https://doi.org/10.1007/978-3-319-94914-7_43.
19. Virches A, Miyazaki ET, dos Santos Junior R, Duca WJ, da Silva Fucuta P, da Silva RF, da Silva RDCMA, Basso BP, Domingos NAM, Miyazaki MCdOS. Burden, stress, and depression in informal caregivers of patients pre and post liver transplant. Transplant Proc. 2021;53:233–8. https://doi.org/10.1016/j.transproceed.2020.02.072.
20. Pol SJ, Snyder J, Anthony SJ. "Tremendous financial burden": crowdfunding for organ transplantation costs in Canada. PLoS One. 2019;14(12):e0226686. https://doi.org/10.1371/journal.pone.0226686.
21. DiMartini AF, Golden E, Matz A, Dew MA, Crone C. Post-transplant psychosocial and mental health care of the liver recipient. In: Sher Y, Maldonado J, editors. Psychosocial care of end-stage organ disease and transplant patients. Cham: Springer; 2019. https://doi.org/10.1007/978-3-319-94914-7_15.
22. Ufere NN, Satapathy N, Philpotts L, Lai JC, Serper M. Financial burden in adults with chronic liver disease: a scoping review. Liver Transpl. 2022;28(12):1920–35. https://doi.org/10.1002/lt.26514.
23. Ladin K, Daniels A, Osani M, Bannuru RR. Is social support associated with post-transplant medication adherence and outcomes? A systemic review and meta-analysis. Transplant Rev. 2017;32:16–28. https://doi.org/10.1016/j.trre.2017.04.001.
24. Bajaj JS, Wade JB, Gibson DP, Heuman DM, Thacker LR, Sterling RK, Stravitz RT, Luketic V, Fuchs M, White MB, Bell DE, Gilles H, Morton K, Noble N, Puri P, Sanyal AJ. The multidimensional burden of cirrhosis and hepatic encephalopathy on patients and caregivers. Am J Gastroenterol. 2011;106(9):1646–53. https://doi.org/10.1038/ajg.2011.157.
25. Nash R, Golden E, Dew MA, DiMartini AF. Mental health in chronic and end-stage liver disease. In: Sher Y, Maldonado J, editors. Psychosocial care of end-stage organ disease and transplant patients. Cham: Springer; 2019. https://doi.org/10.1007/978-3-319-94914-7_12.

26. Peretz D, Van Iderstine MG, Bernstein M, Minuk GY. The psychological and financial impact of long-distance travel for liver transplantation. Transplant Direct. 2020;6:e558. https://doi.org/10.1097/TXD.0000000000001005.
27. Nguyen DL, Chao D, Ma G, Morgan T. Quality of life and factors predictive of burden among primary caregivers of chronic liver disease patients. Ann Gastroenterol. 2015;28(1):124–9.
28. Jones JB, Egan M. The transplant experience of liver recipients: ethical issues and practice implications. In: Rosenberg G, Weissman A, editors. Behavioral social work in health care settings. The Haworth Press; 2000.
29. Ufere N, Lago-Hernandez C, Alejandro-Soto A, Walker T, Li L, Schoener K, Keegan E, Gonzalez C, Bethea E, Singh S, El-Jawahri A, Nephew L, Jones P, Serper M. Health care-related transportation insecurity is associated with adverse health outcomes among adults with chronic liver disease. Hepatol Commun. 2023;8:e0358. https://doi.org/10.1097/HC9.0000000000000358.
30. Lago-Hernandez C, Nguyen N, Khera R, Loomba R, Asrani S, Singh S. Cost-related non-adherence to medications among US adults with chronic liver diseases. Mayo Clin Proc. 2021;96(10):2639–50. https://doi.org/10.1016/j.mayocp.2021.02.026.
31. Guimaro MS, Lacerda SS, Karam CH, Ferraz-Neto BH, Andreoli PBA. Psychosocial profile of patients on the liver transplant list. Transplant Proc. 2008;40(3):782–4.
32. Telles-Correia D, Barbosa A, Mega I, Monteiro E. Adherence correlates in liver transplant candidates. Transplant Proc. 2009;14:1731–4. https://doi.org/10.1016/transproceed.2009.02.067.
33. Matthews LA, Musto JA, Deiss-Yehiely N, Daniel KE, Lightbourn C, Garvey M, Osman F, Foley DP, Rice JR, Lucey MR. Psychosocial assessment in liver transplant (LT): an analysis of short-term outcomes. Hepatol Commun. 2023;7:e0017. https://doi.org/10.1097/HC9.0000000000000017.

Evaluation of Living Donors for Liver Transplantation

12

Taylor M. Coe and Anand Ghanekar

Introduction

Living donor liver transplantation (LDLT) is an excellent treatment option for most patients with indications for liver transplantation [1–3]. The use of a partial liver graft relies on the regenerative capacity of the liver and allows for a healthy donor to donate a portion of their liver safely. A comprehensive medical, surgical, and psychosocial evaluation of donors is critical to protect donor safety and identify factors that may compromise excellent donor and recipient outcomes [4]. Donor assessment protocols and acceptance criteria vary between centers that perform LDLT. These variations are related to center experience, the availability of deceased donor organs, and sociocultural norms, and have shown evolution over time [5–7]. In this chapter, we will outline the important elements of the evaluation of living donors for liver transplantation and highlight areas of ongoing discussion. Figure 12.1 provides an example of our center's approach to the evaluation of potential living liver donors.

Development of a Multidisciplinary Team

Evaluation of living liver donors for transplantation requires a multidisciplinary team. Most programs require donor medical evaluation to be completed by both a hepatologist and a liver transplant surgeon, both of whom specialize in LDLT. Psychosocial evaluation should be performed by a professional in this field with experience in transplantation, such as a psychiatrist, psychologist, or social worker. Ideally, the donor evaluation team should not be involved in the care of the

T. M. Coe · A. Ghanekar (✉)
Department of Surgery, University of Toronto, Toronto, Canada
e-mail: Anand.Ghanekar@uhn.ca

B. Eghtesad et al. (eds.), *Liver Transplantation*,
https://doi.org/10.1007/978-3-032-07072-2_12

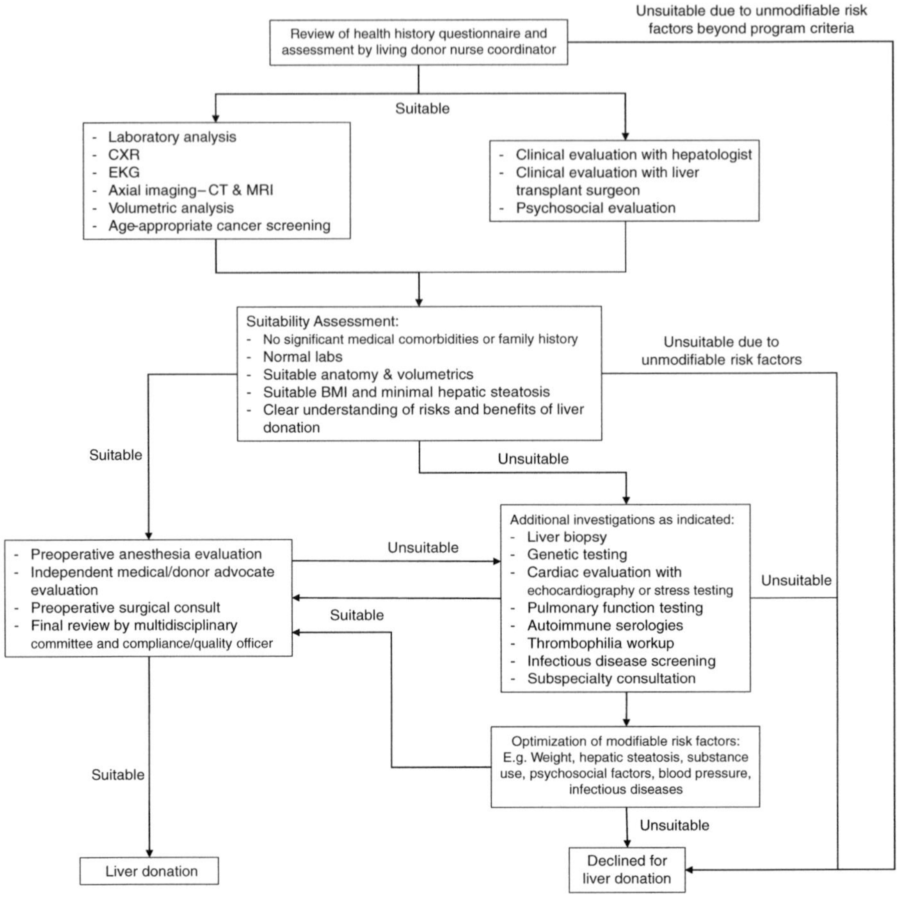

Fig. 12.1 Evaluation pathway for potential living liver donors at the University of Toronto

intended recipient to avoid a conflict of interest when determining the donor's suitability. Furthermore, an independent living donor advocate fully distinct from the transplant team should be available to donors at every step of the evaluation process [8]. The development of a multidisciplinary team committed to LDLT results in opportunities for quality improvement and continued growth.

Donor Workup

A full history and physical exam should be completed for all potential donors. This should outline a patient's past medical and surgical history, mental health history, substance use history (tobacco, alcohol, and recreational drugs), social support network (family, friends, and employment), family history with particular attention to hereditary liver diseases and clotting or bleeding disorders, medications, and allergies. A complete physical exam should include a patient's height, weight, body mass index (BMI), blood pressure, cardiopulmonary, and abdominal examination with particular attention to stigmata of liver disease such as hepatomegaly, splenomegaly, ascites, or edema. Prior abdominal surgery is not a contraindication for donation.

Basic laboratory analysis should include determination of ABO blood group, complete blood count, liver and renal biochemistries, prothrombin time, international normalized ratio (INR), and partial thromboplastin time. Metabolic testing includes blood glucose, cholesterol levels, and a fasting lipid profile. Endocrine testing should include a screening TSH. In patients with personal or family history of hereditary liver disease or bleeding/clotting disorders, further laboratory analyses may include iron studies, alpha 1 antitrypsin level and phenotype, smooth muscle antibody, anti-mitochondrial antibody, antinuclear antibody, antiphospholipid antibody, ceruloplasmin, von Willebrand Factor and a coagulation profile including factor 5 Leiden, antithrombin III, prothrombin II gene mutation, protein C and S. Premenopausal women should complete an HCG quantitative pregnancy test. Genetic testing may also be warranted for first-degree relatives of patients with defined genetic syndromes (e.g., Alagille syndrome and urea cycle disorders). Screening for sickle cell disease and G6PD deficiency should also be considered.

Screening for transmissible infectious diseases should include hepatitis viruses, human immunodeficiency virus, cytomegalovirus, herpes, rapid plasma reagin test for syphilis, Epstein-Barr virus, and Human T lymphotropic virus. In selected cases, screening for tuberculosis, West Nile virus, and Lyme disease may be indicated.

Chest X-Ray and electrocardiogram should be obtained for all potential donors. Echocardiogram and cardiac stress testing should be performed for donors over age 50 or those with established risk factors for coronary artery disease [9]. Age-appropriate cancer screening for cervical, breast, prostate, colon, and skin cancer is necessary. Additional imaging required for anatomic evaluation will be outlined below.

Preoperative liver biopsy is not required but rather performed selectively by most centers [5]. Laboratory or imaging findings suggestive of hepatic steatosis, fibrosis, or hepatitis are common indications for liver biopsy.

Donor Characteristics

Donor age is typically between 18 and 60 years, though some groups have accepted donors over 60 years of age [5]. The minimum age reflects when donors are deemed legally competent by society and capable of autonomous decision-making. The upper age limit reflects concerns related to age-related comorbidities, an increased risk of perioperative complications, and a reduction in the regenerative capacity of both the remnant liver and transplanted liver graft [10].

Increasing donor BMI can lead to increased donor surgical risk and acts as a surrogate marker for hepatic steatosis. Many centers have a lower limit of BMI between 16 and 20 and an upper limit between 30 and 33 [5].

Centers have variable protocols related to management of donors with evidence of hepatic steatosis on noninvasive imaging or with an elevated BMI [11]. Biopsy is frequently used to quantify the degree of macrovesicular steatosis, accepting donors below an upper limit of 10–20% [5, 7]. Most centers have protocols in place related to weight loss strategies for donors, as many can become fit for donation with weight reduction and evidence of improvement of steatosis on imaging or biopsy.

Donor Anatomic Considerations

Donor hepatic arterial, portal venous, hepatic venous, and biliary anatomy must be clearly evaluated to ensure that donation can occur safely for the donor with a high probability of successful vascular and biliary reconstruction of the liver graft in the recipient. Preoperative donor anatomic evaluation is accomplished through axial imaging with contrast-enhanced, triple-phase computed tomography (CT), and magnetic resonance imaging (MRI). Intraoperative cholangiography is used as an adjunct to confirm biliary anatomy and minimize the risk of bile duct injury during division of the biliary plate [12]. The potential impact of anatomic variations on both donor safety and recipient outcome should be considered when determining donor suitability.

Vascular Anatomy

Variant hepatic arterial anatomy can be present in as many as 50% of cases and CT angiography can clearly elucidate these findings preoperatively [13]. The presence of replaced or accessory right or left hepatic arteries, the origin of the segment 4 artery, and the number of separate arterial branches supplying the planned liver graft may impact the suitability of a donor and should be well understood prior to donation [14].

Variant portal vein anatomy is estimated to occur in 35% of cases and can be appreciated on both contrast-enhanced CT and MRI [15]. Common variations include portal vein trifurcation, separate origins of the anterior and posterior right portal veins, or the anterior portal vein arising from the left portal vein [14]. Some variants may preclude donation, while others may be technically feasible with appropriate reconstruction. These variants are essential to be aware of prior to donation to ascertain the risk to both donor and recipient and ensure the appropriateness of donation.

Variant hepatic venous anatomy occurs in roughly 40% of cases and is evident on contrast-enhanced CT and MRI. Optimizing venous outflow is important for graft regeneration and to prevent graft hyperperfusion and the risk of small for size syndrome (SFSS). Typical hepatic venous anatomy involves a right hepatic vein and a common trunk of the middle and left hepatic veins. Variations may include accessory segment VI and VII draining veins, which may alter the intrahepatic dominant drainage between the right and middle hepatic veins. Centers have varying practices related to the inclusion of the middle hepatic vein with a right lobe graft, as well as reconstruction practices related to segment V and VIII tributaries. The International

Liver Transplant Society Guidelines on Living Liver Donation suggest reconstruction of venous branches greater than 5 mm when present in segments V, VI, or VIII [16].

Biliary Anatomy

The anatomy of the biliary confluence of the right and left ducts can be variable in as many as 50% of cases. This is best evaluated in the preoperative setting with MRI using hepatobiliary contrast agents [17]. For right lobe donation, it is imperative to understand the drainage of the anterior and posterior ducts, as there can commonly be variations such as trifurcation of the left, right anterior, and right posterior ducts or insertion of the right posterior duct to the left or common duct. The biliary anatomy is typically further delineated intraoperatively with a cholangiogram obtained by cannulation of the cystic duct. Variant biliary anatomy does not necessarily preclude donation; however, it should be assessed in the context of donor and recipient risk factors, as it has known implications on both recipient and donor outcomes [18, 19].

Parenchymal Evaluation

The hepatic parenchyma should be evaluated for both focal lesions (e.g., cysts, adenomas, and hemangiomas) and diffuse processes (e.g., steatosis) that could impact donor safety or recipient outcomes. Hepatic steatosis is most accurately assessed by MRI proton density fat fraction (PDFF) [17].

Liver Volumes

Volumetric analysis of the potential donor's liver is necessary to calculate the future liver remnant (FLR) for the donor and the graft:recipient weight ratio (GRWR) for the recipient. The typical accepted FLR is >30% to mitigate the risk of postoperative liver insufficiency and ensure donor safety. A GRWR >0.8 is a common cutoff to ensure adequate liver volume for the recipient to avoid SFSS, though good outcomes have been demonstrated with smaller grafts [20].

Psychosocial Considerations

A thorough psychosocial evaluation of potential donors is critical to identify risk factors that may complicate a donor's short- or long-term recovery or place the donor at risk of a poor psychosocial outcome [21]. There is significant variation in how centers conduct this evaluation, as well as the long-term follow-up practices, but it is a required part of the preoperative assessment [8]. The psychosocial evaluation should include review of a patient's mental health history, substance use behaviors, understanding of the risks of donation, ability to provide informed consent, confirmation of a lack of coercion or undue pressure, and the ability to cope with the social, emotional, and financial aspects of donation [22]. Aspects of this evaluation are typically incorporated into each clinical encounter the potential donor has with the LDLT team, in addition to being performed by a professional in this field such as a social worker, psychiatrist, or psychologist. It is important that donors are aware that the process of donation is entirely voluntary and can be halted at any time during the evaluation process without repercussions. Concerns identified during the psychosocial evaluation can be reason for exclusion from donation.

Reasons for Exclusion

The rate of donor acceptance varies per center and has been reported to range from 27% to 63% [23]. Donors may be excluded for any condition that may jeopardize donor safety or recipient outcomes. Common reasons for exclusion from donation include identification of prohibitive medical problems, withdrawal of consent, anatomic concerns, hepatic steatosis, insufficient FLR or GRWR, hypercoagulability risk, or the availability of a superior liver for transplantation into the recipient [6, 11]. Examples of prohibitive medical problems include coronary artery disease, prior stroke, or active malignancy.

In summary, a thorough evaluation of all potential liver donors is required to ensure donor safety and optimal donor and recipient outcomes. The evaluation should be multidisciplinary in nature and seek to identify any possible medical, anatomic, or psychosocial findings that may preclude donation. As illustrated in Fig. 12.1, the donor evaluation process may identify health issues that require further investigation and management before donation may safely proceed, while other issues may arise that prevent donation altogether. While many centers have variable protocols and donor acceptance criteria, all are committed to donor safety above all else.

References

1. Jackson WE, Malamon JS, Kaplan B, et al. Survival benefit of living-donor liver transplant. JAMA Surg. 2022;157(10):926–32.
2. Magyar CTJ, Li Z, Aceituno L, et al. Temporal evolution of living donor liver transplantation survival—a United Network for organ sharing registry study. Am J Transplant. 2025;25(2):406–16.
3. Li Z, Jones O, Magyar CTJ, et al. Living donor availability improves patient survival in a North American center: an intention-to-treat analysis. Ann Surg. 2024; https://doi.org/10.1097/SLA.0000000000006451.
4. Guidance for the Medical Evaluation of Potential Living Liver Donors. Organ Procurement and Transplantation Network. https://optn.transplant.hrsa.gov/professionals/by-topic/guidance/guidance-for-the-medical-evaluation-of-potential-living-liver-donors/. Accessed 9 March 2025.
5. Soin AS, Chaudhary RJ, Pahari H, Pomfret EA. A worldwide survey of live liver donor selection policies at 24 centers with a combined experience of 19 009 adult living donor liver transplants. Transplantation. 2019;103(2):e39–47.
6. Trotter JF, Wisniewski KA, Terrault NA, et al. Outcomes of donor evaluation in adult-to-adult living donor liver transplantation. Hepatology. 2007;46(5):1476–84.
7. Brandhagen D, Fidler J, Rosen C. Evaluation of the donor liver for living donor liver transplantation. Liver Transpl. 2003;9(10C):S16–28.

8. OPTN Policies, Policy 14: Living Donation. 14.1 Psychosocial evaluation requirements for living donors. Organ Procurement and Transplantation Network. https://optn.transplant.hrsa.gov/media/eavh5bf3/optn_policies.pdf. Accessed 9 March 2025.
9. Thompson A, Fleischmann KE, Smilowitz NR, et al. 2024 AHA/ACC/ACS/ASNC/HRS/SCA/SCCT/SCMR/SVM guideline for perioperative cardiovascular management for noncardiac surgery: a report of the American College of Cardiology/American Heart Association Joint Committee on Clinical Practice Guidelines. Circulation. 2024;150(19):e351–442.
10. Patel S, Orloff M, Tsoulfas G, et al. Living-donor liver transplantation in the United States: identifying donors at risk for perioperative complications. Am J Transplant. 2007;7(10):2344–9.
11. Nugroho A, Kim OK, Lee KW, et al. Evaluation of donor workups and exclusions in a single-center experience of living donor liver transplantation. Liver Transpl. 2017;23(5):614–24.
12. Borhani AA, Elsayes KM, Catania R, et al. Imaging evaluation of living liver donor candidates: techniques, protocols, and anatomy. Radiographics. 2021;41(6):1572–91.
13. Hiatt JR, Gabbay J, Busuttil RW. Surgical anatomy of the hepatic arteries in 1000 cases. Ann Surg. 1994;220(1):50–2.
14. Goldaracena N, Vargas PA, McCormack L. Pre-operative assessment of living liver donors' liver anatomy and volumes. Updates Surg. 2024; https://doi.org/10.1007/s13304-024-01806-6.
15. Sureka B, Patidar Y, Bansal K, Rajesh S, Agrawal N, Arora A. Portal vein variations in 1000 patients: surgical and radiological importance. Br J Radiol. 2015;88(1055):20150326.
16. Miller CM, Durand F, Heimbach JK, et al. The international liver transplant society guideline on living liver donation. Transplantation. 2016;100(6):1238.
17. Cahalane AM, Mojtahed A, Sahani DV, Elias N, Kambadakone AR. Pre-hepatic and pre-pancreatic transplant donor evaluation. Cardiovasc Diagn Ther. 2019;9(S1):S97–S115.
18. Baker TB, Zimmerman MA, Goodrich NP, et al. Biliary reconstructive techniques and associated anatomic variants in adult living donor liver transplantations: the adult-to-adult living donor liver transplantation cohort study experience. Liver Transpl. 2017;23(12):1519–30.
19. Takagi K, Umeda Y, Yoshida R, et al. Short-term and long-term outcomes in living donors for liver transplantation: cohort study. Int J Surg. 2020;84:147–53.
20. Fujiki M, Hashimoto K, Quintini C, et al. Living donor liver transplantation with augmented venous outflow and splenectomy: a promised land for small left lobe grafts. Ann Surg. 2022;276(5):838–45.
21. Dew MA, Butt Z, Liu Q, et al. Prevalence and predictors of patient-reported long-term mental and physical health after donation in the adult-to-adult living-donor liver transplantation cohort study. Transplantation. 2018;102(1):105–18.
22. Zimbrean PC, Rubman S, Andacoglu O, et al. Psychosocial evaluation of living liver donors-state of current practices in the United States. Liver Transpl. 2024;30(5):505–18.
23. Kasiske BL, Ahn YS, Conboy M, et al. Outcomes of living liver donor candidate evaluations in the living donor collective pilot registry. Clin Transpl. 2021;35(9):e14394.

Part II

Transplant Process

The Liver Transplant Procedure

13

John J. Fung, Arielle Cimeno, Bijan Eghtesad, John LaMattina, and Rolf Barth

Introduction

Orthotopic liver transplantation (LTX) has become the gold-standard means for the treatment of end-stage liver disease (ESLD). Although the technique of LTX has been refined to a relatively standardized approach, the operation still remains a formidable surgical challenge. As such, LTX is associated with numerous potential surgical complications, in which the recipient's pretransplant condition, anatomy, and diagnosis, as well as donor and immunologic factors, all contribute. These risks can be minimized by fully appreciating anatomic variations, performing appropriate ABO matching, size matching of the donor liver to the recipient habitus, adequate maintenance of donor liver function, attention to organ procurement, and minimization of cold ischemic time. Application of "technical variant" liver allografts, such as split liver and living donor liver transplantation, require additional modifications to the recipient operation. The purpose of this chapter is to review both the donor and recipient operative procedures and to highlight some of the more important intraoperative and early and late postoperative complications.

J. J. Fung (✉) · A. Cimeno · J. LaMattina · R. Barth
University of Chicago, Department of Surgery, Chicago, IL, USA
e-mail: jfung@surgery.bsd.uchicago.edu; cimenoa@bsd.uchicago.edu; jlamatti@bsd.uchicago.edu; Rolf.Barth@bsd.uchicago.edu

B. Eghtesad
Cleveland Clinic, Digestive Disease and Surgery Institute, Cleveland, OH, USA

B. Eghtesad et al. (eds.), *Liver Transplantation*,
https://doi.org/10.1007/978-3-032-07072-2_13

Terminology

Orthotopic LTX replaces the removed liver with the transplanted allograft liver in the anatomically correct position. Heterotopic LTX places the liver allograft in an extrahepatic site, usually at the root of the mesentery, but it is of historical significance only, due to poor outcomes. Auxiliary LTX is the placement of the donor liver in the presence of the native liver. Such auxiliary transplants can be either orthotopic, after removal of part of the native liver, or heterotopic, with placement of a portion of the donor liver in a heterotopic position.

Segmental LTX places only a portion of the donor liver into the recipient—this utilizes a reduced-size liver allograft, sometimes referred to as a "technical variant" liver allograft. The source of segmental grafts can be cadaveric, living donor, or both (in the case of dual donor segmental transplants). In the case of cadaveric segments, the graft can be a split liver graft, where the cadaveric whole liver is reduced to one or two smaller grafts. In each case, the segmental allograft maintains its own venous drainage, portal-venous inflow, hepatic artery inflow, and biliary drainage. In practice, these structures must be partitioned in a way so as to maximize the likelihood of survival, but this entails added risk compared with a whole cadaveric graft. Living donor segmental LTX is similar to split livers in terms of technical issues and complications related to recipient outcomes, but introduces the risk of complications in the donor.

Historical Background

Although attempts at orthotopic liver transplantation were performed in large animals as early as 1952 by Vittorio Staudacher at the University of Milan [1], the technical aspects of the operation, including the critical need for portal-venous blood flow, were first elucidated by Thomas Starzl in 1960 [2] prior to the first attempt at clinical LTX in 1963 [3]. The 3-year-old boy with biliary atresia ultimately died of hemorrhage and coagulopathy. This was followed by six more unsuccessful LTXs in Denver, Boston, and Paris [3–5]. The poor outcomes of the first human LTX attempts resulted in a moratorium that extended into the summer of 1967 when a child finally underwent successful LTX in Denver [6]. This was followed in 1968 by the opening of an LTX unit in Cambridge, United Kingdom, by Roy Calne [7]. The first 33 LTX, of which 25 were performed in Denver and four in Cambridge, were later summarized in 1969 in a book entitled *Experience in Hepatic Transplantation* [8].

To overcome severe donor shortage, LTX using partial grafts was introduced in 1980s. Bismuth first described the reduction of an adult liver to transplant a small pediatric recipient [9]. This technique subsequently evolved to a new concept of "splitting" a whole liver to simultaneously transplant two recipients [10]. In split liver transplantation (SLT), whole livers from deceased donors are most commonly split into a smaller left lateral segment (Couinaud Segments II and III) for children and a larger right trisegment (Segments I, IV–VIII) for adults (Fig. 13.1a). This

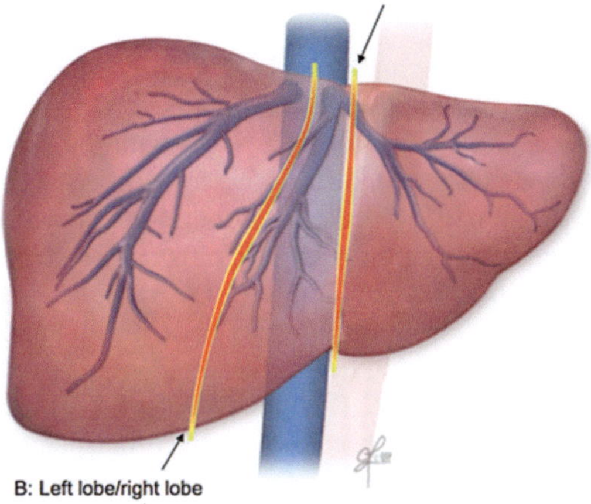

Fig. 13.1 Line of transection to create a segmental or partial graft. (**a**) division along the right side of the falciform ligament, creating a smaller left lateral segment (Couinaud Segments II and III) and a larger extended right trisegment (Segments 1, IV–VIII); and (**b**) division along Cantlie's line, creating a full left lobe (Segments II–IV with or without Segment I) and a full right lobe (Segments V–VIII with or without Segment I)

technique contributed to the reduction of pediatric waiting list mortality [11]. The indication was further expanded to create two hemiliver grafts, a left lobe (Segments I–IV) and a right lobe (Segments V–VIII), for two adults (Fig. 13.1b). Although SLT was initially characterized by higher rates of recipient morbidity and mortality [12, 13], various advancements in patient selection, surgical techniques, and postoperative management have helped increase the use of split grafts with improved outcomes [14, 15].

In 1989, the first successful LDLT was performed in Australia with a left lateral segment graft following a failed attempt in Brazil [16], while the longest survivor of a living donor graft was transplanted at the University of Chicago [17]. The first successful application of adult-to-adult LDLT was done by Makuuchi using a left lobe graft in 1993 [18]. To overcome size mismatch issues, the right lobe graft has become a dominant type in adult-to-adult LDLT [19, 20]. Despite excellent outcomes, right lobe donation is associated with an increased risk of morbidity and mortality compared to the left-sided graft [21].

With public awareness of several living donor deaths, the left lobe graft has become the preferred choice for adults at many centers. Less frequently, the extended right lobe including the middle hepatic vein is used to gain more liver volume for recipients [21]. The right posterior segment (segments VI and VII) graft can be used when the donor has a disproportionately small left lobe with a rare anatomical variant of the portal vein and bile duct. However, this graft requires very complex surgical techniques and has higher risks of recipient complications [22]. Finally, dual LDLT combinations have been utilized with good outcomes [23].

Donor Considerations

As noted by Starzl in 1967: *"The provision of a viable and minimally damaged homograft is undoubtedly the most important single factor in the determinant of success"* [8]. Thus, the key to successful LTX starts with the procurement of an optimally functioning donor liver allograft. As noted earlier, the source for donor organs can be from living donors or deceased donors. The nuances of options in both are complex; for example, living donor allografts can be segmental (as noted above) or whole grafts (in the case of a domino liver transplant). The options for sources of liver allografts will differ according to the age and size of the recipient, diagnosis, geographic location, waiting list size, and technical expertise.

Living donor liver transplantation (LDLT) has emerged as a partial solution to the current shortage of allografts for those awaiting liver transplantation. The adoption of this innovative approach, along with other technical variant livers, to address the organ shortage in the pediatric ESLD population has significantly reduced waiting list deaths in this historically high mortality while waiting group with outcomes that match those of using whole pediatric grafts [9, 11, 24]. However, with the increasing mortality in adult candidates, the development of living adult-to-adult lobar donation has generated greater interest due to a potentially larger beneficiary pool. The principal concern is the demand for a larger volume of functional transplanted liver and the added technical skill and experience needed to minimize the risk to both the living donor and recipient. Since the institutional adoption of adult-to-adult LDLT by the University of Hong Kong in 1996, an increasingly clearer assessment of the risk to the donor, using a standardized approach to the collection and categorization of complications, has been achieved [19, 21, 26]. Partitioning a liver into two parts, with one portion used to rescue a dying recipient and the other to maintain a previously healthy donor, requires considerable surgical expertise. There are limitations on the smallest amount of liver that can be effectively transplanted in the face of a hostile recipient physiology with hyperdynamic cardiac output and markedly increased mesenteric blood flow; this is particularly evident in adult recipients. Consequently, physiologic and anatomic considerations dictate that adult LDLT operations use a larger donor liver mass, usually the right lobe, which also increases the risk of donor complications [19, 21, 25–27]. In addition, any other factors that negatively influence liver regeneration, such as older age [28, 29] and steatosis [30], can negatively influence the outcome for both the donor and recipient. In essence, a better understanding of the underlying biology can minimize both the risk of failure for the recipient and complications in the donor and thus lessen or eliminate some of the ethical concerns.

In LDLT, there are two important concepts to understand better graft and recipient selection: future liver remnant (FLR) and graft-to-recipient body weight ratio (GRWR). The FLR is the proportion of the donor liver that will be left in the donor after living donation. An FLR of 30–35% is generally considered as a lower limit that living donor hepatectomy can be safely done [25]. The GRWR is the ratio between the donor liver weight and the recipient body weight. A GRWR of 0.6–0.8% is acceptable to avoid size mismatch-related complications after LDLT, but the minimum volume varies according to a variety of factors, the most important being the severity of recipient portal hypertension.

In spite of dependence on the use of living donors in many parts of Asia, the overwhelming contribution of liver allografts in Europe and North and South America is from deceased donors. The majority of livers are from brain-dead donors (referred to as donation after brain death or DBD), although the use of classic, non-heart-beating donors (currently referred to as donation after circulatory death or DCD) is increasing. For DBD, following the declaration of death and consent for donation, careful management of donor physiologic parameters optimizes allograft function and thus recipient outcomes following LTX. The goal is to maintain adequate circulation, oxygenation, and metabolism prior to organ procurement [31]. This can be difficult in the face of cardiac instability, neurogenic shock, volatile intravascular fluid status, loss of the normal hormonal milieu, and depletion of high-energy stores for liver function.

As the number of waiting list patients exceeds the number of livers available for transplantation, the utilization of donors that in the past were not considered has been reassessed. "Expanded criteria donor" (ECD) category encompasses donors in whom certain characteristics impart either real or perceived short- and/or long-term risks to the recipient. In particular, efforts have focused on identifying and defining ECDs [32]. Although there is no universally accepted definition of the ECD donor, the following criteria include a list of some possible characteristics of an expanded criteria liver donor:

- A medical history of systemic malignancy in the donor, particularly lung, central nervous system, and melanoma.
- A pre-donation course of hemodynamic instability, reflected by high donor serum sodium, high levels of vasopressor use, prolonged cardiac arrest, or anoxia.
- Donation after circulatory death (DCD).
- High-risk social behavior (e.g., incarceration, multiple sex partners, prostitution, active intravenous drug use) with or without serologic and molecular evidence of active viral infection, e.g., Hepatitis B, Hepatitis C, and Human immunodeficiency virus.
- Evidence of less than optimal liver function prior to surgical recovery, including liver biopsy findings of significant steatosis.
- Adverse intraoperative recovery events, including iatrogenic surgical injury during procurement.
- Advanced donor age.
- Cause of death other than traumatic.
- Long cold-ischemia time.
- Technical variant (reduced and split liver transplant).

Details on the techniques of deceased liver procurement, optimal preservation of the deceased donor graft, evolving approaches to optimizing function and utilization of donation after circulatory death livers, considerations in splitting the liver allograft, and considerations and techniques of living donor hepatectomy will be covered in detail in other chapters of this book.

Recipient Operation

The technique of LTX has been progressively refined since its introduction in humans in 1963, with several variations that are applied selectively according to the patient's specific situation and/or the transplant center's routine practice. The initially described conventional LTX involves resection of the recipient native liver (hepatectomy) along with the retrohepatic inferior vena cava (IVC) and a short anhepatic phase, followed by the implantation of a whole deceased donor liver graft with the interposed donor IVC. Restoration of venous continuity during the implantation is achieved by an upper subdiaphragmatic and a lower suprarenal end-to-end donor-to-recipient IVC anastomosis. The donor-to-recipient portal vein and hepatic artery anastomoses are also performed in an end-to-end fashion. The biliary continuity is reestablished using either a primary duct-to-duct technique or the performance of a hepaticojejunostomy (Fig. 13.2).

Hepatectomy

The "standard incision" for LTX has historically been a bilateral subcostal incision with or without an upper midline extension to the xiphoid (sometimes called an inverted Y or Mercedes incision) (Fig. 13.3). Other incisions have been used; however, the principle in determining the type of incision is to gain adequate exposure to the liver and to other intra-abdominal structures, such as the infrarenal aorta, should the need arise. The type of incision is of paramount importance, and choosing the wrong incision can make the operation difficult. The presence of previous

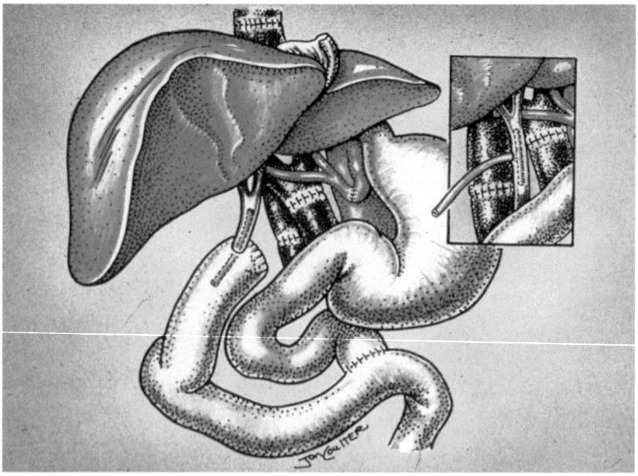

Fig. 13.2 Illustration of the standard orthotopic liver transplant as described by Starzl [6]. The figure demonstrates a bicaval anastomosis, portal venous and hepatic artery reconstruction with the biliary reconstruction as a hepaticojejunostomy over a biliary stent or choledocholedochostomy over a T tube (inset). Reproduced with permission [33]

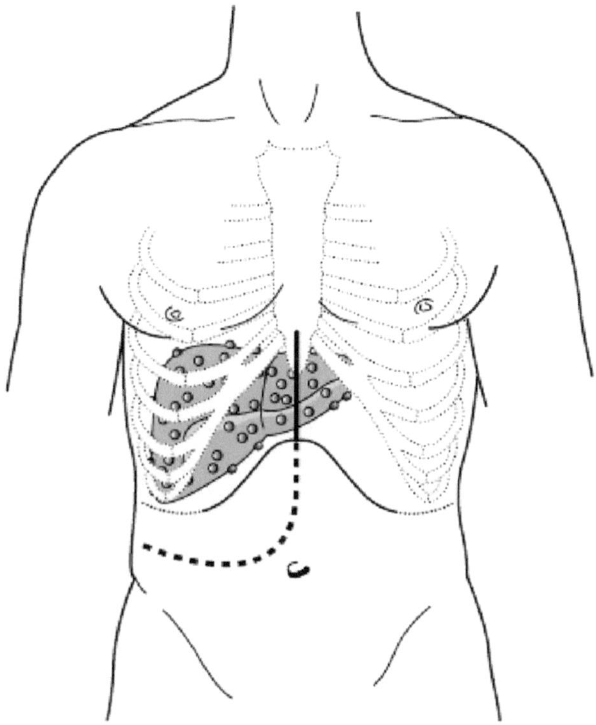

Fig. 13.3 Types of incisions utilized in liver transplantation, classically utilizing a bilateral subcostal incision with or without an upper midline incision. Alternatively, a bilateral subcostal incision without an upper midline incision, or right subcostal with an upper midline extension, can be utilized

incisions may require modification to the planned incision in order to avoid flap necrosis from devascularization.

In the case of preceding surgery in the LTX recipient, particular attention must be paid upon entering the abdominal cavity, as the presence of vascular adhesions can lead to both significant blood loss and/or violation of the gastrointestinal tract.

Usually, the hepatectomy is the most difficult part of the LTX procedure. Consequently, technical misadventures during this phase of the operation may result in significant complications. This is particularly true during the hepatectomy in patients with previous upper abdominal surgery, with excessive bleeding being the most common complication. This can be the result of carelessness, massive portal hypertension, and the presence of unusual collaterals (especially in the presence of portal vein thrombosis) and/or vascularized adhesions. Deliberate, methodic, and bloodless dissection translates to a much smoother operation and, ironically, a considerably shorter total case time. It is particularly difficult to perform surgical hemostasis once the allograft is in place, especially if there is any degree of post-reperfusion coagulopathy and if the graft is relatively large compared with the recipient's abdominal compartment. In addition, early portal decompression with the veno-venous bypass (see below) may aid in reducing the risk of massive bleeding.

Careful dissection of the hilum of the liver is critical during the hepatectomy. This is true especially in the case of hepatectomy for segmental LTX, in cases of previous surgical procedures in the hilum of the liver (including retransplantation), when there is portal vein thrombosis (due to collaterals), and in cases where there are anatomic variants. The goal in hepatectomy is preservation of the hilar structures, especially the hepatic artery and portal vein needed to revascularize the new liver allograft, as well as preservation of a sufficient length of the common bile and hepatic ducts for biliary reconstruction. Approaches to the hilum can commence either from the right side with dissection of the cystic duct and common bile duct or from the left with dissection of the hepatic artery. After identification of the common bile duct, it is good practice to preserve the surrounding soft tissue so as not to cause damage to the bile duct blood supply (Fig. 13.4). This is important to prevent postoperative bile duct ischemia and necrosis or stricture formation. An important technical issue in the dissection of the hepatic artery is to start dissection of the artery at the level of the right and left branches and to proceed to the confluence, and then to the gastroduodenal artery, and finally to the common hepatic artery. The surgeon should avoid too much traction of the artery to prevent intimal dissection in the artery, which can predispose the artery to postoperative thrombosis. Dissection of the branches of the common hepatic artery will allow the surgeon to select which part of the artery will provide a better size match with the donor hepatic artery, especially when using a technical variant allograft. In addition, recognition of variations in the recipient anatomy of the hepatic artery is helpful in the event that alternative inflow for hepatic artery reconstruction is required.

Portal vein dissection is usually done after division of the hepatic artery and bile duct. All the soft tissue around the portal vein should be dissected and removed from the hilar plate to the level of the head of the pancreas. The avulsion of small pancreatic branches entering the portal vein or injury to the left gastric vein can cause massive bleeding in light of portal hypertension.

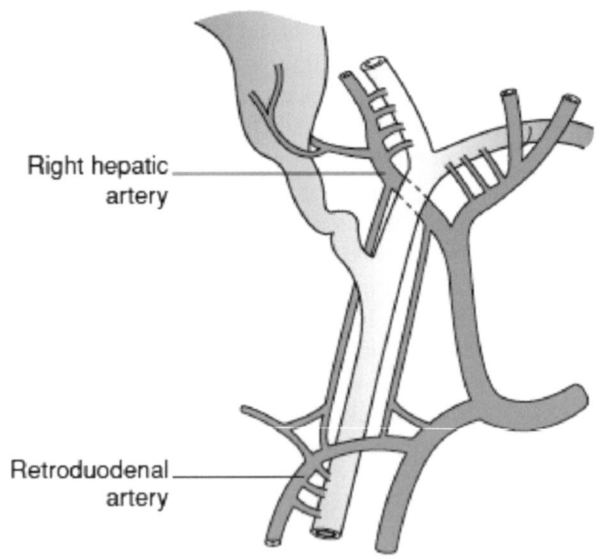

Fig. 13.4 Blood supply of the biliary system. The unique nature of the blood supply for the bile duct depends solely on a hepatic artery blood supply via a vascular plexus to assure bile duct viability. This is true for both the donor and recipient bile ducts

A potentially serious complication during hepatectomy is injury to the right adrenal gland, which results in severe bleeding that is difficult to control and may require adrenalectomy. Another feared complication is injury to the right renal vein during mobilization of the infrahepatic vena cava. Dissection of the vena cava at too low a level must be avoided. Injury of the suprahepatic vena cava is an uncommon but potentially disastrous complication. Rarely, injury of the suprahepatic vena cava, with a resulting cuff that is too short, in patients with Budd–Chiari syndrome or in patients undergoing liver retransplantation in the face of a previous suprahepatic vena caval stenosis, may require control of the vena cava at the level of the diaphragm or within the pericardium. This allows placement of the vascular clamp close to or at the level of the right atrium. If necessary, the suprahepatic vena cava may need to be sutured closed, and venous outflow of the hepatic allograft may require a caval–atrial anastomosis.

Another potential complication is injury to the right phrenic nerve. This occurs when an excessive amount of diaphragm is included in the suprahepatic vascular clamp, particularly in the pediatric patient. This injury is usually reversible, but on occasion it can lead to permanent paralysis of the right hemidiaphragm. In addition, excessive diathermy to the right diaphragm may lead to necrosis and subsequently result in a diaphragmatic hernia.

Anhepatic Phase

During the classic LTX procedure, simultaneous complete occlusion of the recipient IVC and portal vein can lead to hemodynamic instability (Fig. 13.5). As a result, veno-venous bypass was developed to allow diversion of blood from the recipient

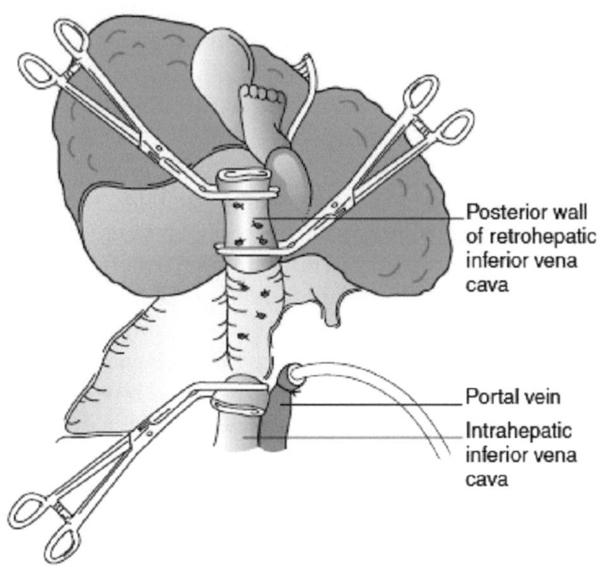

Fig. 13.5 Requirement for infrahepatic vena cava and portal vein clamping during classic standard liver transplantation. In this case, a veno-venous bypass is being utilized, as evidenced by the portal-venous cannulae in place to decompress the mesenteric venous system

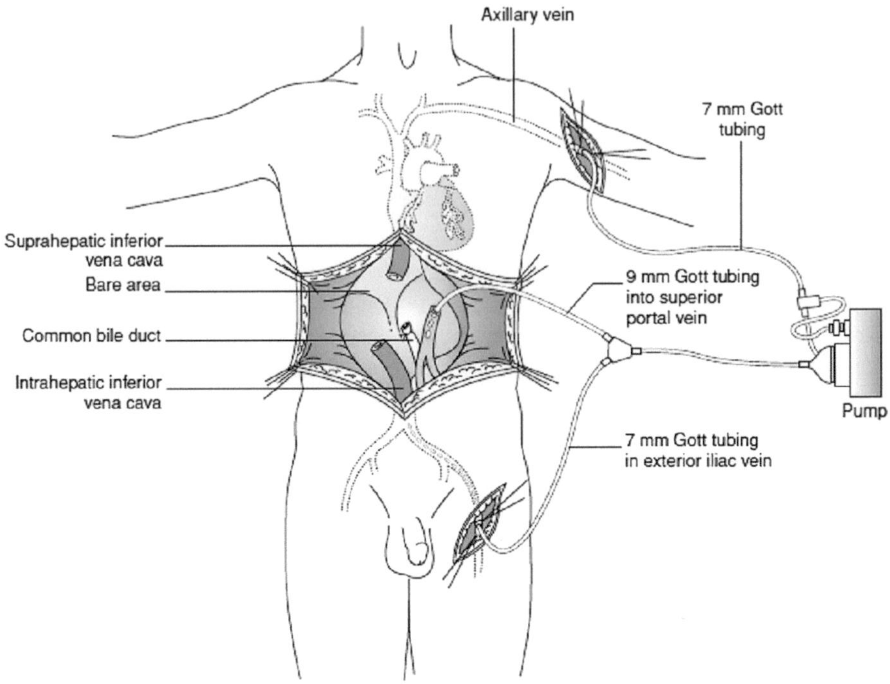

Fig. 13.6 Veno-venous bypass in liver transplantation, shown in the anhepatic phase with removal of the recipient vena cava using the right axillary vein as the inflow. Alternatively, the bypass may utilize percutaneously placed cannulae through the common femoral vein and internal jugular vein

IVC and portal vein directly to the patient's superior vena cava during the anhepatic phase, using heparin-bonded cannulae and a motor-driven bypass system (Fig. 13.6) [34]. Veno-venous bypass can be used either routinely or selectively in patients showing hemodynamic instability after a trial of clamping the IVC and portal vein, prior to the total removal of the recipient liver [35].

Advantages of veno-venous bypass include the following:

- The avoidance of cardiovascular instability resulting from reduced venous return to the heart during venous cross-clamping, particularly in patients with acute liver failure or in patients with noncirrhotic indications for LTX who have not developed portosystemic venous collaterals.
- The reduction of blood loss due to decompression of the portal circulation, minimizing transfusion and volume requirements.
- The avoidance of mesenteric stasis and bowel edema, and the subsequent development and release of anaerobic metabolic products and bacterial translocation into the circulation after reperfusion.
- The protection of renal function by avoiding renal-venous hypertension with a reduction of renal perfusion.

- Decompression of the portal system pressures and the avoidance of hemodynamic instability thus allowing a safe prolongation of the anhepatic phase. This allows meticulous hemostasis and any necessary dissection as well as facilitating the correction of any complications arising during this phase of the operation.

Another advantage of the veno-venous bypass is to allow a methodic approach to teaching trainees the complex procedure of LTX. However, the veno-venous bypass can cause complications, some of them fatal. Complications associated with veno-venous bypass have been described as occurring in 10–30% of cases [36–38]. These include seroma at the site of cannulae insertion, hematoma, wound infection, deep venous thrombosis, femoral artery injury and femoral nerve injury. The most frequent complications are wound lymphoceles, both in the inguinal and axillary incisions. They can be avoided by careful dissection and ligation of all lymphatics. Lymphoceles are usually self-limiting and self-healing, but occasionally chronic lymphorrhea can be quite disabling and requires surgical correction. Newer approaches to percutaneous cannulation of the femoral vein and internal jugular vein may obviate wound complications associated with cutdowns [39]; however, the risk of hematoma formation or venous perforation exists with these techniques. Mortality has also been described with an air embolus at the time of decannulation as well as intracircuit clots and a subsequent pulmonary embolus, the latter having occurred mainly when nonheparin-bonded tubing was used [40].

Over the past two decades, there has been a trend toward avoiding the use of veno-venous bypass entirely [41, 42]. This is due in part to the improved intraoperative hemodynamic management of the patient by the anesthesiology team and in part to the improved technical skills of the surgeons. The preservation of the entire retrohepatic vena cava and anastomosis of the new liver to a cuff formed from one or more of the main suprahepatic veins (end-to-side cavocavostomy) or as a side-to-side cavocavostomy has been advocated as a method of avoiding veno-venous bypass. The advantages of preserving the vena cava can be significant, but this technique (also known as the "piggyback technique") requires additional skills and complete knowledge of and confidence with standard LTX with veno-venous bypass [43]. Essentially, the technique consists of the dissection of the caudate process and right lobe of the liver from the retrohepatic vena cava, until only the right, middle, and left hepatic veins remain. Subsequently, the major hepatic veins are clamped and interconnected, thus forming a cuff that can then be anastomosed to the suprahepatic vena cava of the donor liver, in an end-to-side fashion (Fig. 13.7). After flushing the liver to clear the preserving solution, the infrahepatic cava of the allograft can be simply ligated. The new liver will then lie on top of the recipient's vena cava, but can also result in compression of the recipient's vena cava with the development of thrombosis [44, 45].

There are several potential advantages of the piggyback technique, including less bleeding, less chance of adrenal gland and renal vein injury, shortening the anhepatic phase by eliminating the lower caval anastomosis, protection of the renal-venous outflow and function, and potentially less hemodynamic instability. In this

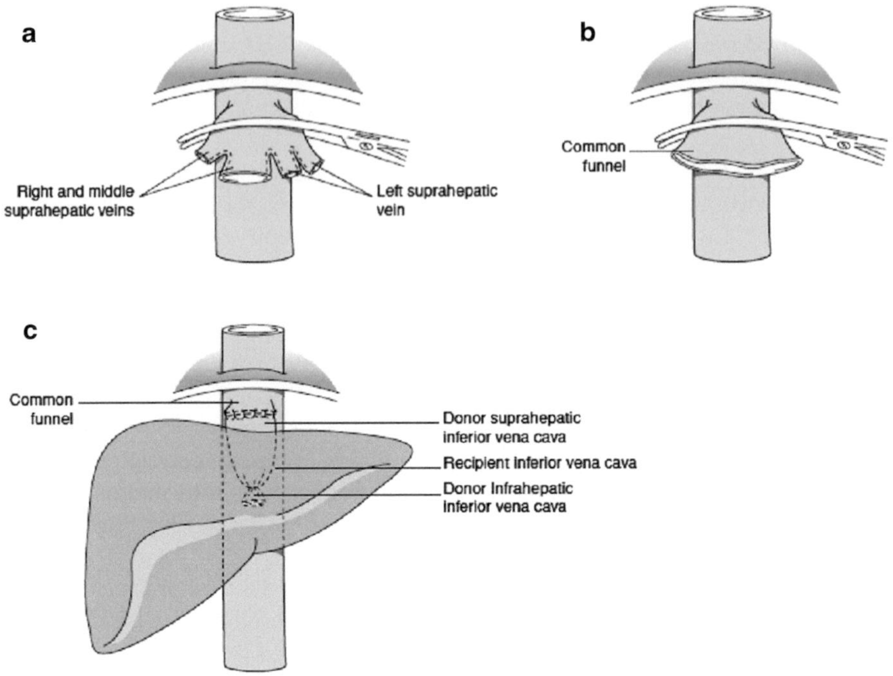

Fig. 13.7 The "Classical Piggyback Technique" of recipient hepatectomy preserving the intrahepatic vena cava for liver allograft implantation utilizing end-to-side cavo-hepatic venous anastomosis. (**a**) Following removal of the liver with origins of individual hepatic veins; (**b**) creating a common orifice by dividing the septa between individual hepatic veins; (**c**) end-to-side cavo-cavostomy using suprahepatic vena cava of the donor to the common funnel orifice of the recipient hepatic veins

situation, if portal cross-clamping in the patient with existing portal hypertension is well tolerated, it may be appropriate not to utilize a veno-venous bypass.

If portal vein clamping is not tolerated, it is still possible to avoid veno-venous bypass by the creation of a temporary portacaval shunt to decompress the mesenteric system in the anhepatic phase, so long as the recipient's own vena cava remains patent. This is particularly true in cases without preexisting portal hypertension (e.g., fulminant hepatitis) (Fig. 13.8) [46]. There have been many modifications to the caval-preserving methods used in different conditions and indications at the time of transplantation. The essential part of all these methods is to preserve the inferior vena cava with or without the use of veno-venous bypass. In addition, modifications to implantation, using a side-to-side cavo-cavostomy, either handsewn [47, 48] or by stapler [49], have been described.

It is important to take advantage of the anhepatic phase and perform a thorough hemostatic survey of the operative area. At times, after the implantation of the new liver, there is not enough exposure to get a good hemostasis in the retrohepatic

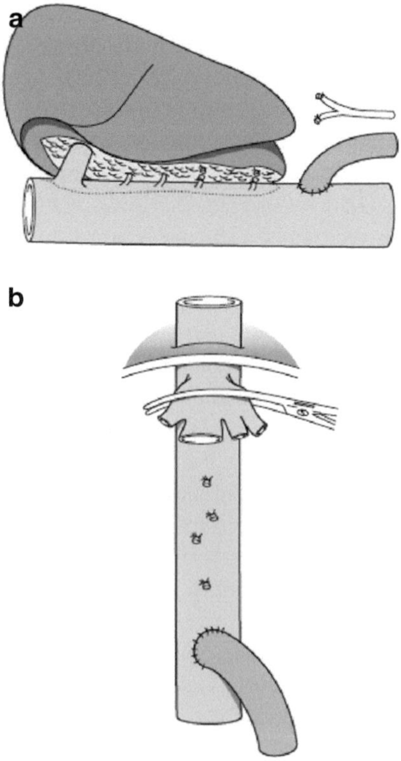

Fig. 13.8 Use of a temporary portacaval shunt with piggyback vena caval preservation. (**a**) Lateral view of portocaval shunt prior to mobilization of liver from short hepatic veins; (**b**) frontal illustration of recipient inferior vena cava with portocaval shunt after removal of liver

space. This is especially true in cases when the allograft is large and difficult to mobilize.

Implantation

Implantation of the liver allograft consists of several vascular anastomoses, reperfusion of the liver with the recipient's blood, and biliary reconstruction. The conventional method of implanting the new liver consists of end-to-end anastomoses of the supra- and infrahepatic vena cava of the donor liver to the corresponding vena caval cuffs in the recipient, followed by end-to-end anastomosis of the portal vein of the donor liver to the recipient portal vein. Usually, after completion of these anastomoses, the liver is reperfused with the recipient's blood and the clamps are removed, and the recipient's venous circulation is reestablished through the new liver—this helps to decompress the venous beds. Reperfusion of the liver can be one of the more unstable parts of the procedure. This is mainly due to the potential risk of cardiac arrhythmias, hypotension, and pulmonary edema secondary to the release of effluent from the liver allograft, which contains relatively high concentrations of potassium, necrotic debris, and cytokines, into the circulation, also known as "post-reperfusion syndrome" [50]. The use of preservative solutions with a high potassium content, such as the University of Wisconsin solution, and the use of livers from expanded criteria donors (including steatotic grafts) or livers with a prolonged cold ischemia time can exaggerate the magnitude of these complications and add to morbidity and mortality [51]. To potentially lessen or prevent these problems, many surgeons flush the liver with lactated Ringer solution, 5% albumin, or recipient portal blood before full reperfusion.

In describing the surgical techniques involved in LTX, variations in the approach to recipients with preexisting underlying portal vein thrombosis should be mentioned. The incidence of portal vein thrombosis in patients with cirrhosis has been reported to vary between 0.6% and 64.1% depending upon the diagnostic study used and on the patient population [52, 53]. The presence of portal vein thrombosis was previously considered a relative contraindication for LTX, a viewpoint that has since changed. Therapeutic options in the approach during LTX to preexisting portal vein thrombosis include eversion thromboendartectomy of the recipient portal vein (Fig. 13.9), the use of either interposition or jump venous grafts between the donor portal vein and the recipient portal or superior mesenteric vein (Fig. 13.10); cavoportal hemitransposition [54]; anastomosis of the donor portal vein to an alternative recipient vein or venous collateral [53]; recipient left renal vein to donor portal vein (usually requiring a venous interposition graft), i.e., renoportal anastomosis [55]; and rarely arterialization of the portal vein [56]. Cavoportal hemitransposition is an option utilized when extensive thrombosis of the recipient portomesenteric venous system is present and its use is rarely indicated. Finally, a careful search for retroperitoneal and retrogastric collaterals should be undertaken, as failing to interrupt them after restoring portal venous flow following successful endovenectomy can lead to portal venous "steal," with subsequent ischemia to the newly transplanted liver [57].

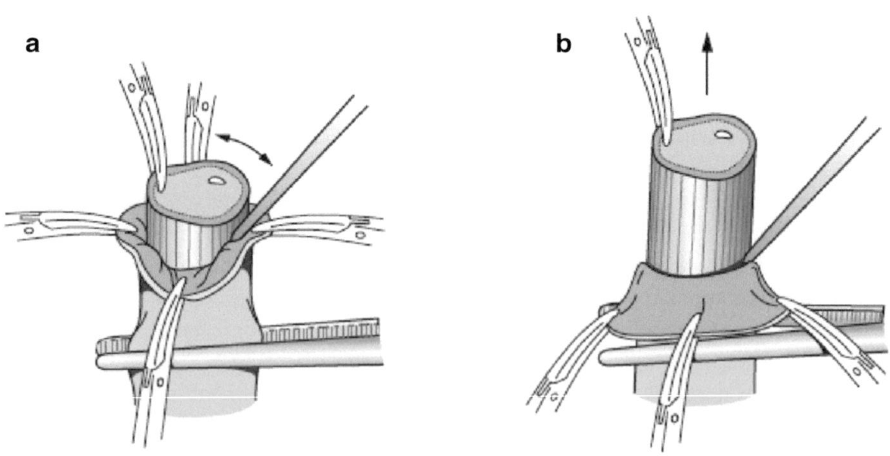

Fig. 13.9 Eversion portal-venous thromboendarterectomy to reestablish the blood flow in portal vein thrombosis

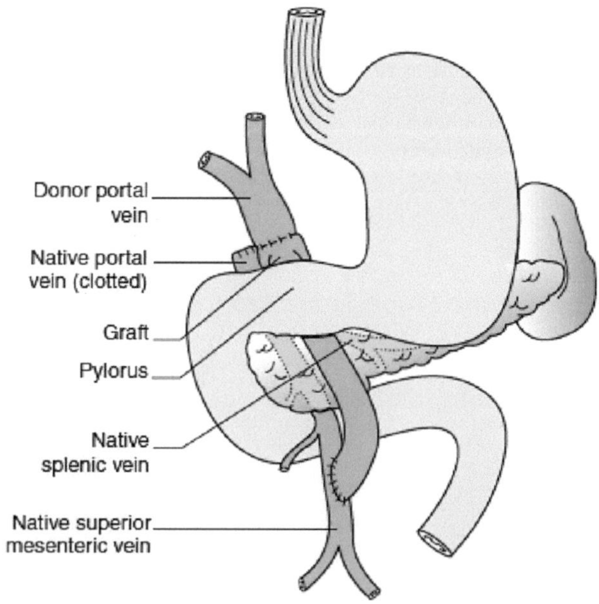

Fig. 13.10 Use of an interposition vein graft from the recipient's superior mesenteric vein to the allograft portal vein in the setting of portal vein thrombosis

Arterial anastomosis between the donor and recipient arteries is usually end-to-end, and the site usually varies depending on the arterial anatomy of the donor and recipient and the surgeon's preference. One must recognize that patients with an anomalous hepatic arterial anatomy may not have a large enough common hepatic artery to use as inflow. Patients with celiac axis stenosis may also have inadequate inflow. The median arcuate ligament syndrome has been described as affecting arterial inflow in LTX [58]. In these circumstances, the use of a donor iliac arterial conduit from the infrarenal aorta (Fig. 13.11) or supraceliac aorta (Fig. 13.12) to the allograft may be necessary. Artificial conduits, e.g., polytetrafluoroethylene (PTFE) (Gortex®) grafts, can be used, but have been associated with a higher risk of thrombosis and infection.

The biliary anastomosis has been referred to as the "Achilles heel" of the LTX operation [59]. There are currently two commonly practised biliary reconstructions after LTX. The most common is the choledochocholedochostomy (duct-to-duct anastomosis) and the other is the hepaticojejunostom/ choledochojejunostomy (to a Roux-en-Y defunctionalized intestinal limb) (Fig. 13.13). The duct-to-duct anastomosis is usually done over a T tube, which remains as a stent in the duct for a few months (Fig. 13.13, insert). The advantages of leaving a T tube are the ability to quantify and characterize bile production as an early sign of hepatic allograft function, and to provide ready cholangiographic access to the biliary system in cases of abnormal liver function tests to rule out biliary problems. The disadvantage of the T tube is the risk of bile leak after removal of the tube, requiring emergent endoscopic retrograde cholangiopancreatography (ERCP) and decompression of the duct. Over time, transplant surgeons have abandoned the use of a T tube in duct-to-duct anastomosis [60–62], some using a catheter inserted into the recipient cystic duct remnant to retain access to the biliary system [63].

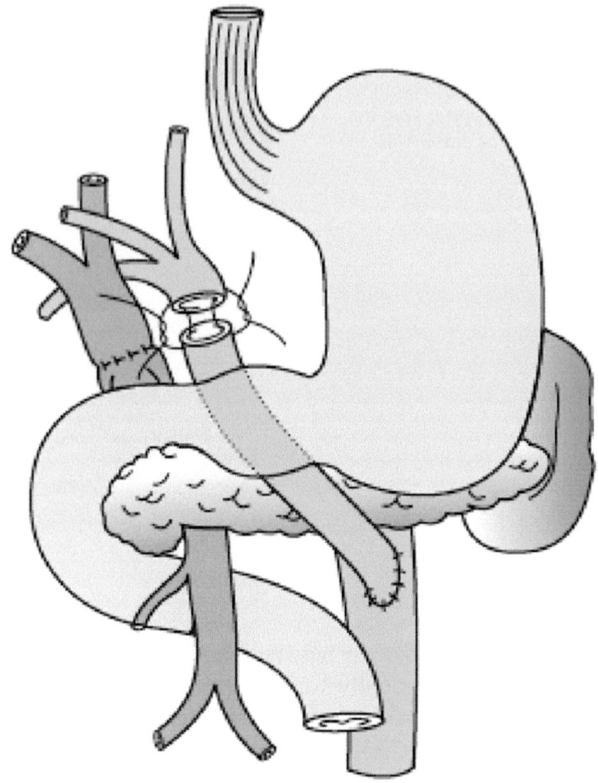

Fig. 13.11 Use of an interposition arterial graft from the infrarenal aorta to the allograft hepatic artery in the setting of inadequate recipient hepatic artery inflow

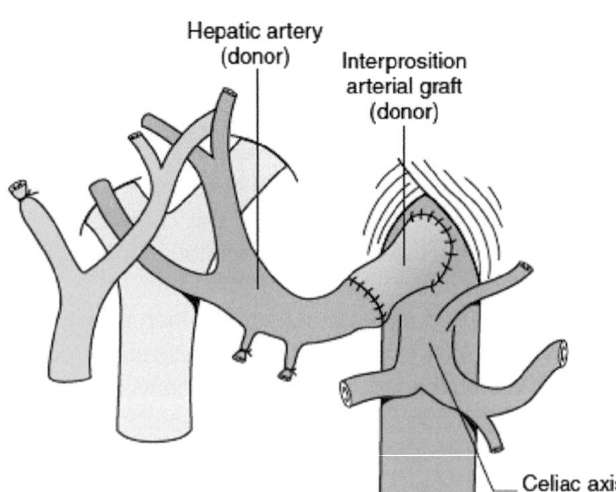

Fig. 13.12 Use of an interposition arterial graft from the supraceliac aorta to the allograft hepatic artery in the setting of inadequate recipient hepatic artery inflow

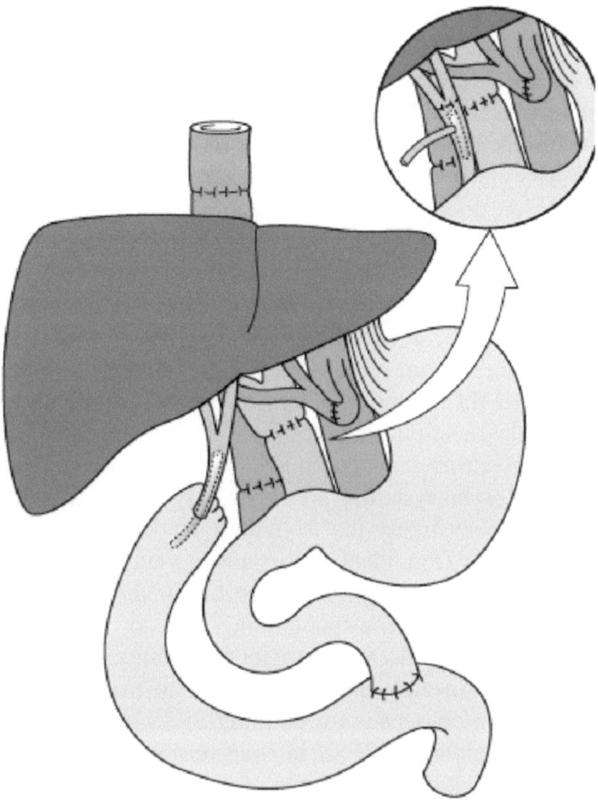

Fig. 13.13 Options for establishing biliary continuity using a hepaticojejunostomy over a temporary indwelling biliary stent or alternatively a primary duct-to-duct technique over a T tube (insert)

The use of stents in Roux-en-Y choledochojejunostomy is also a matter of controversy, and some surgeons have stopped using them because of complications such as retention of the stent and obstruction of the biliary system. Other "historic" types of biliary reconstructions include choledochoduodenostomy and the now defunct cholecystoduodenostomy (the "Wadell–Calne" biliary reconstruction) [64].

Complications

Complications after LTX have a significant impact on the outcome and cost of the procedure. The postoperative course in patients can range from straightforward to extremely complicated, and the outcome depends on the status of the recipient, the donor organ, and the technical conduct of the operation. Timely diagnosis of alterations in the normal postoperative course is the critical factor to minimize morbidity and mortality and to improve outcomes.

Primary Nonfunction

Primary nonfunction (PNF) is characterized by encephalopathy, coagulopathy, minimal bile output, and progressive renal and multisystem failure with increasing serum lactate levels and rapidly rising liver enzymes and histologic evidence of hepatocyte necrosis in the absence of any vascular complications. With better deceased donor management and selection, improved operative techniques, and newer preservation solutions, the risk of PNF has decreased but still occurs in somewhere between 2% and 4% of deceased donor LTX procedures. Various donor risk factors can be implicated in primary graft dysfunction; these include prolonged cold ischemia time, an unstable donor, high level of steatosis in the liver allograft, older donor, high serum sodium level in the donor, preformed lymphocytotoxic antibodies, ABO incompatibility, and recovered organs from DCD donors. Patients with initial dysfunction may recover with support but those who progress to show evidence of extrahepatic complications such as hemodynamic instability, renal failure, or other organ system dysfunction may require urgent retransplantation [65–67].

It has been argued that PNF does not occur in living donor liver transplants, since the livers are from ideal donors under controlled circumstances. Nevertheless, early graft loss and graft dysfunction occur in approximately 2–5% of adult-to-adult living donor liver transplantation, due to complications from "Small-for-Size Syndrome" (SFSS). SFSS is a recognizable clinical syndrome occurring in the presence of an insufficient mass of liver to maintain normal liver function [68–71]. Although a consensus for defining SFSS has yet to be fully defined, the common clinical features of SFSS include postoperative liver dysfunction with prolonged cholestasis and coagulopathy portal hypertension, and ascites. The underlying pathophysiology is excessive portal venous perfusion of the remnant liver, leading to endothelial cell damage, hemorrhage, and extreme intrahepatic manifestation of the hepatic artery buffer response, in which the inverse relationship between hepatic artery blood flow and portal venous blood flow, leads also to functional dearterialization of the remnant liver graft [72, 73]. Similar pathophysiological consequences can be seen with other small-for-size allografts, including deceased small pediatric-sized allografts and split liver allografts into larger adult recipients.

Hepatic Artery Stenosis/Thrombosis

Angiographic evidence of a greater than 50% reduction in the caliber of the lumen of the hepatic artery is defined as hepatic artery stenosis. This is reported in about 5% of cases after LTX. Clinically, these patients may show an increase in liver numbers or be entirely asymptomatic. Sonographically, the presence of a low resistive index of less than 0.5 with an increase in focal peak velocity is suggestive of this pathology [74–76]. The detection of hepatic artery stenosis early after LTX can usually be managed by surgical intervention, when the risk for anastomotic disruption by angioplasty is highest [77]. Percutaneous angioplasty is generally reserved for stenosis occurring several weeks after the transplant procedure, with over 90% success rate [78, 79].

Intimal dissection of the artery can result from too vigorous manipulation during surgery, either in the donor or the recipient, or from direct trauma to the artery from too forceful clamping. If not recognized early, intimal flaps will lead to arterial thrombosis. Complete thrombosis of the hepatic artery (HAT) is usually symptomatic and can be quite dramatic, especially when it occurs early in the posttransplant period and when it occurs in adults, more so than in children. Clinical presentations include: acute, massive necrosis with liver failure; the formation of a central biloma secondary to intrahepatic duct necrosis; multiple intrahepatic biliary structures; and/or intermittent bacteremia [80–82]. Occasionally, rarely in adults but more often in children, HAT can be asymptomatic. The factors that determine whether a liver fails or survives in the face of complete HAT are not known; however, the presence of collateral circulation (e.g., from the phrenic artery via vascularized adhesions to the liver) is usually associated with a more benign course after HAT. Segmental or lobar HAT has also been described—left HAT (usually associated with an injury to an unrecognized anomalous left hepatic artery arising from the left gastric artery) is generally benign. However, right HAT (usually associated with an injury to an unrecognized anomalous right hepatic artery arising from the superior mesenteric artery, or from technically imperfect reconstruction of the anomalous right hepatic artery at the back table) is associated with the development of biliary strictures, due to the dependence of biliary viability on hepatic artery blood flow. Angiography is the gold standard for diagnosis, but given clinical suspicion and early intervention of HAT with urgent revascularization, restoration of arterial patency may salvage the allograft [83, 84]. In addition, if available, the use of hyperbaric oxygen has been shown to rescue or delay the onset of necrosis in livers with HAT and is particularly effective in the smaller pediatric population [85]. However, the success of revascularization falls quickly when the period from thrombosis to revascularization is several days or longer, and a significant number of patients treated in this manner may still require retransplantation due to biliary complications and persistent biliary sepsis [86, 87].

Portal Vein Stenosis/Thrombosis

Portal vein stenosis can present shortly after LTX characterized by an increased production of ascites and liver allograft dysfunction. The cause is usually technical in nature, due to kinking or failure to incorporate a growth factor during the portal vein anastomosis, but may also be due to unrecognized proximal partial portal vein thrombosis or atresia of the portal vein, thus more frequently encountered in children with biliary atresia [88]. Ultrasonography and computed tomography (CT) angiography are usually diagnostic [89], while superior mesenteric artery angiography with late films is occasionally required for confirmation and subsequent planning for intervention. Treatment is by surgical intervention in early posttransplantation or by percutaneous transhepatic or transsplenic dilatation or stenting of the stricture later after LTX [90]. If left untreated, it can progress to complete thrombosis of the vein or severe graft dysfunction and hemodynamic instability secondary to a massive production of ascites, as well as the redevelopment of esophageal varices.

Portal vein thrombosis (PVT) is an uncommon but significant complication after adult LTX, but it is more common following pediatric LTX [88]. The incidence of PVT is also increased in patients in whom portal vein thrombectomy was performed as part of the original LTX. PVT can manifest by rapid graft dysfunction with the production of massive ascites. The differential diagnosis of portal-venous insufficiency includes technical errors such as kinking or redundancy of the portal vein, poor mesenteric flow secondary to the open collateral venous system (steal syndrome), and anastomotic stricture or twist. Treatment is immediate surgical revascularization of the graft by thrombectomy and correction of the technical problem, ligation of large collaterals in the portal-venous system, bypass grafting via the superior mesenteric vein, or percutaneous portal vein stenting. Otherwise, retransplantation may be the only therapeutic option.

Hepatic Venous Outflow Obstruction

Complications associated with vena caval stenosis include a 2.5–6% incidence of venous outflow obstruction (iatrogenic Budd–Chiari syndrome) caused by either rotation of the liver graft or anastomotic stricture [90]. Stenosis of the suprahepatic cava anastomosis can present with hepatic outflow obstruction in the form of liver allograft dysfunction, ascites formation, and impairment of renal function. The problem carries a high risk for morbidity and mortality. Although hepatic outflow obstruction occurs following both standard and piggyback techniques, it is more common with the piggyback procedure. One study showed a reduction in the incidence of venous outflow obstruction from 6% to 1% when the caval anastomosis was performed using a common orifice of the three native hepatic veins rather than an orifice created from only two hepatic veins [45]. Others have adopted a side-to-side cavo-cavoplasty in order to reduce the risk of stenosis [46, 47].

The diagnosis of hepatic vein outflow obstruction can be made by cavagram and measurements of the venous pressure gradients proximal and distal to the anastomosis. Treatment options are by angioplasty, stent placement, or surgical correction of the strictured area [91–96]. Anastomosis between the infrahepatic donor cava and the recipient cava with the piggyback technique can decompress the liver in patients with outflow obstruction secondary to anastomotic narrowing between the suprahepatic donor cava and the confluence of the hepatic vein in the recipient [49]. When all these measures fail, retransplantation may be the only option.

Biliary Complications

Biliary complications continue to pose a major area for complications after LTX, with an overall incidence of about 15–20% [97–99]. These complications range from early anastomotic leak to late stricture and obstruction, both in the extrahepatic or intrahepatic biliary system. The associated mortality rate with biliary complications is about 10% and this is mainly due to delays in diagnosis or misdiagnosis of the problem, secondary infectious complications, and graft dysfunction [100]. The biochemical abnormalities with elevation of bilirubin and canalicular enzymes (alkaline phosphatase and γ-glutamyltransferase) are not specific. These indicators of biliary obstruction are also seen in ischemic graft injury, rejection, recurrent hepatitis C virus (HCV), and sepsis. In order to make an accurate diagnosis, it is helpful to use imaging modalities like cholangiography, both transhepatic and endoscopic, to evaluate strictures, obstruction, or leak; ultrasonography for the detection of biliary dilatation; and radioisotope studies to evaluate anastomotic or cut surface leaks [101–103]. The use of magnetic resonance cholangiopancreatography (MRCP) has also proven to be of use in experienced centers [104].

The most common biliary complication is biliary stenosis. This is the result of either an imperfect anastomotic technique or ischemia of the bile duct, which, as it heals, leads to a stenotic area in the common bile duct, either at or slightly proximal to the biliary anastomosis, with proximal biliary dilatation. Recurrent bouts of cholangitis or persistent abnormal liver function tests may indicate an obstruction to bile outflow. In these cases, endoscopic or percutaneous balloon dilatation of the bile duct stricture and stenting have been successful [105–107]. In cases with no response, revision of the choledochojejunostomy or conversion of the duct-to-duct anastomosis to a choledochojejunostomy with a Roux-en-Y loop is the treatment of choice.

The papilla of Vater is innervated by fibers coursing through the hepatic branch of the vagus, and during hepatectomy, interrupting these branches can result in a syndrome known as "ampullary dysfunction" or "Sphincter of Oddi dysfunction" [108]. The radiologic examination of the biliary tree reveals dilatation of both the donor and recipient bile ducts, distal to the ampulla, many times with a "beak" sign. The treatment consists of endoscopic papillotomy, or conversion to a choledochojejunostomy.

Intrahepatic strictures of the biliary tree have been associated with a variety of risk factors [109]. In many cases, the strictures seem to be associated with a hepatic artery thrombosis or stenosis, and ischemia of the biliary tree is probably the etiology, especially in DCD [110]. Preservation damage of the allograft may result in multiple intrahepatic biliary strictures, with or without biliary sludge and casts. An immunologic association with a positive lymphocytotoxic-positive crossmatch has also been hypothesized as a cause of intrahepatic strictures. In some patients who were originally transplanted for primary sclerosing cholangitis, recurrence of the disease is a possibility [111–115]. While some patients with multiple intrahepatic strictures eventually need to be retransplanted, others can live for years with minimal difficulties, especially if they receive chronic antibiotic prophylaxis and appropriate dilatation of major strictures is performed. Recently, a grading system for intrahepatic biliary strictures and their projections for outcomes based on a large number of DCD liver transplant recipients was described [116].

The most feared complication of the biliary anastomosis is an anastomotic biliary leak. This complication can be lethal in choledochojejunostomies since the bile collection is rapidly infected with enteric organisms, which results in inflamed and friable tissues, making attempted repair more tenuous. The presence of continued enteric leak may result in mycotic rupture of the hepatic artery anastomosis. In choledochocholedochostomy, the leak usually occurs at the exit site of the T tube. In order to avoid this, a purse-string suture should be placed around the exit site. Leakage at the T tube exit site is usually self-containing, and no treatment is necessary so long as the distal bile duct empties well. Some surgeons have advocated not using any stenting following choledochocholedochostomy in an attempt to avoid the risk of T tube site leakage [60–62].

When a Roux-en-Y loop is used, bleeding can occur at the jejunojejunostomy anastomosis. In about half of the cases, this is a self-limiting problem; however, in the other half, endoscopic intervention with a pediatric colonoscope with a heater probe or epinephrine injection or the need for surgical exploration for hemostasis may be necessary. This complication can be avoided by using a hemostatic running suture to approximate the mucosa and submucosa. Another potentially lethal complication of Roux-en-Y biliary drainage, generally occurring late after LTX, is an unrecognized internal herniation of bowel through the mesentery at the jejunojejunostomy, leading to unexplained abdominal distention and pain-out-of-proportion to physical findings, related to small bowel volvulus that can progress to vascular compromise and loss of intestinal viability. Prompt recognition is critical, and CT scans may reveal findings of a closed-loop obstruction. Careful closure of the defect in the mesentery at the time of LTX can reduce this complication [117].

Bleeding

Poor graft function, coagulopathy, imperfect hemostasis, or slippage of a tie may result in postoperative bleeding requiring reexploration. Postoperative bleeding is reported to occur between 7% and 15% of patients and requires reexploration in approximately half of them [118]. Even if easily controlled, postoperative bleeding leads to increased cost, morbidity, and mortality. Thus, meticulous attention to intraoperative hemostasis and correction of coagulopathy will reduce the likelihood of postoperative hemorrhage. Early reexploration is indicated when the volume of blood transfusions exceeds 4 units within 24 h.

Survey of Liver Transplantation Practices

An international survey of the practice of performing deceased donor LTX was conducted by Cherqui and coworkers and reported in 2011 [119]. This survey, Survey on Adult Liver Transplantation (SALT), encompassed 50 centers in Europe, eight centers in North America, two in South America, one in South Africa, and three in the Middle East. As shown in Table 13.1, there is considerable

Table 13.1 Summary of the SALT survey on the practice of liver transplantation

Technique used	World	United States	Europe
IVC preservation (piggyback):			
Always		4%	29%
Never		0%	4%
Selectively		4%	18%
Temporary portacaval shunt used:			
Yes		0%	58%
Type of caval anastomosis:			
Piggyback—three hepatic veins		22%	36%
Piggyback—two hepatic veins		33%	13%
Side-to-side		22%	38%
Other		23%	13%
Placement of aortic conduit:			
Supraceliac		17%	30%
Infrarenal		33%	49%
Either		50%	41%
Biliary anastomosis			
Use of stents			
Duct-to-duct without T tube	75%	86%	72%
Duct-to-duct with T tube	24%	14%	26%
Suture technique:			
Posterior running and anterior interrupted	16%	10%	14%
Interrupted	47%	50%	46%
Running	37%	40%	40%
Use of drains:			
None	10%		
One drain	20%		
Two drains	43%		
Three drains	18%		
Other	9%		
Closure:			
Full thickness		25%	10%
By layer		75%	90%

intercontinental variation in some specific aspects of the LTX procedure outlined in this chapter.

Of note was that preservation of the IVC (for piggyback implantation) was the most frequently used technique—used routinely by 57% of the teams and selectively by 38%. The use of venous bypass was in 15% of cases of IVC preservation and in 58% when the IVC was resected. Several types of venous outflow reconstruction were used—the most common being piggyback on the stump of two or three hepatic veins, followed by a side-to-side caval anastomosis. Lastly, the duct-to-duct biliary anastomosis was most often used as the standard biliary reconstructive technique, with a T tube being used in 25% of the programs on a routine basis.

Given the excellent outcomes obtained around the world, it suggests that these modifications are rather insignificant in the hands of experienced surgeons in the current era of LTX.

Conclusions

While the results of LTX have improved dramatically over the past 60 years, many of the same technical considerations have plagued the procedure since its inception. With the increasing complexity of candidates undergoing LTX, an improved understanding of the pathophysiology of donor organ preservation, reperfusion injury, improved immunosuppression, more effective diagnostic tools, and new anti-infective agents have all contributed to a smoother posttransplant course. The application of ex vivo machine perfusion has increased the utilization of expanded criteria donors and has positively impacted the posttransplant course with improved function, reduced LOS and complications. Nevertheless, all of these advances cannot negate a poorly performed technical procedure. Modifications of the standard LTX, with adoption of segmental allografts, emphasize even more the impact to which technical complications play in short- and long-term outcomes.

References

1. Staudacher V. Trapianti di Organi con Anostomosi Vascolari. Riforma Med. 1952;66(39): 1060.
2. Starzl TE, Kaupp HA, Brock DR, Lazarus RE, Johnson RV. Reconstructive problems in canine homotransplantations with special reference to the postoperative role of hepatic venous flow. Surg Gynecol Obstet. 1960;111:733–43.
3. Starzl TE, Marchioro TL, von Kaulla KN, Hermann G, Brittain RS, Waddell WR. Homotransplantaion of the liver in humans. Surg Gynecol Obstet. 1963;117:659–76.
4. Moore FD, Dagher F, Veith F, et al. Immunosuppression and vascular insufficiency in liver transplantation. Ann N Y Acad Sci. 1964;102:729–38.
5. Kuss R, Bourget P. An illustrated history of organ transplantation. Rueil–Malmaison: Sandoz; 1992.
6. Starzl TE, Groth CG, Brettschneider L, et al. Orthotopic homotransplantation of the human liver. Ann Surg. 1968;168:392–415.
7. Calne RY, Williams R. Liver transplantation in man. I. Observations of technique and organization in five cases. Br Med J. 1968;4:535–40.
8. Starzl TE, Putnam CW. Experience in hepatic transplantation. Philadelphia: WB Saunders; 1969. p. 131–5.
9. Bismuth H, Houssin D. Reduced-sized orthotopic liver graft in hepatic transplantation in children. Surgery. 1984;95:367–70.
10. Pichlmayr R, Ringe B, Gubernatis G, et al. Transplantation of a donor liver to 2 recipients (splitting transplantation): a new method in the further development of segmental liver transplantation. Langenbecks Arch Chir. 1988;373:127–30.
11. Diamond IR, Fecteau A, Millis JM, Losanoff JE, Ng V, Anand R, Song C. SPLIT Research Group: Impact of graft type on outcome in pediatric liver transplantation: a report from Studies of Pediatric Liver Transplantation (SPLIT). Ann Surg. 2007;246:301–10.

12. Bismuth H, Morino M, Castaing D, Gillon MC, Descorps Declere A, Saliba F, Samuel D. Emergency orthotopic liver transplantation in two patients using one donor liver. Br J Surg. 1989;76:722–4.
13. Emond JC, Whitington PF, Thistlethwaite JR, Cherqui D, Alonso EA, Woodle IS, Vogelbach P, Busse-Henry SM, Zucker AR, Broelsch CE. Transplantation of two patients with one liver. Analysis of a preliminary experience with 'split-liver' grafting. Ann Surg. 1990;212:14–22.
14. Lee WC, Chan KM, Chou HS, et al. Feasibility of split liver transplantation for 2 adults in the model of end-stage liver disease era. Ann Surg. 2013;258:306–11.
15. Hashimoto K, Quintini C, Aucejo FN, et al. Split liver transplantation using Hemiliver graft in the MELD era: a single center experience in the United States. Am J Transplant. 2014;14:2072–80.
16. Strong RW, Lynch SV, Ong TH, Matsunami H, Koido Y, Balderson GA. Successful liver transplantation from a living donor to her son. N Engl J Med. 1990;322:1505–7.
17. Millis JM, Cronin DC, Brady LM, Newell KA, Woodle ES, Bruce DS, Thistlethwaite JR, Broelsch CE. Primary living-donor liver transplantation at the University of Chicago: technical aspects of the first 104 recipients. Ann Surg. 2000;232(1):104–11. https://doi.org/10.1097/00000658-200007000-00015. PMID: 10862202; PMCID: PMC1421114.
18. Hashikura Y, Makuuchi M, Kawasaki S, Matsunami H, Ikegami T, Nakazawa Y, Kiyosawa K, Ichida T. Successful living-related partial liver transplantation to an adult patient. Lancet. 1994;343:1233–4.
19. Lo CM, Fan ST, Liu CL, Wei WI, Lo RJ, Lai CL, Chan JK, Ng IO, Fung A, Wong J. Adult-to-adult living donor liver transplantation using extended right lobe grafts. Ann Surg. 1997;226:261–9.
20. Miller CM, Gondolesi GE, Florman S, Matsumoto C, Muñoz L, Yoshizumi T, Artis T, Fishbein TM, Sheiner PA, Kim-Schluger L, Schiano T, Shneider BL, Emre S, Schwartz ME. One hundred nine living donor liver transplants in adults and children: a single-center experience. Ann Surg. 2001;234:301–11.
21. Chan SC, Fan ST, Lo CM, Liu CL, Wei WI, Chik BH, Wong J. A decade of right liver adult-to-adult living donor liver transplantation: the recipient mid-term outcomes. Ann Surg. 2008;248:411–9.
22. Yoshizumi T, Ikegami T, Kimura K, Uchiyama H, Ikeda T, Shirabe K, Maehara Y. Selection of a right posterior sector graft for living donor liver transplantation. Liver Transpl. 2014;20:1089–96.
23. Song GW, Lee SG, Moon DB, Ahn CS, Hwang S, Kim KH, Ha TY, Jung DH. Dual-graft adult living donor liver transplantation: an innovative surgical procedure for live liver donor pool expansion. Ann Surg. 2017;266(1):10–18. https://doi.org/10.1097/SLA.0000000000001776. PMID: 27192349.
24. Colombani P, Dunn S, Harmon W, Magee J, McDiarmid S, Spray T. Pediatric transplantation. Am J Transplant. 2003;3(Suppl 4):53–63.
25. Sakamoto S, Uemoto S, Uryuhara K, Kim I, Kiuchi T, Egawa H, Inomata Y, Tanaka K. Graft size assessment and analysis of donors for living donor liver transplantation using right lobe. Transplantation. 2001;71(10):1407–13.
26. Fan ST. Live donor liver transplantation in adults. Transplantation. 2006;82:723–32.
27. Shimada M, Shiotani S, Ninomiya M, Terashi T, Hiroshige S, Minagawa R, et al. Characteristics of liver grafts in living-donor adult liver transplantation: comparison between right- and left-lobe grafts. Arch Surg. 2002;137(10):1174–9.
28. Shah SA, Cattral MS, McGilvray ID, Adcock LD, Gallagher G, Smith R, et al. Selective use of older adults in right lobe living donor liver transplantation. Am J Transplant. 2007;7(1):142–50.
29. Yoshizumi T, Taketomi A, Soejima Y, Uchiyama H, Ikegami T, Harada N, et al. Impact of donor age and recipient status on left-lobe graft for living donor adult liver transplantation. Transpl Int. 2008;21(1):81–8.

30. Yamamoto K, Takada Y, Fujimoto Y, Haga H, Oike F, Kobayashi N, Tanaka K. Nonalcoholic steatohepatitis in donors for living donor liver transplantation. Transplantation. 2007;83(3):257–62.
31. Marino IR, Doyle HR, Fung JJ. Liver. In: Higgins RSD, Sanchez JS, Lorber MI, Baldwin JC, editors. The multi-organ donor. Selection and management. Oxford: Blackwell Science; 1997. p. 241–64.
32. Feng S, Goodrich NP, Bragg-Gresham JL, et al. Characteristics associated with liver graft failure. The concept of a donor risk index. Am J Transplant. 2006;6:783–90.
33. Eghtesad B, Kadry Z, Fung J. Technical considerations in liver transplantation: what a hepatologist needs to know (and every surgeon should practice). Liver Transpl. 2005;11(8):861–71.
34. Shaw BW, Marquez JM, Kang YG, et al. Venous bypass in clinical liver transplantation. Ann Surg. 1984;200:524–34.
35. Chari RS, Gan TJ, Robertson KM, et al. Venovenous bypass in adult orthotopic liver transplantation. Routine or selective use? J Am Coll Surg. 1998;186:683–90.
36. Khoury GF, Mann ME, Porot MJ, Abdul-Rasool IH, Busuttil RW. Air embolism associated with venovenous bypass during orthotopic liver transplantation. Anaesthesiology. 1987;67:848–51.
37. Navalgund AA, Kang Y, Sarner JB, Jahr JS, Gieraerts R. Massive pulmonary thromboembolism during liver transplantation. Anesth Analg. 1988;67:400–2.
38. Katirji MB. Brachial plexus injury following liver transplantation. Neurology. 1989;39:736–8.
39. Ozaki CF, Langnas AN, Bynon JS, et al. A percutaneous method for venovenous bypass in liver transplantation. Transplantation. 1994;57:472–3.
40. Budd JM, Isaac JL, Bennet J, Freeman JW. Morbidity and mortality associated with large-bore percutaneous venovenous bypass cannulation for 312 orthotopic liver transplantations. Liver Transpl. 2001;7:359–62.
41. Wall WJ, Grant DR, Duff JH, Kutt JL, Ghent CN, Bloch MS. Liver transplantation without venous bypass. Transplantation. 1987;43:56–61.
42. Stock PG, Payne WD, Ascher NL, et al. Rapid infusion technique as a safe alternative to veno-venous bypass in orthotopic liver transplant. Transplant Proc. 1989;21:2322–5.
43. Tzakis A, Todo S, Starzl TE. Orthotopic liver transplantation with preservation of the inferior vena cava. Ann Surg. 1989;210:649–52.
44. Parrilla P, Sánchez-Bueno F, Figueras J, et al. Analysis of the complications of the piggyback technique in 1,112 liver transplants. Transplantation. 1999;67:1214–7.
45. Robles R, Parrilla P, Acosta F, et al. Complications related to hepatic venous outflow in piggyback liver transplantation. Two versus three suprahepatic vein anastomosis. Transplant Proc. 1999;31:2390–1.
46. Belghiti J, Noun R, Sauvanet A. Temporary portocaval anastomosis with preservation of caval flow during orthotopic. Am J Surg. 1995;169:277–9.
47. Bismuth H, Castaing D, Sherlock DJ. Liver transplantation by face-a-face vena cavaplasty. Surgery. 1992;111:151–5.
48. Belghiti J, Panis Y, Sauvanet A, Gayet B, Fékété F. A new technique of side to side caval anastomosis during orthotopic hepatic transplantation without inferior vena caval occlusion. Surg Gynecol Obstet. 1992;175:270–2.
49. Quintini C, Miller CM, Hashimoto K, et al. Side-to-side cavocavostomy with an endovascular stapler. Rescue technique for severe hepatic vein and/or inferior vena cava outflow obstruction after liver transplantation using the piggyback technique. Liver Transpl. 2009;15:49–53.
50. Aggarwal S, Kang Y, Freeman J, DeWolf AM, Begliomini B. Is there a post-reperfusion syndrome? Transplant Proc. 1989;21(3):3497–9.
51. Paugam-Burtz C, Kavafyan J, Merckx P, Dahmani S, Sommacale D, Ramsay M, Belghiti J, Mantz J. Postreperfusion syndrome during liver transplantation for cirrhosis: outcome and predictors. Liver Transpl. 2009;15(5):522–9.
52. Yerdel MA, Gunson B, Mirza D, et al. Portal vein thrombosis in adults undergoing liver transplantation. Risk factors, screening, management, and outcome. Transplantation. 2000;69:1873–81.

53. Stieber AC, Zetti G, Todo S, et al. The spectrum of portal vein thrombosis in liver transplantation. Ann Surg. 1991;213(3):199–206.
54. Tzakis AG, Kirkegaard P, Pinna AD, et al. Liver transplantation with cavoportal hemitransposition in the presence of diffuse portal vein thrombosis. Transplantation. 1998;65(5):619–24.
55. Kato T, Levi DM, DeFaria W, Nishida S, Tzakis AG. Liver transplantation with renoportal anastomosis after distal splenorenal shunt. Arch Surg. 2000;135(12):1401–4. https://doi.org/10.1001/archsurg.135.12.1401. PMID: 11115340.
56. Erhard J, Lange R, Giebler R, Rauen U, de Groot H, Eigler FW. Arterialization of the portal vein in orthotopic and auxiliary liver transplantation. A report of three cases. Transplantation. 1995;60:877–9.
57. Sanada Y, Mizuta K, Urahashi T, Wakiya T, Ihara Y, Okada N, Yamada N, Nakata M, Yasuda Y. Impact of posttransplant portosystemic shunts on liver transplantation. World J Surg. 2012;36(10):2449–54. https://doi.org/10.1007/s00268-012-1692-z. PMID: 22744218.
58. Jurim O, Shaked A, Kiai K, Millis JM, Colquhoun SD, Busuttil RW. Celiac compression syndrome and liver transplantation. Ann Surg. 1993;218:10–2.
59. Calne RY. A new technique for biliary drainage in orthotopic liver transplantation utilizing the gall bladder as a pedicle graft conduit between the donor and recipient common bile ducts. Ann Surg. 1976;184:605–9.
60. Koivusalo A, Isoniemi H, Salmela K, Edgren J, von Numers H, Höckerstedt K. Biliary complications in one hundred adult liver transplantations. Scand J Gastroenterol. 1996;31:506–11.
61. Shimoda M, Saab S, Morrisey M, et al. A cost effectiveness analysis of biliary anastomosis with or without T-tube after orthotopic liver transplantation. Am J Transplant. 2001;1:157–61.
62. Scatton O, Meunier B, Cherqui D, et al. Randomized trial of choledochocholedocostomy with or without T-tube in orthotopic liver transplantation. Ann Surg. 2001;233:432–7.
63. Sawyer RG, Punch JD. Incidence and management of biliary complications after 291 liver transplants following the introduction of transcystic stenting. Transplantation. 1998;66(9):1201–7. https://doi.org/10.1097/00007890-199811150-00015. PMID: 9825818.
64. Busuttil RW, Tanaka K. The utility of marginal donors in liver transplantation. Liver Transpl. 2003;9:651–63.
65. González FX, Rimola A, Grande L, et al. Predictive factors of early postoperative graft function in human liver transplantation. Hepatology. 1994;20:565–73.
66. Bezeizi KI, Jalan R, Plevris JN, Hayes PC. Primary graft dysfunction after liver transplantation. From pathogenesis to prevention. Liver Transpl. 1997;3:137–48.
67. Olthoff KM, Kulik L, Samstein B, Kaminski M, Abecassis M, Emond J, Shaked A, Christie JD. Validation of a current definition of early allograft dysfunction in liver transplant recipients and analysis of risk factors. Liver Transpl. 2010;16(8):943–9.
68. Lo CM, Fan ST, Chan JK, Wei W, Lo RJ, Lai CL. Minimum graft volume for successful adult-to-adult living donor liver transplantation for fulminant hepatic failure. Transplantation. 1996;62:696–8.
69. Kiuchi T, Kasahara M, Uryhara K, Inomata Y, Uemoto S, Asomuma K. Impact of graft size mismatching on graft prognosis in liver transplantation from living donors. Transplantation. 1999;67:521–7.
70. Nishizaki T, Ikegami T, Hiroshige S, Hashimoto K, Uchiyama H, Yoshizumi T, Kishikawa K, Shimada M, Sugimachi K. Small graft for living donor liver transplantation. Ann Surg. 2001;233:575–80.
71. Kelly DM, Demetris AJ, Fung JJ, Marcos A, Zhu Y, Subbotin V, Yin L, Totsuka E, Ishii T, Lee MC, Gutierrez J, Costa G, Venkataraman R, Madariaga JR. Porcine partial liver transplantation: a novel model of the “small-for-size” liver graft. Liver Transpl. 2004;10(2):253–63.
72. Kelly D, Zhu X, Shiba H, Irefin S, Trenti L, Cocieru A, Quintini C, Diago-Uso T, Nakagawa S, Fung J. Adenosine restores the hepatic artery buffer response (HABR) and improves survival in a porcine model of the small-for-size syndrome (SFSS). Liver Transpl. 2009;15:1448–57.
73. Demetris AJ, Kelly DM, Eghtesad B, Fontes P, Wallis Marsh J, Tom K, Tan HP, Shaw-Stiffel T, Boig L, Novelli P, Planinsic R, Fung JJ, Marcos AJ. Pathophysiologic observations and

histopathologic recognition of the portal hyperperfusion or small-for-size syndrome. Am J Surg Pathol. 2006;30:986–93.
74. Stange BJ, Glanemann M, Nuessler NC, Settmacher U, Steinmuller T, Neuhaus P. Hepatic artery thrombosis after adult liver transplantation. Liver Transpl. 2003;9:612–20.
75. Dodd GD 3rd, Memel DS, Zajko AB, Baron RL, Santaguida LA. Hepatic artery stenosis and thrombosis in transplant recipients. Doppler diagnosis with resistive index and systolic acceleration time. Radiology. 1994;192:657–61.
76. Nolten A, Sproat IA. Hepatic artery thrombosis after liver transplantation. Temporal accuracy of diagnosis with duplex-US and the syndrome of impending thrombosis. Radiology. 1996;198:553–9.
77. Sheiner PA, Varma CV, Guarrera JV, et al. Selective revascularization of hepatic artery thrombosis after liver transplantation improves patient and graft survival. Transplantation. 1997;64:1295–9.
78. Mondragon RS, Karani JB, Heaton ND, et al. The use of percutaneous transluminal angioplasty in hepatic artery stenosis after liver transplantation. Transplantation. 1994;57:228–31.
79. Orons PD, Zajko AB, Bron KM, Trecha GT, Selby RR, Fung JJ. Hepatic artery angioplasty after liver transplantation. Experience in 21 allografts. J Vasc Interv Radiol. 1995;6:523–9.
80. Tzakis AG, Gordon RD, Shaw BW Jr, Iwatsuki S, Starzl TE. Clinical presentation of hepatic artery thrombosis after liver transplantation in the cyclosporine era. Transplantation. 1985;40:667–71.
81. Bhattacharjya S, Gunson BK, Mirza DF, et al. Delayed hepatic artery thrombosis in adult orthotopic liver transplantation. A 12-year experience. Transplantation. 2001;71:1592–6.
82. Tzakis AG. The dearterialized liver graft. Semin Liver Dis. 1985;5:375–6.
83. Pinna AD, Smith CV, Furukawa H, Starzl TE, Fung JJ. Urgent revascularization of liver allografts after early hepatic artery thrombosis. Transplantation. 1996;62:1584–7.
84. Yanaga K, Lebeau G, Marsh JW. Hepatic artery reconstruction for hepatic artery thrombosis after liver transplantation. Arch Surg. 1990;125:628–31.
85. Mazariegos GV, O'Toole KO, Mieles LA, Dvorchik I, Meza M, Briassoulis G, Arzate J, Osorio G, Fung JJ, Reyes J. Hyperbaric oxygen therapy for hepatic artery thrombosis after liver transplantation in children. Liver Transplant Surg. 1999;5(5):429–36.
86. Rabin JM, Roof SL, Cordless CL, et al. Hepatic allograft abscess with hepatic arterial thrombosis. Am J Surg. 1998;175:354–9.
87. Tarzan K, Shacked A, Although KM. Etiology and management of symptomatic adult hepatic artery thrombosis after orthotopic liver transplantation. Am Surg. 1996;62:237–40.
88. Vasavada B, Chen CL. Vascular complications in biliary atresia patients undergoing living donor liver transplantation: analysis of 110 patients over 10 years. J Indian Assoc Pediatr Surg. 2015;20(3):121–6.
89. Crossing JD, Mirada D, Wilson SR. Ultrasound of liver transplants: normal and abnormal. Radiographic. 2003;23:1093–114.
90. Ohm JY, Ko GY, Sung KB, Gwon DI, Ko HK. Safety and efficacy of transhepatic and transsplenic access for endovascular management of portal vein complications after liver transplantation. Liver Transpl. 2017;23(9):1133–42. https://doi.org/10.1002/lt.24737. PMID: 28152572.
91. Settmacher U, Nussler NC, Glanemann M, et al. Venous complications after orthotopic liver transplantation. Clin Transpl. 2000;14:235–41.
92. Tsiotos GG, Nagorney DM, de Groen PC. Selective management of hepatic venous outflow obstruction. J Gastrointest Surg. 1997;1:377–85.
93. Althaus SJ, Perkins JD, Soltes G, Glickerman D. Use of a Wallstent in successful treatment of IVC obstruction following liver transplantation. Transplantation. 1996;61:669–72.
94. Simó G, Echenagusia A, Camúñez F, et al. Stenosis of the inferior vena cava after liver transplantation. Treatment with Gianturco expandable metallic stent. Cardiovasc Interv Radiol. 1993;18:212–6.
95. Stieber AS, Gordon RD, Bassi N. A simple solution to a technical complication in "piggy back" liver transplantation. Transplantation. 1997;64:654–5.

96. Gunasekaran G, Bencsath K, Hupertz V, Fung JJ, Pettersson G, Miller C. Deep hypothermia with circulatory arrest to aid in the management of suprahepatic vena cava stenosis after liver transplantation. Liver Transpl. 2010;16:1434–6.
97. O'Connor TP, Lewis WD, Jenkins RL. Biliary tract complications after liver transplantation. Arch Surg. 1995;130:312–7.
98. Qian YB, Liu CL, Lo CM, Fan ST. Risk factors for biliary complications after liver transplantation. Arch Surg. 2004;139:1101–5.
99. Nemec P, Ondrásek J, Studeník P, Hökl J, Cern J. Biliary complications in liver transplantation. Ann Transplant. 2001;6:24–8.
100. Greif F, Bronsther OL, Van Thiel DH, et al. The incidence, timing, and management of biliary tract complications after orthotopic liver transplantation. Ann Surg. 1994;219:40–5.
101. Kurzawinski TR, Selves L, Farouk M. Prospective study of hepatobiliary scintigraphy and endoscopic cholangiography for the detection of early biliary complications after orthotopic liver transplantation. Br J Surg. 1997;84:620–3.
102. Sung RS, Campbell DA Jr, Rudich SM, et al. Long-term follow-up of percutaneous transhepatic balloon cholangioplasty in the management of biliary strictures after liver transplantation. Transplantation. 2004;77:110–5.
103. Thuluvath PJ, Atassi T, Lee J. An endoscopic approach to biliary complications following orthotopic liver transplantation. Liver Int. 2003;23:156–62.
104. Xu YB, Min ZG, Jiang HX, Qin SY, Hu BL. Diagnostic value of magnetic resonance cholangiopancreatography for biliary complications in orthotopic liver transplantation: a meta-analysis. Transplant Proc. 2013;45(6):2341–6.
105. Shah S, Dooley J, Agarwal R, et al. Routine endoscopic retrograde cholangiography in the detection of early biliary complications after liver transplantation. Liver Transpl. 2002;8:491–4.
106. Mata A, Bordas JM, Llach J, et al. ERCP in orthotopic liver transplanted patients. Hepato-Gastroenterology. 2004;51:1801–4.
107. Rizk RS, McVicar JP, Emond MJ, et al. Endoscopic management of biliary strictures in liver transplant recipient: effect on patient and graft survival. Gastrointest Endosc. 1998;47:128–35.
108. Douzdjian V, Abecassis MM, Johlin FC. Sphincter of Oddi dysfunction following liver transplantation. Screening by bedside manometry and definitive manometric evaluation. Dig Dis Sci. 1994;39(2):253–6.
109. Nakamura N, Nishida S, Neff GR, et al. Intrahepatic biliary strictures without hepatic artery thrombosis after liver transplantation. An analysis of 1113 liver transplants at a single center. Transplantation. 2005;79:427–32.
110. Abt P, Crawford M, Desai N, Markmann J, Olthoff K, Shaked A. Liver transplantation from controlled non-heart-beating donors. An increased incidence of biliary complications. Transplantation. 2003;75:1659–63.
111. Khettry U, Keaveny A, Goldar-Najafi A, et al. Liver transplantation for primary sclerosing cholangitis. A long-term clinicopathologic study. Hum Pathol. 2003;34:1127–36.
112. Gopal DV, Corless CL, Rabkins JM, Olyaei AJ, Rosen HR. Graft failure from severe recurrent primary sclerosing cholangitis following orthotopic liver transplantation. J Clin Gastroenterol. 2003;37:344–7.
113. Balan V, Abu-Elmagd K, Demetris AJ. Autoimmune liver disease. Recurrence after liver transplantation. Surg Clin North Am. 1999;79:147–52.
114. Neuberger J. Recurrence of primary biliary cirrhosis, primary sclerosing cholangitis and autoimmune hepatitis. Liver Transpl. 1995;1:109–15.
115. Vera A, Moledina S, Gunson B, et al. Risk factors for recurrence of primary sclerosing cholangitis of liver allograft. Lancet. 2002;360:1943–4.
116. Lee HW, Suh KS, Shin WY, et al. Classification and prognosis of intrahepatic biliary stricture after liver transplantation. Liver Transpl. 2007;13:1736–42.
117. Khanna A, Newman B, Reyes J, Fung JJ, Todo T, Starzl TE. Internal hernia and volvulus of the small bowel following liver transplantation. Transpl Int. 1997;10:133–6.

118. Ozaki CF, Katz SM, Monsour HP. Surgical complications of liver transplantation. Surg Clin North Am. 1994;74:1155–67.
119. Kluger MD, Memeo R, Laurent A, Tayar C, Cherqui D. Survey of adult liver transplantation techniques (SALT): an international study of current practices in deceased donor liver transplantation. HPB. 2011;13(10):692–8.

Deceased Donation and Liver Transplantation

14

Alicia Pérez-Blanco, Eduardo Miñambres, and Beatriz Domínguez-Gil

Abbreviations

DC	Donor Coordinator
DCDD	Donation after the circulatory determination of death
DNDD	Donation after the neurological determination of death
EAD	Early Allograft Dysfunction
ECMO	Extracorporeal Membrane Oxygenation
ICOD	Intensive Care to Facilitate Organ Donation
LT	Liver Transplantation
MAiD	Medical Assistance in Dying
NRP	Normothermic Regional Perfusion
OPO	Organ Procurement Organization
PNF	Primary Non-Function
SRR	Standard Rapid Recovery
WLST	Withdrawal of Life-Sustaining Therapies

A. Pérez-Blanco · B. Domínguez-Gil (✉)
Organización Nacional de Trasplantes, Madrid, Spain
e-mail: bdominguez@mscbs.es

E. Miñambres
Transplant Coordination Unit & Service of Intensive Care, University Hospital Marqués de Valdecilla-IDIVAL. School of Medicine, Universidad de Cantabria, Santander, Spain

B. Eghtesad et al. (eds.), *Liver Transplantation*,
https://doi.org/10.1007/978-3-032-07072-2_14

Introduction

Since Thomas Starzl performed the first human liver transplant (LT) in 1963, this therapy has undergone remarkable evolution, now delivering exceptional outcomes in both quality and length of life for patients with no other viable treatment options. According to data from the Global Observatory on Organ Donation and Transplantation, over 41,000 LT procedures were conducted worldwide in 2023 [1].

LT differs from other health interventions because it demands not only technical expertise and material resources, but also access to a donated organ, sourced either from a deceased or a living individual. LT activity levels vary significantly across countries (Fig. 14.1) [1]. While some regions have achieved high LT rates through the use of live donor organs, the majority of LT procedures worldwide rely on organs from deceased donors [2]. Consequently, the overall LT activity in a given area is closely tied to the availability and frequency of deceased organ donation.

Deceased donation rates also vary across jurisdictions, as shown in Fig. 14.2. While a minimum level of development seems necessary to facilitate deceased donation, disparities persist even among countries with high levels of human development. Several factors have been proposed to explain these variations. One widely discussed factor is the consent policy in place. Some scholars argue that an opt-out system, also known as presumed consent—where individuals are considered organ donors unless they have explicitly opted out during their lifetime—has a positive impact on donation rates. However, studies examining the relationship between the type of consent policy and donation rates have produced conflicting results [3, 4]. Furthermore, no country has demonstrated a sustained increase in deceased donation rates solely due to the adoption of an opt-out system [5]. Another theory is that higher mortality rates associated with organ donation (such as those from traffic accidents or cerebrovascular diseases) could correlate with higher donation rates. Yet, in European countries, a steady decline in these mortality rates has been observed alongside a consistent increase in the number of donors, only interrupted by the COVID-19 pandemic [6]. Additionally, a 2007 survey conducted by the European Commission found no correlation between the population's willingness to donate organs and the actual rate of deceased donation activities [7]. Disparities in deceased donation are more likely attributed to differences in the organizational approaches to managing the deceased donation pathway—a highly complex process that extends from the identification of possible organ donors (persons who have died or are about to die in conditions consistent with organ donation) to the successful recovery of organs usable for transplantation [8].

This chapter examines the pathway of deceased donation, detailing how it unfolds depending on the circumstances of an individual's death. It also highlights the critical role of donor coordinators in managing and streamlining this intricate process. Special emphasis is placed on the importance of integrating organ donation into end-of-life care and of engaging the critical care community to routinely consider organ donation as a fundamental component of their professional practice.

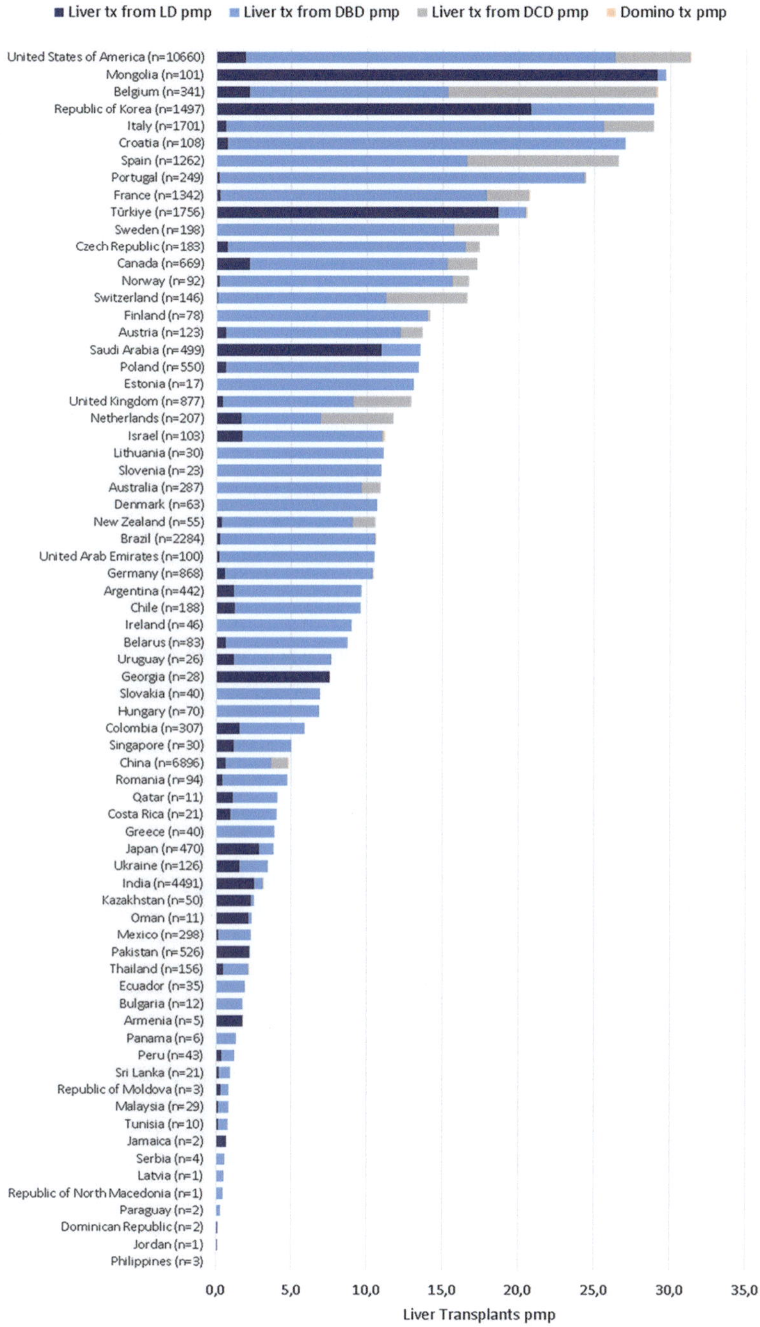

Fig. 14.1 Liver transplantation activity per million population (pmp) in countries reporting to the Global Observatory on Organ Donation and Transplantation (GODT); 71 out of 93 countries participating in the GODT reported 41,099 liver transplants. Liver transplants from living, DNDD and DCDD donors, and domino liver transplants pmp. In brackets, absolute number of liver transplants. Year 2023. (Source: http://www.transplant-observatory.org/)

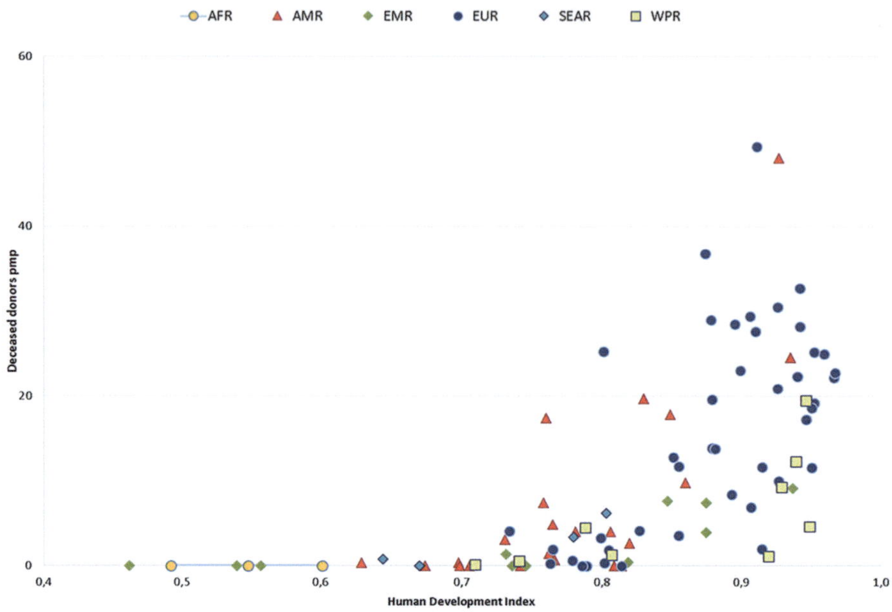

Fig. 14.2 Deceased donors per million population (pmp) and human development index in countries reporting to the Global Observatory on Organ Donation and Transplantation. Year 2023. (Source: http://www.transplant-observatory.org/)

Deceased Donation Pathways and Their Impact on Liver Transplantation

Deceased organ donation usually begins with identifying patients who have suffered a devastating brain injury or lesion and can be declared dead based on neurological criteria [9]. This activates the process of DNDD. Alternatively, donation may commence when a decision is made to withdraw life-sustaining therapies (WLST) that are deemed no longer beneficial to the patient. This initiates the pathway of controlled donation after the circulatory determination of death (cDCDD). In jurisdictions where medical assistance in dying (MAiD) is legally permitted, this latest pathway can also be activated in such context of death [10]. Lastly, uncontrolled donation after the circulatory determination of death (uDCDD) applies to cases where a patient dies following an unexpected cardiac arrest that resuscitation efforts fail to reverse. Currently, DCDD is implemented in a limited number of countries [1, 11]. Barriers to its development include legal-ethical concerns, insufficient technical or organizational capacity, and a lack of professional or public confidence in the program [12].

Donor identification relies on the treating physician or care team recognizing donation opportunities when a patient dies or is expected to die in conditions compatible with organ donation [13, 14]. Following identification, the potential donor must be referred to the donor coordinator (DC) or the relevant organ procurement organization (OPO). A failure to systematically identify and refer possible organ donors is the primary reason for disparities in deceased donation rates among hospitals, regions, and countries. End-of-life decisions significantly influence the pool of possible organ donors. Decisions to withhold or WLST on grounds of futility eliminate donation opportunities. Conversely, extending life-sustaining therapies beyond futility allows time for confirming poor prognoses, providing optimal palliative care, and integrating organ donation into the end-of-life care plan [15]. This practice, known as intensive care to facilitate organ donation (ICOD), can substantially expand the donor pool, but is applied in a reduced number of countries [16, 17].

Once a deceased donation process is initiated, several phases ensue. While donation pathways differ (Fig. 14.3), a critical shared phase is the *family approach*. Surrogates must be informed about their loved one's death or ominous prognosis and, when appropriate, the futility of further curative treatment. Discussions should then explore whether organ donation aligns with the patient's values and wishes. A study of 67 hospitals across 15 European countries revealed that families declined donation authorization in 24% of DNDD cases and 33% of cDCDD cases [14].

The *determination of death*—whether by neurological or circulatory criteria—must be performed by professionals who do not participate in organ recovery or transplantation, and in accordance with national regulations [18]. Potential DNDD donors may not become eligible because death by neurological criteria cannot be confirmed, often due to a lack of necessary technical or human resources. In some countries, up to 30% of patients who meet clinical conditions consistent with brain death cannot be confirmed dead by these criteria, which eliminates DNDD as an option [19]. In such cases, the cDCDD pathway might be considered, but prioritizing cDCDD over DNDD should be avoided when possible. This is because the conversion rate from potential to actual donation is currently lower in cDCDD, and organ (including liver) utilization rates are also reduced compared to DNDD, even with advanced preservation techniques. Potential cDCDD donors may also become ineligible if circulatory death is not determined within the timeframe required for organ recovery. For liver donation, this timeframe is particularly critical due to the organ's susceptibility to warm ischemia [11, 12].

Another essential phase of the deceased donation process is *evaluating the medical suitability of potential donors*. While absolute contraindications to organ donation are rare, perceived medical unsuitability often results in missed referrals. Audits in Spain revealed that 11% of decisions not to refer potential DNDD donors due to medical concerns were unjustified [20]. This underscores the importance of donor eligibility being assessed by trained DC or OPO staff, alongside transplant professionals. Their evaluations should balance the safety and quality of the organ against the risks faced by patients on the waiting lists.

Finally, the deceased donation process requires seamless *logistical coordination for organ recovery, preservation, transportation, and communication with suprahospital organ-sharing offices* to ensure strict adherence to allocation criteria.

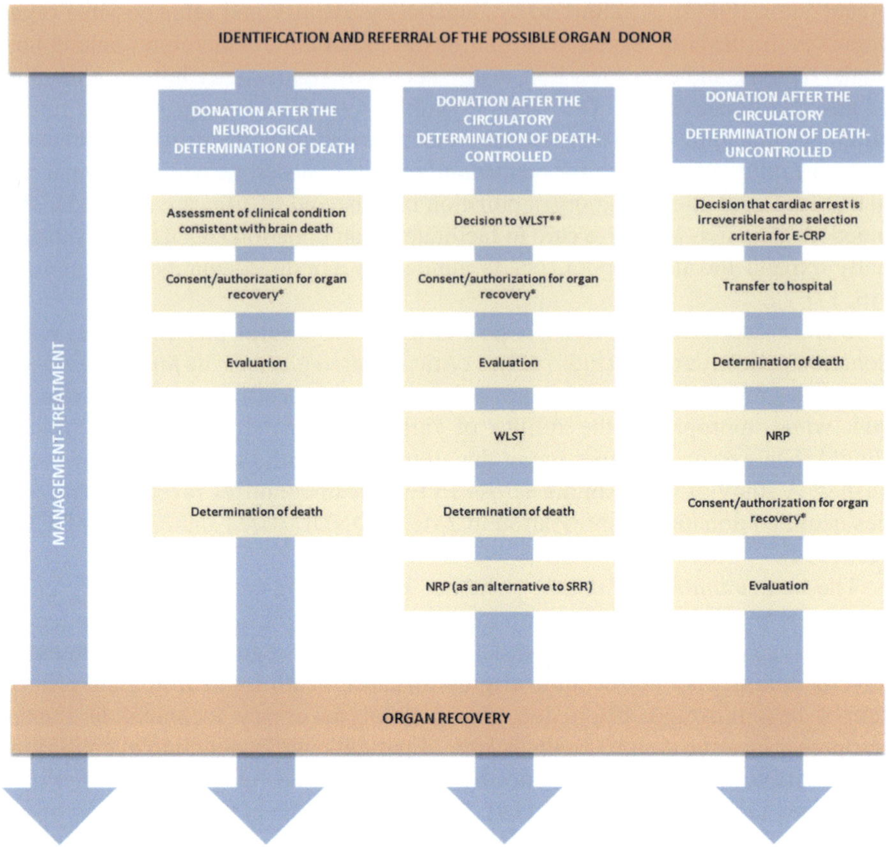

Fig. 14.3 Deceased donation pathways
*The potential cDCDD donor may be a person with a devastating brain injury or lesion, or a person with another disease or condition in whom the decision is made to WLST because they are no longer deemed beneficial. In countries where legally possible, the potential cDCDD donor can also be a person in whom authorization has been granted for medical assistance in dying. **This phase of the process can take place at different moments in the pathway, attending to the circumstances and the emotional situation of the family, along with elements established in the national regulatory framework
E-CPR Extracorporeal-assisted cardiopulmonary resuscitation, NRP Normothermic Regional Perfusion, WLST Withdrawal of life-sustaining therapies

The following sections explore the distinct features of each deceased donation pathway, with a particular focus on strategies to enhance the quantity and quality of livers available for transplantation.

Donation After the Neurological Determination of Death

Brain death triggers pathophysiological changes that may require aggressive use of fluids, vasopressors, and hormone therapy. Managing a multiorgan donor requires striking a delicate balance between interventions that may benefit one organ while potentially compromising another. Nevertheless, optimal donor management benefits all organs eligible for transplantation, maximizing their viability [21]. A potential DNDD donor should be treated as a "critical patient," an approach proven to be the most effective way to maximize the number of transplantable organs, including livers. This requires donor care to be directed by an expert in critical care with deep knowledge of respiratory and circulatory physiology, as well as the mechanics of ventilation [22].

In the DNDD context, the liver faces particular challenges stemming from complications such as hypotension and diabetes insipidus, both of which can lead to hypoperfusion and subsequent liver injury [21]. Hypernatremia can also have a deleterious effect on the liver. Table 14.1 outlines key targets for managing potential DNDD donors to mitigate these risks.

Strategies to Increase Liver Availability from DNDD Donors

Efforts to expand the availability of transplantable livers from DNDD donors include the following strategies:

1. *Utilizing Livers from Older Donors*

   As populations age, so does the pool of potential organ donors. Though associated with worse posttransplant outcomes, livers from DNDD donors of advanced age can help to better meet the transplantation needs of patients. Successfully utilizing these organs requires a meticulous assessment of graft quality to ensure viability. Advanced techniques such as ex situ machine perfusion have shown significant promise in preserving and rehabilitating these grafts, particularly in cases involving severe steatosis [23].

Table 14.1 Targets in the management of the potential DNDD donor

1. Central body temperature 36–37 °C
2. Invasive mean arterial pressure 60–75 mm Hg
3. Heart rate 70–100/min
4. Urine output 0.5–1.5 mL/kg/h
5. Central venous pressure 6–12 mm Hg
6. Peripheral arterial oxygen saturation >95%
7. Arterial blood gas, pH 7.35–7.45
8. Na 135–145 mmol/L
9. K 3.5–4.5 mmol/L
10. Blood glucose <180 mg/dL
11. Calcium level within normal range
12. Hemoglobin ≥7 g/dL
13. Platelets >50 G/L
14. Prothrombin time/partial thromboplastin time within an acceptable range to avoid bleeding
15. Magnesia level within normal range
16. When monitoring with a Swan-Ganz catheter, pulmonary wedge pressure 10–12 mm Hg
17. When monitoring with PICCO®, systemic resistance index within the normal range (1800–2400 units), extravascular lung water index <10 mL/kg, and systolic volume variation index <15%.

2. *Improving Liver Assessment During Recovery*
   One of the primary reasons for discarding livers during organ recovery is the subjective evaluation of the organ by the recovery team. To address this, liver recovery should be entrusted to experienced surgeons capable of making accurate assessments under challenging conditions. In addition, emerging technologies are expected to play a transformative role in liver validation, offering objective and standardized evaluation criteria that enhance decision-making and reduce unnecessary discard rates [24].

Controlled Donation After the Circulatory Determination of Death

Over the past decade, cDCDD has undergone substantial growth [11]. This pathway is primarily considered for patients with devastating brain injuries or terminal conditions (e.g., end-stage cardiac, pulmonary, or neurodegenerative diseases) when a decision is made to WLST on grounds of futility, which is becoming common practice worldwide [25]. In some instances, the decision to discontinue such therapies is initiated by the patient or their surrogates, based on unacceptable prognoses or personal values [26]. Additionally, in jurisdictions where MAiD is legally permissible, cDCDD can also be activated under similar circumstances.

Once cDCDD is contemplated, discussions must confirm that organ donation aligns with the patient's wishes and values. If *ante-mortem interventions* such as heparin administration or vascular cannulation are planned, explicit informed consent is required [11].

The timeline of warm ischemia begins at the moment of WLST. The *functional warm ischemic time (FWIT)* starts with significant hypoperfusion, though definitions vary across countries, relying on parameters like systolic or mean blood pressure and oxygen saturation [27]. FWIT ends when organ preservation measures commence. Death is declared following a mandatory period of complete absence of circulation and respiration, known as the *no-touch period*. The duration of the no-touch period differs between countries, though it typically lasts five minutes [11, 12]—this 5 min period is now supported by evidence from a multicenter study, confirming that spontaneous return of circulation does not occur beyond this timeframe once death is declared following the WLST [28].

Challenges and Strategies to Optimize cDCDD Outcomes—Normothermic Regional Perfusion

An *extended withdrawal period* negatively affects graft viability. An FWIT exceeding 30 min is generally deemed a contraindication for LT, but the strict upper limit of FWIT remains controversial and can be influenced by the availability of novel organ preservation strategies [29]. The liver is particularly vulnerable to warm ischemia, and its effects are further exacerbated during subsequent cold ischemia. These conditions have historically led to higher incidences of *primary non-function (PNF), early allograft dysfunction (EAD)*, graft loss, and biliary complications in cDCDD compared to DNDD [30]. However, advances in organ preservation techniques are transforming cDCDD LT outcomes. The opportunities brought by ex situ machine perfusion are beyond the scope of this chapter, where we only briefly revise *normothermic regional perfusion (NRP)* that can be deemed a form of donor treatment.

Spanish experiences with NRP in uDCDD (see below) have spurred growing interest in its application to cDCDD. Based on the use of extracorporeal membrane oxygenation (ECMO) or extracorporeal circulation, NRP restores blood flow to ischemic organs following the diagnosis of death and prior to organ recovery. This technique replenishes cellular energy reserves, enhances organ quality, and allows pretransplant graft assessment [31]. Although there are no randomized controlled trials available, there is an overwhelming body of evidence on the benefits of NRP versus standard rapid recovery (SRR) in cDCDD LT, to the extent that donor age can be safely expanded (Table 14.2). Initial single-center studies demonstrated that *abdominal NRP (A-NRP)* reduced PNF and biliary complications compared to SRR [32–34]. Subsequent multicenter analyses have reinforced these findings [35–38]. In Spain, a comparison of 545 cDCDD livers retrieved with A-NRP versus 258 with SRR showed significant reductions in EAD, hepatic artery thrombosis, biliary complications, ischemic-type biliary lesions, graft loss, and patient mortality [36]. In the United Kingdom, Watson et al. undertook a retrospective analysis of 43 cDCDD livers recovered with the A-NRP approach compared with 187 subject to SRR at two British centers [37]. The study revealed that A-NRP significantly decreased EAD, graft loss, and biliary complications, including ischemic cholangiopathy and anastomotic strictures. Nationwide data in the United Kingdom confirmed a 51% lower adjusted risk of liver failure in recipients of A-NRP livers [38]. De Beule et al. conducted a systematic review and meta-analysis to evaluate the efficacy of A-NRP compared to SRR in cDCDD LT [39]. Their analysis included eight primary studies. While the results indicated that A-NRP did not significantly reduce the incidence of EAD or mortality, it demonstrated a substantial reduction in biliary complications, decreasing the risk of ischemic cholangiopathy by 75% and anastomotic strictures by 65%.

Another relevant experience has been that reported by France, where A-NRP is mandatory in case the liver is recovered from cDCDD donors. Savier et al. undertook a multicenter retrospective study where recipients of cDCDD livers obtained with A-NRP (n = 50) were matched to 100 recipients of DNDD livers [40]. The authors did not observe increased rates of EAD or biliary complications in the cDCDD group and graft and patient survival rates were similar up to 2 years. Such

Table 14.2 Limits for accepting an uncontrolled DCDD liver for transplantation in Spain

Donor age ≤65 years
Length of cardiac arrest prior to advanced life support <20 min
Total length of warm ischemia (time from arrest to initiation of A-NRP) <150 min
Length of A-NRP < 4 h, though NRP can be maintained for up to 6 h as long as biochemical, gasometric, and hematological parameters remain stable.
Transaminase evolution during A-NRP: Initial AST/ALT levels: <4xULN
Final AST/ALT: <5xULN

comparable outcomes of recipients of cDCDD livers obtained with A-NRP versus recipients of DNDD livers have been confirmed by others [41].

Thoraco-abdominal NRP (TA-NRP) has emerged in recent years to allow the recovery and validation of the DCDD heart. The first series on liver transplantation with grafts obtained from cDCDD donors subject to TA-NRP describes appropriate utilization rates and posttransplant outcomes [42–44].

Comparisons between *A-NRP* and *ex situ preservation strategies* such as normothermic machine perfusion (NMP) and hypothermic oxygenated perfusion (HOPE) have yielded variable results. For instance, a single-center study showed that both A-NRP and NMP improved early liver function, but A-NRP provided superior biliary system preservation [45]. In contrast, a multicenter study found comparable outcomes between HOPE and A-NRP, even though the HOPE group faced higher graft risk factors [46].

One of the main concerns in the initial experiences with A-NRP was the simultaneous recovery of the liver and the lungs. Several experiences have shown that, though technically complex, this combined retrieval is safe for both types of grafts with optimal posttransplant outcomes [47, 48].

The use of NRP in smaller centers lacking specialized resources presents logistical challenges. Portable ECMO devices offer potential solutions, as early experiences demonstrate success in such settings [49]. Ethical concerns surrounding NRP, particularly the potential for unintentional brain perfusion after death determination, have prompted safeguards. Measures such as aortic balloon occlusion or surgical clamping are employed to prevent cerebral blood flow during A-NRP [11]. *TA-NRP*, which enables cDCDD heart recovery, necessitates ligating supra-aortic vessels and implementing additional safeguards to divert collateral circulation to the brain [50, 51]. In addition, measures are required to ensure that no technical failure occurs, which should immediately lead to halting the NRP procedure [34, 52].

With robust evidence supporting the benefits of NRP in cDCDD LT, its application is likely to expand, enabling the safe inclusion of older donors and grafts previously deemed marginal. Its combination with ex situ machine perfusion promises to improve outcomes and broaden the scope of cDCDD programs globally.

Uncontrolled Donation After Circulatory Death—Uncontrolled

uDCDD involves donors who experience sudden cardiac arrest, often outside of a hospital setting. When advanced cardiopulmonary resuscitation efforts have been exhausted and deemed unsuccessful, uDCDD can be activated in individuals meeting eligibility criteria, Table 14.2 transferring the patient to the nearest center equipped for uDCDD [53]. Upon arrival at the hospital, death is declared based on the absence of circulation and spontaneous respiration, following a mandatory *non-touch period* of 5 min, as practiced in most countries. In some jurisdictions, chest compressions and mechanical ventilation may be resumed after a death declaration to maintain organ viability. Subsequently, the femoral vessels are rapidly cannulated to initiate *A-NRP*. This procedure is carried out concurrently with obtaining consent, completing authorization requirements, and conducting donor evaluations [54].

Despite the immense theoretical potential of uDCDD—given the global incidence of sudden cardiac arrests—it remains limited to a small number of countries and centers. This is largely due to its *logistical and technical complexities*, including the need for specialized equipment, trained personnel, and rapid activation protocols [11].

A successful uDCDD program hinges on meticulous planning to streamline the activation pathway once a donation opportunity is identified. The cornerstone of these programs is the reduction of warm ischemic injury before organ preservation begins at the hospital.

The low conversion rate of potential uDCDD donors into utilized liver donors and the relatively high rates of *PNF* are major challenges [55]. Consequently, while promising, LT outcomes from uDCDD donors—particularly graft survival—still lag behind those achieved with standard DNDD livers [31, 56].

The increasing adoption of NRP for cDCDD donors offers a potential avenue for expanding expertise in using ECMO devices, which could enhance the viability and utilization of uDCDD livers. Several strategies may help improve outcomes:

1. *Selective Donor Criteria*: Avoiding the simultaneous use of expanded criteria for uDCDD liver acceptance could enhance graft viability and recipient outcomes.
2. *Ex Situ Machine Perfusion*: Applying this technique to uDCDD livers may expand the pool of viable grafts, offering the potential for improved posttransplant outcomes [57].
3. *Logistical Optimization*: Developing streamlined protocols to minimize warm ischemic times and ensure rapid cannulation and preservation could significantly improve graft quality.

As expertise with NRP grows and ex situ machine perfusion becomes more widely available, the feasibility and success of uDCDD LT are likely to improve. With targeted efforts to address logistical, technical, and donor selection challenges, uDCDD could become a more prominent source of viable organs, helping to meet the growing demand for liver transplants.

The Role of the Donor Coordinator in Ensuring a Successful Development of the Deceased Donation Process

Deceased organ donation is a highly complex process that demands the coordination and interaction of professionals from diverse disciplines, often operating across multiple locations, settings, and organizations. To manage this intricate system, the role of the DC was created. While many systems rely on organ procurement organizations, the most successful countries in organ donation have adopted models centered on in-hospital DCs [8, 58, 59].

The background, level of dedication, and organizational alignment of DCs vary across countries, but their core responsibilities are widely recognized and consistent. A primary role of the DC is to ensure that possible organ donors are systematically identified and referred by treating teams. This necessitates fostering a culture of *routine referral* among critical care professionals. DCs play a vital role in educating the critical care community on the importance of routinely considering donation opportunities. This involves advocating for a decision-making framework at the end of life that encompasses not only medical aspects but also *social, moral, and ethical considerations* [60]. Incorporating organ donation as a standard component of end-of-life care aligns with the patient's wishes and values, ensuring donation opportunities are identified and facilitated [61–64].

To streamline referrals, clinical triggers must be clearly defined, easy to interpret, and readily accessible. Effective communication systems for contacting the DC and regular feedback sessions with critical care units also enhance engagement. Importantly, DCs should adopt proactive donor identification strategies, such as monitoring patients with severe brain injuries to anticipate donation possibilities.

Internationally, *engaging the critical care community* has been acknowledged as essential for successful donor identification and management [65, 66]. Different organizational models support this engagement. In Spain, donor coordination units are led directly by critical care professionals [67], while in countries like Australia, Canada, or the United Kingdom, the figure of the donation physician with a critical care background has been incorporated to foster the culture of organ donation at national, regional, or hospital levels [68, 69]. These initiatives have significantly contributed to improvements in donation rates and organ availability in various jurisdictions.

DCs are typically the best-qualified professionals to lead *conversations with donor families*. Evidence suggests that consent rates for organ recovery are higher when these discussions are facilitated by DCs [70]. This role becomes particularly nuanced in cases where *ICOD* is considered [16, 17]. A deep understanding of neurocritical care is crucial for suggesting ICOD only when brain death is likely to occur within a short timeframe [71]. Once it is confirmed that donation aligns with the patient's wishes and values, the DC should provide continuous support to the family, ensuring a compassionate and informed process.

DCs are also responsible for ensuring a *thorough evaluation of donor and organ suitability*, maintaining high standards of quality and safety. The increasing acceptance of donors with advanced age or comorbidities has made this evaluation more complex, requiring meticulous assessment to minimize risks of disease transmission (e.g., infections or neoplasias) while avoiding the unnecessary loss of viable organs. Donor evaluation involves differentiating acute from chronic organ impairments, addressing incidental findings during imaging or organ recovery or deciding on the need for biopsies based on donor characteristics and macroscopic findings.

Adhering to intensive care principles in *donor management* has proven effective in increasing both the quantity and quality of organs (and livers) for transplantation. When donor care is led by critical care experts, the number of recovered organs *per* donor significantly rises [22]. Conversely, nonexpert care often leads to technical errors and complications that can jeopardize the process. Similarly, in DCDD, the use of *NRP* adds procedural complexity. DCs must therefore be trained in donor management and in overseeing advanced preservation strategies like NRP.

While DCs should not participate in *diagnosing death* to avoid conflicts of interest, they must ensure that those responsible for the diagnosis are adequately trained and have access to ancillary tests when necessary. This requires comprehensive knowledge of both neurological and circulatory death criteria, including the application and limitations of ancillary tests.

Efficient timing management is another critical aspect of the DC's role. Balancing sensitivity toward the donor's family with the logistical demands of organ sharing and recovery requires careful planning. DCs must ensure timely reporting of possible donors to the organ sharing office and be familiar with all steps in the donation process, including differences between DNDD and DCDD, and addressing judicial, religious, or spiritual considerations that could affect the process.

In conclusion, the role of the DC is indispensable in deceased organ donation. From proactive donor identification and family engagement to meticulous donor management and collaboration with transplant teams, DCs ensure the success of a highly intricate process. By fostering interdisciplinary coordination, adhering to ethical practices, and embracing advanced preservation technologies, DCs can contribute significantly to improving organ donation outcomes.

Conclusions

LT activities are intrinsically tied to the successful realization of the deceased donation process. Deceased donation can occur under various circumstances of death, activating distinct pathways (DNDD, cDCDD, and uDCDD). The failure to identify organ donation opportunities remains the leading cause of low donation rates in many jurisdictions. To address this, it is essential that all possible organ donors are systematically referred to DCs or OPO staff by the treating healthcare teams. Once a possible organ donor is identified, the process moves through subsequent critical phases—family approach, donor evaluation, diagnosis of death, and logistical aspects. At each stage, there is a risk of losing donation opportunities due to procedural inefficiencies or a lack of coordination. However, targeted interventions can significantly enhance both the availability of livers and the quality of donated organs. These include proactive donor identification strategies, streamlined referral processes, and improved training for professionals involved in the pathway. Undoubtedly, the designation of qualified and well-trained professionals to lead and oversee the process is fundamental to its success. Their active engagement not only ensures the seamless progression through each phase but also plays a critical role in maintaining the quality and safety of deceased donor livers for transplantation.

References

1. Global Observatory on Organ Donation and Transplantation. Available at: http://www.transplant-observatory.org/. Accessed Dec 2024.
2. Gardiner D, McGee A, Kareem Al Obaidli AA, Cooper M, Lentine KL, Miñambres E, et al. Developing and expanding deceased organ donation to its maximum therapeutic potential: an actionable global challenge from the 2023 Santander Summit. Transplantation. 2025;109(1):10–21. https://doi.org/10.1097/TP.0000000000005234.
3. Ahmad MU, Hanna A, Mohamed AZ, Schlindwein A, Pley C, Bahner I, et al. A systematic review of opt-out versus opt-in consent on deceased organ donation and transplantation (2006–2016). World J Surg. 2019;43(12):3161–71. https://doi.org/10.1007/s00268-019-05118-4.
4. Arshad A, Anderson B, Sharif A. Comparison of organ donation and transplantation rates between opt-out and opt-in systems. Kidney Int. 2019;95(6):1453–60. https://doi.org/10.1016/j.kint.2019.01.036.
5. Matesanz R, Domínguez-Gil B. Opt-out legislations: the mysterious viability of the false. Kidney Int. 2019;95(6):1301–3. https://doi.org/10.1016/j.kint.2019.02.028.
6. Eurostat. Available at: https://ec.europa.eu/eurostat/data/database. Accessed Dec 2024.
7. Organ donation and transplantation facts, figures and European Union action. Available at: https://www.europarl.europa.eu/RegData/etudes/BRIE/2020/649363/EPRS_BRI(2020)649363_EN.pdf. Accessed Dec 2024.
8. Matesanz R, Domínguez-Gil B, Coll E, de la Rosa G, Marazuela R. Spanish experience as a leading country: what kind of measures were taken? Transpl Int. 2011;24(4):333–43. https://doi.org/10.1111/j.1432-2277.2010.01204.x.
9. Domínguez-Gil B, Delmonico FL, Shaheen FA, Matesanz R, O'Connor K, Minina M, et al. The critical pathway for deceased donation: reportable uniformity in the approach to deceased donation. Transpl Int. 2011;24(4):373–8. https://doi.org/10.1111/j.1432-2277.2011.01243.x.
10. Mulder J, Sonneveld H, Van Raemdonck D, Downar J, Wiebe K, Domínguez-Gil B, et al. Practice and challenges for organ donation after medical assistance in dying: a scoping review including the results of the first international roundtable in 2021. Am J Transplant. 2022;22(12):2759–80. https://doi.org/10.1111/ajt.17198.
11. Lomero M, Gardiner D, Coll E, Haase-Kromwijk B, Procaccio F, Immer F, et al. Donation after circulatory death today: an updated overview of the European landscape. Transpl Int. 2019; https://doi.org/10.1111/tri.13506.
12. Smith M, Dominguez-Gil B, Greer DM, Manara AR, Souter MJ. Organ donation after circulatory death: current status and future potential. Intensive Care Med. 2019;45(3):310–21. https://doi.org/10.1007/s00134-019-05533-0.
13. Domínguez-Gil B, Murphy P, Procaccio F. Ten changes that could improve organ donation in the intensive care unit. Intensive Care Med. 2016;42(2):264–7. https://doi.org/10.1007/s00134-015-3833-y.
14. Manara A, Procaccio F, Domínguez-Gil B. Expanding the pool of deceased organ donors: the ICU and beyond. Intensive Care Med. 2019;45(3):357–60. https://doi.org/10.1007/s00134-019-05546-9.
15. Manara AR, Thomas I, Harding R. A case for stopping the early withdrawal of life sustaining therapies in patients with devastating brain injuries. J Intensive Care Soc. 2016;17(4):295–301. https://doi.org/10.1177/1751143716647980.
16. Martín-Delgado MC, Martínez-Soba F, Masnou N, Pérez-Villares JM, Pont T, Sánchez Carretero MJ, et al. Summary of Spanish recommendations on intensive care to facilitate organ donation. Am J Transplant. 2019;19(6):1782–91. https://doi.org/10.1111/ajt.15253.
17. Domínguez-Gil B, Coll E, Elizalde J, Herrero JE, Pont T, Quindós B, et al. Expanding the donor pool through intensive care to facilitate organ donation: results of a Spanish multicenter study. Transplantation. 2017;101(8):e265–72. https://doi.org/10.1097/TP.0000000000001701.

18. WHO Guiding Principles on human cell, tissue and organ transplantation. Available at: https://www.who.int/transplantation/Guiding_PrinciplesTransplantation_WHA63.22en.pdf?ua=1. Accessed Dec 2024.
19. de Groot YJ, Wijdicks EF, van der Jagt M, Bakker J, Lingsma HF, Ijzermans JN, Kompanje EJ. Donor conversion rates depend on the assessment tools used in the evaluation of potential organ donors. Intensive Care Med. 2011;37(4):665–70. https://doi.org/10.1007/s00134-011-2131-6.
20. de la Rosa G, Domínguez-Gil B, Matesanz R, Ramón S, Alonso-Álvarez J, Araiz J, et al. Continuously evaluating performance in deceased donation: the Spanish quality assurance program. Am J Transplant. 2012;12(9):2507–13. https://doi.org/10.1111/j.1600-6143.2012.04138.x.
21. European Directorate for the Quality of Medicines and Healthcare, editor. Chapter 5: Management of the potential donor. In: Guide to the quality and safety of organs for transplantation. Council of Europe (8th Edition); 2022.
22. Singbartl K, Murugan R, Kaynar AM, Crippen DW, Tisherman SA, Shutterly K, et al. Intensivist-led management of brain-dead donors is associated with an increase in organ recovery for transplantation. Am J Transplant. 2011;11(7):1517–21. https://doi.org/10.1111/j.1600-6143.2011.03485.x.
23. Schlegel A, Mergental H, Fondevila C, Porte RJ, Friend PJ, Dutkowski P. Machine perfusion of the liver and bioengineering. J Hepatol. 2023;78(6):1181–98. https://doi.org/10.1016/j.jhep.2023.02.009.
24. Gómez-Gavara C, Bilbao I, Piella G, Vazquez-Corral J, Benet-Cugat B, Pando E, et al. Enhanced artificial intelligence methods for liver steatosis assessment using machine learning and color image processing: liver color project. Clin Transpl. 2024;38(10):e15465. https://doi.org/10.1111/ctr.15465.
25. Avidan A, Sprung CL, Schefold JC, Ricou B, Hartog CS, Nates JL, et al. Variations in end-of-life practices in intensive care units worldwide (Ethicus-2): a prospective observational study. Lancet Respir Med. 2021;9(10):1101–10. https://doi.org/10.1016/S2213-2600(21)00261-7.
26. Domínguez-Gil B, Ascher N, Capron AM, Gardiner D, Manara AR, Bernat JL, et al. Expanding controlled donation after the circulatory determination of death: statement from an international collaborative. Intensive Care Med. 2021;47(3):265–81. https://doi.org/10.1007/s00134-020-06341-7.
27. Jochmans I, Hessheimer AJ, Neyrinck AP, Paredes D, Bellini MI, Dark JH, et al. Consensus statement on normothermic regional perfusion in donation after circulatory death: report from the European Society for Organ Transplantation's transplant learning journey. Transpl Int. 2021;34(11):2019–30. https://doi.org/10.1111/tri.13951.
28. Dhanani S, Hornby L, van Beinum A, Scales NB, Hogue M, Baker A, et al. Resumption of cardiac activity after withdrawal of life-sustaining measures. N Engl J Med. 2021;384(4):345–52. https://doi.org/10.1056/NEJMoa2022713.
29. Hessheimer AJ, Gastaca M, Miñambres E, Colmenero J, Fondevila C. Donation after circulatory death liver transplantation: consensus statements from the Spanish Liver Transplantation Society. Transpl Int. 2020;33(8):902–16. https://doi.org/10.1111/tri.13619.
30. Jay C, Ladner D, Wang E, Lyuksemburg V, Kang R, Chang Y, et al. A comprehensive risk assessment of mortality following donation after cardiac death liver transplant – an analysis of the national registry. J Hepatol. 2011;55(4):808–13. https://doi.org/10.1016/j.jhep.2011.01.040.
31. Hessheimer AJ, García-Valdecasas JC, Fondevila C. Abdominal regional in-situ perfusion in donation after circulatory determination of death donors. Curr Opin Organ Transplant. 2016;21:322–8. https://doi.org/10.1097/MOT.0000000000000315.
32. Rojas-Peña A, Sall LE, Gravel MT, Cooley EG, Pelletier SJ, Bartlett RH, Punch JD. Donation after circulatory determination of death: the university of Michigan experience with extracorporeal support. Transplantation. 2014;98(3):328–34. https://doi.org/10.1097/TP.0000000000000070.

33. Oniscu GC, Randle LV, Muiesan P, Butler AJ, Currie IS, Perera MT, et al. In situ normothermic regional perfusion for controlled donation after circulatory death—the United Kingdom experience. Am J Transplant. 2014;14:2846–54. https://doi.org/10.1111/ajt.12927.
34. Miñambres E, Suberviola B, Domínguez-Gil B, Rodrigo E, Ruiz-San Millán JC, Ballesteros MA. Improving the outcomes of organs obtained from controlled donation after circulatory death donors using abdominal normothermic regional perfusion. Am J Transplant. 2017;17:2165–72. https://doi.org/10.1111/ajt.14214.
35. Hessheimer AJ, Coll E, Torres F, Ruíz P, Gastaca M, Rivas JI, et al. Normothermic regional perfusion vs. super-rapid recovery in controlled donation after circulatory death liver transplantation. J Hepatol. 2019;70(4):658–65. https://doi.org/10.1016/j.jhep.2018.12.013.
36. Hessheimer AJ, de la Rosa G, Gastaca M, Ruíz P, Otero A, Gómez M, et al. Abdominal normothermic regional perfusion in controlled donation after circulatory determination of death liver transplantation: outcomes and risk factors for graft loss. Am J Transplant. 2022;22(4):1169–81. https://doi.org/10.1111/ajt.16899.
37. Watson CJE, Hunt F, Messer S, Currie I, Large S, Sutherland A, et al. In situ normothermic perfusion of livers in controlled circulatory death donation may prevent ischemic cholangiopathy and improve graft survival. Am J Transplant. 2019;19(6):1745–58. https://doi.org/10.1111/ajt.15241.
38. Oniscu GC, Mehew J, Butler AJ, Sutherland A, Gaurav R, Hogg R, et al. Improved organ utilization and better transplant outcomes with in situ normothermic regional perfusion in controlled donation after circulatory death. Transplantation. 2023;107(2):438–48. https://doi.org/10.1097/TP.0000000000004280.
39. De Beule J, Vandendriessche K, Pengel LHM, Bellini MI, Dark JH, Hessheimer AJ, et al. A systematic review and meta-analyses of regional perfusion in donation after circulatory death solid organ transplantation. Transpl Int. 2021;34(11):2046–60. https://doi.org/10.1111/tri.14121.
40. Savier E, Lim C, Rayar M, Orlando F, Boudjema K, Mohkam K, et al. Favorable outcomes of liver transplantation from controlled circulatory death donors using normothermic regional perfusion compared to brain death donors. Transplantation. 2020;104(9):1943–51. https://doi.org/10.1097/TP.0000000000003372.
41. Ruiz P, Valdivieso A, Palomares I, Prieto M, Ventoso A, Salvador P, et al. Similar results in liver transplantation from controlled donation after circulatory death donors with normothermic regional perfusion and donation after brain death donors: a case-matched single-center study. Liver Transpl. 2021;27(12):1747–57. https://doi.org/10.1002/lt.26281.
42. Brubaker AL, Sellers MT, Abt PL, Croome KP, Merani S, Wall A, et al. US liver transplant outcomes after normothermic regional perfusion vs standard super rapid recovery. JAMA Surg. 2024;159(6):677–85. https://doi.org/10.1001/jamasurg.2024.0520.
43. Secanella L, Alconchel F, López-Monclús J, Toledo-Martínez E, Barrios O, Ramírez P, et al. Outcomes of liver transplantation with thoracoabdominal normothermic regional perfusion: a matched-controlled initial experience in Spain. Front Transplant. 2023;2:1280454. https://doi.org/10.3389/frtra.2023.1280454.
44. Wall AE, Adams BL, Brubaker A, Chang CWJ, Croome KP, Frontera J, et al. The American Society of Transplant Surgeons Consensus Statement on normothermic regional perfusion. Transplantation. 2024;108(2):312–8. https://doi.org/10.1097/TP.0000000000004894.
45. Gaurav R, Butler AJ, Kosmoliaptsis V, et al. Liver transplantation outcomes from controlled circulatory death donors: SCS vs in situ NRP vs ex situ NMP. Ann Surg. 2022;275(6):1156–64. https://doi.org/10.1097/SLA.0000000000005428.
46. Muller X, Mohkam K, Mueller M, et al. Hypothermic oxygenated perfusion versus normothermic regional perfusion in liver transplantation from controlled donation after circulatory death: first international comparative study. Ann Surg. 2020;272(5):751–8. https://doi.org/10.1097/SLA.0000000000004268.
47. Miñambres E, Ruiz P, Ballesteros MA, Álvarez C, Cifrián JM, Atutxa L, Ventoso A, Castillo F, Gastaca M. Combined lung and liver procurement in controlled donation after circulatory

death using normothermic abdominal perfusion. Initial experience in two Spanish centers. Am J Transplant. 2020;20:231–40.
48. Campo-Cañaveral de la Cruz JL, Miñambres E, Coll E, Padilla M, Antolín GS, de la Rosa G, et al. Outcomes of lung and liver transplantation after simultaneous recovery using abdominal normothermic regional perfusion in donors after the circulatory determination of death versus donors after brain death. Am J Transplant. 2023;23(7):996–1008. https://doi.org/10.1016/j.ajt.2023.04.016.
49. Pérez-Villares JM, Lara-Rosales R, Fernández-Carmona A, Fuentes-Garcia P, Burgos-Fuentes M, Baquedano-Fernández B. Mobile ECMO team for controlled donation after circulatory death. Am J Transplant. 2018;18:1293–4. https://doi.org/10.1111/ajt.14656.
50. Manara A, Shemie SD, Large S, Healey A, Baker A, Badiwala M, et al. Maintaining the permanence principle for death during in situ normothermic regional perfusion for donation after circulatory death organ recovery: a United Kingdom and Canadian proposal. Am J Transplant. 2020;20(8):2017–25. https://doi.org/10.1111/ajt.15775.
51. Domínguez-Gil B, Miñambres E, Pérez-Blanco A, Coll E, Royo-Villanova M. Sustained absence of perfusion to the brain must be ensured during thoracoabdominal normothermic regional perfusion. Transplantation. 2025;109(1):e78. https://doi.org/10.1097/TP.0000000000005230.
52. Pérez-Villares JM, Rubio JJ, Del Río F, Miñambres E. Validation of a new proposal to avoid donor resuscitation in controlled donation after circulatory death with normothermic regional perfusion. Resuscitation. 2017;117:46–9. https://doi.org/10.1016/j.resuscitation.2017.05.030.
53. Coll E, Miñambres E, Sánchez-Fructuoso A, Fondevila C, Campo-Cañaveral de la Cruz JL, Domínguez-Gil B. Uncontrolled donation after circulatory death: a unique opportunity. Transplantation. 2020;104(8):1542–52. https://doi.org/10.1097/TP.0000000000003139.
54. Miñambres E, Rubio JJ, Coll E, Domínguez-Gil B. Donation after circulatory death and its expansion in Spain. Curr Opin Organ Transplant. 2018;23:120–9. https://doi.org/10.1097/MOT.0000000000000480.
55. Domínguez-Gil B, Duranteau J, Mateos A, Núñez JR, Cheisson G, Corral E, et al. Uncontrolled donation after circulatory death: European practices and recommendations for the development and optimization of an effective programme. Transpl Int. 2016;29:842–59. https://doi.org/10.1111/tri.12734.
56. Savier E, Dondero F, Vibert E, Eyraud D, Brisson H, Riou B, et al. First experience of liver transplantation with type 2 donation after cardiac death in France. Liver Transpl. 2015;21:631–43. https://doi.org/10.1002/lt.24107.
57. De CR, Di SS, Lauterio A, Botta F, Ferla F, Andorno E, et al. Liver grafts from donors after circulatory death on regional perfusion with extended warm ischemia compared with donors after brain death. Liver Transpl. 2018;24:1523–35. https://doi.org/10.1002/lt.25312.
58. Salim A, Berry C, Ley EJ, Schulman D, Desai C, Navarro S, et al. In-house coordinator programs improve conversion rates for organ donation. J Trauma. 2011;71:733–6. https://doi.org/10.1097/TA.0b013e31820500e6.
59. Caramiciu JA, Adams JP, McKown BT, French CD, Ruggieri ER, Heard SO. Effects of an in-house coordinator and practitioner referral rather than proxy referral on tissue donation rates. Transplant Proc. 2014;46:1274–80. https://doi.org/10.1016/j.transproceed.2014.03.005.
60. Committee on Bioethics (DH-BIO) of the Council of Europe. Guide on the decision-making process regarding medical treatment in end-of-life situations. Available at: http://www.coe.int/en/web/bioethics/guide-on-the-decision-making-process-regarding-medical-treatment-in-end-of-life-situations. Accessed Dec 2024.
61. Truog RD, Campbell ML, Curtis JR, Haas CE, Luce JM, Rubenfeld GD, et al. Recommendations for end-of-life care in the intensive care unit: a consensus statement by the American College [corrected] of Critical Care Medicine. Crit Care Med. 2008;36(3):953–63. https://doi.org/10.1097/CCM.0B013E3181659096.
62. Mentzelopoulos SD, Couper K, Voorde PV, Druwé P, Blom M, Perkins GD, et al. European Resuscitation Council Guidelines 2021: ethics of resuscitation and end of life decisions. Resuscitation. 2021;161:408–32. https://doi.org/10.1016/j.resuscitation.2021.02.017.

63. Hernández-Tejedor A, Peñuelas O, Sirgo Rodríguez G, Llompart-Pou JA, Palencia Herrejón E, Estella A, et al. Recommendations of the Working Groups from the Spanish Society of Intensive and Critical Care Medicine and Coronary Units (SEMICYUC) for the management of adult critically ill patients. Med Intensiva. 2017;41(5):285–305. https://doi.org/10.1016/j.medin.2017.03.004.
64. Domínguez-Gil B, López-Fraga M, Muller E, Potena L, Martin DE, Pérez Blanco A, et al. Santander global summit in transplantation: supporting global convergence in the shared goals of sufficiency, transparency, and oversight. Transplantation. 2025;109(1):2–6. https://doi.org/10.1097/TP.0000000000005222.
65. Resolution CM/Res(2015)10 on the role and training of critical care professionals in deceased donation. Available at: https://search.coe.int/cm#{%22CoEIdentifier%22:[%2209000016805c2b4a%22],%22sort%22:[%22CoEValidationDate%20Descending%22]}. Last accessed Dec 2024.
66. The Madrid resolution on organ donation and transplantation: national responsibility in meeting the needs of patients, guided by the WHO principles. Transplantation 2011; 91 Suppl 11: S29–S31. doi: https://doi.org/10.1097/01.tp.0000399131.74618.a5.
67. Matesanz R, Domínguez-Gil B, Coll E, Mahíllo B, Marazuela R. How Spain reached 40 deceased organ donors per million population. Am J Transplant. 2017;17(6):1447–54. https://doi.org/10.1111/ajt.14104.
68. MacDonald SI, Shemie S. Ethical challenges and the donation physician specialist: a scoping review. Transplantation. 2017;101(5S Suppl 1):S27–40. https://doi.org/10.1097/TP.0000000000001697.
69. Clinical Lead for Organ Donation (CLOD) review—summary September 2017. Available at: https://nhsbtdbe.blob.core.windows.net/umbraco-assets-corp/5829/clod-review-summary.pdf. Last accessed Dec 2024.
70. Domínguez-Gil B, Coll E, Pont T, Lebrón M, Miñambres E, Coronil A, et al. End-of-life practices in patients with devastating brain injury in Spain: implications for organ donation. Med Intensiva. 2017;41(3):162–73. https://doi.org/10.1016/j.medin.2016.07.011.
71. Pérez-Blanco A, Acevedo M, Padilla M, Gómez A, Zapata L, Barber M, et al. Assessing outcomes of patients subject to intensive care to facilitate organ donation: a Spanish multicenter prospective study. Transpl Int. 2024;37:12791. https://doi.org/10.3389/ti.2024.12791.

Liver Transplantation from Partial Livers: Living Donor, Split and Reduced-Size Transplantation

15

Sadhana Shankar, Ashwin Rammohan, and Mohamed Rela

Introduction

Following the success of liver transplantation with whole liver grafts, the main impediments to its progress were the shortage of deceased donor organs and the technical difficulty encountered while transplanting pediatric patients. This led to the evolution of techniques using partial liver (PL) grafts such as split liver transplantation (SLT), reduced liver transplantation (RLT), and living donor liver transplantation (LDLT). Smith et al. were the first to advocate the idea of a partial liver allograft for pediatric transplantation [1]. Subsequently, Bismuth and Broelsch simultaneously reported successful RLT, wherein an adult liver was surgically reduced to a left lobe (LL) or left lateral segment (LLS) graft to fit the abdominal cavity of a pediatric recipient, discarding the remaining liver [2, 3]. Although this technique reduced pediatric waiting list mortality, it placed adult recipients at a relative disadvantage, which in turn led to the evolution of SLT, wherein a whole liver was split into two allografts for transplantation to two different recipients. Pichlmayr et al. were the first to split a liver into right and left lobes for transplantation to adult and pediatric recipients, respectively [4].

Given the disparity between deceased donor organ availability and the increasing number of patients requiring LT, LDLT was the logical extension of RLT. Further, it also helped overcome the sociocultural bias against deceased donation in the eastern part of the world. Notwithstanding its major ethical conundrum of placing a healthy donor at risk, LDLT provided the potential advantages of using an ideal donor liver, allowing optimization of the recipient and scheduling the transplant appropriately, to maximize outcomes and minimize complications. The evolution of hepato-biliary surgery further strengthened the concept of using PL grafts, as surgeons could

S. Shankar · A. Rammohan · M. Rela (✉)
The Institute of Liver Disease & Transplantation, Dr. Rela Institute & Medical Centre, Bharath Institute of Higher Education & Research, Chennai, India

B. Eghtesad et al. (eds.), *Liver Transplantation*,
https://doi.org/10.1007/978-3-032-07072-2_15

effectively transfer their skills to splitting the liver for transplantation. SLT and LDLT are widely practiced and have significantly reduced waiting list mortality among both adult and pediatric recipients.

Fundamental to the success of PLT is choosing an appropriate liver allograft and avoiding technical complications in both the donor and recipient. This, in turn, is largely dependent on the anatomical knowledge and technical acumen of the surgeon. In this chapter, we aim to describe liver anatomy, donor selection for retrieving partial grafts, and important technical concepts in LDLT and SLT, with a view to provide a better understanding of their clinical application.

Functional Anatomy of Liver

Transplantation using partial liver grafts evolved from the principle that a component of liver with a vascular pedicle, venous drainage, and bile duct, along with sufficient hepatocyte mass, can sustain the function of the entire organ in an individual. Morphologically, the liver is divided into right and left lobes by Cantlie's line, which overlies the position of the middle hepatic vein (MHV) [5]. The Brisbane 2000 terminology, based on Couinaud's system, is widely accepted and commonly used for describing segmental anatomy of the liver (Fig. 15.1) [6, 7]. It describes three orders of division of liver—first order division into right and left lobes; second order division of each lobe into anterior and posterior, or medial and lateral sections; and third order division of each section into individual segments or sectors.

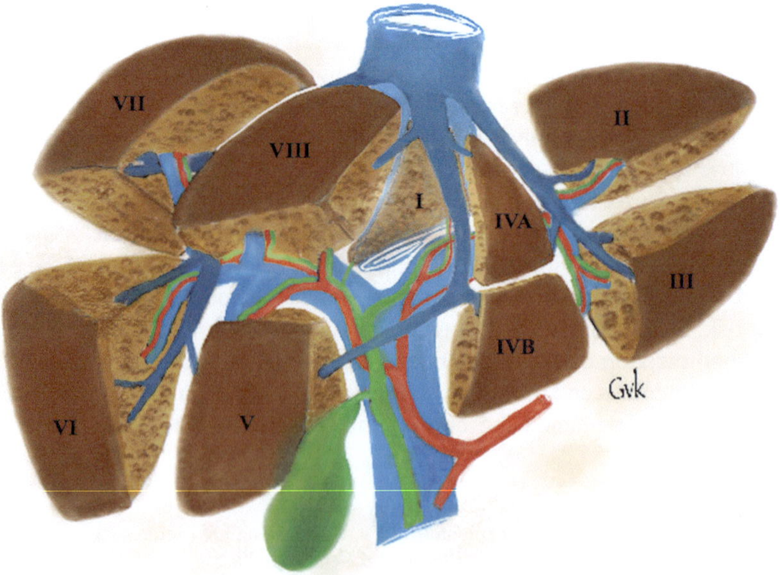

Fig. 15.1 Schematic representation of Couinaud segments of liver

Each segment of the liver receives a "portal triad" consisting of a portal venous branch, hepatic arterial branch, and bile duct radicle, and is drained by a dedicated hepatic vein branch. This functional classification permits the use of partial liver grafts in transplantation, derived either from living donors or by splitting a deceased donor liver.

Anatomical variations in hepatic vasculature and biliary tree are encountered in 50–60% of the population. The most commonly followed anatomical classification systems are the Michels et al. [8] for hepatic artery, Nakamura et al. [9] for portal vein (PV), and Huang et al. [10] and Okhubo et al. [11] for biliary system. A thorough knowledge of these variations is sine qua non for successful PLT. The proper hepatic artery is a continuation of the common hepatic artery (CHA) after the origin of the gastro-duodenal artery (GDA) and branches into the right and left hepatic arteries (RHA and LHA) (Fig. 15.2a). Segment IV artery, historically called the middle hepatic artery, may sometimes arise from the RHA. The commonest variation (25%) seen is an aberrant (replaced or accessory) LHA that arises from the left gastric artery and runs through the hepatogastric ligament to enter the umbilical fissure (Fig. 15.2b) [8]. An aberrant RHA is found in 17% of cases and arises from the superior mesenteric artery (Fig. 15.2b) [8]. This artery has a more posterior course lying behind the main PV in the porta hepatis, before coursing anterolaterally to enter the liver. The main portal vein (MPV) is formed by the confluence of the splenic and superior mesenteric veins behind the neck of the pancreas. At the hilum of the liver, it divides into right and left branches. The right portal vein (RPV) in turn divides into branches for the anterior (RAPV) and posterior (RPPV) sectors of the right lobe (Fig. 15.3a). However, trifurcation of the MPV (type B) and anomalous origin of the RAPV from the left portal vein (LPV) (type C) is also frequently encountered (Fig. 15.3b, c) [9]. The left portal vein (LPV) has a long extra-hepatic

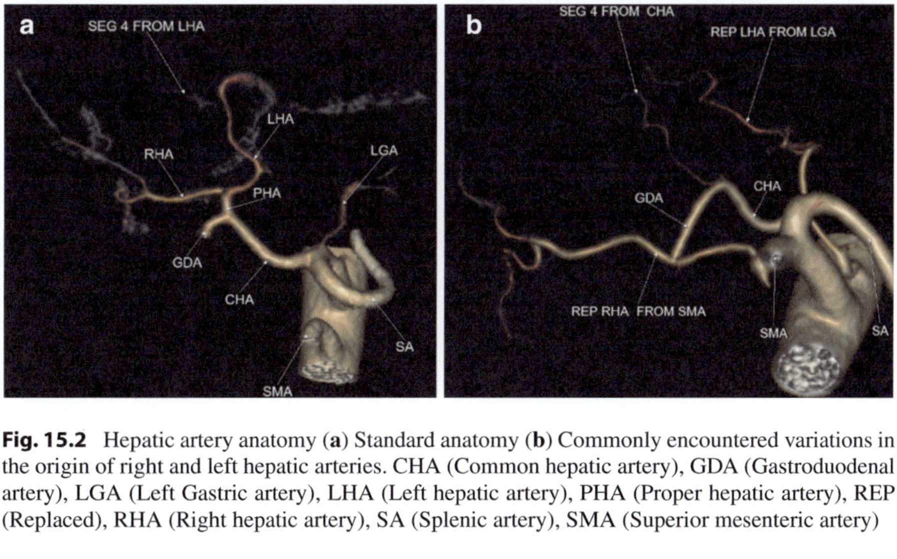

Fig. 15.2 Hepatic artery anatomy (**a**) Standard anatomy (**b**) Commonly encountered variations in the origin of right and left hepatic arteries. CHA (Common hepatic artery), GDA (Gastroduodenal artery), LGA (Left Gastric artery), LHA (Left hepatic artery), PHA (Proper hepatic artery), REP (Replaced), RHA (Right hepatic artery), SA (Splenic artery), SMA (Superior mesenteric artery)

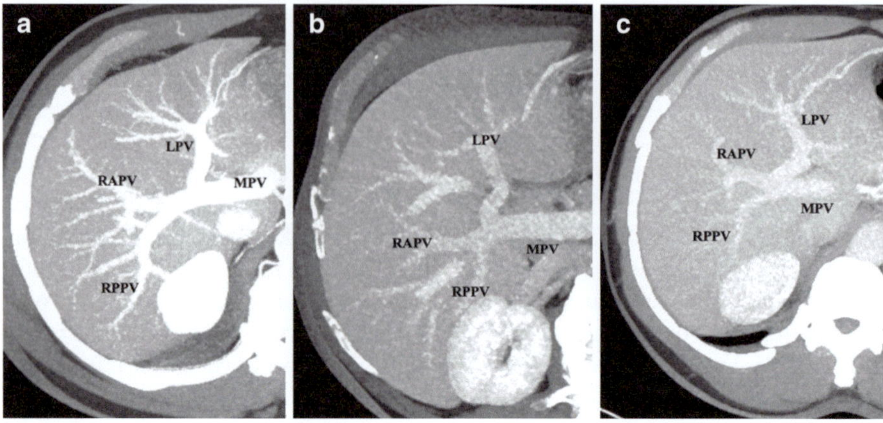

Fig. 15.3 Reconstructed computed tomographic (CT) image showing Nakamura classification of portal veins: (**a**) Type A with normal anatomy, (**b**) type B, and (**c**) type C. Both type B and C portal veins produce two orifices in right lobe liver grafts, which need reconstruction to facilitate implantation. LPV left portal vein, MPV main portal vein, RAPV right anterior portal vein, RPPV right posterior portal vein

course divided into two parts: the transverse part along the base of segment IV and the vertical part running through the umbilical fissure.

The hepatic veins are more constant in position, although variations may exist in dominant segments drained by them. The right hepatic vein (RHV) drains segments V, VI, VII, and VIII, and the size of its main trunk determines the presence of additional inferior right hepatic veins (IRHV) which usually drain the posteroinferior segments of the right lobe (Fig. 15.4). The middle hepatic vein is formed by the union of segment V and IVb veins and drains segments V, VIII, and IV. In 70–84% of cases, the MHV joins left hepatic vein (LHV) to form a common trunk, before draining into the inferior vena cava (IVC) [12–15]. The LHV drains segments II, III

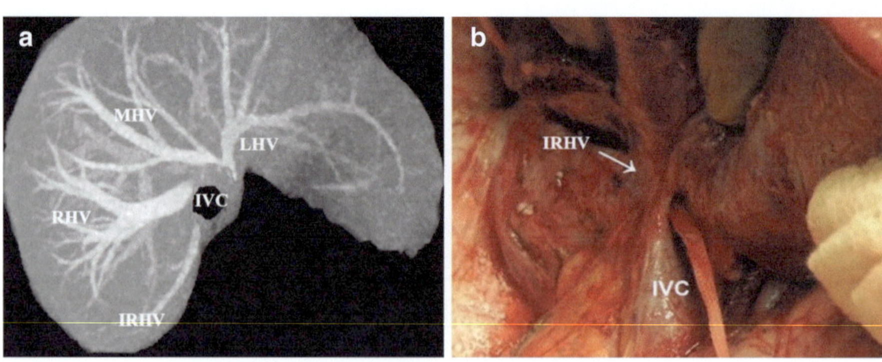

Fig. 15.4 Anatomy of hepatic Veins (**a**) CT scan showing the right (RHV), middle (MHV), left (LHV), and inferior right hepatic vein (IRHV). (**b**) Intraoperative image in a live donor operation showing the IRHV (white arrow) draining into the IVC.

and may show considerable variations in its drainage pattern in up to 15% of individuals, where segments II and III veins may open separately into the IVC, or segment III vein joins the MHV [15]. A tributary called the umbilical fissural vein (UFV) often drains segments IV and III. It drains into the LHV in 87.5% of cases, whereas in others it joins the MHV [16–18].

The intra-hepatic segmental bile ducts follow a remarkably similar course as the portal inflow due to their common embryological origin. On the right side, the right hepatic duct (RHD) is formed by the confluence of the right anterior (RASD) and right posterior sectoral ducts (RPSD). On the left side, the segment II and III ducts join together in the umbilical fissure and this common duct is then joined by the segment IV duct to form the left hepatic duct (LHD). The right and left hepatic ducts join extra-hepatically to form the common hepatic duct (CHD), which as it descends down, is joined by the cystic duct to form the common bile duct (CBD). Variations in biliary anatomy are very common and can contribute to significant morbidity if not meticulously identified and addressed (Fig. 15.5) [10, 11].

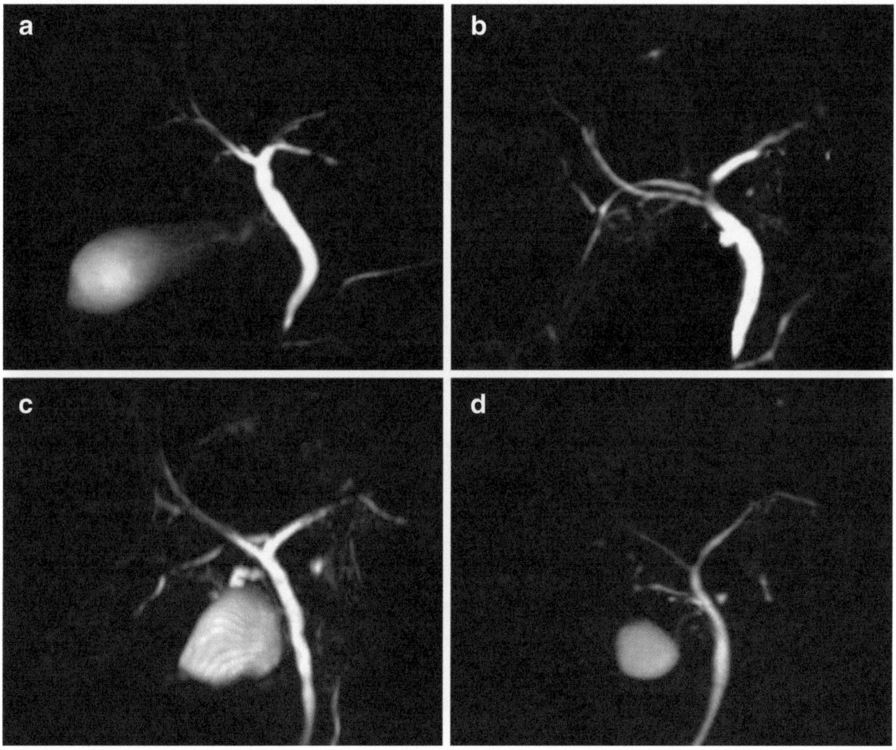

Fig. 15.5 Magnetic resonance cholangio-pancreaticogram (MRCP) images showing biliary anatomy: (**a**) normal anatomy, (**b**) trifurcation of ducts, (**c**) right posterior duct joining left hepatic duct, and (**d**) right posterior duct joining common hepatic duct. **b**, **c**, and **d** give rise to two ducts in a right lobe graft

The caudate lobe of liver (segment I) is divided into three parts: the Spiegel lobe (to the left of IVC), the paracaval portion (anterior to IVC), and the caudate process (to the right of IVC). It is unique in that it derives blood supply from both sides and drains by 1 to 3 individual veins and multiple smaller venules, directly into the IVC. There are 1 to 3 bile ducts draining individual parts of the caudate into either side of the biliary tree and care should be taken to identify and suture these ducts during transection in donors to prevent bile leak. The caudate may sometimes wrap around the IVC and requires careful dissection during explant surgery to minimize blood loss.

Living Donor Liver Transplantation

The first successful LDLT was performed from an adult to a pediatric recipient in 1989 using a left lateral segment (LLS) graft [19]. It was followed by the use of extended LLS graft and left lobe (LL) grafts with MHV, as the indication moved to transplanting older children, with the same small risk to the living donor. For adult-to-adult LDLT, the technique evolved to utilizing a right lobe, which is currently the most common graft used [20].

Donor Selection

A living donor may be related, unrelated, or altruistic. In many countries, due to ethical reasons, only close relatives are permitted to donate. An ideal donor should be between 18 and 50 years of age, free from comorbidities, and have a compatible blood group. However, experienced centers may use donors up to 55 years or those with milder and well-controlled comorbidities, depending upon their physical fitness and liver quality. ABO incompatible LDLT and paired exchange donation is also feasible if a blood group compatible donor is unavailable [21–24]. A prospective donor should undergo careful evaluation to assess their medical risks, suitability of the potential liver graft, and remnant donor liver. Clinical evaluation is done to identify comorbidities, previous surgery, and risk factors such as smoking, alcohol intake, and substance abuse. In addition to routine investigations, comprehensive laboratory tests are done to exclude transmissible viral infections, pro-thrombotic, hemolytic, and autoimmune conditions in the donor. In case of transplantation for metabolic liver diseases, additional genetic tests may be necessary prior to donation. Psychological evaluation is also done to rule out coercion and to ensure that the donor understands the risk of donation.

For evaluation of the donor liver, most centers utilize a contrast-enhanced triphasic computed tomography (CT) scan along with a magnetic resonance imaging (MRI) scan. The liver as a graft is assessed with regard to its quality, size, vascular, and biliary anatomy. Hepatic steatosis, especially macrovascular steatosis, increases cold ischemic injury, reduces rate of hepatic regeneration, and increases the risk of primary nonfunction (PNF) and early allograft dysfunction (EAD), thereby contributing to morbidity and mortality following transplantation [25, 26]. The degree of steatosis can be estimated by several noninvasive tests such as fibroscan (transient elastography), measurement of liver attenuation index (LAI) on a plain CT scan, or by MRI fat estimation. An ideal donor should have an LAI ≥ +6 as this reliably corelates with a steatosis of <20%. LAI between −5 and + 5 requires donor optimization and liver biopsy for assessment of graft steatosis. Studies have shown that living donor grafts with mild degrees of steatosis (up to 30%) can be safely transplanted without increased risk of graft dysfunction and morbidity to the recipient [27, 28].

Both graft volume and remnant volume must be calculated and taken into consideration while assessing suitability. For volume calculation, software-assisted image processing is commonly used. Obtaining an accurate estimate is critical to ensure that both the graft and remnant contain sufficient liver mass to maintain function individually in the recipient and donor, respectively. Kiuchi et al. described the widely followed concept of graft-recipient body weight ratio (GRWR) to determine the minimal volume of graft liver needed to prevent "small for size syndrome" (SFSS) [29]. Tanaka et al. showed that GRWR ≥0.8% was ideal to minimize SFSS and improve survival after adult LDLT [30]. Recent studies show that among selected adult transplant recipients with Child A cirrhosis, grafts with GRWR as low as 0.6% can be safely used [31, 32]. In pediatric recipients, GRWR is usually maintained between 2 and 4, as larger grafts may be a size mismatch to the recipient's abdominal cavity. In case of "large for size" grafts, reduction (anatomical or non-anatomical) may be necessary depending upon the volume, anteroposterior thickness, and length of the graft to facilitate abdominal closure [33].

For donor safety, a remnant volume of 40% of standard liver volume (SLV) is optimal. However, Fan et al. showed that even a 30% remnant can be safely tolerated by the donor, provided there is the absence of steatosis [34]. The choice of graft depends upon both the recipient's status, the remnant volume in the donor, quality, and the vascular and biliary anatomy of the graft. In general, smaller children can be safely transplanted with LLS grafts, whereas larger children (over 25 kgs), adolescents, and adults may need left or right lobes. In a large adult, when even a right lobe graft is insufficient, dual grafts from two separate donors can also be transplanted to provide sufficient hepatic mass [35].

Surgical Principles of Graft Retrieval

Living donor liver retrieval can be done by open, laparoscopic, or robotic techniques. Following mobilization of the lobe that is to be retrieved, meticulous hilar dissection is done to identify the blood vessels supplying it. Dissection around the bile duct is kept to a minimum to preserve its blood supply and minimize the risk of stenosis. Particular attention is given to identify anomalous vascular supply and biliary anatomy, as they would require appropriate reconstruction to minimize complications for both the donor and the recipient.

For right and left lobe retrieval, a cholecystectomy is routinely done. The plane of transection is along the right border of MHV and can be identified by temporarily occluding the inflow to mark the line of demarcation. The anatomy of the MHV is the cornerstone of right lobe (RL) donation as it drains parts of both right and left lobes (Fig. 15.6). Traditionally, the MHV was taken with the RL graft. However, there is a center-to-center variation and more recently, there has been a decisive shift toward retaining the MHV with the donor to improve safety. This leads to congestion of segments V and VIII and troublesome bleeding in the recipient after reperfusion, as well as a decrease in the functional graft volume. Hence, outflow from these segments is reconstructed on the backbench using prosthetic material or cadaveric vessel grafts to restore the anterior sector outflow (Fig. 15.7) [36–38]. IRHV of size >5 mm when encountered in the RL graft is implanted separately onto the recipient's IVC. In RL donation, type B and C portal anatomy will give rise to two portal vein stumps in the graft. These are reconstructed in the backbench, using either the recipient's portal vein retrieved from the explanted liver (Y graft) or with a cadaveric vein patch (combined unification venoplasty). It is crucial to ensure that the lumen and direction of either of the orifices is not compromised during reconstruction in order to avoid stenosis later [39–42]. Type E PV is an absolute contraindication to donation.

Hepatic arterial anomalies should be promptly identified, as their reconstruction is more difficult in LDLT. Double arteries are more commonly encountered in the left lobe (LL) graft when the segment 4 artery arises from the RHA. Similarly, the presence of accessory right or left hepatic artery and extra-hepatic branching of the RHA forming a girdle around the bile duct may also result in 2 arteries in the graft. In such cases, both arteries are reconstructed in the recipient, if there is an absence of pulsatile backflow after division of the smaller artery, indicating a lack of intraparenchymal arterial overlap (Fig. 15.8) [39]. Anomalous biliary anatomy is present in almost half the population and is an important contributor to biliary complications postoperatively. With RL donation, pre-donation imaging helps define the anatomy, allowing for safe division of the RHD. Some centers also use intraoperative cholangiogram to further elucidate the anatomy before division, as it is crucial to maintain the continuity of the donor's biliary system. Particular care must be taken while transecting the caudate lobe, as failure to identify transected ducts here may lead to troublesome bile leaks and collections adjacent to the biliary anastomosis, resulting in inflammatory strictures. To ensure vascularity of the bile duct, it is isolated and divided with an intact hilar plate, flush with the liver parenchyma. In case of multiple ducts which are close to each other in the graft, a single anastomosis can be done. Whereas, if they are far apart, then two or more anastomosis are done onto the recipient duct or a roux loop of jejunum.

In left lateral sector (LLS) donation for pediatric liver transplantation, the line of transection is 1 cm to the right of the falciform ligament. The portal and arterial inflow to the LLS graft is divided in the umbilical fissure, where they have a long extra-hepatic course. Care should be taken while dividing LHV, as variations in the outflow from segments 2 and 3 are often found, with each of them opening separately into the IVC, or segment 3 outflow joining the MHV [15]. In both these

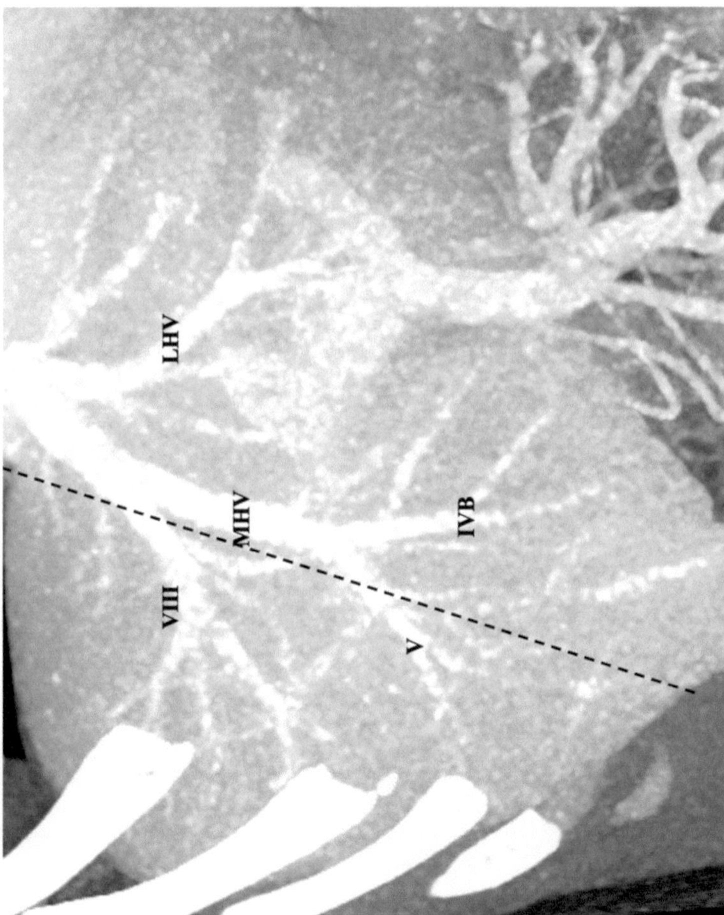

Fig. 15.6 CT image showing formation of the middle hepatic vein (MHV) from segment V and segment IVB veins. Segment VIII tributary is also seen draining into MHV, which in turn joins the left hepatic vein (LHV) before draining into the inferior vena cava. The dotted line represents the line of transection for retrieval of a right lobe graft

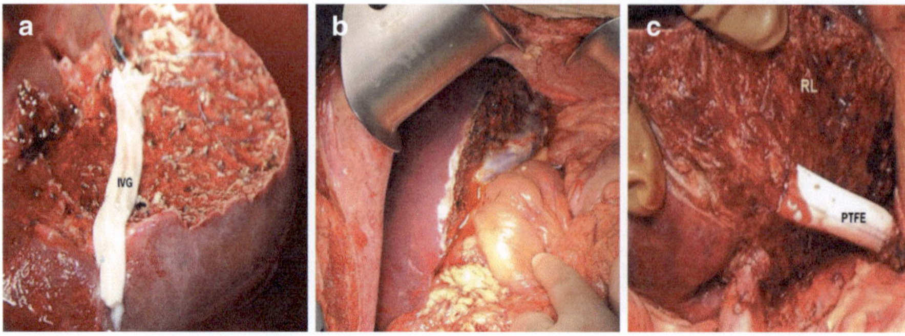

Fig. 15.7 (**a**) Right lobe (RL) graft showing segment 5 outflow reconstruction using cadaveric iliac vein graft (IVG), (**b**) graft following implantation showing a well-drained anterior sector, and (**c**) RL graft with segment 5 outflow reconstructed using synthetic polytetrafluoroethylene (PTFE) graft

scenarios, there will be two outflow orifices in the graft, which need reconstruction in the backbench prior to implantation (Fig. 15.9). Meticulous care is taken while anastomosing the hepatic artery and portal vein as thrombosis is common due to the small caliber of vessels in the recipient. An atretic portal vein is often encountered in children with biliary atresia, which may require reconstruction using an interposition graft or a jump graft from the SMV to ensure adequate portal flow to the graft (Fig. 15.10). Similarly, ligation of large collaterals may also help augment the portal inflow to the graft. In very young pediatric recipients, as the size of the abdominal cavity may be small, attention is given to the thickness and volume of the LLS graft. Long, flat grafts may be accommodated within the abdomen easily, whereas in the case of large, thick grafts, nonanatomical reduction, either in situ or in the backbench, may be necessary to facilitate abdominal closure. Alternatively,

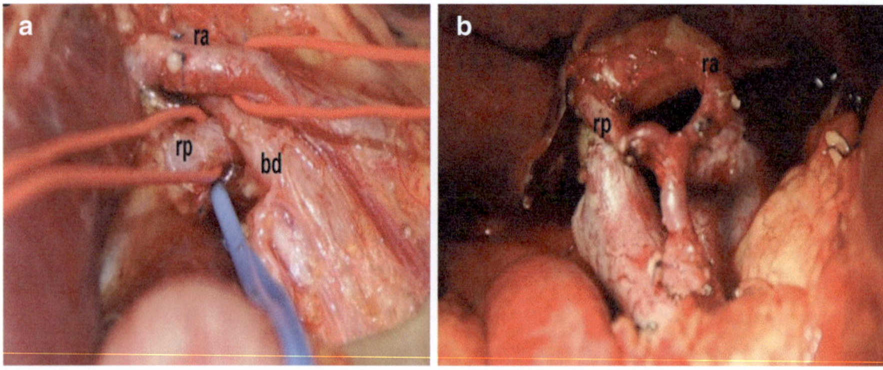

Fig. 15.8 (**a**) Intraoperative view showing extrahepatic bifurcation of right hepatic artery into its anterior (ra) and posterior (rp) divisions coursing on either side of the common bile duct (bd). This variation leads to two arteries in a right lobe graft. (**b**) Both arteries (ra and rp) reconstructed in the recipient

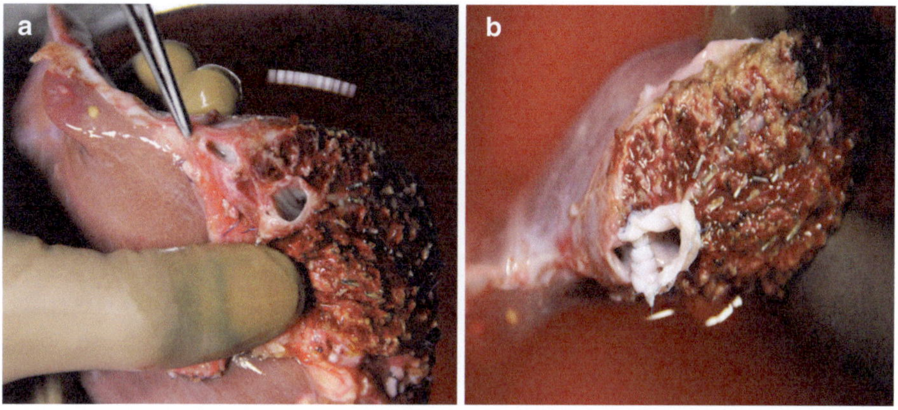

Fig. 15.9 (**a**) Left lateral segment graft showing two separate hepatic venous outflows from segments 2 and 3. (**b**) Conjoint unification venoplasty done using a cadaveric venous graft to create a single outflow for implantation

monosegment grafts can also be retrieved to avoid large for size syndrome, which carries a significant risk of allograft dysfunction [43–45].

Portal Inflow Modulation

Following graft implantation and reperfusion, portal pressure is ideally maintained between 10 and 15 mm Hg and portal flow between 100 and 250 ml/min/100 grams of liver tissue [46–49]. When this is not achieved, portal inflow modulation (PIM) may become necessary to either augment or reduce portal flow to minimize early allograft dysfunction. Several other factors are also taken into account prior to modulation, such as the GRWR, spleen size, and presence of large collaterals (coronary vein or spleno-renal collateral) in the recipient. In case of hypoperfusion (indicated

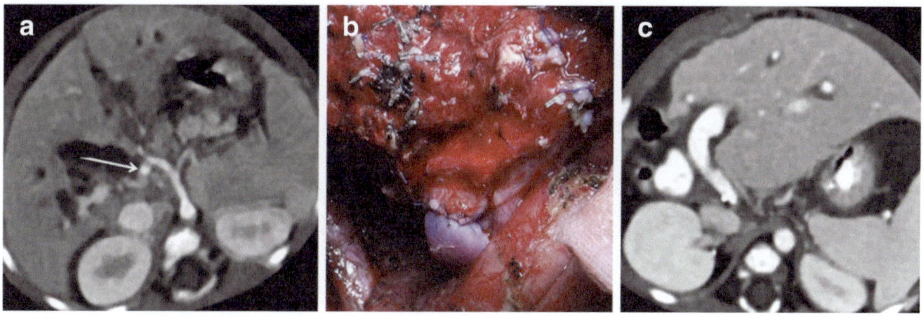

Fig. 15.10 (**a**) CT scan showing atretic portal vein (arrow) in an infant with biliary atresia. Note the size of the vein in comparison to the artery next to it. (**b**) Intraoperative picture showing portal vein reconstruction using a cadaveric vein interposition graft, (**c**) Postoperative CT scan showing widely patent interposition graft

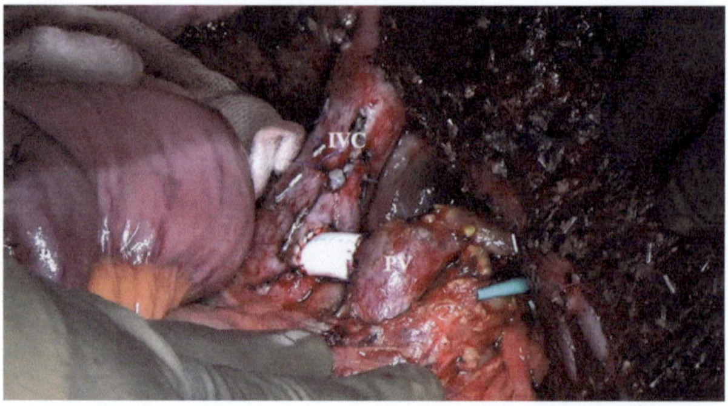

Fig. 15.11 Partial portacaval shunt created using a synthetic 8 mm PTFE graft between the portal vein (PV) and inferior vena cava (IVC)

by low portal pressure and flow) caused by large collaterals shunting blood away from the liver, ligating them becomes necessary to augment the portal flow. In case of a large spleno-renal shunt, left renal vein ligation can also be done as a safe alternative [50]. A contrasting situation, when collateral ligation is preferably done, is when the portal pressure is acceptable, yet is associated with poor portal flow. In this scenario, it is crucial to exclude hepatic vein outflow obstruction (HVOO) and once affirmed, the other possibilities are a stiff graft or a small for size graft, both of which can further increase sinusoidal hypertension, which in turn will enlarge pre-existing collaterals and cause significant portal steal. Hence, collateral ligation is done to prevent SFSS. If portal pressure is over 15 mm Hg, splenic artery ligation is a safe technique to reduce the pressure by up to 2–3 mmHg. If greater decompression is necessary, then partial portacaval shunt (PPCS) or splenectomy can be done. PPCS (Fig. 15.11) should be used selectively as it carries a higher risk of causing severe portal steal and even graft necrosis, if there is an undetected HVOO. Splenectomy on the other hand offers excellent reduction in portal flow without the danger of portal steal or encephalopathy. However, due to increased risk of blood loss and postoperative infection, many centers do not routinely practice it. Pharmacological PIM is also commonly used as an adjunct; however, its effects on portal flow may be short-lived.

Split Liver Transplantation

With SLT, a whole adult deceased donor liver is split into two functioning grafts. The rationale for splitting is to increase the donor pool and reduce waiting time mortality, and subsequently to benefit pediatric recipients. Pichlmayr and Bismuth initially advocated SLT as an ex vivo procedure [4, 51]. However, this lengthens the cold ischemia time and potentially exposes the graft to rewarming during manipulation. Broelsch and Busuttil introduced in situ splitting at the donor hospital, with surgical division completed in the heart-beating donor immediately prior to aortic cross clamp and organ cold perfusion [3, 52]. In situ SLT reduces cold ischemia, simplifies identification of biliary and vascular structures, eliminates unintentional graft rewarming during ex vivo manipulation, and reduces hemorrhage upon graft reperfusion. However, it requires specialized skills and equipment at the donor institution.

Donor Selection

Successful SLT requires thorough consideration and evaluation whenever a donor organ is available. The decision to split an organ depends upon donor status, anatomical considerations and quality of the graft, recipient characteristics, and logistic parameters. The ideal liver for splitting would be from a young donor (less than 50 years), with no history of liver disease, acceptable liver enzymes (AST and ALT less than twice the normal value, GGT < 50 U/L), serum sodium <160 mmol/dL, and a short intensive care unit stay with hemodynamic stability before and during organ retrieval

[52–54]. Macroscopically, the liver should have a soft consistency with sharp edges, macroscopic steatosis <20% and a good size LLS for splitting [53, 54]. For optimal logistics, the donor should be available in the transplant center itself for in situ splitting. If not, it is important to keep the cold ischemia time as short as possible (less than 12 h) during ex situ splitting and transportation of the organ to the transplanting center. The prospective recipients are also of relevance while making a decision about splitting an organ. If the potential recipient is a sick adult with a high Model for End stage Liver Disease (MELD) score or requiring urgent transplantation, or is undergoing retransplantation, splitting is contraindicated. On the contrary, in case of high urgency in a pediatric recipient, splitting is beneficial to provide a size-matched organ. In an elective situation, the size and quality of the organ should aid in deciding the potential recipients, ensuring that a graft with a minimum GRWR of 0.8% can be provided for an adult recipient.

Surgical Principles of Splitting

In the commonest form of SLT, the liver is split into an extended right lobe graft (Segments I, IV–VIII) for implantation into an adult recipient and a left lateral segment graft (Segments II and III) for implantation into a pediatric recipient. In less common cases, the liver is split into right (Segments I, V–VIII) and left (Segments II–IV) lobes for two adult recipients. The key to successful procurement of partial allografts is to maintain vascular and biliary supply to both sides of the liver without sabotaging either. Hence, it is imperative to have a thorough knowledge of the surgical anatomy of the hilar structures and the relationship of the middle and right hepatic veins, in order to safely execute these procedures and to minimize both donor and recipient postoperative complications.

In SLT, the hilar structures are first evaluated thoroughly to identify the presence of variant anatomy. The technique of splitting the vasculature varies between different centers [52, 55–58]. However, the most common method involves preserving the main trunk of the common hepatic artery with the right lobe graft, by dividing the

LHA at the level of its confluence (Fig. 15.12). Similarly, the main trunk of the PV is allocated to the right lobe graft, as the LPV has a longer extra-hepatic course, which provides sufficient length for anastomosis to the recipient. Probing the CBD helps in identifying the confluence to ensure safe division of the ducts. The common bile duct is given to the right lobe graft, and the left hepatic duct is sectioned just away from the hilum and retained with the LL or LLS. The plane of parenchymal transection is just to the right of the umbilical fissure in the RL and LLS split. The LHV is retained with the LLS graft whereas the RHV and MHV along with the IVC are allocated to the extended right lobe. There is persisting controversy regarding retaining a necrotic segment IV with the right side. Some centers prefer to discard it, as it may lead to bile leak postoperatively, whereas others retain it to reduce cut surface bleeding [54–57]. In RL and LL split, the plane of transection starts in the gallbladder fossa, and as the parenchymal dissection continues superiorly, the venous outflow from segment 5 is used as a signpost to identify the origin of MHV, which is then retained with the LL graft by progressing the transection along its right border. Parenchymal transection is done by the Kelly-clysis technique or using the cavitron ultrasonic suction and aspiration (CUSA) device. During ex situ split, care should be taken to ensure that the graft is kept immersed in ice-cold preservative solution, to minimize mitochondrial damage caused by rewarming (Fig. 15.13). During transection, care is taken to ligate all vessels and major pedicles along the cut surface to prevent inadvertent bleeding and bile leak following reperfusion. Such bleeding can be addressed later by application of hemostatic patches or argon beam coagulation to the cut surface. Injection of propofol through the cystic or

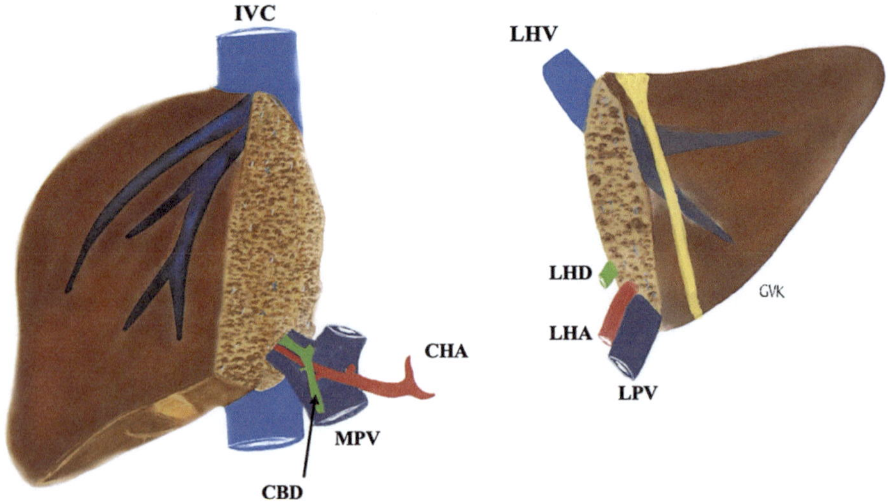

Fig. 15.12 Schematic representation of splitting a whole liver into extended right lobe and left lateral segment grafts. CBD Common bile duct, CHA Common hepatic artery, IVC Inferior vena cava, LHA Left hepatic artery, LHD Left hepatic duct, LHV Left hepatic vein, LPV Left portal vein, MPV Main portal vein

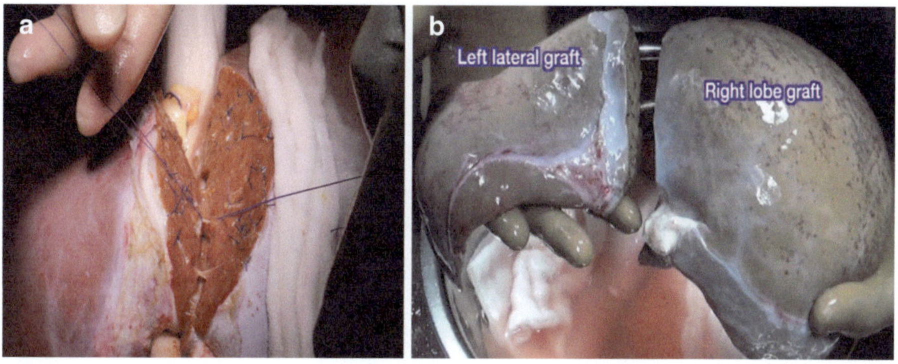

Fig. 15.13 (**a**) Ex situ splitting of whole liver graft; (**b**) graft after splitting

hepatic duct prior to biliary anastomosis also aids in identifying bile leak from open ducts along the cut surface.

Auxiliary Partial Orthotopic Liver Transplantation (APOLT)

APOLT is a technique wherein the left or right lobe of the native liver is resected and replaced by a healthy partial liver graft. This technique was originally introduced for non-cirrhotic metabolic liver diseases (NCMLD) and potentially reversible fulminant hepatic failure. The advantage of APOLT for fulminant hepatic failure is twofold, where it supports the native liver during regeneration and later helps in discontinuation of immunosuppression [58–61]. In NCMLD, it can compensate for enzyme deficiency without complete removal of native liver, which may aid the recipient in case of potential graft failure [62]. It has also been utilized in LDLT with a small for size graft, where a delayed native hepatectomy is performed in order to support regeneration of the implanted partial graft [63]. The concept of APOLT has been further revolutionized to develop the DOMINO-APOLT technique, wherein resected liver from one NCMLD patient is transplanted by an APOLT to another recipient with a different NCMLD, and the resected liver from the latter provides APOLT graft for the former recipient. In this scenario, the metabolic abnormality of each partial liver is compensated by the other, thereby totally avoiding the need for a donor [62].

The current common practice in APOLT is to perform an extended left hepatectomy in the recipient and perform a left APOLT using a LLS graft from a deceased split liver or a living donor liver in case of children (Fig. 15.14). Older children and adults may require a left lobe or even a right lobe graft. Thorough preoperative evaluation of the recipient's CT is done for planning implantation. In the common technique, the blood supply to the native right liver is preserved in continuity. The LHV of the graft is anastomosed perfectly to the MHV/LHV stump of the recipient, as any outflow resistance will further add to portal steal and cause graft atrophy. The LPV of the graft is anastomosed to the left side of the MPV of the recipient as this

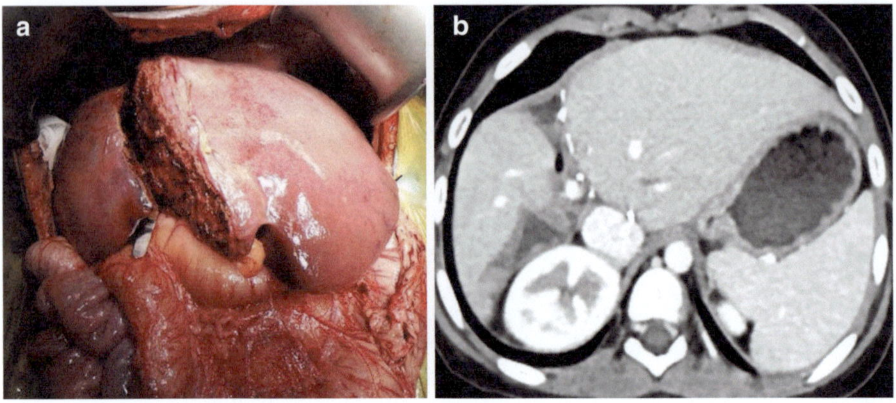

Fig. 15.14 (**a**) Intraoperative picture of auxiliary partial orthotopic liver transplantation (APOLT) using a left lateral segment graft. (**b**) Postoperative CT scan showing significant atrophy of the native right lobe

creates a wider orifice. Portal flow modulation to the native graft is always done by placing a partially occlusive ligature around the native RPV, thereby preferentially directing the flow to the APOLT graft to avoid potential portal steal by the native liver. The recipient CHA is divided proximal to the origin of the GDA after ensuring a patent arcade and the proximal CHA stump is used for anastomosis to the LHA of the graft. A new roux en Y loop is constructed for hepaticojejunostomy to the graft LHD.

Conclusion

Partial liver allografts have successfully increased the donor organ pool and reduced waiting list morbidity and mortality for chronic liver disease patients. Successful use of these grafts mandates a detailed understanding of intra-hepatic anatomy. Meticulous donor evaluation and excellent surgical skills further help to minimize complications. Innovative techniques such as APOLT and evolving minimally invasive techniques such as laparoscopic and robotic donor hepatectomy and recipient transplantation have further revolutionized liver transplantation using partial grafts, with excellent short- and long-term outcomes.

Acknowledgments The authors gratefully acknowledge Dr. Vasanthakumar Gunasekaran, Consultant Liver transplant and Hepato-pancreatico-biliary surgeon, Dr. Rela Institute and Medical Centre, Chennai, India, for contributing his original artwork to this chapter.

Conflict of Interest and Financial Support Disclosure The authors of this manuscript have no conflicts of interest or financial ties to disclose.

Data Availability Statement The datasets generated during and/or analyzed during the current study are available from the corresponding author on reasonable request.

Author Contributions Dr. Sadhana Shankar, Dr. Ashwin Rammohan & Prof. Mohamed Rela contributed to conception, design, acquisition, analysis and interpretation of data. Dr. Sadhana Shankar, Dr. Ashwin Rammohan & Prof. Mohamed Rela drafted the article and revised it critically for important intellectual content and Prof. Mohamed Rela gave the final approval of the version to be published.

References

1. Smith B. Segmental liver transplantation from a living donor. J Pediatr Surg. 1969;4(1):126–32.
2. Bismuth H, Houssin D. Reduced-sized orthotopic liver graft in hepatic transplantation in children. Surgery. 1984;95(3):367–70.
3. Brölsch CE, Neuhaus P, Burdelski M, Bernsau U, Pichlmayr R, Orthotopic transplantation of hepatic segments in infants with biliary atresia. InChirurgisches Forum'84 für experimentelle und klinische Forschung: 101. Kongreß der Deutschen Gesellschaft für Chirurgie, München, 25.–28. 1984. Berlin Heidelberg: Springer; 1984. p. 105–9.
4. Pichlmayr R. Transplantation einer Spenderleber anf zwei Empfanger (splitting transplantation): Eine neue methode in der welterentwicklung der lebersegment. Transplantation. 1988;373:127–30.
5. Cantlie MA. On a new arrangement of the right and left lobes of the liver. Proc Anatom Soc Great Britain Irel. 1898;32:4–9.
6. Strasberg SM, Belghiti J, Clavien PA, Gadzijev E, Garden JO, Lau WY, Makuuchi M, Strong RW. The Brisbane 2000 terminology of liver anatomy and resections. HPB. 2000;2(3):333–9.
7. Couinaud C. Les enveloppes vasculobiliares de foie ou capsule de Glisson. Leur interet dans la chirurgie vesiculaire, les resections hepatiques et l'abord du hile du foie. Lyon Chir. 1954;49:589–615.
8. Michels NA. Newer anatomy of the liver and its variant blood supply and collateral circulation. Am J Surg. 1966;112(3):337–47.
9. Nakamura T, Tanaka K, Kiuchi T, Kasahara M, Oike F, Ueda M, Kaihara S, Egawa H, Ozden I, Kobayashi N, Uemoto S. Anatomical variations and surgical strategies in right lobe living donor liver transplantation: lessons from 120 cases1. Transplantation. 2002;73(12):1896–903.
10. Huang TL, Cheng YF, Chen CL, Chen TY, Lee TY. Variants of the bile ducts: clinical application in the potential donor of living-related hepatic transplantation. In: Transplantation proceedings (Vol. 28, No. 3, pp. 1669–70); 1996.
11. Ohkubo M, Nagino M, Kamiya J, Yuasa N, Oda K, Arai T, Nishio H, Nimura Y. Surgical anatomy of the bile ducts at the hepatic hilum as applied to living donor liver transplantation. Ann Surg. 2004;239(1):82.
12. Nakamura S, Tsuzuki T. Surgical anatomy of the hepatic veins and the inferior vena cava. Surg Gynecol Obstet. 1981;152(1):43–50.
13. Shilal P, Agarwal S, Tuli A, Kakkar S. Variations in the drainage pattern of middle hepatic vein and left hepatic vein in the left lobe of liver. J Clin Diagn Res. 2018;12(9).
14. Hwang S, Lee SG, Choi ST, Moon DB, Ha TY, Lee YJ, Park KM, Kim KH, Ahn CS, Kim KK, Kim YD. Hepatic vein anatomy of the medial segment for living donor liver transplantation using extended right lobe graft. Liver Transpl. 2005;11(4):449–55.

15. Shankar S, Rammohan A, Gunasekaran V, Narasimhan G, Rajalingam R, Palaniappan K, Kanagavelu R, Rajkumar A, Kaliamoorthy I, Rela M. Anatomical variations of left hepatic vein and outflow reconstruction techniques in pediatric living donor liver transplantation. Am J Transplant. 2023;23:786.
16. Tani K, Shindoh J, Akamatsu N, Arita J, Kaneko J, Sakamoto Y, Hasegawa K, Kokudo N. Venous drainage map of the liver for complex hepatobiliary surgery and liver transplantation. HPB. 2016;18(12):1031–8.
17. Honda H, Yanaga K, Onitsuka H, Kaneko K, Murakami J, Masuda K. Ultrasonographic anatomy of veins draining the left lobe of the liver: feasibility of live related transplantation. Acta Radiol. 1991;32(6):479–84.
18. Ortale JR, Bonet C, Prado PF, Mariotto A. Anatomy of the intrahepatic ramification of the intermediate and left hepatic veins in humans. J Morphol Sci. 2017;20(1).
19. Strong RW, Lynch SV, Ong TH, et al. Successful liver transplantation from a living donor to her son. N Engl J Med. 1990;322:1505–7.
20. Yamaoka Y, Washida M, Honda K, Tanaka K, Mori K, Shimahara Y, Okamoto S, Ueda M, Hayashi M, Tanaka A, Morimoto T. Liver transplantation using a right lobe graft from a living related donor. Transplantation. 1994;57(7):1127–9.
21. Raut V, Uemoto S. Management of ABO-incompatible living-donor liver transplantation: past and present trends. Surg Today. 2011;41:317–22.
22. Kozaki K, Egawa H, Kasahara M, Oike F, Yoshizawa A, Fukatsu A, Tanaka K. Therapeutic strategy and the role of apheresis therapy for ABO incompatible living donor liver transplantation. Ther Apher Dial. 2005;9(4):285–91.
23. Kim JM. Increasing living liver donor pools: liver paired exchange versus ABO-incompatible living donor liver transplantation. Transplantation. 2022;106(11):2118–9.
24. Hwang S, Lee SG, Moon DB, Song GW, Ahn CS, Kim KH, Ha TY, Jung DH, Kim KW, Choi NK, Park GC. Exchange living donor liver transplantation to overcome ABO incompatibility in adult patients. Liver Transpl. 2010;16(4):482–90.
25. Diehl AM. Cytokine regulation of liver injury and repair. Immunol Rev. 2000;174(1):160–71.
26. Selzner M, Clavien PA. Failure of regeneration of the steatotic rat liver: disruption at two different levels in the regeneration pathway. Hepatology. 2000;31(1):35–42.
27. Angele MK, Rentsch M, Hartl WH, Wittmann B, Graeb C, Jauch KW, Loehe F. Effect of graft steatosis on liver function and organ survival after liver transplantation. Am J Surg. 2008;195(2):214–20.
28. Cho JY, Suh KS, Kwon CH, Yi NJ, Cho SY, Jang JJ, Kim SH, Lee KU. The hepatic regeneration power of mild steatotic grafts is not impaired in living-donor liver transplantation. Liver Transpl. 2005;11(2):210–7.
29. Kiuchi T, Kasahara M, Uryuhara K, Inomata Y, Uemoto S, Asonuma K, Egawa H, Fujita S, Hayashi M, Tanaka K. Impact of graft size mismatching on graft prognosis in liver transplantation from living donors1, 2. Transplantation. 1999;67(2):321–7.
30. Tanaka K, Ogura Y. "Small-for-size graft" and "small-for-size syndrome" in living donor liver transplantation. Yonsei Med J. 2004;45(6):1089–94.
31. Wong TC, Fung JY, Cui TY, Sin SL, Ma KW, She BW, Chan AC, Chok KS, Dai JW, Cheung TT, Lo CM. The risk of going small: lowering GRWR and overcoming small-for-size syndrome in adult living donor liver transplantation. Ann Surg. 2021;274(6):e1260–8.
32. Kaido T, Mori A, Ogura Y, Hata K, Yoshizawa A, Iida T, Yagi S, Uemoto S. Lower limit of the graft-to-recipient weight ratio can be safely reduced to 0.6% in adult-to-adult living donor liver transplantation in combination with portal pressure control. In: Transplantation proceedings (Vol. 43, No. 6, pp. 2391–2393). Elsevier; 2011.
33. Rammohan A, Gunasekaran V, Reddy MS, Rela M. Graft reduction in pediatric liver transplantation: the myth of 4? Am J Transplant. 2018;18(12):3081–2.
34. Fan ST, Lo CM, Liu CL, Yong BH, Chan JK, Ng IO. Safety of donors in live donor liver transplantation using right lobe grafts. Arch Surg. 2000;135(3):336–40.

35. Lee SG, Hwang S, Park KM, Kim KH, Ahn CS, Lee YJ, Cheon JY, Joo SH, Moon DB, Joo CW, Min PC. Seventeen adult-to-adult living donor liver transplantations using dual grafts. In: Transplantation proceedings (Vol. 33, No. 7–8, pp. 3461–3). Elsevier; 2001.
36. Kasahara M, Takada Y, Fujimoto Y, Ogura Y, Ogawa K, Uryuhara K, Yonekawa Y, Ueda M, Egawa H, Tanaka K. Impact of right lobe with middle hepatic vein graft in living-donor liver transplantation. Am J Transplant. 2005;5(6):1339–46.
37. Ghobrial RM, Hsieh CB, Lerner S, Winters S, Nissen N, Dawson S, Amersi F, Chen P, Farmer D, Yersiz H, Busuttil RW. Technical challenges of hepatic venous outflow reconstruction in right lobe adult living donor liver transplantation. Liver Transpl. 2001;7(6):551–5.
38. Lee SG. Techniques of reconstruction of hepatic veins in living-donor liver transplantation, especially for right hepatic vein and major short hepatic veins of right-lobe graft. J Hepato-Biliary-Pancreat Surg. 2006;13:131–8.
39. Marcos A, Orloff M, Mieles L, Olzinski A, Sitzmann J. Reconstruction of double hepatic arterial and portal venous branches for right-lobe living donor liver transplantation. Liver Transpl. 2001;7(8):673–9.
40. Ha TY, Hwang S, Moon DB, Ahn CS, Kim KH, Song GW, Jung DH, Park GC, Kang SH, Jung BH, Lee SG. Conjoined unification venoplasty for graft double portal vein branches as a modification of autologous Y-graft interposition. Liver Transpl. 2015;21(5):707–10.
41. Hwang S, Lee SG, Ahn CS, Kim KH, Moon DB, Ha TY, Song GW, Jung DH, Ryu JH, Ko KH, Choi NK. Technique and outcome of autologous portal Y-graft interposition for anomalous right portal veins in living donor liver transplantation. Liver Transpl. 2009;15(4):427–34.
42. Hwang S, Ha TY, Song GW, Jung DH, Moon DB, Ahn CS, Kim KH, Park GC, Lee SG. Conjoined unification venoplasty for double portal vein branches of right liver graft: 1-year experience at a high-volume living donor liver transplantation center. J Gastrointest Surg. 2016;20:199–205.
43. Ogawa K, Kasahara M, Sakamoto S, Ito T, Taira K, Oike F, Ueda M, Egawa H, Takada Y, Uemoto S. Living donor liver transplantation with reduced monosegments for neonates and small infants. Transplantation. 2007;83(10):1337–40.
44. Shehata MR, Yagi S, Okamura Y, Iida T, Hori T, Yoshizawa A, Hata K, Fujimoto Y, Ogawa K, Okamoto S, Ogura Y. Pediatric liver transplantation using reduced and hyper-reduced left lateral segment grafts: a 10-year single-center experience. Am J Transplant. 2012;12(12):3406–13.
45. Kasahara M, Sakamoto S, Umeshita K, Uemoto S. Effect of graft size matching on pediatric living-donor liver transplant in Japan. Ratio. 2014;4:8.
46. Reddy MS, Rela M. Portosystemic collaterals in living donor liver transplantation: what is all the fuss about? Liver Transpl. 2017;23(4):537–44.
47. Troisi R, Ricciardi S, Smeets P, Petrovic M, Van Maele G, Colle I, Van Vlierberghe H, De Hemptinne B. Effects of hemi-portocaval shunts for inflow modulation on the outcome of small-for-size grafts in living donor liver transplantation. Am J Transplant. 2005;5(6):1397–404.
48. Kow AW, Liu J, Patel MS, De Martin E, Reddy MS, Soejima Y, Syn N, Watt K, Xia Q, Saraf N, Kamel R. Post living donor liver transplantation small-for-size syndrome: definitions, timelines, biochemical, and clinical factors for diagnosis: guidelines from the ILTS-iLDLT-LTSI consensus conference. Transplantation. 2023;107(10):2226–37.
49. Kirchner VA, Shankar S, Victor DW III, Tanaka T, Goldaracena N, Troisi RI, Olthoff KM, Kim JM, Pomfret EA, Heaton N, Polak WG. Management of established small-for-size syndrome in post living donor liver transplantation: medical, radiological, and surgical interventions: guidelines from the ILTS-iLDLT-LTSI consensus conference. Transplantation. 2023;107(10):2238–46.
50. Shankar S, Rammohan A, Balasubramanian B, Palaniappan K, Rajalingam R, Rela M. Renal implications of left renal vein ligation for portal flow augmentation in liver transplantation. World J Surg. 2021;45(8):2567–71.
51. Bismuth H, Morino M, Castaing D, Gillon MC, Declere AD, Saliba F, Samuel D. Emergency orthotopic liver transplantation in two patients using one donor liver. J Br Surg. 1989;76(7):722–4.
52. Busuttil RW, Goss JA. Split liver transplantation. Ann Surg. 1999;229(3):313.

53. Renz JF, Yersiz H, Reichert PR, Hisatake GM, Farmer DG, Emond JC, Busuttil RW. Split-liver transplantation: a review. Am J Transplant. 2003;3(11):1323–35.
54. Broering DC, Wilms C, Lenk C, Jan Schulte Esch II, Schönherr S, Mueller L, Kim JS, Helmke K, Burdelski M, Rogiers X. Technical refinements and results in full-right full-left splitting of the deceased donor liver. Ann Surg. 2005;242(6):802–13.
55. Rela M, Vougas V, Muiesan P, Vilca-Melendez H, Smyrniotis V, Gibbs P, Karani J, Williams R, Heaton N. Split liver transplantation: King's College Hospital experience. Ann Surg. 1998;227(2):282.
56. Azoulay D, Astarcioglu I, Bismuth H, Castaing D, Majno P, Adam R, Johann M. Split-liver transplantation. The Paul Brousse policy. Ann Surg. 1996;224(6):737.
57. Reyes J, Gerber D, Mazariegos GV, Casavilla A, Sindhi R, Bueno J, Madariaga J, Fung JJ. Split-liver transplantation: a comparison of ex vivo and in situ techniques. J Pediatr Surg. 2000;35(2):283–90.
58. Vagefi PA, Parekh J, Ascher NL, Roberts JP, Freise CE. Outcomes with split liver transplantation in 106 recipients: the University of California, San Francisco, experience from 1993 to 2010. Arch Surg. 2011;146(9):1052–9.
59. Boudjema K, Cherqui D, Jaeck D, Chenard-Neu MP, Steib A, Becmeur F, Brunot B, Simeoni U, Bellocq JP, Tempe JD, Wolf P. Auxiliary liver transplantation for fulminant and subfulminant hepatic failure. Transplantation. 1995;59(2):218–23.
60. Saigal S, Srinivasan P, Devlin J, De Boer B, Thomas B, Portmann B, Heaton ND, O'Grady J, Rela M. Auxiliary partial orthotopic liver transplantation in acute liver failure due to hepatitis B. Transpl Int. 2002;15(7):369–73.
61. Kasahara M, Takada Y, Egawa H, Fujimoto Y, Ogura Y, Ogawa K, Kozaki K, Haga H, Ueda M, Tanaka K. Auxiliary partial orthotopic living donor liver transplantation: Kyoto University experience. Am J Transplant. 2005;5(3):558–65.
62. Reddy MS, Rajalingam R, Rela M. Revisiting APOLT for metabolic liver disease: a new look at an old idea. Transplantation. 2017;101(2):260–6.
63. Inomata Y, Kiuchi T, Kim ID, Uemoto S, Egawa H, Asonuma K, Fujita S, Hayashi M, Tanaka K. Auxiliary partial orthotopic living donor liver transplantation as an aid for small-for-size grafts in larger recipients. Transplantation. 1999;67(10):1314–9.

Machine Perfusion in Liver Transplantation

16

Chase J. Wehrle, Rebecca Panconesi, and Andrea Schlegel

Introduction

Machine perfusion has emerged as an essential tool for transplant programs. Generally speaking, ex situ machine perfusion refers to the use of a device to preserve the liver with perfusate/blood during the preservation phase of transplantation (from procurement of the graft to surgical implantation). In situ machine perfusion refers to reestablishment of circulation during graft procurement. General benefits of machine perfusion include improved logistics/reduced time constraints on transplantation, proposed improvements in graft outcomes, and increased donor utilization rates; detriments are mainly centered on the theoretical cost of this technique [1]. There are two commonly employed types of ex situ perfusion: hypothermic-oxygenated (HOPE) and normothermic machine perfusion (NMP). The two may also be combined, a strategy referred to as "sequential perfusion," in which HOPE is applied first, followed by NMP. Ex situ perfusion may generally be "end-ischemic," occurring at the recipient institution after procurement and transport, or occur during transport to the home institution [2, 3]. At present, only NMP is approved for clinical use in the United States, with the approval of HOPE anticipated in 2024. In situ perfusion consists primarily of normothermic regional

C. J. Wehrle
Transplantation Center, Cleveland Clinic, Cleveland, OH, USA
e-mail: Wehrlec@ccf.org

R. Panconesi
Department of Inflammation and Immunity, Lerner Research Institute, Cleveland, OH, USA
e-mail: panconr@ccf.org

A. Schlegel (✉)
Transplantation Center, Cleveland Clinic, Cleveland, OH, USA

Department of Inflammation and Immunity, Lerner Research Institute, Cleveland, OH, USA
e-mail: Schlega4@ccf.org

B. Eghtesad et al. (eds.), *Liver Transplantation*,
https://doi.org/10.1007/978-3-032-07072-2_16

perfusion (NRP) and is gaining traction in the procurement/preservation of donation after cardiac death (DCD) grafts. Table 16.1 presents an overview, advantages, and disadvantages of current perfusion techniques.

Liver grafts have historically been transported using ice at close to 0 °C, known as Static-Cold Storage (SCS). This approach was historically used to prevent anaerobic metabolism, leading to cell death during the cold-ischemia time (CIT). The graft is rewarmed at the time of reperfusion during implantation, which reintroduces oxygen and restarts aerobic metabolism. This does, however, create a paradoxical graft injury. Specifically, reintroduction of oxygen leads to reactive oxygen species (ROS) generated in the mitochondria of the graft, leading to oxidative stress known as Ischemic-Reperfusion Injury (IRI) [Fig. 16.1]. This damages the graft, sometimes irreparably, and also can lead to systemic hypoperfusion, termed post-reperfusion syndrome (PRS). Generally speaking, perfusion strategies are aimed at reducing IRI by limiting CIT thus reducing the amount of oxidative radicals generated on reperfusion, and also reducing PRS by reintroducing oxygen ex situ rather than in the patient.

Hypothermic-Oxygenated Perfusion

HOPE refers to the circulation of oxygenated perfusate at colder temperatures (generally 8–12 °C), and is usually end-ischemic, or after a period of CIT. HOPE may be conducted in two fashions: traditional HOPE, in which graft inflow comes from the portal vein only, or dual HOPE (D-HOPE), wherein both the hepatic artery and portal vein receive perfusate inflow [4].

Evidence has consistently shown the protective effects of HOPE/D-HOPE on mitochondrial injury in the transplanted grafts. Traditional reperfusion involves rapid reintroduction of oxygen species at normothermic temperatures. Such reintroduction leads to the formation and release of reactive oxygen species (ROS), which are the established instigators of ischemia-reperfusion injury (IRI) [5, 6]. The hypothermic nature of HOPE/D-HOPE seems to have a protective effect on mitochondria in the graft. Specifically, reestablishing aerobic metabolism in the cold protects mitochondrial complex I, limiting the production and release of ROS through a slow but steady mitochondrial complex activity with succinate metabolism, reducing ROS during both HOPE and later normothermic reperfusion on devices or in the recipient [7, 8]. This has led to demonstrated reductions in IRI and improved graft function following transplantation (Fig. 16.1) [7–9]. These effects further translate to improved long-term graft survival, including reductions in ischemic cholangiopathy (IC) and the need for retransplantation [10–12]. Both HOPE and NMP offer logistical benefits, including the capability to perfuse the graft for 12–24 h, subsequently providing potentially much-needed flexibility for transplant teams [1, 13].

It was initially believed that viability assessment was limited in HOPE due to the reduced metabolic activity of the graft during cold perfusion. However, work from the Swiss group has demonstrated that the viability assessment is possible during HOPE. This mostly involves the use of Flavin Mononucleotide (FMN), a marker of

Table 16.1 Summary of perfusion types, including advantages, disadvantages, and relevant clinical trials

	NRP	NMP	HOPE	Sequential
Location	In-Situ	Ex-Situ	Ex-Situ	Ex-Situ
Graft types	DCD	DBD, DCD	DBD, DCD	DBD, DCD
Main advantages	Can treat all abdominal organs Early viability assessment before CIT Relatively less expensive per-organ	Best established viability assessment Future treatments during perfusion Prolongs preservation time	Improves graft survival after transplantation Protection of the biliary tree Reprogram mitochondria with minimal ROS and inflammation Offers viability testing Prolongs preservation time Least expensive technique	Protection of biliary tree due to HOPE Viability assessment during HOPE and NMP Prolongs preservation time
Main disadvantages	Does not prolong preservation capabilities Requires greater donor hospital resources Viability criteria need to be better established and validated No post-CIT viability testing	Expensive No evidence of improvement in biliary complications Validation and modulation of viability tests required to increase predictive value for graft loss and biliary complications	Validation studies needed to confirm viability assessment More pharmacological studies needed assess liver treatments during HOPE/D-HOPE	High personnel cost Perfusate changes required if not using hemopure
Relevant Randomized Controlled Trials	None	Nasralla (2018) [2] Ghinolfi (2019) [61] Markmann (2022) [62] Chapman (2023) [63]	Guarrera (2015) [12] Van Rijn (2021) [7] Czigany (2021, 2024) [64, 65] Ravaioli (2022) [8] Schlegel (2023) [66] Panayotova (2023) [9] Brüggenwirth (2024) [67]	None

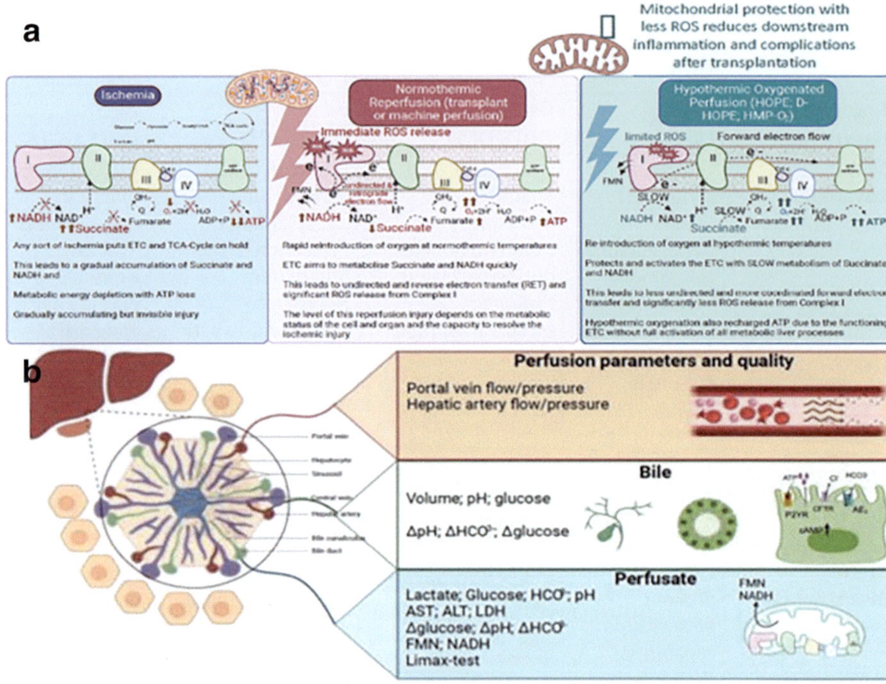

Fig. 16.1 Ischemia-Reperfusion Injury and the Role of Machine Perfusion for Preservation and Viability Assessment in Organ Transplantation. Invisibly, liver injury starts to accumulate right before donation and liver preservation in donors prior to hospital admission. During static cold storage, this proinflammatory status remains invisible until oxygen is reintroduced into such ischemic tissues. The direct response to this reoxygenation can be assessed during all different organ perfusion techniques, where reactive oxygen species are released immediately from complex-I, triggering downstream inflammation and release of various pro- and anti-inflammatory molecules. The level of this ischemia-reperfusion injury (IRI) depends on the metabolic pre-damage of the tissue and the temperature when oxygen is reintroduced. Under normothermic conditions, more injury, more ROS, and more inflammation are caused, compared to hypothermic reoxygenation. Interventions are currently tested for their value to reduce this inflammation and safely increase the number of transplantable organs. COR controlled oxygenated rewarming; HOPE hypothermic oxygenated perfusion; IFOT "Ischemia-free organ transplantation"; IRI ischemia-reperfusion injury, NMP normothermic machine perfusion; NRP normothermic regional perfusion

damage to mitochondria (specifically Complex I) that correlates well with graft loss after liver transplantation [14–16]. Additional viability criteria are somewhat less studied in HOPE and require further validation studies and correlation to posttransplant complications and graft survival [17].

HOPE offers additional advantages with respect to cost. While HOPE/D-HOPE are unsurprisingly more expensive during the perfusion phase compared to SCS, they offer cost savings when compared with NMP [18]. In general, the cost of most HOPE-perfusions in the United States ranges from \$1 to \$10,000, versus \$25–\$80,000 for NMP depending on the approach. As case volume and experience continue to grow, it is likely that the cost-effectiveness of all machine perfusion will improve, supporting increasing utilization of such technology [19, 20].

Normothermic Machine Perfusion

NMP is the perfusion of the liver graft at near-physiologic temperatures prior to transplantation. Unlike HOPE, which requires an artificial perfusion solution, NMP typically employs diluted red blood cell concentrates as the perfusate, which has natural oxygen-carrying effects. In end-ischemic NMP, the liver graft endures a period of traditional static-cold storage followed by warm ex situ perfusion (Fig. 16.1). Other systems, termed "device-to-donor," reduce SCS further by transporting the liver during perfusion. This approach has supposed benefits in avoiding SCS, though this has not yet been definitively linked to improved outcomes, and has potential detriments, the most significant of which is cost. That said, there have been US studies demonstrating that back-to-base NMP did not increase costs considering waitlist costs, transplantation admission itself and the first 3 months after liver transplantation [21]. Longer follow-up and larger cohorts are however required, ideally in comparison with other perfusion techniques.

The widespread clinical utility of NMP was first established in the landmark 2018 Oxford trial, which showed reductions in hepatocellular enzymes and reduced graft discard rates with upfront NMP [2]. Additional trials have also demonstrated reductions in graft injury and reinforced improved graft utilization with NMP [22, 23]. Such perfusion techniques further offer benefits with respect to viability assessment, which can be performed in a metabolically active liver during perfusion, thus allowing prediction of graft function and other outcomes [1, 24–27]. In addition to the use of mitochondrial markers, such as FMN, there are traditionally described viability parameters obtained in the perfusate (including lactate clearance, pH, glucose utilization) and in bile (i.e., pH, HCO3, glucose) and more [3, 28, 29]. At present, each center and, indeed, each surgeon has their own criteria for accepting a graft, and large-scale, multinational studies are necessary to correlate viability assessment and donor risk with outcomes of transplantation.

NMP has been associated with a reduction in overall 3-month complications in early experiences from US practices, reducing certain complications, including the need for renal replacement therapy and/or postoperative bleeding [21]. This same study found that, while back-to-base NMP was more costly specifically during organ preservation/acquisition, downstream reduction in early 3-month complications led to no difference in the cost of medical care with NMP versus cold storage alone [21]. More studies are needed considering higher donor–recipient risk profiles and international environment.

While end-ischemic NMP was found to improve graft utilization, it does appear to have limitations with respect to the protection of the biliary endothelium. Most notably, studies demonstrate an equivalent rate of non-anastomotic strictures with SCS and NMP, possibly relating to ongoing ROS-mediated inflammation during warm reperfusion [22, 30]. The period of pre-NMP cold storage introduces mitochondrial injury as seen in standard SCS-associated IRI [1]. The reintroduction of oxygen reactivates the respiratory chain to build energy (ATP) at the price of ROS release inducing ongoing inflammation, that leads to IC [1, 14, 30]. Interestingly, proteomic analysis of bile from NMP-treated livers demonstrates factors associated with biliary regeneration, supporting the proliferative capability of the biliary tree during NMP, and presenting targets for future work [31].

In addition to HOPE, "ischemia-free liver transplantation" (IFLT) has been proposed as a method of protecting against IRI, and early experiences report reductions in cholangiopathy [32, 33]. The IFLT-concept includes the connection of a liver to a normothermic machine in the donor, bridging the transfer to and implantation in the recipient with reported NMP-times of 6 h [32]. This approach targets the avoidance of any cold flush and CIT-related IRI injury. However, IFLT is quite costly, with current US-based estimates predicting this approach as unsustainable, despite the proposed reductions in complications [18]. Further prospective work is needed comparing the relative approaches in the real world, including cost-benefit analyses that incorporate long-term patient outcomes.

Lastly, the metabolically active graft offers the chance for intervention prior to transplantation. Though still preliminary, reports of potential gene-modulation during NMP and HOPE have been described [34, 35]. Additionally, multiple studies have proposed the "de-fatting" during NMP, though this has not yet been described in a manner ready for routine clinical use [36–38]. An RCT is currently ongoing in the United Kingdom [1]. Emricasan, which inhibits the apoptotic factor caspase, can be delivered during NMP, which may decrease damage-associated molecular patterns (DAMPs) and prevent cellular apoptosis [39]. Finally, Tietjen et al. described the use of nanoparticles to aid anti-inflammatory drug delivery to the endothelium in NMP-treated kidneys, though this has not yet been tested during hepatic NMP [40]. Several other liver-modulating concepts, including ex situ regeneration, are currently tested. To succeed with such techniques, prolonged NMP beyond a few hours is required, with novel devices that replace other "organs" in an ex situ environment, including the kidney with a dialysis circuit and many more [41]. The Wyss team from Zurich has recently presented such a new device with successful NMP for 3 days with subsequent implantation [42].

Sequential Perfusion

Sequential perfusion associates HOPE and NMP with the aim of combining the purported benefits of both approaches. HOPE/D-HOPE is well recognized for its ability to protect against IRI, while NMP is thought to offer improved viability assessment. Thus, HOPE/D-HOPE + sequential NMP or HOPE/D-HOPE + controlled oxygenated rewarming (COR) + NMP have been proposed as protecting the cholangiocytes by reintroducing oxygen in the cold phase, followed by rewarming after reducing succinate and ATP replenishment, knowing this limits ROS-formation and reduces downstream inflammation and complications [43]. Studies in Europe and the United States have demonstrated the utility of viability testing in NMP-after-HOPE [17, 44].

Sequential perfusion can be performed in a "back-to-base" model, without requiring the logistical challenges and added cost of transporting a machine [17, 43, 45]. Though randomized trials have not yet compared back-to-base sequential perfusion with IFLT, isolated HOPE, and NMP, it does seem that the pre-NMP HOPE confers benefit to the biliary tree.

Normothermic Regional Perfusion

NRP involves the circulation of oxygenated donor blood at physiologic temperatures immediately after circulatory arrest during the procurement of DCD livers. This follows the initial donor warm ischemia time (dWIT) and circulatory arrest. The main potential benefit of NRP is to reintroduce oxygen early and assess viability (injury).

Early experiences from Spain and others demonstrated that NRP is associated with reduced biliary complications versus standard ("super-rapid recovery," SRR) procurement with immediate cold flush [46]. Early US experiences support good early allograft function, despite longer functional dWIT's ($\geq$ 30 min) [47]. The proposed mechanism for this improvement is immediate reoxygenation prior to any cold-ischemia time thus preventing compounding injuries of dWIT and long CIT. Indeed, circulating cytokines have been quantified during NRP, demonstrating a reduction of IL-10 and TNFα [48]. Some questions do remain about the true efficacy of NRP. The Spanish cohort was not truly "risky," and the organ discard rate was similarly high in both NRP and SRR groups (34% and 38%, respectively) [49]. More studies are required with higher risk donors comparing NRP with other techniques. Specifically, there are no RCTs yet conducted reporting outcomes of NRP. This is urgently needed.

Authors from France and Spain have demonstrated higher graft loss rates after NRP with prolonged dWIT or CIT of >30 min and > 7–8 h, respectively. This was even more evident when such DCD livers were used for recipients with additional risk factors, including retransplantation [50, 51]. These studies support the clinical approach in Italy, where NRP is always combined with end-ischemic machine perfusion, most often HOPE, to reduce IRI injury [52]. This is of high relevance because Italy is the country with the longest dWIT (>40–50 min) due to a 20 min stand-off period prior to NRP or cold flush [53, 54]. The combined approach of NRP plus CIT and HOPE has demonstrated the lowest biliary complications and graft loss rates despite such high risk [52, 55].

Another benefit of NRP has been described with increasing access to multiorgan transplants from DCD-donors, an approach that may also aid with increased access [56]. This comes secondary to the ability of NRP to treat multiple abdominal organs, rather than the individual treatment of each organ after procurement. Additionally, NRP does require significant operating room time at the donor hospital, as the perfusion circuit runs for an optimal 1–4 h before graft explant [51], thus requiring resources of the donor hospital. Further, NRP has been linked to improved organ utilization rates with simultaneously reduced costs to the recipient transplant program, though costs attributable to the donor hospital or organ-procurement organization (OPO) remain less well understood [57].

NRP does offer the chance for in situ viability testing like the ex situ approaches. Indeed, testing of circulating markers of graft damage during NRP may reflect the degree of inherent early IRI in an entire abdominal compartment of a DCD donor, prior to introducing additional transplant-associated injuries [1, 48]. This does however also include other organs (i.e., intestine and kidneys) contributing to the quantified injury, thereby limiting the specific assessment of an isolated liver. Current markers, i.e., Lactate and Transaminase thresholds, require prospective validation, and bile parameters assessed during ex situ machine perfusion have not yet been established during NRP on a larger scale [58].

NRP also brings unique ethical challenges, as works like Glazier and Capron argue that NRP is not compatible with, for example, US standards for determining death [59]. Advocates maintain that the declaration protocol for DCD-donors is similar regardless of NRP use [60], though opponents maintain that the resumption of circulation is contrary to the accepted definitions of death in the United States. While there is no current national consensus, OPOs are increasingly offering this approach. Ultimately, a national consensus on both the ethics of NRP and its optimal conduct are necessary to avoid ongoing controversy.

Conclusion

Hypothermic oxygenated perfusion (HOPE) and Normothermic Machine Perfusion (NMP) both demonstrate impressive clinical utility in liver transplantation. HOPE offers benefits including costs and improved protection of the biliary tree, which is facilitated by a reduction in mitochondrial-mediated inflammation. NMP offers a range of markers for viability testing at our current level of understanding. Sequential perfusion (HOPE followed by COR and NMP) combines approaches, which may create logistical challenges, but can offset graft-related detriments of both. All techniques aid with logistics, easing the time constraints of traditional SCS. Future prospective, randomized research and large cohort REAL-world data are needed to compare the different approaches, helping elucidate which graft would benefit from each technique.

References

1. Schlegel A, et al. Machine perfusion of the liver and bioengineering. J Hepatol. 2023;78(6):1181–98.
2. Nasralla D, et al. A randomized trial of normothermic preservation in liver transplantation. Nature. 2018;557(7703):50–6.
3. Mergental H, et al. Transplantation of discarded livers following viability testing with normothermic machine perfusion. Nat Commun. 2020;11(1):2939.

4. Schlegel A, Porte R, Dutkowski P. Protective mechanisms and current clinical evidence of hypothermic oxygenated machine perfusion (HOPE) in preventing post-transplant cholangiopathy. J Hepatol. 2022;76(6):1330–47.
5. Teodoro JS, et al. Shaping of hepatic ischemia/reperfusion events: the crucial role of mitochondria. Cells. 2022;11(4).
6. Chouchani ET, et al. Ischaemic accumulation of succinate controls reperfusion injury through mitochondrial ROS. Nature. 2014;515(7527):431–5.
7. van Rijn R, et al. Hypothermic machine perfusion in liver transplantation — a randomized trial. N Engl J Med. 2021;384(15):1391–401.
8. Ravaioli M, et al. Hypothermic oxygenated perfusion in extended criteria donor liver transplantation—a randomized clinical trial. Am J Transplant. 2022;22(10):2401–8.
9. Panayotova GG, et al. Portable hypothermic oxygenated machine perfusion for organ preservation in liver transplantation (PILOTTM): a randomized, open-label, clinical trial. Hepatology. 2023.
10. Dutkowski P, et al. First comparison of hypothermic oxygenated perfusion versus static cold storage of human donation after cardiac death liver transplants. Ann Surg. 2015;262(5):764–71.
11. Guarrera J, et al. Hypothermic machine preservation in human liver transplantation: the first clinical series. Am J Transplant. 2010;10(2):372–81.
12. Guarrera JV, et al. Hypothermic machine preservation facilitates successful transplantation of "orphan" extended criteria donor livers. Am J Transplant. 2015;15(1):161–9.
13. Brüggenwirth IMA, et al. Prolonged preservation by hypothermic machine perfusion facilitates logistics in liver transplantation: a European observational cohort study. Am J Transplant. 2022;22(7):1842–51.
14. Schlegel A, et al. Hypothermic oxygenated perfusion protects from mitochondrial injury before liver transplantation. EBioMedicine. 2020;60:103014.
15. Eden J, et al. Screening for mitochondrial function before use-routine liver assessment during hypothermic oxygenated perfusion impacts liver utilization. EBioMedicine. 2023;98:104857.
16. Muller X, et al. Novel real-time prediction of liver graft function during hypothermic oxygenated machine perfusion before liver transplantation. Ann Surg. 2019;270(5):783–90.
17. van Leeuwen OB, et al. Hypothermic machine perfusion before viability testing of previously discarded human livers. Nat Commun. 2021;12(1):1008.
18. Zimmermann J, Carter AW. Cost-utility analysis of normothermic and hypothermic ex-situ machine perfusion in liver transplantation. Br J Surg. 2022;109(2):e31–2.
19. Boteon YL, Boteon A, Martins PN. Comment on: cost-utility analysis of normothermic and hypothermic ex-situ machine perfusion in liver transplantation. Br J Surg. 2022;109(11):e123.
20. Boteon YL, et al. The economic impact of machine perfusion technology in liver transplantation. Artif Organs. 2022;46(2):191–200.
21. Wehrle CJ. Impact of back-to-base normothermic machine perfusion on complications and costs: a multi-center, real-world risk-matched analysis. Ann Surg. 2024;280:300.
22. Gaurav R, et al. Liver transplantation outcomes from controlled circulatory death donors: SCS vs in situ NRP vs ex situ NMP. Ann Surg. 2022;275(6):1156–64.
23. Quintini C, et al. Transplantation of declined livers after normothermic perfusion. Surgery. 2022;171(3):747–56.
24. van Beekum CJ, et al. Normothermic machine perfusion (NMP) of the liver - current status and future perspectives. Ann Transplant. 2021;26:e931664.
25. Parente A, et al. Machine perfusion techniques for liver transplantation - a meta-analysis of the first seven randomized-controlled trials. J Hepatol. 2023;79:1201.
26. Watson CJ, et al. Observations on the ex situ perfusion of livers for transplantation. Am J Transplant. 2018;18(8):2005–20.
27. Watson CJE, Jochmans I. From “gut feeling” to objectivity: machine preservation of the liver as a tool to assess organ viability. Curr Transplant Rep. 2018;5(1):72–81.
28. Weissenbacher A, et al. Perfusate enzymes and platelets indicate early allograft dysfunction after transplantation of normothermically preserved livers. Transplantation. 2022;106(4):792–805.

29. Mergental H, et al. Introduction of the concept of diagnostic sensitivity and specificity of normothermic perfusion protocols to assess high-risk donor livers. Liver Transpl. 2022;28(5):794.
30. Beetz O, et al. Interleukin-18 and high-mobility-group-protein B1 are early and sensitive indicators for cell damage during normothermic machine perfusion after prolonged cold ischemic storage of porcine liver grafts. Transpl Int. 2022;35.
31. Thorne AM, et al. Bile proteome reveals biliary regeneration during normothermic preservation of human donor livers. Nat Commun. 2023;14(1):7880.
32. Guo Z, et al. Ischaemia-free liver transplantation in humans: a first-in-human trial. Lancet Reg Health West Pac. 2021;16.
33. Guo Z, et al. A randomized-controlled trial of ischemia-free liver transplantation for end-stage liver disease. J Hepatol. 2023;79(2):394–402.
34. Staubli SM, Ceresa CDL, Pollok JM. The current role and future applications of machine perfusion in liver transplantation. Bioengineering (Basel). 2023;10(5):593.
35. Stimmeder S, et al. Genetic modulation: future trends toward graft optimization during machine perfusion. Transplantation:9900.
36. Mazilescu LI, Selzner M, Selzner N. Defatting strategies in the current era of liver steatosis. JHEP Reports. 2021;3(3):100265.
37. Sousa Da Silva RX, et al. Defatting of human livers during long-term e x situ normothermic perfusion: novel strategy to rescue discarded organs for transplantation. Ann Surg. 2023;278(5):669–75.
38. Goumard C, et al. Ex-vivo pharmacological defatting of the liver: a review. J Clin Med. 2021;10(6).
39. Raigani S, et al. Pan-caspase inhibition during normothermic machine perfusion of discarded livers mitigates ex situ innate immune responses. Front Immunol. 2022;13:4062.
40. Tietjen GT, et al. Nanoparticle targeting to the endothelium during normothermic machine perfusion of human kidneys. Sci Transl Med. 2017;9(418):eaam6764.
41. Eshmuminov D, et al. An integrated perfusion machine preserves injured human livers for 1 week. Nat Biotechnol. 2020;38(2):189–98.
42. Clavien PA, et al. Transplantation of a human liver following 3 days of ex situ normothermic preservation. Nat Biotechnol. 2022;40(11):1610–6.
43. van Leeuwen OB, et al. Sequential hypothermic and normothermic machine perfusion enables safe transplantation of high-risk donor livers. Am J Transplant. 2022;22(6):1658–70.
44. Liu Q, et al. Sequential hypothermic and normothermic perfusion preservation and transplantation of expanded criteria donor livers. Surgery. 2023;173(3):846–54.
45. van Leeuwen OB, et al. Excellent long-term outcomes after sequential hypothermic and normothermic machine perfusion challenges the importance of functional donor warm ischemia time in DCD liver transplantation. J Hepatol. 2023;79(6):e244–5.
46. Hessheimer AJ, et al. Normothermic regional perfusion vs. super-rapid recovery in controlled donation after circulatory death liver transplantation. J Hepatol. 2019;70(4):658–65.
47. Brubaker AL, et al. Early patient and liver allograft outcomes from donation after circulatory death donors using thoracoabdominal normothermic regional: a multi-center observational experience. Front Transpl. 2023;2.
48. Baroni S, et al. Cytokine mass balance levels in donation after circulatory death donors using hemoadsorption: case series report. Int J Artif Organs. 2022;45(7):642–6.
49. Schlegel A, Muiesan P, Dutkowski P. Normothermic regional perfusion—what is the benefit? J Hepatol. 2019;71(2):441–3.
50. Hessheimer AJ, et al. Abdominal normothermic regional perfusion in controlled donation after circulatory determination of death liver transplantation: outcomes and risk factors for graft loss. Am J Transplant. 2022;22(4):1169–81.
51. Barbier L, et al. Impact of the duration of normothermic regional perfusion on the results of liver transplant from controlled circulatory death donors: a retrospective, multicentric study. Clin Transpl. 2022;36(2):e14536.
52. De Carlis R, et al. Current practice of normothermic regional perfusion and machine perfusion in donation after circulatory death liver transplants in Italy. Updat Surg. 2022;74(2):501–10.

53. Panconesi R, et al. Viability assessment in liver transplantation-what is the impact of dynamic organ preservation? Biomedicine. 2021. 9(2).
54. Panconesi R, et al. Mitochondria and ischemia reperfusion injury. Curr Opin Organ Transplant. 2022;27(5):434–45.
55. Schlegel A, et al. A multicentre outcome analysis to define global benchmarks for donation after circulatory death liver transplantation. J Hepatol. 2022;76(2):371–82.
56. Brubaker AL, et al. Heart-liver-kidney transplantation for AL amyloidosis using normothermic recovery and storage from a donor following circulatory death: short-term outcome in a first-in-world experience. Am J Transplant. 2023;23(2):291–3.
57. Bakhtiyar SS, et al. Association of Procurement Technique with organ yield and cost following donation after circulatory death. Am J Transplant. 2024;24:1803.
58. Schurink IJ, et al. Donor eligibility criteria and liver graft acceptance criteria during normothermic regional perfusion: a systematic review. Liver Transpl. 2022;28(10):1563–75.
59. Glazier AK, Capron AM. Normothermic regional perfusion and US legal standards for determining death are not aligned. Wiley Online Library; 2022. p. 1289–90.
60. Wall AE, et al. Applying the ethical framework for donation after circulatory death to thoracic normothermic regional perfusion procedures. Am J Transplant. 2022;22(5):1311–5.
61. Ghinolfi D, et al. Pilot, open, randomized, prospective trial for Normothermic machine perfusion evaluation in liver transplantation from older donors. Liver Transpl. 2019;25(3):436–49.
62. Markmann JF, et al. Impact of portable Normothermic blood-based machine perfusion on outcomes of liver transplant: the OCS liver PROTECT randomized clinical trial. JAMA Surg. 2022;157(3):189–98.
63. Chapman WC, et al. Normothermic machine perfusion of donor livers for transplantation in the United States: a randomized controlled trial. Ann Surg. 2023;278(5):e912–21.
64. Czigany Z, et al. Hypothermic oxygenated machine perfusion reduces early allograft injury and improves post-transplant outcomes in extended criteria donation liver transplantation from donation after brain death: results from a multicenter randomized controlled trial (HOPE ECD-DBD). Ann Surg. 2021;274(5):705–12.
65. Czigany Z, et al. Improved outcomes after hypothermic oxygenated machine perfusion in liver transplantation-long-term follow-up of a multicenter randomized controlled trial. Hepatol Commun. 2024;8(2).
66. Schlegel A, et al. A multicenter randomized-controlled trial of hypothermic oxygenated perfusion (HOPE) for human liver grafts before transplantation. J Hepatol. 2023;78(4):783–93.
67. Brüggenwirth IMA, et al. Prolonged hypothermic machine perfusion enables daytime liver transplantation - an IDEAL stage 2 prospective clinical trial. eClinicalMedicine. 2024;68.

17 Histocompatibility Tests for Liver Transplantation: An Immunological Aspect

Qignyong Xu and Adriana Zeevi

Introduction

Although there is an evolving literature, there is still controversy regarding the role of allo-sensitization and the impact of preformed and de novo donor-specific antibodies (DSAs) to human leukocyte antigen (HLA) on liver allografts [1–5]. The liver is considered an immunologically privileged and tolerogenic organ resistant to alloimmune injury. Several mechanisms are proposed that may contribute to resistance to cellular and humoral injury: (1) dilution of cell-based antigen-antibody binding, partially due to the liver's large microvascular surface area and dual blood supply; (2) secretion of soluble HLA molecules capable of forming immune complexes with anti-donor antibodies; (3) phagocytic activities of Kupffer and liver sinusoidal endothelial cells, which express abundant Fcγ receptors able to clear different immune complexes, complement-fixing DSA and platelet aggregates; (4) decreased availability of Class II DSA targets due to variable hepatic microvascular HLA Class II expression; and (5) the liver's ability to heal and regenerate [6]. However, these tolerance-promoting properties do not always protect liver allografts from cellular and humoral-mediated injury. Preformed and de novo DSA have short- and long-term impacts on liver allografts and are associated with (1) increased risk of T cell-mediated rejection (TCMR) and antibody-mediated rejection (AMR); (2) decreased 5-year patient and graft survival; and (3) graft inflammation, fibrosis, and chronic rejection [2, 3].

Although HLA antibodies have been associated with a broad spectrum of allograft damage, not all HLA antibodies are equal. Solid-phase Luminex-based single antigen bead (SAB) assays have improved detection sensitivity and specificity and enabled the functional characterization of DSA. Additionally, the

Q. Xu (✉) · A. Zeevi
Department of Pathology, University of Pittsburgh, Pittsburgh, PA, USA
e-mail: xuq5@upmc.edu

B. Eghtesad et al. (eds.), *Liver Transplantation*,
https://doi.org/10.1007/978-3-032-07072-2_17

introduction of molecular HLA genotyping has allowed for better discrimination of donor antigens and has improved our ability to risk-stratify candidates before transplant. These advances in HLA antibody testing, including interpretation and limitations of various techniques, have been summarized in several consensus publications [7–10]. Characteristics associated with the pathogenesis and deleterious effects of DSA in solid organ transplants include HLA-DQ specificity, high titer, and the ability to bind complement. Circulating DSA has recently been incorporated into the diagnostic criteria for AMR in liver transplantation [11]. The few studies evaluating paired DSA assessment and concomitant biopsy histology have shown that DSA is associated with inflammation and a unique pattern of fibrosis despite normal liver function tests [1].

This chapter may be a guiding tool for hepatologists and liver surgeons. Here, we discuss the basics of various assays and the interpretations that can be provided by the histocompatibility laboratory experts. In addition, we describe two cases that illustrate the application of HLA testing and the potential impact on early posttransplant outcomes in patients with preformed DSA in liver transplants and the kinetics of de novo DSA in combined liver/kidney transplant recipients.

Pretransplantation Tests

The literature regarding the utility of pretransplant tests in liver recipients for anti-HLA antibodies has been mixed [1, 2, 12–15]. Thus, many liver transplant programs do not routinely test for anti-HLA antibodies before surgery. Early studies were limited to using the complement-dependent cytotoxicity crossmatch (CDC XM) method to assess the presence of preformed donor-specific antibodies. The CDC XM is performed by mixing donor lymphocytes with recipient serum collected pretransplant. Liver transplants with a positive CDC XM pretransplantation exhibited elevated risk for early (< 3 weeks posttransplant) cellular rejection and antibody-mediated injury, such as positive C4d staining on endothelial cells of liver allograft biopsies [16]. Recently, histocompatibility laboratories have applied a rather sensitive method to detect circulating HLA-specific antibodies using an SAB assay on a multiplex platform such as Luminex. Along with detecting overall DSA presence and specificity, this platform can be modified to test for complement-fixing antibodies (C1q assay) or the presence of antibodies to specific isotypes, such as IgG3. In large cohorts of >1000 liver transplants, O'Leary et al. found that preformed DSAs, specifically complement-fixing with high mean fluorescence intensity (MFI), were associated with an increased risk of patient death [17, 18]. Furthermore, up to 10% of unexplained early (< 3-month posttransplant) graft loss may be attributed to AMR caused by the presence of strong preformed DSAs before surgery [19]. Thus, considering the scarcity of liver donors and high mortality on the liver candidate waiting list, the comprehensive assessment of histocompatibility between donor and recipient is justified for risk stratification and improving patient management posttransplantation. The recommended test protocols before liver transplantation are detailed below.

Tests at the Time of Candidate Evaluation

The histocompatibility evaluation of a liver transplant candidate includes the assessment of the strength and specificity of circulating anti-HLA antibodies. Class I and Class II anti-HLA antibodies are determined with an SAB assay. It is also recommended that serum be tested with multi-antigen panel-reactive antibody (PRA) beads, which present HLA antigens in configurations similar to those on the cell surface. The prozone effect in some Luminex SAB assays often causes false negative results; thus, a mitigation approach, such as treating serum with EDTA, is strongly recommended. Due to the limited amount of antigen on the beads, the SAB assay is also subject to bead saturation when an excessive anti-HLA antibody is present in the serum. Serum dilutions are the only approach to address the bead saturation issue, which often occurs for strong antibodies with MFI > 10,000 in undiluted serum [20]. In these scenarios, a few dilutions (e.g., 1:16, 1:64, 1:128) should be performed to evaluate the antibody level and to risk-stratify the patient when transplantation is performed in the presence of DSA. In addition, a SAB C1q assay may be informative in detecting complement-fixing antibodies associated with an elevated risk [20]. It has been shown that antibodies with MFI > 4000 at 1:16 dilution are often complement-binding.

Serum samples from patients waiting for a transplant should be collected periodically (every 3–6 months), for storage and testing as needed prior to transplantation. Anti-HLA antibody testing is highly recommended after allo-sensitization events such as transfusions.

HLA genotyping for the recipient candidate, minimally at the low-intermediate level, is also highly recommended. Knowing self-HLA is informative for determining the specificity of anti-HLA antibodies, which often have some false positivity and high background binding. Many labs have adopted high-resolution typing using next-generation sequencing methods, whose cost is now similar to that of the routine low-intermediate typing methods. High-resolution HLA typing also offers opportunities to refine the immunological risk stratification posttransplantation using various molecular mismatch algorithms.

Testing at the Time of Transplant

For deceased donor liver transplantation, a cell-based crossmatch and antibody testing by SAB on the most recent stored serum is done retrospectively, often on the next working day after surgery. The donor may need to be HLA genotyped if not previously done. The cell-based crossmatch can be either CDC XM or Flow XM. CDC XM lacks sensitivity and is prone to false positivity. Hence, many labs have applied a strong positive flow XM result as a surrogate or equivalent for a positive CDC XM [21]. However, in some cases, Flow XM may also be prone to false reactivity. The best interpretation of XM results requires the identification and characterization of the DSA specificity.

For living donor liver transplants, the SAB test on recipient serum, donor HLA genotyping, and XM are often performed before transplantation at the time of donor assessment. If the planned surgery date is more than six months after the initial assessment, XM and SAB tests may need to be updated with a fresh serum sample from the patient.

Currently, the presence of preformed DSA to a donor is not an absolute contraindication to liver transplantation. However, knowing the recipient and donor HLA genotypes, along with the characterization of preformed DSA, facilitates better clinical management of the recipient after transplantation. In addition, this information is used to perform a virtual crossmatch to risk-stratify a patient transplanted across DSA.

Tests for Combined Transplantation with Other Organs

The liver allograft is known to be able to absorb Class I DSA and, to a lesser extent, Class II DSA [2, 13]. Thus, the protection provided by the liver allograft to combined organs, such as the kidney, heart, and intestinal graft, is limited, especially for Class II DSAs [22, 23]. Currently, in the United States organ allocation system, the United Network for Organ Sharing (UNOS), no unacceptable antigens are usually listed for liver-alone candidates to prevent the automatic exclusion of any deceased liver offers. However, when the transplant includes a combined organ, such as a kidney, some unacceptable antigens may be listed to avoid an offer with a strong Class II DSA. Usually, complement-fixing Class II antibodies, indicated by either a positive C1q test or MFI > 4000 at 1:16 serum dilution, should be listed as an avoidance in UNOS. Before accepting a donor offer, an HLA expert usually performs a virtual XM to evaluate positive DSAs with MFI > 1000 or 2000 in undiluted serum, based on the laboratory's established cutoff. Transplantation across multiple DSAs should be considered a higher risk because of potential synergy in vivo. Although Class I HLA antibodies are significantly absorbed and removed by the liver allograft, high-titer Class II DSA might sometimes persist after transplantation, especially for the split liver, which may be insufficient to absorb the DSA.

For a combined liver-heart transplantation, the heart graft is usually placed before the liver graft; thus, the protection from the liver graft is less potent. For highly sensitized candidates, placing the liver before the heart is beneficial for taking advantage of the liver's protective effect [21]. For liver-inclusive intestinal transplants, either liver-intestinal or full multi-visceral grafts, the liver's protective effect is also more prominent for Class I DSAs than Class II DSAs [24].

Posttransplantation Testing

Antibody-mediated rejection was first introduced into Banff liver allograft pathology in 2016, and the criteria for diagnosing AMR included the presence of circulating DSA [11]. Therefore, a DSA test is often performed when a biopsy indicates possible AMR. The literature well documents the negative impact of de novo DSA on liver grafts and patient survival [18, 19, 25]. Although not consistently associated with changes in liver function tests, the presence of circulating DSA after liver transplantation is associated with liver allograft injuries such as fibrosis, inflammation, and TCMR, and is a biomarker for under-immunosuppression [4, 26]. Despite improvement in one-year survival, long-term patient survival of liver transplant recipients has stagnated in the past three decades [27]. In a recent Banff liver group meeting report [4], it has been recommended to include DSA monitoring posttransplantation. Based on the literature review [1, 3, 28] and the practice at our institution, the protocol below summarizes recommendations for monitoring DSA after liver transplantation:

1. Test DSA anytime during a for-cause liver allograft biopsy.
2. Test DSA before and after immunosuppression minimization.
3. Test DSA annually posttransplantation.
4. Perform more intensive DSA monitoring in the scenarios below:
   (a) Patients with a history of preformed/de novo DSA;
   (b) Patients with a history of AMR, steroid-resistant rejection, or biopsy with unexplained inflammation/fibrosis;
   (c) Following treatment of AMR;
   (d) For DSAs with MFI > 10,000 in undiluted serum, perform serum dilutions and/or test for complement-fixing antibodies.

A Case of Preformed DSA in a Living Donor Liver Transplant

In case #1, a 71-year-old female was evaluated for a living donor liver transplant from her son. Patient HLA typing: A2,26; B62,39; Cw9; DR12,13; DQ7, 6; DP4,19; donor HLA typing: A2,**3**; B62,**35**; Cw4,**9**; DR**1**,13; DQ**5**,6; DP**2**,19 (mismatched antigens are highlighted in bold). The patient was broadly sensitized, with 100% calculated PRA (cPRA), and preformed Class I and II DSA to the donor's paternal haplotype. Pretransplant CDC XM showed strong positive reactivity to both T and B cells. The transplant was performed, and the patient experienced early AMR with macrophage margination, C4d positivity, and liver allograft dysfunction. The DSA pre- (day-1) and posttransplant day 7 were summarized in Fig. 17.1. The patient had antibodies to Class I HLA-A3 and Cw4, as well as Class II HLA-DR1 and DP2 (Fig. 17.1a). On posttransplant day 7, the Class I DSA had significantly decreased, while the Class II DSA persisted (Fig. 17.1a). The Class II DSAs were also C1q-reactive, with antibody to DR1 still strongly positive on posttransplant day 7 (Fig. 17.1b). This case illustrates that preformed strong Class I & Class II DSAs with high MFI (Fig. 17.1a) and C1q-positivity (Fig. 17.1b) may have deleterious effects on the liver allograft. The persistence of both Class I and Class II DSAs posttransplant also indicates that the liver allograft could not absorb/remove the preformed DSA, especially Class II, which remained high titer and C1q-positive.

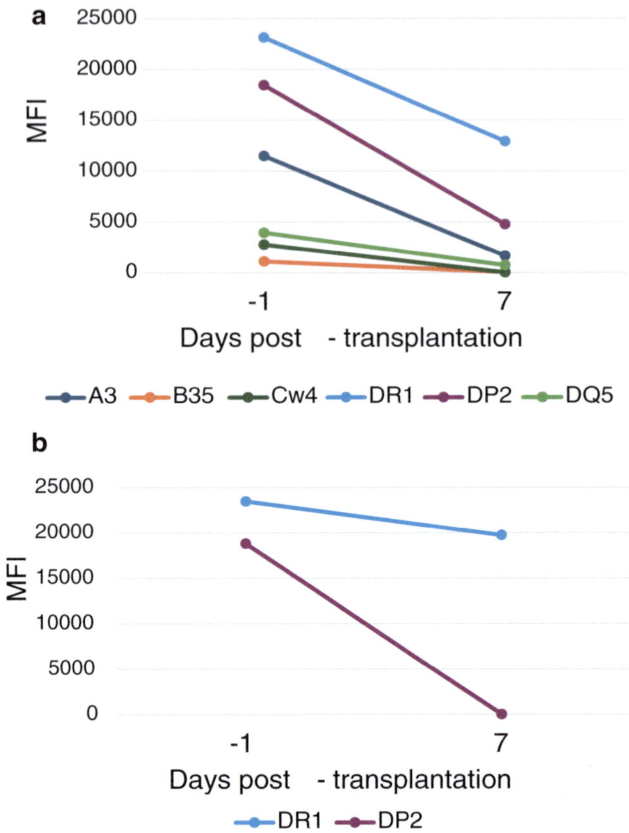

Fig. 17.1 Case #1, the pre/posttransplant course of preformed DSA in a living donor liver transplant recipient. (**a**) IgG DSA, undiluted serum. (**b**) C1q DSA

A Case of De Novo Class II DSA in a Combined Liver-Kidney Transplant Recipient

In case #2, a 16-year-old nonsensitized female received a liver/kidney combined transplant in 2013. Nine years later, the patient was admitted following an elevated liver function test. The immunosuppression drug level was low as a consequence of noncompliance. Strong DSAs to DQ7/DQA1*05 (24,330 MFI), DQ6 (27,869 MFI), and DR51 (16,815 MFI) were detected in the patient's serum (Fig. 17.2a, denoted as week 0 post-DSA detection). The DQ7/DQA1*05 and DQ6 DSA were strongly positive at 1:64 serum dilution (Fig. 17.2b) and in the C1q assay (Fig. 17.2c). The liver allograft biopsy one week later showed acute cellular rejection (ACR) with a pattern of hepatic injury, and the patient was treated with steroids. One week after treatment (denoted as week 2 in Fig. 17.2), DSAs were reduced, and a liver biopsy showed resolved ACR. However, a kidney allograft biopsy at the same time showed

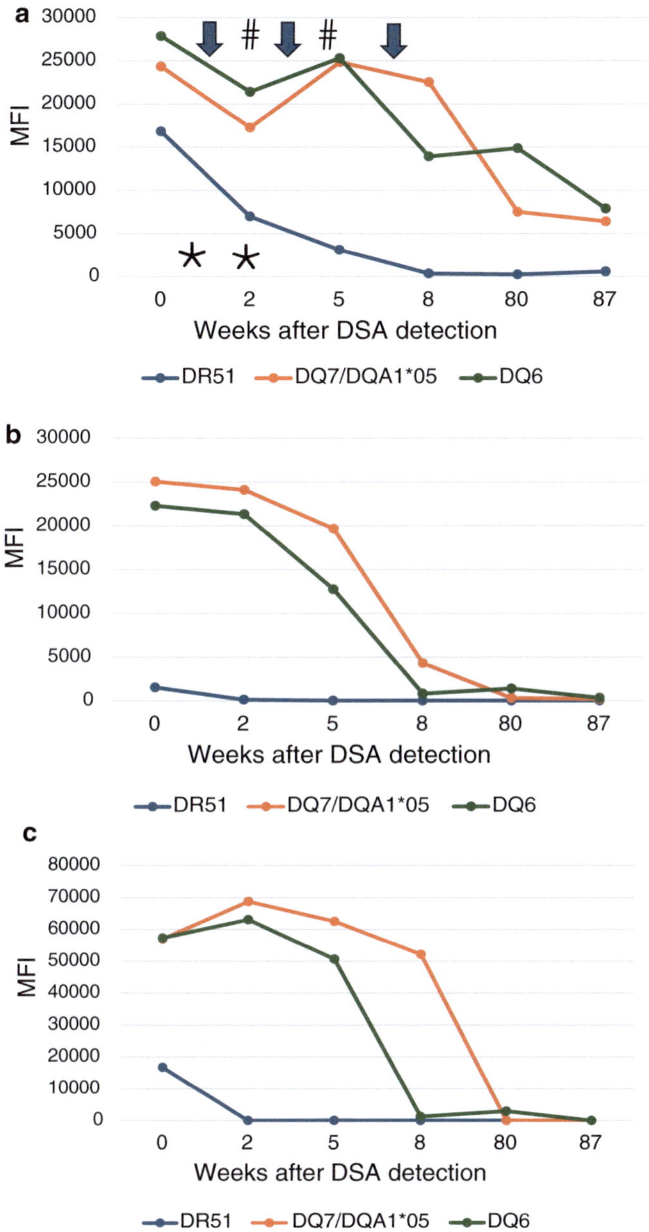

Fig. 17.2 The treatment course of de novo DSAs following liver/kidney combined transplantation. The time of detecting peak DSA was denoted as week 0. (**a**) IgG DSA, undiluted serum. (**b**) IgG DSA, 1:64 serum dilution. (**c**) C1q DSA. The asterisk denotes liver biopsy, the pound sign denotes kidney biopsy, and the arrow denotes treatments for rejection

AMR, ACR, diffused C4d, and early chronic transplant glomerulopathy, despite normal creatinine. In considering the strong DSA and pathological features of AMR, the patient was treated with steroids and intravenous Immunoglobulin (IVIG). Three weeks after treatment (denoted as week 5 in Fig. 17.2), all DSAs were reduced at 1:64 serum dilution and in the C1q assay, albeit antibodies to DQ6 and DQ7/DQA1*05 remained high in undiluted serum and strongly positive in the C1q assay. A new kidney allograft biopsy (week 5 in Fig. 17.2) showed resolved ACR but ongoing AMR, with diffused C4d and early chronic transplant glomerulopathy. The patient then received steroids, rituximab, and IVIG for three days, followed by four cycles of plasmapheresis, IVIG, and bortezomib treatment every other day. Three weeks after the intensive AMR treatment (denoted as week 8 in Fig. 17.2), DQ6 and DQ7/DQA1*05 DSAs maintained positivity in undiluted serum but were greatly reduced at 1:64 serum dilution. The DQ7/DQA1*05 DSA remained positive in the C1q assay until 80 weeks post-DSA detection.

Conclusions

In summary, antibodies to mismatched donor HLA can be detrimental to liver allografts. The impact is more pronounced for Class II antibodies, especially DQ-specific antibodies, which are not efficiently absorbed by the liver graft and thus could persist for a long time. Histocompatibility tests are important in assessing the immunological risk before and after liver transplantation. Incorporating histocompatibility testing into risk assessment and patient management may improve the long-term survival of liver transplant recipients. Personalized medicine and immunosuppression minimization protocols often require monitoring for de novo DSA as a biomarker of immune activation. Thus, a multidiscipline team that includes histocompatibility experts is highly recommended for providing state-of-the-art patient care.

Acknowledgments We sincerely thank Mrs. Marilyn Marrari for editing and proofreading this manuscript.

References

1. Lefaucheur C, Louis K, Morris AB, Taupin JL, Nickerson P, Tambur AR, et al. Clinical recommendations for posttransplant assessment of anti-HLA (Human Leukocyte Antigen) donor-specific antibodies: a Sensitization in Transplantation: Assessment of Risk consensus document. Am J Transplant. 2023;23(1):115–32.
2. O'Leary JG, Demetris AJ, Friedman LS, Gebel HM, Halloran PF, Kirk AD, et al. The role of donor-specific HLA alloantibodies in liver transplantation. Am J Transplant. 2014;14(4):779–87.
3. Demetris AJ. Longterm outcome of the liver graft: the pathologist's perspective. Liver Transpl. 2017;23(S1):S70–S5.
4. Bellamy COC, O'Leary JG, Adeyi O, Baddour N, Batal I, Bucuvalas J, et al. Banff 2022 liver group meeting report: monitoring long-term allograft health. Am J Transplant. 2024;24(6):905–17.

5. Taner T, Stegall MD, Heimbach JK. Antibody-mediated rejection in liver transplantation: current controversies and future directions. Liver Transpl. 2014;20(5):514–27.
6. Demetris AJ, Zeevi A, O'Leary JG. ABO-compatible liver allograft antibody-mediated rejection: an update. Curr Opin Organ Transplant. 2015;20(3):314–24.
7. Tambur AR, Bestard O, Campbell P, Chong AS, Barrio MC, Ford ML, et al. Sensitization in transplantation: assessment of risk 2022 working group meeting report. Am J Transplant. 2023;23(1):133–49.
8. Tambur AR, Campbell P, Chong AS, Feng S, Ford ML, Gebel H, et al. Sensitization in transplantation: Assessment of risk (STAR) 2019 Working Group Meeting Report. Am J Transplant. 2020;20:2652.
9. Tambur AR, Campbell P, Claas FH, Feng S, Gebel HM, Jackson AM, et al. Sensitization in transplantation: Assessment of risk (STAR) 2017 Working Group Meeting Report. Am J Transplant. 2018.
10. Tait BD, Susal C, Gebel HM, Nickerson PW, Zachary AA, Claas FH, et al. Consensus guidelines on the testing and clinical management issues associated with HLA and non-HLA antibodies in transplantation. Transplantation. 2013;95(1):19–47.
11. Demetris AJ, Bellamy C, Hübscher SG, O'Leary J, Randhawa PS, Feng S, et al. 2016 comprehensive update of the Banff Working Group on liver allograft pathology: introduction of antibody-mediated rejection. Am J Transplant. 2016;16(10):2816–35.
12. Del Bello A, Neau-Cransac M, Lavayssiere L, Dubois V, Congy-Jolivet N, Visentin J, et al. Outcome of liver transplant patients with preformed donor-specific anti–human Leukocyte antigen antibodies. Liver Transpl. 2019.
13. Taner T, Gandhi MJ, Sanderson SO, Poterucha CR, De Goey SR, Stegall MD, et al. Prevalence, course and impact of HLA donor-specific antibodies in liver transplantation in the first year. Am J Transplant. 2012;12(6):1504–10.
14. Badawy A, Kaido T, Yoshizawa A, Yagi S, Fukumitsu K, Okajima H, et al. Human leukocyte antigen compatibility and lymphocyte cross-matching play no significant role in the current adult-to-adult living donor liver transplantation. Clin Transpl. 2018;32(4):e13234.
15. Xu Q, Shrum B, Leckie S, Skaro A, McAlister VC. The impact of alloantibodies directed against the second donor on long-term outcomes of repeat liver transplantation. Hepatobiliary Surg Nutr. 2019;8(3):246–52.
16. Lunz J, Ruppert KM, Cajaiba MM, Isse K, Bentlejewski CA, Minervini M, et al. Re-examination of the lymphocytotoxic crossmatch in liver transplantation: can C4d stains help in monitoring? Am J Transplant. 2012;12(1):171–82.
17. O'Leary JG, Kaneku H, Jennings LW, Bañuelos N, Susskind BM, Terasaki PI, et al. Preformed class II donor-specific antibodies are associated with an increased risk of early rejection after liver transplantation. Liver Transplant. 2013;19(9):973–80.
18. O'Leary JG, Kaneku H, Banuelos N, Jennings LW, Klintmalm GB, Terasaki PI. Impact of IgG3 subclass and C1q-fixing donor-specific HLA alloantibodies on rejection and survival in liver transplantation. Am J Transplant. 2015;15(4):1003–13.
19. O'Leary JG, Kaneku H, Demetris AJ, Marr JD, Shiller SM, Susskind BM, et al. Antibody-mediated rejection as a contributor to previously unexplained early liver allograft loss. Liver Transplant. 2014;20(2):218–27.
20. Tambur AR, Herrera ND, Haarberg KM, Cusick MF, Gordon RA, Leventhal JR, et al. Assessing antibody strength: comparison of MFI, C1q, and titer information. Am J Transplant. 2015;15(9):2421–30.
21. Daly RC, Rosenbaum AN, Dearani JA, Clavell AL, Pereira NL, Boilson BA, et al. Heart-after-liver transplantation attenuates rejection of cardiac allografts in sensitized patients. J Am Coll Cardiol. 2021;77(10):1331–40.
22. O'Leary JG, Gebel HM, Ruiz R, Bray RA, Marr JD, Zhou XJ, et al. Class II alloantibody and mortality in simultaneous liver-kidney transplantation. Am J Transplant. 2013;13(4):954–60.
23. Dar W, Agarwal A, Watkins C, Gebel HM, Bray RA, Kokko KE, et al. Donor-directed MHC class I antibody is preferentially cleared from sensitized recipients of combined liver/kidney transplants. Am J Transplant. 2011;11(4):841–7.

24. Xu Q, Zeevi A, Ganoza A, Cruz RJ, Jr., Mazariegos GV. Current approaches for risk assessment of intestinal transplant patients: a view from the histocompatibility laboratory. Hum Immunol. 2024:110768.
25. Kaneku H, O'Leary JG, Banuelos N, Jennings LW, Susskind BM, Klintmalm GB, et al. De novo donor-specific HLA antibodies decrease patient and graft survival in liver transplant recipients. Am J Transplant. 2013;13(6):1541–8.
26. Jucaud V, Shaked A, DesMarais M, Sayre P, Feng S, Levitsky J, et al. Prevalence and impact of De novo donor-specific antibodies during a multicenter immunosuppression withdrawal trial in adult liver transplant recipients. Hepatology. 2019;69(3):1273–86.
27. Rana A, Ackah RL, Webb GJ, Halazun KJ, Vierling JM, Liu H, et al. No gains in long-term survival after liver transplantation over the past three decades. Ann Surg. 2019;269(1):20–7.
28. Neuberger JM, Bechstein WO, Kuypers DR, Burra P, Citterio F, De Geest S, et al. Practical recommendations for long-term management of modifiable risks in kidney and liver transplant recipients: a guidance report and clinical checklist by the consensus on managing modifiable risk in transplantation (COMMIT) group. Transplantation. 2017;101(4S Suppl 2):S1–S56.

Combined Organ Transplantation

18

Sangeeta Satish and Alejandro Pita

Introduction

Since the early years in the development of solid organ transplantation, the use of multiorgan transplant has increased steadily to treat a wide variety of diseases. Since the first simultaneous double-organ transplant in 1983, a combined liver and kidney transplant (CLKT), the number of these combined procedures has dramatically increased within the last decade, with over 938 simultaneous liver and second-organ transplants performed in 2024 in the United States alone [1, 2]. The work of Dr. Thomas Starzl laid the foundations for many developments in this field. The first simultaneous liver and thoracic transplant was a combined heart and liver transplant (CHLT) performed by Starzl in 1984 in a 6-year-old patient with homozygous familial hypercholesterolemia [3], followed by the first combined lung and liver transplant (CLLT) in the 1990s [4].

Combined transplants are used to treat disorders that impact multiple organs to the severity that transplantation with one organ alone will not suffice. A disorder can cause synchronous damage to multiple organs. Alternatively, the presence of end-stage disease in one organ may result in the ongoing injury of a second organ system. Lastly, combined transplants may also be utilized to prevent recurrence of disease within the new graft. As combined transplants require extensive technical expertise and collaboration among multiple disciplines, it remains a non-ubiquitous entity only performed by a few highly experienced centers across the globe.

Herein, we provide an overview of the current medical literature on CLKT, CHLT, and CLLT, focusing on the indications, selection criteria, preoperative considerations, surgical technique, postoperative management, and patient outcomes.

S. Satish · A. Pita (✉)
Department of General Surgery, Digestive Disease and Surgery Institute, Cleveland Clinic, Cleveland, OH, USA
e-mail: pitaa@ccf.org

B. Eghtesad et al. (eds.), *Liver Transplantation*,
https://doi.org/10.1007/978-3-032-07072-2_18

Combined Liver and Kidney Transplant

Indications

Hepatorenal syndrome (HRS) accounts for 15–30% of acute kidney injury (AKI) in cirrhotic patients and is associated with 50–80% 90-day mortality [5]. Renal dysfunction occurs secondary to hypoperfusion, due to compensatory release of vasodilatory agents in response to portal hypertension, as well as decreased circulating volume secondary to low oncotic pressure in cirrhotic patients. Ultimately, kidney function declines to the volume-unresponsive renal failure of HRS, which can manifest in two ways. HRS-AKI presents with rapidly progressing kidney failure in response to an inciting event such as spontaneous bacterial peritonitis, acute on chronic liver failure, or gastrointestinal bleeding. HRS-CKD has a more indolent course and develops over time.

Cirrhotic patients can also develop non-HRS kidney injury due to hypovolemia from bleeding, acute tubular necrosis from septic shock, or from nephrotoxic agents such as antibiotics and diuretics. Patients with metabolic-associated steatotic liver disease (MASLD) have several co-morbidities such as diabetes and hypertension that can result in concomitant kidney dysfunction. MASLD can also result in oxidative damage and dysregulation of the renin-angiotensin-aldosterone system, causing renal hypertrophy and fibrosis [6]. Hepatitis B and C patients can deposit immune complexes within the glomeruli and renal parenchyma, causing nephritic and nephrotic syndromes that may progress to CKD. Other conditions that may result in the need for CLKT include polycystic kidney and liver disease in adults, and inherited metabolic and structural abnormalities such as primary hyperoxaluria type 1 in the pediatric population.

Selection Criteria

The Model for End Stage Liver Disease (MELD) score was implemented in 2002 as the basis to guide liver allocation. Since then, a drastic increase in CLKT has been observed as the MELD score accounts for serum creatinine and pre-transplant renal replacement therapy (RRT). Initially, there was significant variation in selection criteria among different transplant centers. As the kidneys are allocated with the liver, high-quality kidney grafts with a kidney donor profile index (KDPI; a prognostic score that utilizes donor factors to estimate risk of graft failure) less than 35% were utilized in almost 50% of CLKT [7]. This led to the development of medical eligibility criteria for simultaneous liver-kidney transplants (SLK) in 2017 (Table 18.1). Safety net criteria were also established for kidney after liver transplant (KALT) to prioritize patients who did not meet SLK criteria and underwent liver transplant (LT) alone with unimproved or worsening kidney function during the first year following liver transplant. Since the implementation of these criteria, transplant volume for SLK has decreased with no change in 1-year survival, and wait-list mortality has decreased with safety net prioritization [8].

Table 18.1 Medical eligibility criteria for SLK and safety net prioritization for liver transplant patients with worsening or unimproved kidney function according to KDPI sequence

Diagnosis confirmed by transplant nephrologist	*Additional associated criteria that must be present prior to transplant*
CKD with eGFR ≤60 ml/min for 90 consecutive days	Patient has ESRD with initiation of dialysis **OR** Patient's most recent CrCl or eGFR ≤35 ml/min at time of listing
Sustained AKI	Need for dialysis at least once every 7 days for the last 6 weeks **AND/OR** CrCl or eGFR ≤25 ml/min at least once every 7 days for the last 6 weeks
Metabolic disease	Diagnosis of at least one of the following: Hyperoxaluria aHUS from mutations in factor H or factor I Familial non-neuropathic systemic amyloidosis Methylmalonic aciduria

Safety net criteria
2–12 months post-LT: registered on kidney transplant wait list with (1) ESRD on dialysis OR (2) eGFR ≤20 ml/min

Sequence A *KDPI ≤ 20%*	*Sequence B* *20% < KDPI ≤ 35%*	*Sequence C* *35% < KDPI ≤ 85%*	*Sequence B* *KDPI > 85%*
Safety net patients not considered	Highly sensitized Zero antigen mismatch Prior living donor Local pediatrics *Local safety net* Local adults Regional pediatrics Regional adults National pediatrics National adults	Highly sensitized Zero antigen mismatch Prior living donor *Local safety net* Local candidates Regional candidates National candidates	Highly sensitized Zero antigen mismatch *Local safety net* Local and regional candidates National candidates

AKI acute kidney injury, *aHUS* atypical hemolytic uremic syndrome, *CKD* chronic kidney disease, *CrCl* creatinine clearance, *ESRD* end-stage renal disease, *eGFR* estimated glomerular filtration rate, *KDPI* kidney donor profile index, *LT* liver transplantation

Pretransplant Considerations

AKI in cirrhotic patients must be promptly recognized and intervened upon. As a first step, all nephrotoxic agents should be discontinued, and volume expansion should be attempted. On initial presentation, all patients should undergo urine analysis to differentiate between etiologies of kidney disease. Low urinary sodium and low fractional excretion of sodium are usually related to HRS, whereas the presence of microscopic hematuria, proteinuria, and casts indicates acute tubular necrosis. Proteinuria on urine analysis may also indicate the development of CKD. Renal ultrasound should be obtained to rule out any structural disease, and a kidney biopsy may be needed to further identify the etiology of kidney dysfunction. Patients with HRS tend to have normal renal ultrasound and histology.

HRS does not resolve with fluid resuscitation, and while transplant is the only definitive treatment, medical therapy is utilized to mitigate the vasodilatory effect of cirrhosis. Terlipressin is a vasopressin analog that results in vasoconstriction of the splanchnic vasculature and has been found to increase HRS reversal and decrease the need for RRT [5]. Norepinephrine, midodrine, and octreotide with albumin are other pharmacological options for HRS treatment. If patients show no response to treatment after 14 days, medical therapy is stopped and evaluation for transjugular intrahepatic portosystemic shunt (TIPS) and RRT is considered. Although TIPS has been shown to improve renal function and 1-year survival in patients with HRS, it may also exacerbate liver failure and worsen HRS. RRT can result in several complications within cirrhotic patients and has not been shown to improve survival in HRS patients [6]. Both therapies are currently used as a bridging therapy for patients listed for transplant.

Surgical Technique

During SLK, the liver and kidney are often procured from the same donor and implanted in the recipient under the same anesthesia setting. The liver is transplanted first, followed by the kidney. The liver is transplanted in an orthotopic fashion, replacing the old liver with the allograft. The recipient's native kidneys are not usually removed during transplant. In most cases, the kidney allograft is implanted in the right or left lower abdomen in an extraperitoneal approach, using the iliac vessels and allowing for ease of ureteral implantation to the bladder due to its close proximity. Some centers utilize the en bloc technique to minimize operative time and cold ischemia time (CIT) [9], where the liver and kidney are implanted through the same incision and share the same blood supply. While the en bloc technique may confer some advantages, postoperative complications such as arterial thrombosis may impact both organs. In addition, reoperation may be particularly difficult due to the proximity of the two organs.

Sequential transplant describes the separate implantation of the liver and kidney under different anesthesia settings. The Indiana approach [10] is a short interval sequential transplant where the liver is implanted first, with the kidney transplant taking place sometime between postoperative days 2 through 5. During this time, the kidney allograft is maintained via continuous pulsatile hypothermic machine perfusion. The Indiana approach has been utilized in patients with a positive crossmatch, with improved graft function and survival and decreased rejection [11]. KALT falls under the category of sequential transplants and involves two separate donors for the two organs.

Postoperative Management

Immunosuppression regimens vary between centers. Induction immunosuppression with lymphocyte-depleting rabbit antithymocyte globulin (r-ATG) or interleukin 2 receptor antagonist (IL2RA) has been historically used to decrease the incidence of acute rejection. However, a recent study showed that use of r-ATG or IL2RA did not lower the risk of liver or kidney rejection rates compared to no induction, with an associated increased risk in mortality with r-ATG use. Maintenance immunosuppression consists of a calcineurin inhibitor (CNI), such as tacrolimus, and an antimetabolite such as mycophenolate mofetil (MMF). Steroids have also been used for maintenance immunosuppression; however, use of steroids has been decreasing with a recent study showing decreased mortality with steroid-sparing regimens [12].

SLK has been associated with decreased rates of kidney graft rejection compared to KT alone [13, 14], due to the liver's role in mediating immunotolerance through several mechanisms (Fig. 18.1). For instance, chimerism is defined as the migration of donor leukocytes to recipient organs, increasing immunotolerance towards the graft. The unique structure of the hepatic sinusoids allows the liver to encounter alloreactive T-cells and eliminate them [15]. Inactivation of CD8+ T-cells, neutralization or passive absorption of preexisting antibodies, and generation of anti-inflammatory cytokines all contribute to the immunoprotection observed with combined liver transplants. As KALT patients receive organs from two different donors, there is no immunotolerance observed.

Outcomes

Kidney delayed graft function (K-DGF) is defined as the need for dialysis within the first week post-transplant and is noted in 16–49% of CLKT patients [16]. Risk factors include older age, history of hypertension and diabetes, DCD donors, higher KDPI, longer CIT, and higher recipient MELD [16]. Use of machine perfusion has been noted to decrease the incidence of K-DGF [16]. K-DGF has been associated with increased mortality, liver graft failure, and kidney graft failure. Other postoperative renal-specific complications include renal artery stenosis, renal artery thrombosis, renal vein thrombosis, urinary leakage, ureteral obstruction, and hematoma formation, all of which may impact graft and patient survival.

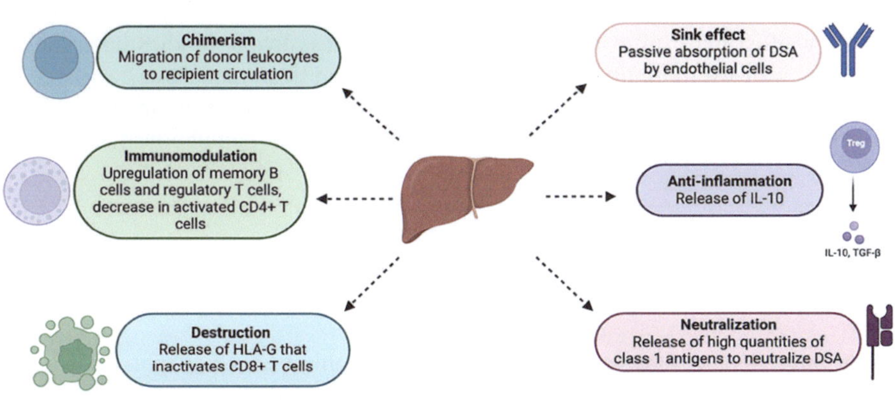

Fig. 18.1 Liver's role in immunotolerance in combined transplant. HLA-G human leukocyte antigen G, DSA donor-specific antibody, IL-10 interleukin 10. (Figures created with Biorender.com)

CLKT patients have good long-term post-transplant outcomes with 1-year survival ranging from 83–96% [8, 17, 18]. As mentioned above, the implementation of SLK criteria has helped control the rise in CLKT, and safety net prioritization has improved waitlist mortality [8]. Deciding which patients should be listed for SLK or KALT remains challenging. More than 50% of patients who undergo SLK are estimated to recover native kidney function to some degree. and up to one-third of SLK-listed patients who receive LT alone may have recovery of eGFR to >60 mL/min, with less than 5% needing subsequent renal transplant within one year [7]. However, SLK offers superior outcomes in patients where native renal function does not improve after SLK, highlighting the importance of choosing the combined approach when criteria are met. While standardization of guidelines has helped guide CLKT, the interplay between different techniques and risk factors needs to be refined to determine the best treatment strategies for different patient populations.

Combined Thoracic-Liver Transplant

Combined thoracic and liver transplants require a comprehensive multidisciplinary approach in the pretransplant workup, proficient surgical and anesthesia teams in the intraoperative phase, and experienced intensivist, medical, and surgical teams for the immediate postoperative and long-term management of these patients. These transplants are usually performed at a few high-volume centers, and the highest-volume CHLT center in the US has only performed 56 transplants to date (OPTN data as of August 2024). Due to the overall low patient volumes and variability in practice among centers, standardized selection criteria, surgical approaches, and post-transplant management have not been universally adopted. This variability makes it difficult to compare outcomes and determine the best management of these patients. Postoperative survival for combined thoracic-liver transplants [19–21] may be similar to outcomes in isolated thoracic transplants, but lower survival is observed in combined organ transplants compared to LT alone. In addition, as combined thoracic cases take liver allografts from the donor pool, there is concern that sicker patients on the LT waitlist may suffer from the allocation of these livers. Studies have shown increased wait-list mortality for combined thoracic and liver transplants compared to isolated organ transplants and a survival benefit with receiving a combined transplant from these waitlists, indicating utility within certain patient populations [21].

Combined Heart and Liver Transplant

Indications

Congestive hepatopathy is the leading etiology behind CHLT. Right-sided heart dysfunction causes a systemic back flow of blood, resulting in increased central venous pressure (CVP) (Fig. 18.2). The resulting vascular congestion in the

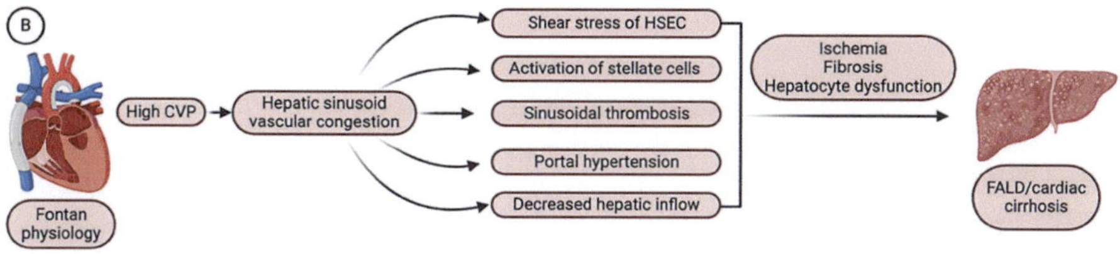

Fig. 18.2 Development of cardiac cirrhosis. HTN hypertension, SVR systemic vascular resistance, HSEC hepatic sinusoidal endothelial cells, RAAS renin-angiotensin-aldosterone system, SNS sympathetic nervous system, CVP central venous pressure, FALD Fontan-associated liver disease. (Figure created with Biorender.com)

hepatic sinusoids causes liver dysfunction through increased pressure and shear stress within the hepatic sinusoidal endothelial cells, resulting in decreased vasodilator release and activation of hepatic stellate cells, causing fibrosis [22]. Sinusoidal thrombosis can develop, causing ischemia and worsening fibrosis. High sinusoidal pressure impairs portal flow, resulting in subsequent portal hypertension. The cumulative hepatic dysfunction can result in cirrhosis and associated sequelae such as ascites, encephalopathy, and hepatocellular carcinoma (HCC).

The prevalence of adults with single ventricle congenital heart disease has increased over time due to the success of pediatric cardiac surgery. The Fontan procedure is part of a series of palliative surgeries for patients with single ventricle anatomy. The purpose of these surgeries is to direct systemic venous return to the pulmonary artery bypassing the heart to decrease intracardiac mixing of oxygenated and deoxygenated blood, allowing the single functioning ventricle to solely focus on providing cardiac output for the systemic circulation [23]. Fontan-associated liver disease (FALD) is a chronic sequela of this physiology. In these patients, the liver experiences ischemia from birth due to the abnormal fetal circulation. Following the Fontan procedure, the liver is constantly exposed to high, non-pulsatile CVP, resulting in hepatic congestion. As the Fontan circulation fails with time, cardiac output decreases and there is an increase in pulmonary shunt-related hypoxia [24]. FALD can progress to cirrhosis with the development of HCC and portal hypertension. It is estimated that almost all adults with Fontan physiology will develop some level FALD. While a heart transplant (HT) alone can be performed in patients with failing Fontan physiology and mild FALD, CHLT is necessary for patients with cirrhotic sequelae.

Familial amyloid polyneuropathy (FAP), which accounts for 24% of CHLT cases in the US, is an autosomal dominant mutation in the transthyretinin gene that results in the production of misfolded protein within the liver [25]. Cardiac deposition of misfolded protein results in arrythmias, heart block, and restrictive cardiomyopathy, while accumulation within the peripheral nerves results in severe dysautonomia. LT has been used to treat the underlying disease process, improving 10-year survival to 80% [26]. Interestingly, the liver from FAP patients can be subsequently used in domino transplants as living donor grafts with no recurrence of disease in the recipient [27].

Selection Criteria

Patients with abnormal LFTs or anomalies on imaging undergo a transjugular liver biopsy with measurement of hepatovenous pressure gradient (HVPG) to assess for cirrhosis and portal hypertension. Those with biopsy-proven cirrhosis or elevated HVPG gradient (>5–6 mmHg) should be considered and evaluated for CHLT [28, 29]. Allocation is primarily driven by the degree of heart dysfunction [30]. High MELD-XI scores, a modification of the MELD score excluding international normalized ratio (INR), are associated with worse post-HT outcomes. Within Fontan patients, Varices, Ascites, Splenomegaly, and Thrombocytopenia is another prognostic score utilized to estimate the level of liver dysfunction, with a score ≥ 2 associated with worse post-HT outcomes and increased risk of HCC or death [31].

Anesthesia Considerations

CHLT patients have limited physiologic reserve due to concurrent heart and liver dysfunction. As patients are awaiting transplant, preoperative optimization of cardiac function is attempted through the placement of pacemakers and ventricular assist devices. Patients with worsening hemodynamics or evidence of end-organ malperfusion are admitted for further preoperative optimization, which can vastly improve intraoperative hemodynamic stability and decrease the duration of cardiopulmonary bypass (CPB).

Anesthesia management is extremely important during CHLT and requires collaboration between cardiac and liver transplant anesthesia teams to maintain the hemodynamic status during the operation [32]. CHLT can be broken down into several stages from an anesthesia perspective, each with its own unique challenges [32, 33] (Table 18.2). For instance, reperfusion of the liver graft can result in several hemodynamic changes that must be diagnosed and treated quickly [33]. Patients with Fontan physiology have special considerations to keep in mind. In the pre-CPB phase, Fontan patients require a high CVP to maintain pulmonary circulation and provide cardiac output. While high CVP is necessary to maintain circulation, it will result in higher blood loss due to the presence of portosystemic collaterals. In addition, pulmonary vascular resistance should be minimized with pulmonary vasodilators and management of hypoxia and hypercarbia.

Surgical Technique

The most common technique for CHLT is the combined orthotopic approach, where the heart is implanted first, followed by the liver, as the donor heart is more susceptible to ischemic injury. Another method is en bloc transplant, where the heart and liver are procured and implanted simultaneously. Advantages include fewer anastomotic sites and protection of the new cardiac graft from hemodynamic changes during hepatectomy and reperfusion. However, cardiac CIT is increased, and the

Table 18.2 Goals, potential complications, and recommended interventions during each phase of CHLT

Anesthesia phase	Goals	Potential complications	Interventions
Preoperative	Reprogram cardiac devices Establish invasive monitoring RSI induction Reversal of anticoagulation Crossmatched blood products	Hypotension during anesthesia induction	Inotropes and vasopressors during induction Induction immunosuppression with MMF/methylprednisone Initiation of preoperative antibiotics
Pre-CPB	MAP 65–85 mmHg TEGs to correct coagulopathy Lower SBP 100 mmHg prior to CPB cannulation	Shearing aortic injury or intimal dissection during initiation of CPB Bleeding	Heparin prior to CPB induction to achieve ACT >450 s
Separation from CPB	TEE evaluation of graft function EKG shows extra nonfunctioning P-wave Heparin reversed for ACT <120 s Hgb $\geq$ 8 g/dL TEG for coagulopathy	Intracardiac air RV dysfunction Arrythmias, Bradycardia Hypothermia	Trendelenberg to assist with de-airing Pulmonary vasodilators and inotropes Epicardial pacing or direct acting agents like epinephrine Protamine to reverse heparin Blood products
Anhepatic	MAP 65–85 mmHg CVP < 10 mmHg CI > 2.2 L/min/m^2 Correct electrolyte abnormalities TEG for coagulopathy TEE-guided fluid resuscitation	Hypotension Decreased cardiac output	Vasopressors, inotropes VVB, VA-ECMO Optimize electrolytes and acidbase status Blood products
Reperfusion	TEE evaluation of graft function MAP 65–85 mmHg CVP < 10 mmHg CI > 2.2 L/min/m^2 Correct electrolyte abnormalities	Reperfusion syndrome RV dysfunction Dynamic LVOT obstruction Intracardiac thrombus/PE Takotsubo cardiomyopathy	Inotropes, vasopressors Pulmonary vasodilators Mechanical support (RVAD, LVAD, VA ECMO) Anticoagulation Optimize electrolytes and acid base status

MMF mycophenolate mofetil, *CPB* cardiopulmonary bypass, *MAP* mean arterial pressure, *TEG* thromboelastography, *SBP* systolic blood pressure, *ACT* activated clotting time, *TEE* transesophageal echocardiogram, *EKG* electrocardiogram, *Hgb* hemoglobin, *RV* right ventricle, *CVP* central venous pressure, *CI* cardiac index, *VVB* veno-venous bypass, *VA-ECMO* veno-arterial extracorporeal membrane oxygenation, *LVOT* left ventricle outflow tract, *PE* pulmonary embolism, *RVAD* right ventricle assist device, *LVAD* left ventricle assist device presence of the heart and liver transplant teams at the same time can be logistically challenging [34]. The liver first approach has been described in sensitized patients to protect the cardiac allograft from donor-specific antibodies, but it would only be applicable in select patients due to potential post-reperfusion related complications [35].

Postoperative Management

In the immediate postoperative period, patients may be at increased risk for the development of thromboembolic events or intracranial hemorrhage. Hypoperfusion and inadequate resuscitation may result in kidney injury, with potential need for RRT. Arrhythmias can be treated with direct acting agents (e.g., epinephrine) as the cardiac allograft maintains autonomic receptors despite being denervated from the autonomic system. There is no standardized induction regimen for CHLT. One center describes induction with MMF followed by methylprednisone after cardiac implantation, while another utilizes methylprednisolone and r-ATG. Maintenance immunosuppression consisted of tacrolimus (variable trough 8–15 ng/ml), MMF, and taper of steroids to end 4–6 months after transplant [31]. Patients with stable graft function with no evidence of rejection were converted to rapamycin (trough 8–12 ng/mL) and weaned off CNIs [36]. Endomyocardial biopsy, echocardiogram, and angiogram are performed at regular intervals to assess allograft function and rejection.

Patient Outcomes

Cardiac allograft vasculopathy (CAV) is a major cause of post-cardiac transplant morbidity and mortality, and it is thought to be an immune-mediated process that damages endothelial cells during allograft rejection [37]. Compared to HT alone, CHLT has a decreased incidence of CAV [36]. CHLT patients have comparable survival outcomes to LT and HT, with 1-year survival ranging from 85% to 100% [27, 38]. CHD patients who underwent CHLT had improved 5-year and 10-year survival at 83% compared to 63% and 39% with HT alone [39]. This has been replicated in several other studies that show improvement in survival with CHLT in non-CHD patients. Rates of cardiac rejection are significantly improved with CHLT compared to heart transplant alone [36, 40].

Combined Liver and Lung Transplant

Indications

Cystic fibrosis is the most common indication for CLLT [41, 42]. It is characterized by a defect within the cystic fibrosis transmembrane regulator (CFTR) gene that impacts the movement of sodium and chloride ions. Approximately 40% of CF patients experience liver dysfunction. Alpha-1-antitrypsin deficiency (AATD) is another indication for CLLT that results in emphysematous lung disease deposition of misfolded AAT within the liver. CLLT may also be considered when pulmonary function deteriorates in cirrhotic patients through hepatopulmonary syndrome (HPS). HPS leads to a ventilation-perfusion mismatch through the presence of intrapulmonary vascular dilation (IPVD) and arteriovenous shunts, causing hypoxia. HPS may be present to some degree in 10–30% of LT patients and is associated with increased mortality [43]. Patients with portal hypertension can also develop pulmonary hypertension over time, resulting in porto-pulmonary hypertension (POPH). While the exact pathophysiology of POPH is unknown, it is hypothesized that the increased circulating volume and the proinflammatory state in cirrhotic patients result in damage to the pulmonary vessels. POPH is diagnosed by RHC with increased mean pulmonary artery pressure and vascular resistance in the presence of normal pulmonary capillary wedge pressure (PCWP). While vasomodulator agents can be used to treat POPH and improve prognosis after LT, POPH may become resistant to treatment and the presence of severe POPH (mPAP >45 mmHg) is a contraindication for liver transplant [44, 45]. Common indications for lung transplant such as chronic obstructive pulmonary disease (COPD) and idiopathic pulmonary fibrosis (IPH) have been associated with an increased risk for liver disease (Table 18.3).

Selection Criteria

While there are no generalized selection criteria for CLLT, the International Society for Heart and Lung Transplantation (ISHLT) recommends that patients meet lung transplant disease-specific criteria and have biopsy-proven evidence of cirrhosis or HVPG greater than 10 mmHg [49]. Relative contraindications to CLLT include severe ascites and encephalopathy, INR >1.8, and albumin <2 g/dL, although

Table 18.3 Indications for CLLT with associated pathophysiology, diagnosis, presentation, and strategies for preoperative optimization

Disease	Pathophysiology resulting in lung and liver dysfunction	Diagnostic testing	Presentation	Preoperative optimization
Systemic diseases				
Cystic fibrosis [46]	Defect in the CFTR gene that impacts the movement of sodium and chloride Impairs mucous clearance in lungs Impacts biliary composition	Positive newborn screening Pilocarpine Sweat [Cl] $\geq$ 60 mmol/L Genetic testing for CF variants	Recurrent sinus and pulmonary infections Steatorrhea Malnutrition Bronchiectasis Biliary cirrhosis Diabetes	Chronic colonization with P. aeruginosa or B. cepacia: pre-transplant antibiotics Parenteral nutrition or tube feeding Tight glycemic control

(continued)

Table 18.3 (continued)

Disease	Pathophysiology resulting in lung and liver dysfunction	Diagnostic testing	Presentation	Preoperative optimization
Alpha-1 antitrypsin deficiency [47]	Point mutation in SERPINA gene Accumulation of misfolded AAT protein in the liver Lung parenchyma destruction with uninhibited protease	Serum AAT phenotype Genetic testing Liver biopsy with PAS-positive globules	Cirrhosis Portal Hypertension Emphysema Bronchiectasis Splenomegaly	Bronchodilator treatment Avoidance of NSAIDs and alcohol Supplementation with fat-soluble vitamins
Liver diseases resulting in lung dysfunction				
HPS [43]	Intrapulmonary vascular dilation and arteriovenous shunts	TTE with agitated saline Tc-MAA lung perfusion scan Supine ABG	Digital clubbing Platypnoea Orthodexia Progressive hypoxia	Embolization of AVM Oxygen therapy, pulmonary vasodilators
POPH [45]	Pulmonary vasculature damage from increased circulating volume and pro-inflammatory cytokines	RHC: increased PAP and resistance, normal PCWP TTE	Dyspnea on exertion Hypoxia Right ventricle hypertrophy	Pulmonary vasodilators Supplemental oxygen
Lung disease resulting in liver dysfunction				
COPD, IPH [48]	Multifactorial secondary to comorbidities	LFTs RUQ US Abdominal CT HVPG Transjugular biopsy	Elevated liver enzymes Hepatosplenomegaly Thrombocytopenia	Optimization of comorbidities Avoidance of hepatotoxic agents

CFTR cystic fibrosis transmembrane regulator, *[Cl]* chloride concentration, *CF* cystic fibrosis, *AAT* alpha-1-antitrypsin, *PAS* periodic acid-Schiff, *NSAIDs* non-steroidal anti-inflammatory drugs, *HPS* hepatopulmonary syndrome, *TTE* transthoracic echocardiogram, *Tc-MAA* 99mTechnetium-labeled macro-aggregated albumin, *ABG* arterial blood gas, *AVM* arteriovenous malformations, *POPH* portopulmonary hypertension, *RHC* right heart catheterization, *PAP* pulmonary artery pressure, *PCWP* pulmonary capillary wedge pressure, *COPD* chronic obstructive pulmonary disease, *IPH* idiopathic pulmonary fibrosis, *LFTs* liver function tests, *RUQ US* right upper quadrant ultrasound, *CT* computed tomography, *HVPG* hepatic venous pressure gradient

practices are usually center-specific. The UNOS Lung Allocation Score (LAS) is a multifactorial score that accounts for recipient co-morbidities, functional status, liver and kidney function, and cardiopulmonary testing measures. As the lung is often the organ with the most dysfunction, the LAS score is used to determine status on the waiting list. Once a patient has become eligible to receive lungs from a specific donor, the donor liver is also allocated to the patient for CLLT. Use of the LAS score to allocate organs for CLLT has been associated with decreased waitlist times and mortality, as well as improved overall survival after transplant [50].

Preoperative Considerations

The degree of pulmonary hypertension is assessed with TTE and RHC. Severity of HPS is quantified based on PaO2 levels—mild: PaO2 $\geq$ 80 mmHg; severe: PaO2 $\geq$ 50–<60 mmHg with A-aO2 $\geq$ 15 mmHg while breathing room air. Preoperative optimization of lung function is attempted with mucolytics, nebulizers, antibiotics, and vaso-modulatory agents [51]. Nutritional optimization and tight glycemic control are necessary in CF patients, who may develop pancreatic insufficiency. Another concern is chronic colonization with organisms such as Pseudomonas aeruginosa and Burkholderia cepacia, requiring infectious disease assessment for consideration of pretransplant antibiotics [42].

Surgical Technique

Transplant of the lung and liver usually occurs in a sequential orthotopic fashion, with the lungs implanted first, followed by the liver. As pulmonary edema is a major concern, some centers elect to perform the abdominal dissection prior to implantation of either organ to minimize the need for fluids or blood products in the presence of the new lung allograft [52]. Several centers have reported a liver-first strategy in CF patients with improvement in overall survival and decreased incidence of lung graft dysfunction and rejection [53, 54]. Although lung CIT is prolonged, this approach minimizes exposure of the new lungs to fluid shifts during liver implantation, decreasing pulmonary edema. With the development of ex situ machine perfusion techniques for the lung and liver, CIT can be minimized, allowing for more flexibility in choosing which organ to transplant first [55, 56].

Postoperative Management

Fluid restriction is important to prevent pulmonary edema, and vasopressors are used to titrate MAP above 65 mmHg [42]. Low oxygen concentrations are used during mechanical ventilation to prevent primary graft failure, and ventilatory volume and pressure are carefully titrated to minimize trauma. There are no generalized immunosuppression regimens for CLLT, although it is often based on the lung transplant regimen. Induction immunosuppression can be performed with steroids and T-cell targeting monoclonal antibodies (e.g., daclizumab, basiliximab) or MMF and ATG [42]. Maintenance is achieved with steroid taper, MMF, and CNIs. Lower rates of rejection are observed in combined liver and lung transplant, although a recent study described 75% of CLLT patients experienced some level of lung allograft rejection, with 25% developing bronchiolitis obliterans syndrome (BOS), a form of chronic lung rejection [57]. Sepsis is the most common postoperative complication in CLLT, especially within CF patients [52]. As mentioned above, CF patients may be colonized and experience postoperative infection from these organisms. They are also susceptible to common nosocomial infections due to a combination of lengthy hospital stays and immunosuppression. However, there is no generalized consensus on postoperative antibiotic management in CF patients.

Patient Outcomes

CLLT patient survival at 1-year ranges from 56% to 100% in the literature. Recent studies have highlighted lower CLLT survival rates compared to LT alone, with no improvement in re-transplantation and acute rejection rates [20]. These finding brings into question the benefit of CLLT, and low patient census, lack of standardization, and variable postoperative management make evaluation of outcomes challenging. The implementation of scoring systems such as MELD and LAS in selection criteria has improved patient outcomes compared to historical cohorts [50], indicating that certain populations may benefit from CLLT.

Conclusion

Combined transplants have been increasing over the last decade and will likely continue to rise as patient disease complexity increases. Standardization of selection criteria and postoperative management is necessary for CHLT and CLLT. CLKT may benefit from fine-tuning patient selection for the different operative approaches. In the current state of high organ demand and a large number of patients in need of transplantation, with the increased organ utilization for combined transplant, appropriate patient selection remains paramount. In addition, the immunotolerance provided by the liver is an important benefit, and future research should focus on elucidating the mechanisms behind this protective effect. While further studies are needed to define optimal outcomes, combined transplants are and will likely remain essential in the treatment of these unique disease processes.

References

1. Margreiter R, et al. Combined liver and kidney transplantation. Lancet. 1984;1(8385):1077–8.
2. OPTN UNOS data. Available from: https://optn.transplant.hrsa.gov/data/view-data-reports/build-advanced/.
3. Starzl TE, et al. Heart-liver transplantation in a patient with familial hypercholesterolaemia. Lancet. 1984;1(8391):1382–3.
4. Couetil JP, et al. Combined lung and liver transplantation in patients with cystic fibrosis. A 4 1/2-year experience. J Thorac Cardiovasc Surg. 1995;110(5):1415–22.
5. Belcher JM. Hepatorenal syndrome. Med Clin North Am. 2023;107(4):781–92.

6. Gupta K, et al. Acute kidney injury and hepatorenal syndrome in cirrhosis. World J Gastroenterol. 2021;27(26):3984–4003.
7. Nair G, Nair V. Simultaneous liver–kidney transplantation. Clin Liver Dis. 2022;26(2):313–22.
8. Wilk AR, et al. Developing simultaneous liver-kidney transplant medical eligibility criteria while providing a safety net: a 2-year review of the OPTN's allocation policy. Am J Transplant. 2021;21(11):3593–607.
9. Nguyen MC, et al. En bloc liver-kidney transplantation with renal artery variation using donor splenic artery and left gastric artery as inflow to the kidney: case report. Int J Surg Case Rep. 2018;53:13–6.
10. Ekser B, et al. A novel approach in combined liver and kidney transplantation with long-term outcomes. Ann Surg. 2017;265(5):1000–8.
11. Goggins WC, et al. Combined liver–kidney transplantation with positive crossmatch: role of delayed kidney transplantation. Surgery. 2021;170(4):1240–7.
12. Weeks SR, et al. Steroid-sparing maintenance immunosuppression is safe and effective after simultaneous liver-kidney transplantation. Clin Transpl. 2020;34(10):e14036.
13. Kim J-Y, et al. Immunoprotective effect of liver allograft on patients with combined liver and kidney transplantation. Ann Transpl. 2023;29.
14. Taner T, et al. Decreased chronic cellular and antibody-mediated injury in the kidney following simultaneous liver-kidney transplantation. Kidney Int. 2016;89(4):909–17.
15. Ortega-Legaspi JM, Hoteit M, Wald J. Immune benefit of combined heart and liver transplantation. Curr Opin Organ Transplant. 2020;25(5):513–8.
16. Swanson KJ, et al. Kidney delayed graft function after combined kidney-solid organ transplantation: a review. Transplant Rev. 2022;36(3):100707.
17. AbdulRahim N, et al. Lack of benefit and potential harm of induction therapy in simultaneous liver-kidney transplants. Liver Transpl. 2019;25(3):411–24.
18. Pita A, et al. Outcomes of liver transplantation in patients on renal replacement therapy: considerations for simultaneous liver kidney transplantation versus safety net. Transplant Direct. 2019;5(10):e490.
19. Cheng XS, Wall A, Teuteberg J. Ethical decision-making in simultaneous heart–liver transplantation. Curr Opin Organ Transplant. 2020;25(5):519–25.
20. Freischlag K, et al. A propensity-matched survival analysis: do simultaneous liver-lung transplant recipients need a liver? Transplantation. 2019;103(8):1675–82.
21. Wolf JH, et al. Simultaneous thoracic and abdominal transplantation: can we justify two organs for one recipient? Am J Transplant. 2013;13(7):1806–16.
22. Fortea JI, et al. Congestive hepatopathy. Int J Mol Sci. 2020;21(24):9420.
23. Gordon-Walker TT, Bove K, Veldtman G. Fontan-associated liver disease: a review. J Cardiol. 2019;74(3):223–32.
24. Tracy KM, Matsuoka LK, Alexopoulos SP. Update on combined heart and liver transplantation: evolving patient selection, improving outcomes, and outstanding questions. Curr Opin Organ Transplant. 2023;28(2):104–9.
25. Gong T, Hall S. Considerations and experience driving expansion of combined heart–liver transplantation. Curr Opin Organ Transplant. 2020;25(5):496–500.
26. Lebray P, Varnous S. Combined heart and liver transplantation: state of knowledge and outlooks. Clin Res Hepatol Gastroenterol. 2019;43(2):123–30.
27. Sickels A, et al. Combined heart-liver and domino liver transplantation in familial amyloidosis. Am Surg. 2021;88(9):2267–73.
28. Kittleson MM, et al. Dual-organ transplantation: indications, evaluation, and outcomes for heart-kidney and heart-liver transplantation: a scientific statement from the American Heart Association. Circulation. 2023;148(7):622–36.
29. Kobashigawa J, et al. Summary of a consensus conference on heart-liver transplantation. Am J Transplant. 2024;24(3):380–90.
30. Mehra MR, et al. The 2016 International Society for Heart Lung Transplantation listing criteria for heart transplantation: a 10-year update. J Heart Lung Transplant. 2016;35(1):1–23.

31. Lee JTC, Sarode D, Emamaullee JA. Review of pediatric combined heart-liver transplantation: a roadmap to success. Pediatr Transplant. 2023;27(8):e14633.
32. Van Loon K, et al. Anesthesia for combined heart-liver transplantation: a narrative review. J Cardiothorac Vasc Anesth. 2024;38:2059.
33. Smeltz AM, Kumar PA, Arora H. Anesthesia for combined heart and liver transplantation. J Cardiothorac Vasc Anesth. 2021;35(11):3350–61.
34. Hill AL, et al. Pediatric combined heart–liver transplantation performed en bloc: a single-center experience. Pediatr Transplant. 2012;16(4):392–7.
35. Daly RC, et al. Combined heart and liver transplantation: protection of the cardiac graft from antibody rejection by initial liver implantation. Transplantation. 2013;95(2):e2–4.
36. Wong TW, et al. Liver allograft provides immunoprotection for the cardiac allograft in combined heart–liver transplantation. Am J Transplant. 2016;16(12):3522–31.
37. Laks JA, Dipchand AI. Cardiac allograft vasculopathy: a review. Pediatr Transplant. 2022;26(3):e14218.
38. Alexopoulos SP, et al. Adult combined heart-liver transplantation: the United States experience. Transpl Int. 2022;35:10036.
39. Bryant R, et al. Contemporary outcomes of combined heart-liver transplant in patients with congenital heart disease. Transplantation. 2018;102(2):e67–73.
40. Zhao K, et al. Incidence of acute rejection and patient survival in combined heart–liver transplantation. Liver Transpl. 2022;28(9):1500–8.
41. Connor AA, et al. Progress in combined liver–lung transplantation at a single center. Transplant Direct. 2023;9(5):e1482.
42. Han JL, et al. Combined liver-lung transplantation: indications, outcomes, current experience and ethical issues. Transplant Rev. 2019;33(2):99–106.
43. Raevens S, Boret M, Fallon MB. Hepatopulmonary syndrome. JHEP Reports. 2022;4(9):100527.
44. Grannas G, et al. Indications for and outcomes after combined lung and liver transplantation: a single-center experience on 13 consecutive cases. Transplantation. 2008;85(4):524–31.
45. Raevens S, et al. Pulmonary abnormalities in liver disease: relevance to transplantation and outcome. Hepatology. 2021;74(3):1674–86.
46. Dickinson KM, Collaco JM. Cystic fibrosis. Pediatr Rev. 2021;42(2):55–67.
47. Suri A, Patel D, Teckman JH. Alpha-1 antitrypsin deficiency liver disease. Clin Liver Dis. 2022;26(3):391–402.
48. Hyzny EJ, et al. A review of liver dysfunction in the lung transplant patient. Clin Transpl. 2021;35(8):e14344.
49. Weill D, et al. A consensus document for the selection of lung transplant candidates: 2014—an update from the Pulmonary Transplantation Council of the International Society for Heart and Lung Transplantation. J Heart Lung Transplant. 2015;34(1):1–15.
50. Freischlag K, et al. Improved survival in simultaneous lung-liver recipients and candidates in the modern era of lung allocation. J Surg Res. 2018;231:395–402.
51. Yager A, et al. Combined thoracic and abdominal organ transplantation: special considerations. Semin Cardiothorac Vasc Anesth. 2020;24(1):84–95.
52. Yi SG, et al. Combined lung and liver transplantation: analysis of a single-center experience. Liver Transpl. 2013;20(1):46–53.
53. Aburahma K, et al. Liver-first strategy for a combined lung and liver transplant in patients with cystic fibrosis. Eur J Cardiothorac Surg. 2021;60(4):822–30.
54. Salman J, et al. The liver-first approach for combined lung and liver transplantation. Eur J Cardiothorac Surg. 2018;54(6):1122–7.
55. Shamaa TM, et al. The use of normothermic liver preservation in combined liver and lung transplantation: a single-center experience. Am J Transplant. 2022;22(9):2261–4.
56. van Leeuwen OB, et al. Machine perfusion of donation after circulatory death liver and lungs before combined liver-lung transplantation. Transplant Direct. 2021;7(7):e718.
57. Freischlag KW, et al. Single-center long-term analysis of combined liver-lung transplant outcomes. Transplant Direct. 2018;4(5):e349.

Part III

Post-transplant Care

19 Interpretation of Blood Work After Liver Transplantation

William Carey

Introduction

The goal of orthotopic liver transplantation (OLT) is to restore normal liver function. A principal marker that this has been accomplished is the presence of normal standard liver tests, including bilirubin, aspartate transferase (AST), alanine transaminase (ALT), gamma-glutamyl-transpeptidase (GGTP), and alkaline phosphatase.

It is customary and useful to categorize liver diseases into three broad categories: *Hepatocellular*, in which primary injury is to the hepatocytes; *cholestatic*, in which primary injury is to the bile ducts; and *infiltrative*, in which the liver is invaded or replaced by non-hepatic substances, such as neoplasm or amyloid. Although there is a great deal of overlap in liver test result abnormalities seen in these three categories, particularly in cholestatic and infiltrative disorders, an attempt to characterize an otherwise undifferentiated clinical case as hepatocellular, cholestatic, or infiltrative often makes subsequent evaluation faster and more efficient. The AST, ALT, and alkaline phosphatase tests are most useful to make the distinction between hepatocellular and cholestatic disease.

A word of caution: when there is elevation of only a single "liver" enzyme, non-hepatic causes must be considered (Table 19.1). Further information about liver tests is available [1, 2].

In both the non-transplant and post-transplant setting, liver enzymes are never, by themselves, diagnostic. Awareness of probable causes is essential. A probable cause varies as a function of time after surgery. Accordingly, time after transplantation provides a useful scaffolding for discussion (Table 19.2). Severe immediate graft dysfunction requires expedited evaluation and management (Table 19.3).

W. Carey (✉)
Cleveland Clinic Lerner College of Medicine of Case Western Reserve University School of Medicine, Cleveland, OH, USA
e-mail: careyw@ccf.org

B. Eghtesad et al. (eds.), *Liver Transplantation*,
https://doi.org/10.1007/978-3-032-07072-2_19

Table 19.1 Possible alternative sources of isolated "liver" tests

Test	Nonhepatic source
Bilirubin	Red blood cells (e.g., hemolysis, intra-abdominal bleed, hematoma)
AST	Skeletal muscle, cardiac muscle, red blood cells
ALT	Skeletal muscle, cardiac muscle, kidneys
LDH	Heart, red blood cells (e.g., hemolysis)
Alkaline phosphatase	Bone, first trimester placenta, kidneys, intestines

AST aspartate aminotransferase, *ALT* alanine aminotransferase, *LDH* lactate dehydrogenase

Table 19.2 Timing of liver enzyme elevations after liver transplantation

Immediate	Days 0–7	Preservation, perfusion Vascular Primary graft non-function Hemodynamic
Early	<1 month	Abscess, fluid collections Hepatic artery thrombosis Biliary strictures Bile leak/cholangitis, DILI
Intermediate	1–12 months	Infection, biliary, infection, rejection, DILI
Late	>12 months	Rejection, infection, recurrent disease, biliary strictures, DILI

DILI drug-induced liver injury

Table 19.3 Features of severe immediate graft dysfunction suggesting primary graft dysfunction or thrombosis of hepatic artery, portal vein, IVC

AST	>3000 within 7 days of transplantation
Prothrombin time INR	>2.5
Arterial pH	<7.3
Lactate	>4 mm/L

AST aspartate aminotransferase, *INR* prothrombin time International Normalized Ratio, *IVC* inferior vena cava

Immediate: Major disequilibrium introduced by liver transplant creates perturbations in liver, cardiac, and renal function. Liver tests may be abnormal because of the effects of organ preservation. In this case, the pattern of liver test abnormality is hepatocellular. Most often, this is mild. And in most cases, the maximum abnormalities are seen within 48 h and then decline.

Suspicion of primary graft dysfunction, occurring in less than 5% of liver transplants, may be heralded by immediate marked elevation of AST and ALT. Vascular thrombosis immediately after liver transplantation also produces profound perturbation in blood testing. Hepatic artery thrombosis is always in the differential diagnosis of severe liver test abnormalities soon after transplant. Laboratory test abnormalities similar to those seen in primary graft dysfunction are typical. Definitive diagnosis is not based on blood testing but on angiography.

Early After Transplant

Biliary complications are still surprisingly frequent after liver transplantation. Any obstruction to the flow of bile is most often manifest in blood testing as an elevation of alkaline phosphatase and GGT. Clinical signs and symptoms are usually present and predominate.

Although the liver is an immunologically privileged organ, immunologic rejection is commonly seen, especially in individuals whose native liver was injured by immunologic disease. Acute T-cell-mediated rejection may occur early or late, sometimes within the first week or two after engraftment. The pattern of abnormal liver test is usually cholestatic. Liver biopsy is required for diagnosis. This will be discussed further, as follows.

Infection

Bacterial infections are common in the early transplant period, often but not always accompanied by leukocytosis and fever. Bacterial infections may affect the surgical site, bloodstream, or lungs. Liver test abnormalities may be absent. When severe, bacterial infections may trigger sepsis syndrome, in which case elevated lactate levels may be seen in addition to clinical signs such as difficulty breathing, fever, tachycardia, and low blood pressure.

Bacterial liver abscess and bacterial ascending cholangitis are usually accompanied by fever and abdominal pain. Liver test abnormalities are common, and alkaline phosphatase tends to predominate.

Viral Infections

Hepatitis C, hepatitis B, cytomegalovirus, and Epstein–Barr virus infections are noteworthy viral infections in the context of OLT.

Hepatitis C

In the era before highly effective antiviral therapies were available, liver transplantation for those with HCV was accompanied by recurrent HCV viremia, liver engraftment, and chronic liver disease. While liver transplant for end-stage liver disease as a consequence of HCV is still common, most often the virus has been eliminated before surgery; in such cases, recurrence after transplant is not expected.

In the case of a HCV viremic recipient, HCV will occur soon after transplantation and be manifest by mild-moderate AST and ALT elevations. An exception to this is in fibrosing cholestatic hepatitis, discussed separately.

It is common practice in many transplant centers to employ HCV-positive donors even for hepatitis C naïve recipients (HCV D+/R-). In this circumstance, HCV will occur in nearly all, usually within days or weeks. Frequent monitoring of HCV RNA PCR after transplant will discover its presence even before liver tests become abnormal. Prompt institution of antiviral therapy is given before liver enzymes surge.

Hepatitis B

Hepatitis B after transplantation is distinctly uncommon in countries with low-HBV prevalence because hepatitis B-infected organs are not used, and recipients who harbor hepatitis B are recognized before surgery and effective preemptive strategies to suppress infection are widely employed. Finally, de novo hepatitis B is uncommon because most recipients will have been immunized prior to surgery.

In the rare case of hepatitis B after OLT, the AST and ALT become elevated. In severe cases, the enzymes may be very high and jaundice may occur.

Fibrosing cholestatic hepatitis In both hepatitis B and C, recurrence of infection after OLT may trigger a distinct and aggressive form of liver injury, fibrosing cholestatic hepatitis. In this disorder, cholestatic liver enzymes predominate with elevated bilirubin in severe cases. It can result in rapid progression and graft loss. There are no diagnostic blood tests, so a liver biopsy is useful. Expected findings include hepatocyte damage, severe cholestasis, and absence of significant inflammation. It may occasionally be confused with T-cell-mediated rejection [3].

Cytomegalovirus

CMV poses a significant risk after OLT unless preemptive prophylactic antiviral therapy is provided to those at risk. CMV usually becomes manifest within the first 6 months after transplantation. In most cases, symptoms such as fever, myalgia, arthralgia, and malaise are present. Liver test abnormalities may include elevation of AST, ALT, and alkaline phosphatase of a modest degree. Diagnosis depends on the detection of CMV virus, antigen, and/or antibodies (IgG, IgM) [4].

Epstein–Barr Virus

EBV after liver transplantation may present with classical infectious mononucleosis symptoms (fever, pharyngitis, cervical adenopathy, enlarged liver and spleen. In such cases, liver test abnormalities are hepatocellular in pattern.

A more sinister form of EBV infection after transplant is post-transplant lymphoproliferative disorder. Definitive diagnosis depends on EBV-virus-specific blood tests [5].

Fungal Infections

Candida (68–93%), aspergillosis (1–9%), and cryptococcus (0.5–5%) are the most common invasive fungal infections after liver transplantation [6].

Preoperative risk factors for Candida include hospitalization or anti-infective treatment within 90 days before transplantation, MELD score above 30, end-stage renal disease or serum creatinine >2 mg/dl, and fungal pre-colonization. Intraoperative factors include donor-derived infection and split liver transplantation. Prolonged (>10 h) operative time, massive transfusions, high urgency transplantation, and Rou-en-Y choledochojejunostomy. Post-operative features posing risk include renal replacement therapy, re-transplantation within 90 days, re-laparotomy, CMV viremia, biliary leakage, and high-level immune suppression [7].

Standard liver tests are unhelpful in the diagnosis of fungal infections. Diagnosis may be based on blood tests (most often candidemia) but is often based on sampling localized fluid collections or tissue. Diagnostic tests are plagued by lack of sensitivity. Tests such as BDG, Candida PCT, and T2 Candida assays in serum are available [8].

Drugs

After liver transplantation, many drugs are administered. A suspicion of drug-induced liver injury should always be present. LiverTox provides up-to-date, unbiased, and easily accessible information on the diagnosis, cause, frequency, clinical patterns, and management of liver injury attributable to prescription and nonprescription medications and selected herbal and dietary supplements (https://www.ncbi.nlm.nih.gov/books/NBK547852/).

Rejection

Immunologic rejection of a transparent organ is currently divided into three clinical forms: acute T cell-mediated rejection (TCMR, formerly acute cellular rejection), acute antibody-mediated rejection (AMR), and chronic rejection (CR). Rejection may occur at any time after transplantation, but most often within the first 5–7 years. Otherwise unexplained elevation of alkaline phosphatase (less commonly AST or ALT) in the right clinical setting should raise concern for rejection. Recent reduction in the dose of immune suppression drugs and low serum levels of immune suppession drugs are addtional risk factors for immunological rejection.

Serum markers of rejection, in addition to liver enzymes, include an elevated absolute eosinophil count in TCMR. Potential biomarkers are being developed. Donor cell-free DNA may be present in blood in response to TCMR, but may also be seen in other causes of liver injury [9]. Other markers under investigation include determination of extracellular vesicles, exosomes, immunophenotyping, cytokine levels, and microRNA panels [9]. At present, neither routine nor novel laboratory tests or assays are accurate enough to make a confident diagnosis of rejection. Liver biopsy remains the most reliable way to establish rejection.

Chronic rejection has a typical serologic profile of sustained elevation of alkaline phosphatase and/ or bilirubin. When competing etiologies, including recurrent disease and biliary tract strictures, do not explain such elevations, chronic rejection should be strongly considered. Liver biopsy is required. Empirical treatment based on blood test results is discouraged.

Recurrent Disease

Recurrence of original disease occurs, most especially alcoholic liver disease, steatotic liver disease, autoimmune hepatitis, primary biliary cholangitis, PSC, hepatitis B, and hepatitis C. The blood test abnormalities will reflect those seen before transplantation. For those with prior primary biliary cholangitis, and autoimmune hepatitis, autoantibodies present before transplant may not disappear even in the absence of recurrent disease. Accordingly, these cannot be used to make a diagnosis of disease recurrence. Liver biopsy is needed in most cases [10]. Ultimately, blood-based testing can suggest but not establish the diagnosis of recurrent autoimmune hepatitis or PBC; a liver biopsy is recommended.

References

1. Carey W. Liver test interpretation- approach to the patient with live disease: a guide to commonly uses liver tests. https://my.clevelandclinic.org/departments/digestive/medical-professionals/hepatology/liver-tests 2021.
2. Carey W. What's the deal with liver enzymes. podcast June 21 2024. https://my.clevelandclinic.org/podcasts/the-medicine-grand-rounders/whats-the-deal-with-liver-enzymes-with-dr-william-carey-md#:~:text=%2DCommon%20drugs%20associated%20with%20cholestatic,captopril%2C%20erythromycin%2C%20and%20azithromycin.&text=Ritika:%20Q9:%20When%20do%20you,have%20also%20gained%20valuable%20insights.
3. Awan RU, Rashid S, Nabeel A, Samant H. Fibrosing cholestatic hepatitis masquerading acute rejection in hepatitis C virus–positive donor liver graft. ACG Case Rep J. 2023;10(5):e01058. Published online 2023 May 24. https://doi.org/10.14309/crj.0000000000001058.
4. Lizaola-Mayo BC, Rodriguez EA. Cytomegalovirus infection after liver transplantation. World J Transplant. 2020;10(7):183–90. Published online 2020 Jul 29. https://doi.org/10.5500/wjt.v10.i7.183.
5. Nijland ML, Kersten MJ, Pals ST, Bemelman FJ, ten Berge IJM. Epstein-Barr virus–positive posttransplant lymphoproliferative disease after solid organ transplantation: pathogenesis, clinical manifestations, diagnosis, and management. Transplant Direct. 2016;2(1):e48. Published online 2015 15. https://doi.org/10.1097/TXD.0000000000000557.

6. Scolarici M, Jorgenson M, Saddler C, Smith J. Fungal infections in liver transplant recipients. J Fungi. 2021;7:524. https://doi.org/10.3390/jof7070524.
7. Senoner T, Breitkopf R, Treml B, Rajsic S. Invasive fungal infections after liver transplantation. J Clin Med. 2023;12(9):3238. Published online 2023 Apr 30. https://doi.org/10.3390/jcm12093238.
8. Krifors A, Ullberg M, Castegren M, Petersson J, Sparrelid E, Hammarström H, Sjölin J, Özenci V, Blennow O. T2Candida assay in the diagnosis of intraabdominal candidiasis: a prospective multicenter study. J Fungi. 2022;16:86. https://doi.org/10.3390/jof8010086.
9. García-Fernández N, Macher HC, Suárez-Artacho G, Gómez-Bravo MÁ, Molinero P, Guerrero JM, Porras-López M, Rubio A. Donor-specific cell-free DNA qPCR quantification as a noninvasive accurate. J Clin Med. 2022;12(1):36.
10. Montano-Loza A, Rodriguez-Peralvuez M, Pageaux G-P, et al. J Hep. 2023;78:1199–215. Montano-Loza AJ, Bhanji RA, Wasilenko S, Mason AL. Systematic review: recurrence of autoimmune liver diseases after liver transplantation. Aliment Pharm Therap, 2016

Immunosuppression and Treatment of Rejection After Liver Transplantation

20

Geoff McCaughan

Prevention of Allograft Rejection (Table 20.1)

A recent International Liver Transplant Society (ILTS) consensus on immunosuppression for the prevention of acute allograft rejection stated that Tacrolimus-based immunosuppression was superior to Cyclosporine-based therapy [1]. Tacrolimus use results in superior combined outcomes of death, re-transplantation, and steroid resistant rejection. In this setting, Tacrolimus is usually used in conjunction with a sliding dose of corticosteroid. In this phase, less allograft rejection is seen if Tacrolimus trough levels are >7 ng/ml.

Delayed introduction of Tacrolimus (usually because of significant early acute kidney injury) combined with either ATG or Basiliximab have, in some studies, resulted in improved renal function with no increase in acute rejection. Additionally, Mycophenolate is often introduced early in these situations. Its use is associated with less allograft rejection than Azathioprine when using a Cyclosporine-based protocol. Recently there has been an increase in the use of prolonged-release Tacrolimus without any change in outcomes. In some studies, Tacrolimus monotherapy has also been reported to be associated with excellent outcomes, although more allograft rejection is observed. Corticosteroid (CS) free protocols have been advocated in the setting of active HCV replication or MAFLD as steroids enhance HCV replication and exacerbate the metabolic syndrome (hypertension, hyperlipidemic, and obesity) posttransplantation. CS free protocols may use Basiliximab and Tacrolimus as induction therapies. Generally, the use of ATG for induction has not been widely adopted, although strongly advocated by some centres.

G. McCaughan (✉)
Royal Prince Alfred Hospital, Centenary Institute, University of Sydney, Sydney, Australia
e-mail: g.mccaughan@centenary.org.au

B. Eghtesad et al. (eds.), *Liver Transplantation*,
https://doi.org/10.1007/978-3-032-07072-2_20

Table 20.1 Induction immunosuppression [2, 1]

Tacrolimus is superior to Cyclosporin reallograft outcomes
Single daily tacrolimus as a slow release preparation shows similar outcomes to twice daily non-slow release medications
Delayed tacrolimus introduction in combination with other agents may reduce acute kidney injury
Corticosteroid-free regimes can safely be used in patients with significant metabolic risk factors.
TOR inhibitors are not recommended in the first month posttransplant.
Induction with ATG or Basilixumab has no additional beneficial outcomes compared with routine tacrolimus regimes

Patterns of Liver Allograft Rejection and Their Treatment

Acute T-Cell-Mediated Rejection (TCMR) [2]

Diagnosis

The timing of acute T-cell-mediated rejection (TCMR) is variable but may occur as early as day five depending on the levels of early immunosuppressive agents. The diagnosis of allograft rejection usually is triggered by increased levels of liver-specific enzymes indicating allograft dysfunction. However, the pattern is not specific to TCMR. The elevation of liver enzymes usually shows a mixed nature with increases in the four classes of serum liver enzymes, i.e., the alkaline phosphatase (ALP), the gamma-glutamyl transferase (GGT), the alanine aminotransferase (ALT), and the aspartate aminotransferase (AST).

The actual diagnosis of TCMR requires *liver biopsy,* which typically demonstrates damage to the interlobular bile ducts, a mixed leucocyte portal infiltrate, and endothelial damage in the form of endotheliitis. Pathological assessment also includes a grading of severity classified as Banff I (mild), Banff II (moderate), and Banff III (severe) depending on the degree of injury to bile ducts, the endothelium, and the level of immune infiltration, which are graded with scores between 0 and 3 for each category. The Rejection Activity Index (RAI) is an aggregate of these three scores, with a cut-off of ≤4 generally considered "mild" rejection.

TCMR is associated with a range of risk factors. These include (1) the level and nature of the immunosuppression, (2) established CMV infection, (3) sex mismatch (when a female donor liver is transplanted into a male, and (4) age of the Recipient. It is generally thought that older recipients have less allograft rejection, although this is not observed in all studies (5) underlying autoimmune conditions. Patients with autoimmune hepatitis are thought to be more susceptible to acute TCMR and develop more severe episodes of the disease (6). Other nonspecific injury to the liver allograft, such as prolonged cold ischemic times and the occurrence of biliary complications, (7) major histocompatibility complex (MHC) mismatch between the donor and the recipient. Although it does not profoundly influence acute TCMR, transplantation of a donor liver into a biologically related recipient following live donation decreases the severity of acute TCMR, (8) the influence of donor-specific antibodies (DSAs), and (9) treatment with immuno-oncology drugs [3, 4].

Although liver biopsy remains the "gold standard for diagnosis attempts to identify biomarkers for acute TCMR such as measuring serum levels of microRNAs, cell-free DNA, various cytokines/chemokines, and bile acids have been undertaken. Currently, however, no biomarker has yet been adopted into clinical practice either to predict rejection at an earlier stage or diagnose it reliably without performing a liver biopsy.

Treatments (Table 20.2)

The classical *treatment* for established moderate-to-severe acute TCMR is a pulse of methylprednisolone (1 g per day) for three successive days. This is a much more effective protocol than a single one-off dose of methylprednisolone. It has, however, been generally accepted that acute mild TCMR can be treated without pulse steroids by adjusting the doses of the calcineurin inhibitor tacrolimus. This cannot be done using cyclosporine-based therapies, as cyclosporine does not seem to be potent enough to reverse ongoing, even mild, acute TCMR.

Treatment is successful in approximately 80–85% of cases, leaving only 15–20% as nonresponders. In such situations, the addition of third-line immunosuppression, if only dual immunosuppression is in place, together with a second pulse of steroids, usually results in resolution. More powerful agents such as anti-thymocyte globulin (ATG) are used if this is unsuccessful. Such approaches are usually successful, leaving only <5% of cases where acute TCMR is not controlled, leading to chronic allograft rejection. In the early years of liver transplantation, the monoclonal anti-CD3 antibody OKT3 was used in this situation. Although OKT3 treatment was very highly successful in reversing severe acute TCMR, it was withdrawn from the market because of its associated toxicity. This was probably a mistake, as it was a very valuable agent in highly selective cases if used by experienced liver transplant physicians and surgeons.

Outcomes

It is well established that in renal, lung, and heart transplantation, mild-to-moderate acute TCMR is associated with the worse outcomes. This was not thought to be the case in liver transplantation. However, more recent studies, including our own, have shown that significant acute rejection was associated with worse patient outcomes and survival post-liver transplantation [5].

Table 20.2 Treatment regimes [2, 1]

High dose pulse corticosteroids are the basis for the treatment of significant ATCMR
Increases in baseline tacrolimus can be used to treat mild ATCMR

Late Acute TCMR

Although early acute TCMR and later episodes of TCMR share a similar pathological diagnosis of T cell rejection, their outcomes appear different [6]. Late acute TCMR occurs generally (by definition) later, within 3- or 6-months posttransplantation, and is associated with much poorer outcomes. It may have an incidence of up to 25%. Late acute TCMR is often associated with delayed recognition because it occurs in the non-hospital patient setting. The longer the duration since transplantation, the less often liver biochemistry and calcineurin inhibitor drug levels are monitored in recipients. Thus, abnormalities are not picked up in a timely fashion compared to daily in-hospital testing. One scenario in which late acute TCMR occurs is during the attempt to eliminate calcineurin inhibitor therapy due to inhibitor-associated renal toxicity. It has been found that replacing calcineurin inhibitor therapy with everolimus or MMF monotherapy is associated with acute TCMR. Additional low-dose corticosteroid therapy is required to prevent such episodes.

Acute Antibody-Mediated Rejection (ABMR)

ABMR is well described in kidney, heart, lung, and pancreas transplants as antibodies directed against MHC antigens in the allograft result in classical microvascular rejection. In liver allografts, it was first recognized in ABO incompatible grafts, but with more sophisticated techniques for the detection and recognition of donor specific antibodies (particularly against MHC class II antigens), rejection caused by donor specific antibodies has been increasingly recognized and characterized in human liver transplantation [7, 8].

Acute ABMR usually occurs within the first several weeks after transplantation. It is often preceded by an episode of ATCMR but may occur in isolation. It is characterized clinically by the rapid onset of allograft dysfunction, often in the presence of fever and particularly high transaminases associated with progressive jaundice. It has now been characterized by several features, and criteria for its diagnosis have been established [7, 8]. These include:

1. A characteristic histological pattern.
2. Detection of donor-specific antibodies (DSAs) usually requiring a Mean Fluorescence Intensity (MFI) titre of >5000.
3. Diffuse C4d microvascular staining on biopsy.
4. The exclusion of other insults, such as hepatic artery thrombosis and bile duct injury.

A recent consensus proposed that all four components are required for the diagnosis [7].

Features of ABMR may occur in conjunction with acute TCMR. However, the additional features that characterize ABMR are portal tract endothelial cell hypertrophy, microvasculitis or capillaritis of portal tract capillaries, and portal tract inlet venules. These structures may contain intraluminal inflammatory cells, including neutrophils and eosinophils.

As mentioned, acute ABMR may occur as a primary pattern of injury, but may also occur following episodes of acute TCMR that have failed to optimally respond to classical anti-T cell therapies.

Discussion of this entity does require an understanding of current DSA data. DSAs may be present before transplant, but unless present in high titre, tend to spontaneously disappear after transplantation. De novo DSAs posttransplant occur in about 15% of recipients and are directed mainly at MHC class II. Both high titre DSA pre- and posttransplant are associated with decreased allograft survival and allograft fibrosis. However, acute ABMR only occurs in about 5% of patients with high-titre DSAs. Thus, the detection of high-titre DSA alone is not sufficient for the diagnosis of acute ABMR. A recent study confirmed that the highest level of both MHC Class 1 and Class 11 DSAs was seen in biopsies that suggested ABMR—so-called Archetype 6 in a series of 490 pairs of biopsies with DSA testing.

Treatments for acute ABMR are not well defined, but most protocols involve plasmapheresis and IVIg as per renal transplant protocols. In a recent nationwide French study, ABMR was diagnosed in only 44 patients over 12-year period [9]. After treatment, usually with a combination of plasmapheresis and IVI Ig, the 5-year allograft survival was less than 50% at 5 years. The proteasome inhibitor Bortezomib has been used to block plasma cell production of antibodies, but the results and its clinical efficacy are not clear. Other therapies include anti-IL-6 and anti-CD38 monoclonal antibodies, compliment inhibitors such as Imlifidase, a recombinant cysteine protease that cleaves human IgG antibodies and complement inhibitors such as Eculizumab. Experimental therapies against plasma cells and B cells such as anti-BAFF and CAR T cells against CD19 are being tested in autoimmune diseases and may eventually find a place in treating ABMR.

Rituximab (an anti-CD20 monoclonal antibody) has a limited role in this setting, while it is effective at depleting B cells, it has no effect on plasma cell production of antibodies in the acute situation. The role of rituximab as secondary preventative therapy following an episode of acute ABMR remains to be defined.

Plasma Cell Hepatitis/Plasma-Cell Rich Allograft Rejection [10]

This pattern of allograft injury has been previously named "de novo autoimmune hepatitis". It is now increasingly recognized as a form of allograft rejection. Its timing usually occurs later than acute TCMR (>6 months posttransplant). Biochemical findings are similar to acute TCMR, although in some cases, liver transaminases may be quite high. However, the biopsy features are characteristic, with high levels of plasma cells in the portal tract inflammatory infiltrate (>30%). Interestingly, it has been shown that the infiltrate may be enriched in IgG4-positive plasma cells. Features of acute TCMR such as interlobular bile duct damage or portal endotheliitis are not usually present, although centrizonal perivenulitis may occur.

In over 50% of cases, patients have high-level detectable auto-antibodies, antinuclear antibodies (ANA), smooth muscle antibodies (SMA), liver-kidney microsomal antibodies (LKMA), or sometimes anti-glutathione-S-transferase (GST) antibodies. Hypergammaglobulinemia including non-subclass-specific increased serum IgG levels may be present. The pattern may not respond as well to immunosuppressive therapy and can be associated with allograft loss. Treatments similar to those used in ABMR are likely to be considered in the future.

Chronic Ductopenic Allograft Rejection [11, 12]

This occurs months to years after liver transplantation. Persistent allograft rejection responses are aimed at the endothelium and biliary cells of the allograft. Classic liver biochemistry reflects biliary damage and is usually cholestatic in nature (raised ALP and GGT) with jaundice and hyperbilirubinemia in severe cases. Progressive ductal atrophy and ductopenia develop, usually in the presence of failed high-dose immunosuppression. In severe cases, interlobular bile duct loss is often associated with portal fibrosis and a diminished immune infiltrate as the immune targets are no longer present. There is often evidence of lobular ischemia with centrizonal hepatocyte cell loss reflecting arteritis in the vasculature, although overt arterial vascular changes are only rarely seen in liver biopsies. However, when explants of such cases are examined, widespread features of vascular rejection are seen. Unlike heart and lung transplantation and kidney transplantation, chronic allograft rejection resulting in allograft loss is thought to occur in less than 10% of human allografts. There are also rare reported cases of reversal of ductopenia with regrowth of interlobular bile ducts.

Chronic ABMR [7]

The role of ABMR events in the evolution of chronic rejection remains under investigation. The Banff working party suggested that chronic ABMR should be considered when the following are present:

1. The presence of an unexplained portal tract infiltrate with interface hepatitis or perivenular changes.
2. Some portal or perivenular fibrosis.
3. High titre DSAs.
4. Focal C4d microvascular staining.
5. Exclusion of other pathologies.

Idiopathic Chronic Hepatitis [13, 14, 15]

This is also thought to be an unusual form of chronic allograft rejection. It is best described in long-term (>10 years survivors) pediatric recipients undergoing protocol biopsies, although it has been described in adults. The liver biochemistry is usually unremarkable and can be normal. The liver biopsy shows features of a lymphocytic-rich portal tract infiltrate with varying levels of interface hepatitis and fibrosis, including cirrhosis. Transcriptional analysis of such biopsies indicates that when lymphocytic infiltrates are seen, these correlate with acute TCMR profiles, suggesting that these patients may be suffering from subclinical rejection. In contrast, biopsies exhibiting purely fibrosis only have upregulation of fibrosis genes [16]. Idiopathic chronic hepatitis usually occurs in patients on low-level non-tacrolimus-based immunosuppression. The natural history is variable but may be associated with progressive fibrosis in 30% of cases. Severity and staging have been proposed by a 2022 Banff liver group meeting. The response to increases in calcineurin doses and low-dose corticosteroids is unclear.

Other Long-Term Changes in Human Liver Allografts [11]

This was addressed in a 2022 Banff liver group meeting. Apart from long-term fibrosis in patients with idiopathic chronic hepatitis, portal vascular changes with parenchymal micronodular remodeling have been observed. The latter refers to areas in the liver parenchyma that involve areas of lobular atrophy with adjacent sublobular hypertrophy. These changes resemble nodular regenerative hyperplasia described in the nontransplant setting. Whether this is a form of chronic allograft rejection remains unclear and is under further study.

Operational Tolerance [17, 18]

There have been several reports indicating that immunosuppressive therapy can be successfully withdrawn from a subset of adult and pediatric liver transplant recipients. From the time of transplantation, this happens in less than 5% of cases. However, in patients who are already on minimal immunosuppression, successful withdrawal can be achieved between 20% and 40% of recipients. The major feature that predicts operational tolerance is the period from the time of liver transplantation itself, along with the period associated with established minimum immunosuppression.

If withdrawal of immunosuppression is done in a proactive manner, then it is highly recommended that a liver biopsy be performed. Successful operational tolerance patients should have a normal liver biopsy with only minor portal tract immune infiltrates, no evidence of interface hepatitis, no bile duct or endothelial changes, and no fibrosis. Liver biochemistry should be normal with no detectable DSAs. There have been various molecular signatures within the allograft and peripheral blood that are thought to be associated with operational tolerance. However, none of these are yet to be used routinely in clinical practice.

References

1. De Martin E, Londoño MC, Emamaullee J, Lerut J, Potts J, Aluvihare V, Spiro M, Raptis DA, G MC, ERAS4OLT. org Working Group, Niemann C. The optimal immunosuppression management to prevent early rejection after liver transplantation: a systematic review of the literature and expert panel recommendations. Clin Transpl. 2022;36(10):e14614.
2. Choudhary NS, Saigal S, Bansal RK, Saraf N, Gautam D, Soin AS. Acute and chronic rejection after liver transplantation: what a clinician needs to know. J Clin Exp Hepatol. 2017;7(4):358–66.
3. Lee BT, Horwich BH, Chopra S, Ahearn A, Han HH. Checkpoint inhibitor-induced rejection of a liver allograft: a combination of acute T cell-mediated and antibody-mediated rejection. Liver Transpl. 2019; https://doi.org/10.1002/lt.25622.
4. Nordness MF, Hamel S, Godfrey CM, Shi C, Johnson DB, Goff LW, O'Dell H, et al. Fatal hepatic necrosis after Nivolumab as a bridge to liver transplant for HCC—are checkpoint inhibitors safe for the pre-transplant patient? Am J Transplant. 2020; https://doi.org/10.1111/ajt.15617.
5. Levitsky J, Goldberg D, Smith AR, Mansfield SA, Gillespie BW, Merion RM, Lok AS, et al. Acute rejection increases risk of graft failure and death in recent liver transplant recipients. Clin Gastroenterol Hepatol. 2017;15(4):584–593.e2.
6. Nacif LS, Pinheiro RS, Pécora RA, Ducatti L, Rocha-Santos V, Andraus W, D'Albuquerque LC. Late acute rejection in liver transplant: a systematic review. Arq Bras Cir Dig. 2015;28(3):212–5.
7. Demetris AJ, Bellamy C, Hübscher SG, O'Leary J, Randhawa PS, Feng S, Neil D, et al. 2016 comprehensive update of the Banff working group on liver allograft pathology: introduction of antibody-mediated rejection. Am J Transplant. 2016;16(10):2816–35.
8. Demetris AJ, Zeevi A, O'Leary JG. ABO-compatible liver allograft antibody-mediated rejection: an update. Curr Opin Organ Transplant. 2015;20(3):314–24.
9. Dumortier J, Conti F, Hiriart JB, Dharancy S, Duvoux C, Besch C, Houssel-Debry P, Latournerie M, Chermak F, Meszaros M, Pageaux GP. Treatment of donor-specific anti-HLA antibodies-mediated rejection after liver transplantation: a French nationwide retrospective study. Liver Transpl. 2023;29(12):1313–22.
10. Fiel MI, Schiano TD. Plasma cell hepatitis (de-novo autoimmune hepatitis) developing post liver transplantation. Curr Opin Organ Transplant. 2012;17(3):287–92.
11. Bellamy CO, O'Leary JG, Adeyi O, Baddour N, Batal I, Bucuvalas J, Del Bello A, El Hag M, El-Monayeri M, Farris AB III, Feng S. Banff 2022 liver group meeting report: monitoring long term allograft health. Am J Transplant. 2024;24:905.
12. Demir Z, Raynaud M, Aubert O, Debray D, Sebach M, et al. Identification of liver transplant biopsy phenotypes associated with distant liver biological markers and allograft survival. Am J Transpl. 2024;24:954–66.
13. Evans HM, Kelly DA, McKiernan PJ, Hübscher S. Progressive histological damage in liver allografts following pediatric liver transplantation. Hepatology. 2006;43(5):1109–17.
14. Feng S, Bucuvalas JC, Demetris AJ, Burrell BE, Spain KM, Kanaparthi S, Magee JC, et al. Evidence of chronic allograft injury in liver biopsies from long-term pediatric recipients of liver transplants. Gastroenterology. 2018;155(6):1838–1851.e7.
15. Sebagh M, Coilly A, Haïm-Boukobzsa S, Allard M-A, Ballot E, Cunha AS, Roche B, et al. Idiopathic post liver-transplant hepatitis remains obscure with respect to its etiology and relationship with immunosuppressiona. J Gastroenterol Hepatol Res. 2015;4(11):1850–7.

16. Londoño MC, Souza LN, Lozano JJ, Miquel R, Abraldes JG, Llovet LP, Quaglia A, et al. Molecular profiling of subclinical inflammatory lesions in long-term surviving adult liver transplant recipients. J Hepatol. 2018;69(3):626–34.
17. Levitsky J, Feng S. Tolerance in clinical liver transplantation. Hum Immunol. 2018;79(5):283–7.
18. Vionnet J, Sánchez-Fueyo A. Biomarkers of immune tolerance in liver transplantation. Hum Immunol. 2018;79(5):388–94.

The Role of the Clinical Transplant Coordinator in Liver Transplantation

21

Stacy Acevedo and Sandra Chicko

The clinical transplant coordinator plays an essential role in facilitating the transplant process and is the linchpin between the patient, referring physician, and the transplant team. This role is dynamic and evolves as the field changes. There are many roles within the transplant center for a transplant coordinator—pre-transplant, wait-list, post-transplant, and living donation. As the patient progresses through different phases of this process, they will be assigned different coordinators [1–3].

Pre-transplant Coordinator Responsibilities

Coordinate the referral intake.
Facilitate fiscal clearance.
Order and schedule pre-transplant testing.
Collect and interpret test results.
Prepare the patient's file for presentation at the selection committee meeting.
Notify the patient of the selection committee's decision [3, 4].

Wait-List Coordinator Responsibilities

List candidates per the Organ Procurement Transplant Network (OPTN) policy.

S. Acevedo
University of Pittsburgh Medical Center, Pittsburgh, PA, USA
e-mail: acevedosl2@upmc.edu

S. Chicko (✉)
University of Pittsburgh, Thomas E. Starzl Transplantation Institute, Pittsburgh, PA, USA
e-mail: sas75@pitt.edu

B. Eghtesad et al. (eds.), *Liver Transplantation*,
https://doi.org/10.1007/978-3-032-07072-2_21

Collaborate with the patient that all testing is ordered and updated and keep them "ready" for transplant.
Maintain listing status per OPTN policies [4].

Post-transplant Coordinator Responsibilities

Review and analyze lab and test results.
Schedule clinic visits.
Order medication refills.
Verify compliance with medications and prescribed routine [3, 4].

Living Donor Coordinator Responsibilities [5]

Order and schedule pre-evaluation testing on potential donor candidates who are approved and accepted donors.
Notify donor of Selection Committee outcome.
Order and schedule pre-transplant testing on approved and accepted donors.
Consistent surveillance of each donor.
Notify donors when updated testing is required.
Schedule surgery and initiate pre-transplant education and bloodwork.
Follow-up for 2 years.

Referral

Once the patient has an established or suspected diagnosis of liver disease, the physician will make a referral to a transplant center. The acuity and urgency of the patient's medical condition dictates when the patient will be seen.

In certain circumstances, a patient with acute failure will need to be transferred to the transplant center immediately. The referring physician will communicate with the transplant team to determine if a transfer is possible. This transfer will be facilitated by the CTC. An indication for immediate transfer could be determined utilizing the Model for End-Stage Liver Disease (MELD)*. This is a calculated formula used to assign priority to liver transplant candidates. This number is indicative of urgency but needs to be correlated with the current clinical picture to assist in determining the need for priority transfer. It should be noted that patients are often "sicker" than their calculated MELD score. Medical and fiscal acceptance must be done concurrently before the transfer can be initiated [6].

*MELD Score Components

- Serum bilirubin.

- INR.
- Serum creatinine.
- Serum sodium.

*A patient's MELD score may range from 6 to 40. The higher the score, the more severe the liver disease.

A routine evaluation may be considered when the patient has documented liver disease but is clinically stable. The attending physician/hepatologist/gastroenterologist will contact the transplant center by phone or by submitting an electronic referral. The CTC will notify the patient of the referral and determine when and where the patient can be seen.

There may be options to be evaluated at the transplant center or at an outreach clinic. Both outpatient transplant center and outreach evaluations are usually 2–3 days in duration. Many transplant centers offer outreach programs where the transplant hepatologist and the transplant coordinator travel to an out-of-town location. This greatly benefits the patient while providing specialty care in their local area. Since most individuals search the internet or turn to social media for information, tech-savvy patients will occasionally self-refer to the transplant center [5].

The Transplant Evaluation

Following fiscal clearance, the appointment for a transplant evaluation will be scheduled and the CTC will call the patient to introduce themselves, explain what to expect at their visit and answer any questions the patient may have. The CTC will review the medical records to determine what testing will be required for the evaluation and initiate the complex scheduling for each patient.

The transplant education process begins here with an initial introduction about the living donor option, which the patient will learn more about during their evaluation. It also outlines education about a lifetime commitment to a medication regimen. Another important aspect that the patient is made aware of is the identification of a designated caregiver. A designated caregiver is considered mandatory, and the patient cannot be listed without one. Caregivers play an important role as the "patient's personal attache" and will act on behalf of the patient and help to assure compliance and adherence to the post-transplant process.

It is usually at this juncture that the patient is working to accept liver transplantation as a likely reality rather than a vague concept. They have many concerns about how it will impact their personal life, their family, work, finances, and long-term health.[1] The CTC will help by guiding them through the transplant education process and by making a referral for psychosocial counseling [5, 6].

[1] Kiran Bambha, MD "Exploring the Human Side of Liver Transplant Journeys: Qualitative Insights into Patient Experiences" Lecture at the Thomas E. Starzl Transplantation Grand Rounds, UPMC, Pittsburgh, PA. 29 January 2025.

Required Testing

Day One Lab draw (fasting), transplant education, transplant hepatologist visit, TeleMedicine visit. If the visit is an outreach visit, the patient is directly connected to the transplant center personnel via TeleMedicine and each visit is 30 min long. If the visit is at a transplant center, the patient and family will meet in person with each member of the transplant team which includes transplant hepatologist, transplant surgeon, transplant coordinator, transplant social worker, fiscal, behavioral health, nutritionist, pharmacist, and anesthesia [5].

Day Two-Three CXR, ECHO, EKG, CT imaging, ultrasound, MRI, Stress test, pulmonary function, and frailty testing.

In addition to transplant testing, all cancer screenings must be up to date, within normal limits, and documented in the patient's medical record. These include age and gender-specific PAP smear, colonoscopy, and mammogram.

Live Donor Liver Transplantation Discussion and Option

In centers that perform live donor transplantation, the transplant surgeon or the transplant hepatologist will initiate the conversation about living donor liver transplantation with the patient and family members at the initial evaluation visit. After the topic is initially discussed, the CTC assumes primary responsibility for operationalizing the process with the candidate. However, the interested donor must make the initial contact to express their wish to be considered before the transplant center can contact them. Any donors who are identified will be evaluated and worked up by the living donor transplant team. This is a completely separate team from the liver transplant candidate team, and information is kept confidential and is never shared between teams.

Educating the patient and family about the option for living donor liver transplantation is an important and serious consideration. The CTC is well prepared to discuss all aspects of live donation. Who can be a donor is one of the most frequently asked questions. A donor could be a family member, spouse, friend, coworker, or anonymous person. The donor must be healthy, willing to donate, and meet the strict criteria of the living donor team. Another frequently asked question is how to find a donor. Creating social media pages, billboards, signs at large events, or religious organization bulletins are a few ways to bring attention to the need for a donor. In many instances, the CTC will recommend that the family find a volunteer who will be the patient's living donor champion. The Living Donor Champion is someone who is designated by the patient to publicize their need for the gift of life [5].

The advantages of a living donor transplant are shortened waiting times, a planned surgery so that the person waiting for the liver transplant is in the best state of health, quicker recovery times, less warm ischemia time and reduces the number of deaths on the transplant wait-list.

The pre-transplant coordinator (PTC) is responsible for reviewing and compiling all test results. Once all testing is completed, reviewed by the transplant team, and presented at the Transplant Selection Committee meeting, patients will be notified by the PTC of their acceptance, denial, or need for further testing.

Selections Outcomes

Acceptance

If the patient is accepted, they will be listed as active or inactive. If the patient is activated, the PTC will list the patient in the UNOS portal and they will begin accruing wait time. If they are accepted but are inactive, the patient will still accrue wait time until they are activated. Once the patient is activated on the transplant list, they will be required to maintain their insurance coverage and call the CTC with any changes in their caregiver, medical condition, or insurance status.

Denial

A patient may be denied if the patient is too well at the time of evaluation, if there is a lack of social support, recent or active substance use, non-hepatic co-morbidities, advanced age, or is too sick in the setting of advanced liver disease.[2] Patients who require rehabilitation for substance use and adhere to compliance in certain circumstances may be reconsidered. In most situations, the CTC, who has developed a rapport with the patient, is responsible for informing the patient of the committee's decision not to move forward with the transplant. This difficult conversation not only requires transparency but also needs to be delivered with empathy and sensitivity.

The wait-list transplant coordinator (WLTC) will collaborate with the referring hepatologist/gastroenterologist/local medical provider during this phase of the transplant evaluation. The WLTC will provide the transplant candidate with a schedule of testing that is required to remain active on the transplant waiting list. The transplant candidate is expected to remain current with testing in conjunction with their local medical provider. To achieve this, the patient can be seen by their local medical provider or via a TeleMedicine visit with the transplant center. Compliance with routine screening is imperative. This is generally the testing that will be required by the transplant center: bloodwork, cardiac testing, imaging, tumor markers, vaccinations, and HLA for tissue matching. Communication to the transplant

[2] Kiran Bambha, MD "Exploring the Human Side of Liver Transplant Journeys: Qualitative Insights into Patient Experiences" Lecture at the Thomas E. Starzl Transplantation Grand Rounds, UPMC, Pittsburgh, PA. 29 January 2025.

center should include updates about appointments with all specialists, any change in their caregiver status, recent hospitalizations or procedures, and any current illness. This not only impacts the candidate's wait-list status but is an indication of how compliant the patient may be following transplantation.

Ongoing patient education is centered around knowing the signs and symptoms of worsening liver disease. Patients should be advised to always carry, charge, and answer their cell phones. Patients are alerted that organ offers can occur at any time.

Deferred Status

This indicates the candidate is in need of additional testing. The WLTC is responsible for informing the patient of what is required and assisting with scheduling the specific tests.

How the Allocation Process Works

The OPTN is notified of an available organ and will look at specific criteria to implement the match. The patient's MELD score*, blood type, geographic proximity, and donor and recipient size are considered.

Liver Transplantation: The Procedure

Once an organ is matched, the CTC will call the patient and complete a brief prescreen assessment. If the assessment is negative, the patient will be asked to come to the transplant center with their designated caregiver. The patient will be admitted to the transplant service, and the pre-operative prep will begin. The surgery and hospital stay vary for each patient.

After Discharge

The role of the post-transplant coordinator in the post-operative period focuses on rejection, infection, compliance with medications, post-op lab work, and clinic visits, as well as addressing ongoing medical or surgical issues. Each transplant center has a protocol for the amount of time that the patient is required to stay in the vicinity of the transplant center for postoperative outpatient care [2, 3].

The Transition to Home

Establishing care with the local medical provider should begin as soon as the patient is discharged. The post-transplant coordinator will form a partnership with the local medical provider to monitor the lab work and frequency, schedule clinic visits, interval follow-up visits, protocol biopsies (which may be center-specific), adjust medications, and spell out immunosuppression specifics. The patient has the responsibility to inform the transplant program with any changes in his/her general health and medication issues and coverage (Table 21.1) [2–4].

The clinical transplant coordinator will remain involved in every aspect of the patient's care from referral through the post-transplant period. In the complex environment of the liver transplant process, the clinical transplant coordinator is a vital contact and can provide guidance and support to both the patient and the referring physician.

Table 21.1 When the patient should call the transplant coordinator

Fever of 100.4 or greater
Vomiting or diarrhea
Forgot to take their medication
New medications are prescribed by a local medical provider
Immunosuppression medication refills
Insurance change or loss
Wound issues
If they are admitted to their local hospital

Acknowledgement The authors thank Karen Emmett, BSN, RN, CCTN, for reviewing our manuscript.

References

1. Heyl AE, Staschak SM, Folk PG, Fioravanti V. The patient coordinator in a liver transplant program. Gastroenterol Clin N Am. 1988;17(1):195–206.
2. Cupples SA, Ohler L. Transplantation nursing secrets. Philadelphia, PA: Hanley & Belfus, Inc; 2003.
3. Cupples SA, Lerret S, McCalmont V, Ohler L. Core curriculum for transplant nurses. 2nd ed. Philadelphia, PA: Lippincott, Williams & Wilkins; 2016.
4. Staschak S, Zamberlan K. Liver transplantation: nursing diagnosis and management. In: Haggerty L, Sigurdson-Poor K, editors. Nursing care of the transplant recipient. Philadelphia, PA: W.B. Saunders; 1990.: Chapter 7. p. 140–79.
5. Busuttil RW, Klintmalm GBG. Transplantation of the liver. 3rd ed. Philadelphia, PA: Elsevier Saunders; 2015.
6. Makowka L, Sher L, Kahn D, Tzakis AG, Todo S, Marsh JW, Stieber A, Koneru B, Klintmalm GBG, Staschak S, Gordon RD, Van Thiel DH, Starzl TE. Which liver disease patients need a transplant? Diagnosi. 1988;10(6):62–79.

Post-transplant Liver Pathology

22

Nigar Anjuman Khurram

Introduction

Changing Trends in Liver Transplantation

Liver transplantation has undergone significant evolution since its inception, driven by advancements in surgical techniques, immunosuppression, and patient management. Shifts in donor utilization, indications for transplantation, and technological innovations have redefined the field. The introduction of direct-acting antivirals has drastically reduced the need for liver transplantation due to hepatitis C virus-related cirrhosis and hepatocellular carcinoma, transforming the disease into a manageable condition. Non-alcoholic steatohepatitis [1] has emerged as a leading indication for liver transplantation, driven by global obesity and diabetes epidemics, while liver transplants for alcohol-associated liver disease have risen due to changing societal attitudes and expanded eligibility criteria. Living donor liver transplantation has become increasingly utilized, offering a solution to organ shortages with advances in surgical techniques and donor safety protocols. Organs from older donors, those with comorbidities, or marginal grafts are now utilized, supported by improved preservation and perfusion techniques. Donation after circulatory death has contributed significantly to the organ pool, with challenges such as ischemia-reperfusion injury mitigated through normothermic machine perfusion to enhance graft viability.

Ex situ perfusion technologies [2–6] allow for enhanced graft assessment and reconditioning of marginal livers, improving utilization rates and outcomes. Research on bioartificial livers and tissue engineering is advancing, offering potential future alternatives to traditional transplantation. Advances in genomics enable

N. A. Khurram (✉)
University of Pittsburgh, Department of Pathology at the Thomas Starzl Institute of Transplantation, Pittsburgh, PA, USA
e-mail: khurramna@upmc.edu

B. Eghtesad et al. (eds.), *Liver Transplantation*,
https://doi.org/10.1007/978-3-032-07072-2_22

tailored immunosuppression protocols, improving graft survival and patient outcomes while facilitating donor-recipient matching. Efforts to reduce lifelong immunosuppressive burdens focus on minimizing complications such as infections, malignancies, and metabolic disorders, with trials exploring immune tolerance induction showing promise [7–9]. Advances in desensitization protocols and immunosuppression have increased the feasibility of ABO-incompatible liver transplantation, particularly in pediatric and living donor settings. Revisions to allocation policies, such as MELD score prioritization, aim to reduce disparities and improve equity in access to liver transplantation. Access to liver transplantation varies significantly across regions, with financial, infrastructural, and cultural barriers limiting availability in low- and middle-income countries. Expanding donor criteria and living donor programs raise ethical concerns about donor risk and equitable organ allocation, requiring robust oversight. Liver transplantation is advancing through innovations in technology, changing epidemiology of liver diseases, and novel donor utilization strategies. Continued efforts to optimize outcomes, address disparities, and expand access are essential to meet the growing demand for transplantation. The material in this chapter is based on multiple previous publications and book chapters from our group. Therefore, redundancy is difficult to avoid [10–15].

Post-transplant Complications

Pathological complications following liver transplantation encompass a broad spectrum of issues that significantly affect graft and patient outcomes. Early complications include ischemia-reperfusion injury and liver allograft rejection. Recurrent or de novo diseases further complicate outcomes. Hepatitis B and C can recur despite antiviral therapies, while lifestyle and metabolic factors contribute to the redevelopment of MASH and alcohol-related liver disease. Immunosuppression increases the risk of de novo malignancies, such as post-transplant lymphoproliferative disorders, and recurrent hepatocellular carcinoma remains a challenge. Infections due to lifelong immunosuppression vary by post-transplant timing, with opportunistic infections (e.g., cytomegalovirus and fungi) predominant early and community-acquired infections later. Metabolic complications, including diabetes, hyperlipidemia, and obesity, arise due to immunosuppressive therapies, requiring meticulous management. Vascular issues, such as hepatic artery thrombosis and portal vein stenosis, pose severe risks to graft survival, necessitating prompt diagnosis and intervention.

Histopathological Diagnosis of Allograft Dysfunction

Evaluation of the Explanted Liver

The liver transplant operation/surgical intervention and factors contributing to allograft dysfunction: The liver transplantation is a complex process, and accurate biopsy interpretation requires a detailed understanding of the donor and recipient operational procedures, basic transplant immunology, immunosuppression management, and technical complications. This is because many insults that contribute to allograft dysfunction can be traced back to agonal events in the donor and surgical complications. Hence, it's important for a pathologist to recognize and understand the criteria for selection for donors and recipients, indications for transplant, different surgical operations available for liver transplantation in different settings, and newer technologies to assess or improve graft function [16]. Interpretation of post-transplant liver biopsies can be exceptionally challenging. The morphological patterns are often atypical and may reflect multiple simultaneous etiologies, including de novo disease, recurrent primary pathology, drug-related injury, infections, or the effects of immunosuppression. Accurate diagnosis of allograft dysfunction requires not only expert histopathologic evaluation but also a thorough clinicopathologic correlation and a detailed understanding of the temporal context of the biopsy—whether it represents the early, intermediate, or late post-transplant period. These factors, together with knowledge of the surgical procedure, perioperative events, and evolving immunologic milieu, are essential for distinguishing overlapping entities such as rejection, biliary complications, ischemic injury, and recurrent or de novo hepatobiliary diseases.

Timing of Causes of Dysfunction: The spectrum of diseases and processes encountered in the liver allograft is broad and transcends non-transplant-related and post-transplant-related pathology [17]. The presence of graft dysfunction is typically identified on routine liver tests, but the identification of the specific cause often requires knowledge of the original disease, time after transplantation, and liver injury test profile. Traditionally, post-transplant pathology has been divided anatomically or as to early or late occurrence in the post-transplant period (Table 22.1). Needless to say, these are complicated patients and two or more clinicopathological processes may co-exist. Therefore, a thorough clinicopathological evaluation should be carried out before a final histopathological diagnosis is given.

Handling of the Explanted Liver (Recipient's Liver): The gross examination of explant or native hepatectomy specimens is a critical component of post-transplant liver pathology. Ideally, the liver should be sliced at intervals of 1.0 cm or less to ensure adequate sampling and to minimize the risk of missing focal or subtle lesions (Figs. 22.1 and 22.2). This approach prevents the possibility of missing the lesions if present in the explant specimen. Before slicing, it is advisable to correlate with the radiological findings to make sure no lesions are missed. The examination of explant liver is crucial in many ways (1). It confirms histological or radiographic diagnoses that have been made previously (2). It can identify incidental masses not recognized on imaging studies (3). Presence of low-grade biliary dysplasia (BilIN) in end-stage livers even those without biliary diseases such as viral or alcoholic hepatitis (4). It helps unmask the etiology in certain cases of cryptogenic cirrhosis (5). It helps grade efficacy of the pre-transplant treatment. Prior to sectioning, cor-

Table 22.1 Liver transplant complications per expected time of occurrence after surgery (complication in bold indicates most likely time of occurrence)

	0–1 months	1–12 months	>12 months
Vascular complications	Hepatic artery thrombosis (HAT) Portal vein thrombosis (PVT)	*Hepatic artery stenosis (HAS)* HAT PVT PVS	Hepatic vein stenosis Portal vein stenosis (PVS) HAT PVT HAS
Biliary complications	Bile leak	Biliary stricture Biliary sludge and casts	Biliary stones and casts Biliary stricture
Parenchymal complications	Post-op collection (hematoma, seroma) Acute rejection	PTLD Recurrent HCC Rejection	Recurrent HCC Recurrence of primary liver disease Chronic rejection

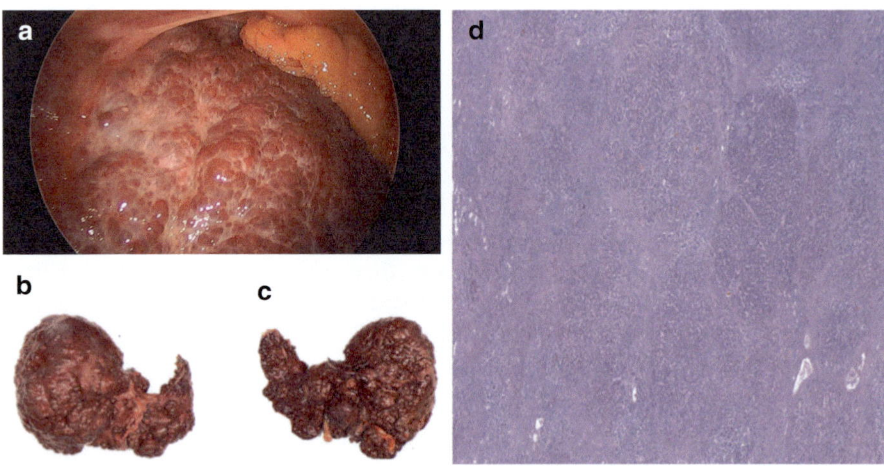

Fig. 22.1 Endoscopic, gross and microscopic evaluation of an explanted liver. (**a**) The endoscopic image of the liver shows nodular surface indicative of end stage cirrhosis secondary to primary biliary cholangitis. (Image provided by Dr. David Geller UPMC). (**b**, **c**) The image is of a cirrhotic liver with micronodules and macro-nodules which is received for further processing in the pathology lab. (**d**) Micronodular cirrhosis with cholestasis and minimal steatosis (H&E, 10X)

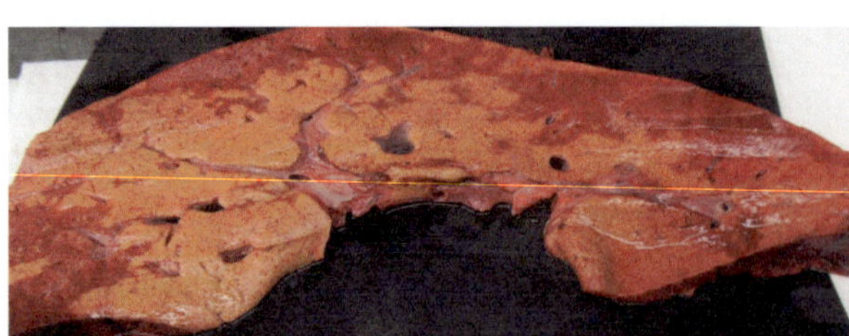

Fig. 22.2 Gross sampling of the hepatectomy specimen. Thin slice of a hepatectomy specimen from a 50-year-old donor which failed due to primary non function of the allograft

relation with preoperative imaging findings is strongly recommended to guide targeted sampling of radiologically identified abnormalities. A meticulous gross and histologic assessment of the explant provides valuable diagnostic and prognostic information. It confirms or refines pre-transplant histologic and radiographic diagnoses, identifies incidental lesions that may have been undetected on imaging, and can uncover biliary intraepithelial neoplasia (BilIN), even in end-stage livers without primary biliary disease such as viral or alcoholic hepatitis. Moreover, explant examination frequently clarifies the etiology in cases previously labeled as cryptogenic cirrhosis and provides an opportunity to assess the efficacy of pre-transplant therapies, including antiviral or oncologic treatment. Together, these insights not only enhance clinicopathologic correlation but also inform post-transplant management and prognostication.

Post-transplant Biopsies

Post-transplant liver biopsy is an essential tool for (1) allograft monitoring, (2) determining the main cause of graft dysfunction in cases of dual pathology (Fig. 22.3), (3) understanding the therapeutic implications, (4) to document the immunological and/or architectural status to help guide chronic IS therapy [18], and (5) assessing the progression of disease to determine the type and timing of intervention.

Tissue triage therefore depends on the reason for biopsy, clinical differential diagnosis, and time after transplantation. Most diagnostically important histopathological stains can be completed on routinely processed, formalin-fixed, paraffin-embedded sections. A clinical differential that includes antibody-mediated rejection (AMR) optimally should include fresh frozen tissue for immunofluorescent staining for immunoglobulin and complement, but less sensitive formalin-fixed paraffin-embedded samples can also be used for C4d staining [19, 20]. For each biopsy, we routinely prepare two H&E-stained slides, each containing two to four step sections, and trichrome, C4d, and CK7 stains. The cytokeratin 7 is used to help localize bile ducts and ductular metaplasia of periportal hepatocytes in cases with suspected cholangiopathic insults. Post-transplant allograft evaluation should include knowledge of the original disease, ABO compatibility, DSA status and related alloantibody information (e.g., C1q activity), time after transplantation, and type of transplant (e.g., standard whole organ deceased, DCD livers, reduced-size deceased, living related). These variables influence the susceptibility to specific complications and consequently affect the histopathological differential diagnosis. A clinical differential diagnosis can also be very helpful in directing the histopathological workup.

Allograft Rejection

Rejection can be simply defined as an immunologic reaction to foreign tissue or organ, which can lead to graft dysfunction and failure if severe [21–23]. In solid organ allografts, rejection has been broadly classified as follows:

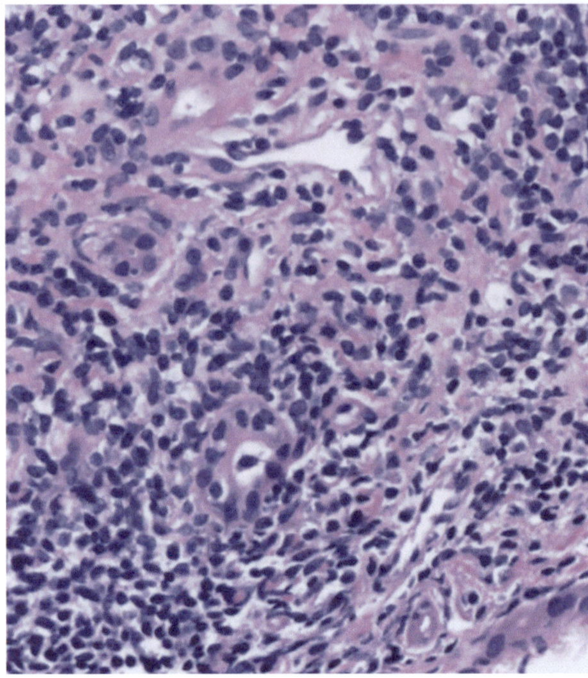

Fig. 22.3 Active T-cell–mediated rejection (TCMR), liver allograft (H&E, ×400). There is dense portal lymphocytic inflammation with extension into the periportal parenchyma (interface activity) and infiltration of bile ducts by activated lymphocytes causing epithelial injury (ductitis). Endothelialitis involving portal venules is also present, characterized by lymphocytes beneath lifting the endothelium. These features are diagnostic of active TCMR according to Banff criteria

hyperacute TCMR, which occurs immediately due to the presence of preformed antibodies; acute TCMR, which develops quickly over a few days; and chronic rejection, which develops gradually over time. Based on predominant pathophysiological mechanisms, rejection can also be classified as antibody-mediated rejection (AMR), T-cell-mediated rejection (TCMR), mixed AMR and TCMR, and chronic rejection (CR), which also often shows a mixed pattern of antibody and T cell-mediated injury. The Banff working group has advised terminology changes in recent years and has advised to prefer the use of the term T-cell-mediated rejection (TCMR) instead of acute cellular rejection (ACR), plasma cell-rich rejection (PCR) for de novo AIH and plasma cell hepatitis (PCH), and antibody-mediated rejection (AMR) for humoral rejection. It is also clear now that many cases that were previously labeled as idiopathic post-transplantation hepatitis occurring late after orthoptic LT (OLT) can now be categorized as late-onset TCMR and/or chronic AMR [24] and chronic hepatitis of unknown cause (hepatitis E) [25–28] (Table 22.2).

T-Cell-Mediated Rejection

TCMR has been defined as "inflammation of the allograft, elicited by a genetic disparity between the donor and recipient, primarily affecting interlobular bile ducts and vascular endothelia, including portal and hepatic veins and occasionally the hepatic artery and its branches" [29]. The Banff Working Group now

Table 22.2 Old versus new Banff recommended terminology

Older terminology	Newer suggested terminology
Acute cellular rejection	T cell–mediated rejection
Humoral rejection	Antibody-mediated rejection
De novo autoimmune or plasma cell-rich hepatitis	Plasma cell–rich rejection
Idiopathic posttransplant hepatitis	More specific terminology when possible Late-onset TCMR Chronic active AMR Chronic hepatitis of known cause (e.g., hepatitis E)

Modified from Demetris et al. [12]

recognizes that TCMR can occur early (within 6 months), likely secondary to direct alloantigen presentation, or late (>6 months), likely secondary to indirect alloantigen presentation [12].

TCMR is characterized histopathologically by (1) predominantly mononuclear but mixed portal inflammation containing blastic or activated lymphocytes, neutrophils, and eosinophils; (2) subendothelial inflammation of portal and/or terminal hepatic venules; and (3) bile duct inflammation and damage [23, 30]. *Minimal diagnostic criteria needed to establish the diagnosis of TCMR include at least two of these histopathological findings.* The diagnosis is strengthened if greater than 50% of the ducts or terminal hepatic veins are damaged or if unequivocal endotheliitis of portal or terminal hepatic vein branches can be identified. Histopathological evidence of severe injury, which is used for histopathological grading, includes perivenular inflammation, centrilobular necrosis, arteritis, and inflammatory, usually central-to-central, bridging inflammation/necrosis (Fig. 22.4a).

Late-onset T-cell-mediated rejection is a form of T-cell-mediated rejection (TCMR) usually occurring 1, 3, or 6 months after transplantation; however, mostly believed to present after 6 weeks of transplantation [31] and leads to worse patient and graft survival after liver transplantation [32]. Histopathological changes include a predominantly mononuclear portal inflammatory infiltrate (contrasting with the mixed population of cells seen in early biopsies), less inflammation of the bile ducts and portal venules, and more prominent interface hepatitis (Fig. 22.4b). The overall appearance thus resembles those seen in chronic hepatitis or AIH. Late TCMR can also present as predominantly or exclusively perivenular lymphohistiocytic inflammation and hepatocyte dropout with minimal or no portal tract changes (isolated central peri-venulitis) [33–36]. Histologically, there are similarities between late TCMR, plasma cell-rich rejection, chronic AMR, and IPTH, suggesting that these conditions may all be part of an overlapping spectrum of late immune-mediated damage in the liver allograft. The Banff working group is currently working to incorporate late allograft changes in the current grading/staging schema (RAI index) so that these late changes are adequately represented while evaluating allografts (Table 22.3).

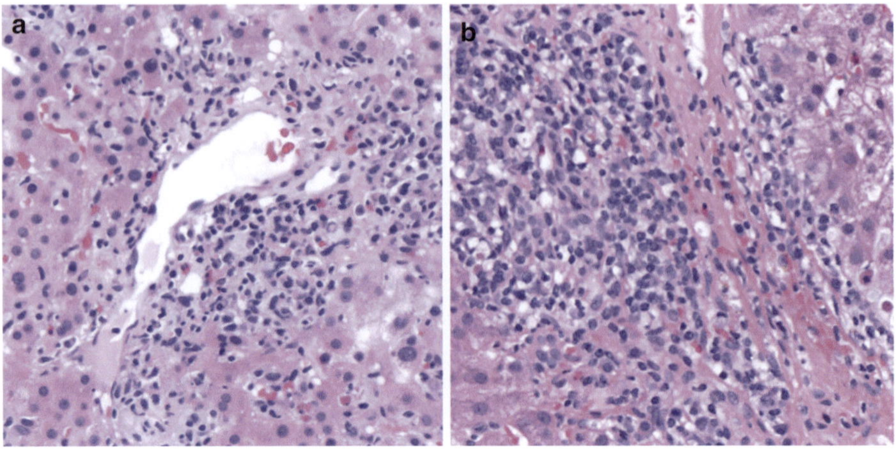

Fig. 22.4 Active T-cell–mediated rejection (TCMR), liver allograft (H&E, ×200). (**a**) Portal tract showing dense lymphocytic infiltration with prominent interface activity and spillover of inflammatory cells into the periportal parenchyma. The infiltrate extends along periportal sinusoids and disrupts the limiting plate, consistent with late TCMR. Occasional plasma cells and eosinophils are present. (**b**) Perivenular inflammation with perivenular drop out

Antibody-Mediated Rejection

AMR can be caused by pre-existing or pre-formed antibodies that are present in the recipient before transplantation or new-onset (de novo) antibodies that develop after transplantation of the donor organ. Two overlapping phenotypic expressions of allograft antibody-mediated rejection are being recognized: acute AMR (Fig. 22.5) and chronic AMR.

Banff criteria for definitive AMR include (1) careful biopsy results review showing changes consistent with a pattern of AMR injury (neutrophilic, eosinophilic, and macrophage-mediated microvasculitis/capillaritis, microvascular endothelial cell hypertrophy, and ductular reaction and hepato-canalicular cholestasis); (2) clinicopathological correlation, which excludes other insults that can cause a similar pattern of injury; (3) serological evidence of DSA; and (4) strong and diffuse complement (C4d) deposition within the injured allograft. Diffuse portal microvascular staining is defined [37] as strong portal vein and capillary and usually periportal sinusoidal endothelial staining involving most portal tracts. In an effort to standardize C4d interpretation, the 2016 Banff Working Group established criteria for C4d-(immune) scoring based on immunohistochemistry performed on formalin-fixed paraffin-embedded tissue [12].

Chronic AMR (cAMR) is less well defined; the exact incidence is not yet clear and is thought to be around 8% at 10-year post-transplant [38]. cAMR is strongly linked to serum class II DSA and associated with late-onset acute TCMR, fibrosis, chronic rejection, and decreased survival. Lesions most strongly associated with persistent DSA include portal, periportal and perivenular lymphoplasmacytic

Table 22.3 Differences between early and late TCMR

	Early or typical TCMR	Late onset TCMR
Timing	Usually ≤6 months, but can occur at anytime especially in inadequately immunosuppressed patients	Usually ≥6 month after transplantation
Liver function Abnormalities	Common and noticeable	Less common; may not be high enough to raise clinical concern
Histopathological Appearance	Typical mixed portal inflammation with lymphocytic cholangitis, subendothelial infiltration of portal or central veins; ± central perivenulitis; usually without fibrosis	Less lymphocytic cholangitis; more interface and perivenular necro-inflammatory activity; resembles chronic hepatitis; variable fibrosis
DSA present	Uncommon	More common than early or typical TCMR
Clinical signs and symptoms	Relatively common	Relatively uncommon
Differential diagnosis	Acute cholangiopathic changes	Other causes of chronic hepatitis and original disease recurrence should be reasonably excluded
Therapy	Increased baseline IS, corticosteroids followed by more aggressive therapy, if not responsive	Clinicians often hesitant to treat because of minor liver function abnormalities; uncertainty as how to treat
Response to therapy	Common and often complete	Often incomplete and follow-up incompletely documented
Banff clinically useful and captures clinicopathological correlation	Yes	Needs updated

inflammation with interface hepatitis, and lobular/perivenular or perivenular necro-inflammatory activity with sub-sinusoidal fibrosis and portal collagenization [25, 26]. Biliary strictures, nodular regenerative hyperplasia, and obliterative arteriopathy are also noted. In cases with double-positive DSA and C4d, Dao et al. [38] demonstrated that peri-venular fibrosis, portal inflammation, and lobular inflammation are significant histological findings. Biliary epithelial senescence and ductopenia can be seen in chronic AMR at lower rates. C4d is an integral element in evaluating biopsies for cAMR, and its positivity is associated with post-transplant DSA, graft fibrosis, and graft loss [25, 39]. At least focal C4d uptake (mostly in portal capillaries in inlet venules) is needed for a diagnosis of probable cAMR [25].

Recent studies suggest that antibody-mediated injury as evidenced by complement deposition, portal endothelial and stromal C4d staining, and serological evidence of DSA might contribute to progressive perivenular and perivenular sub-sinusoidal fibrosis—a form of chronic AMR [40, 41].

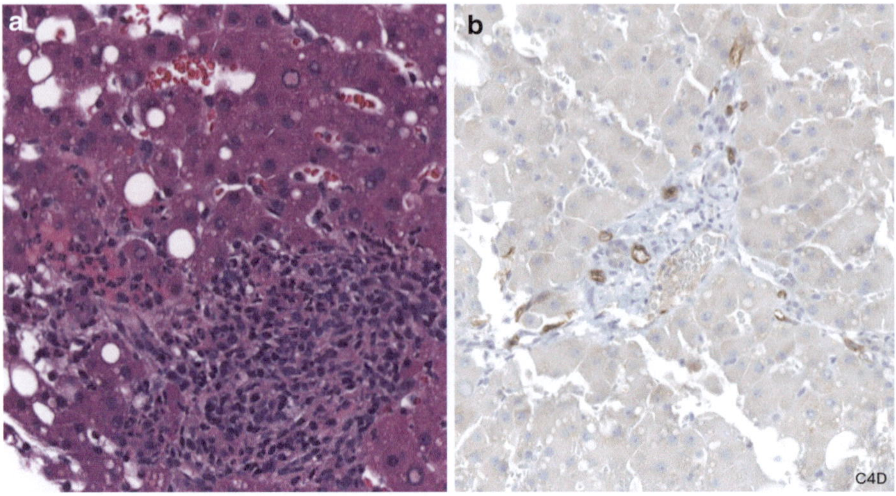

Fig. 22.5 Antibody-mediated rejection (AMR); liver allograft (H&E, x400, C4d, x400). (**a**) Hematoxylin and eosin (H&E) stain showing a portal tract with endothelialitis and perivenular inflammation accompanied by hepatocellular dropout and sinusoidal congestion, typical of microvascular injury in AMR. (**b**) Immunohistochemical stain for C4d demonstrating linear sinusoidal and portal capillary endothelial deposition, confirming complement activation consistent with AMR

Plasma Cell-Rich Rejection

Plasma cell-rich rejection [42, 43] is an uncommon and incompletely understood form of allograft rejection that resembles AIH in the native liver. It is characterized by plasma cell-rich infiltrates, interface and/or centrilobular hepatitis, and perivenular necroinflammatory activity and requirement for corticosteroid-based IS. While evaluating biopsies or resection specimens, a chronic hepatitic pattern of injury with a prominent plasma cell component (>30%) should prompt a complete serological workup to rule out autoimmune hepatitis and exclude other causes of chronic hepatitis. The focus should be to exclude any other possibility with extensive clinicopathological correlation before a diagnosis of plasma cell-rich rejection is made. Native liver AIH, recurrent AIH, and plasma cell-rich rejection are nearly indistinguishable from each other. All are characterized primarily by aggressive, plasma cell-rich necroinflammatory-type interface and variable perivenular necroinflammatory activity.

The Banff working group therefore advocated relatively strict criteria to establish the diagnosis AIH after transplantation and recently further refined specifically by establishing separate diagnostic criteria for plasma cell-rich rejection, which includes portal and/or perivenular plasma cell-rich infiltrates (>30%), lymphocytic cholangitis, and original liver disease other than AIH [12]. Lymphocytic cholangitis is usually present, and a desirable feature for diagnosis is not absolutely needed. Demonstration of increased IgG4-positive plasma cells is also a helpful feature (Fig. 22.6).

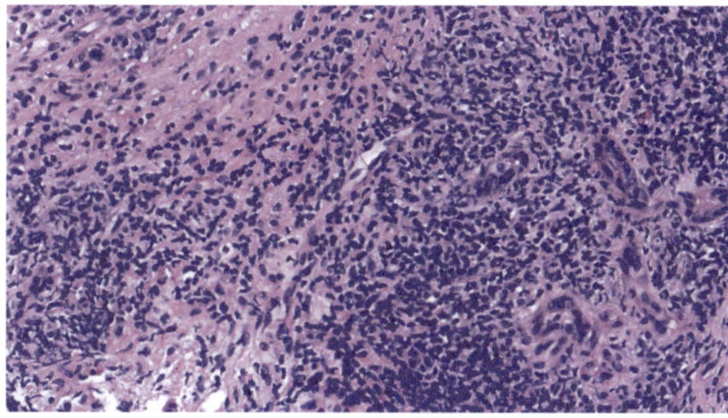

Fig. 22.6 Plasma cell rich rejection (PCR); liver allograft (H&E, ×200). Portal tract with dense, mixed inflammatory infiltrate composed predominantly of plasma cells admixed with lymphocytes and scattered eosinophils. The infiltrate extends into the periportal parenchyma, producing interface activity and hepatocyte dropout

Chronic Rejection

Chronic rejection primarily affects the portal tracts and perivenular regions and is divided into "early" and "late" stages according to the Banff schema [44]. Early chronic rejection findings include mild portal inflammation, lymphocytic cholangitis, and biliary epithelial cell senescence changes involving a majority of small bile ducts, and variable small bile duct loss involving less than 50% of portal tracts. Late allograft rejection is characterized by severe perivenular fibrosis and focal presence of central-to-central bridging fibrosis. There is usually a loss of small hepatic artery branches and small bile ducts, although an occasional biliary epithelial cell can be detected in portal tracts. A final diagnosis of classic chronic rejection (early or late) should be based on a combination of the clinical, radiological, laboratory, and histopathological findings. In a biopsy specimen, *minimal diagnostic criteria for chronic rejection are:* (1) *senescent changes, affecting a majority of the bile ducts, with or without bile duct loss;* (2) *convincing foam cell obliterative arteriopathy; or* (3) *bile duct loss affecting greater than 50% of the portal tracts* [44] (Fig. 22.7).

Bacterial and Fungal Infections

The stress and tissue injury associated with liver transplantation, compounded by the high level of immunosuppression required to prevent acute rejection, predispose recipients to serious opportunistic infections, particularly of bacterial, fungal, and viral origin. A high index of suspicion for infection should therefore be maintained when evaluating post-transplant liver biopsies, as infectious complications can closely mimic rejection, ischemia, or drug-induced injury. Typically, bacterial infections tend to occur beyond six months after transplantation and may result from biliary or vascular complications, abscess formation, or ascending cholangitis. Both bacterial and fungal infections often develop within nonviable or necrotic parenchyma; hence, all necrotic areas should be routinely examined with special stains

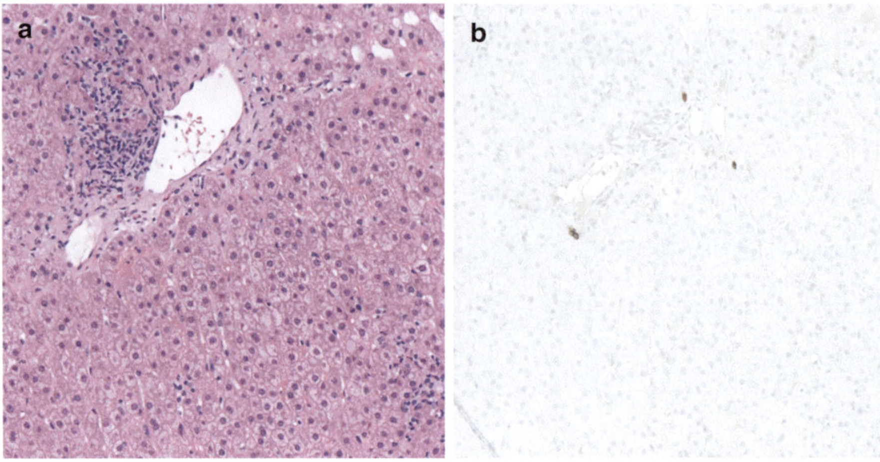

Fig. 22.7 Chronic rejection of a liver allograft; liver allograft (H&E, x100, CK7, x100). (**a**) Hematoxylin and eosin (H&E) stain showing a small portal tract with bile duct loss and mild chronic portal inflammation. The remaining bile duct profiles are shrunken and attenuated, with surrounding hepatocellular cholestasis. (**b**) Immunohistochemical stain for cytokeratin 7 (CK7) highlights residual bile ductules, emphasizing the paucity of native interlobular ducts typical of chronic ductopenic rejection

for organisms, including Gram, PAS, and GMS stains. Histologic clues to infection include coexistent acute, chronic, and granulomatous inflammation, although these features may be attenuated or absent in heavily immunosuppressed recipients. Fungal infections, most frequently due to Candida or Aspergillus species, can exhibit angioinvasive growth with tissue necrosis and thrombosis. While the detailed histopathologic manifestations of deep fungal and bacterial infections are well known to practicing pathologists and are beyond the intended scope of this chapter, awareness of their potential overlap with rejection and other causes of graft dysfunction remains critical for accurate diagnosis and management.

Late Liver Allograft Dysfunction and Protocol Biopsies

Liver allograft biopsy evaluation for late allograft injury and dysfunction is becoming increasingly important, but challenging, because of excellent short-term survival, effective control of recurrent original disease, initiatives to minimize IS, and improved long-term engraftment. Late allograft injury and dysfunction can be caused by a wide variety of insults, and many of them show overlapping clinical, serological, and histopathological features. The Banff working group for liver allograft pathology addressed these issues by spending several years constructing a consensus document 1 to help guide the interpretation of such biopsies [13]. The three most common late allograft insults include recurrence of the original disease (MASH, autoimmune hepatitis, etc.) and obstructive cholangiopathy/suboptimal biliary drainage; and/or classically defined acute and/or chronic TCMR (4% to 38% of late biopsy specimens). Liver allografts are primarily monitored by liver injury test results; in most programs, late biopsies are obtained only when liver injury test results vary from baseline values for that patient, however, protocol biopsies can help in (1) early detection of clinically unapparent disease, (2) identification of recipients that might be successfully weaned from IS, (3) the impact of chronic low-grade injury and alcohol use and consequences of long-term engraftment, (4) monitoring the effects of optimization of IS, [13, 45, 46], and (5) perhaps better recognition of potential consequences of chronic AMR (see earlier), but this area of investigation needs further study.

Recurrent and De Novo Disease in the Allograft

Original disease recurrence and chronic biliary tract strictures are the most common and significant causes of late liver allograft injury and dysfunction in adults. In pediatric recipients, TCMR is more common [28]. Native liver diseases can be classified, for the purpose of studying disease recurrence, as follows: (1) infectious (viral hepatitis A, B, C, D, E, etc.), some of which now mostly of "historical interest"; (2) dysregulated immunity (AIH, PBC, PSC, and overlap syndromes); (3) primary liver malignancies (cholangiocarcinomas and hepatocellular); (4) toxic insults, such as alcohol abuse and drug-induced liver injury; and (5) hepatic-based metabolic diseases (e.g., α1-antitrypsin deficiency and Wilson's disease) and extrahepatic-based metabolic disorders (e.g., metabolic syndrome, Gaucher's disease, hemochromatosis). Uncommon native liver diseases of uncertain etiology have also been shown to recur after liver transplantation [47]. Included are sarcoidosis, idiopathic granulomatous hepatitis, [45] post-infantile giant cell hepatitis, [48] the Budd-Chiari syndrome [48–51]. Liver transplantation can knowingly transmit diseases such as familial amyloidosis polyneuropathy and oxalosis when these genetically diseased, but phenotypically normal, livers are used as "domino" transplants. Discussing all these entities in detail is beyond the permitted word limit of this chapter (Fig. 22.8).

Drug-Induced Liver Injury and Toxic Injury

Hepatic allograft histopathological manifestations of drug-induced liver injury are generally identical to those in native livers. An exception might be drugs that elicit immune-allergic reactions, which might be lessened because of a potent baseline IS. Distinguishing among hepatic-based drug-induced liver injury (DILI) from rejection, recurrent disease, and other complications can be extremely difficult and is rarely encountered [52]. For example, azathioprine use has been associated with centrilobular necrosis and central vein and sub-sinusoidal fibrosis, but similar changes can be seen with late-onset rejection. Nodular regenerative hyperplasia has been attributed to chronic toxicity but is also frequently seen in recipients not treated with this medication and recognized in sensitized recipients [53]. Pseudo–ground-glass cells, composed of abnormal glycogen and closely resembling polyglucosan bodies, are seen with increased frequency in liver allografts and might be related to disturbed glycogen metabolism and polypharmacotherapy (Fig. 22.9).

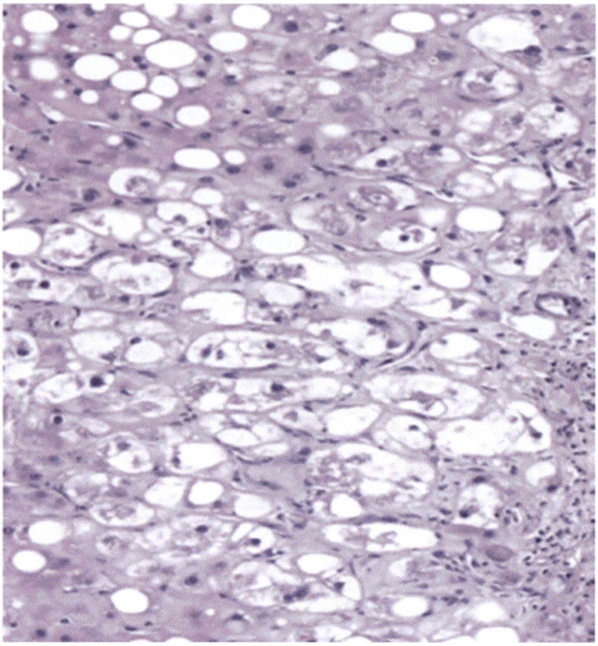

Fig. 22.8 Alcohol induced steatohepatitis. Hepatic parenchyma showing prominent macrovesicular steatosis with ballooned hepatocytes exhibiting rarefied cytoplasm, occasional Mallory–Denk bodies, and mild lobular inflammation. These features are characteristic of steatohepatitis, reflecting hepatocellular injury and inflammatory response associated with metabolic dysfunction or drug-related toxicity

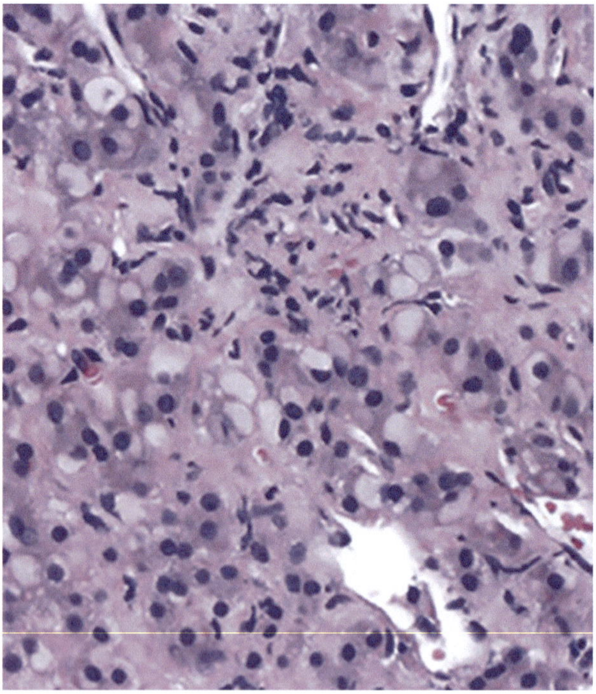

Fig. 22.9 Drug induced injury; liver parenchyma (H&E, x400) Lobular disarray with mixed inflammatory infiltrate, hepatocyte ballooning, and scattered apoptotic (acidophil) bodies. Foci of spotty necrosis and mild cholestasis are present. The injury pattern is consistent with a hepatocellular type of drug-induced injury, which can mimic acute viral or autoimmune hepatitis depending on the drug exposure and immune response

Acknowledgements I extend my sincere thanks to Dr. Jake Demetris who provided invaluable guidance and support for my career path.

References

1. Terrault NA, Francoz C, Berenguer M, Charlton M, Heimbach J. Liver transplantation 2023: status report, current and future challenges. Clin Gastroenterol Hepatol. 2023;21(8):2150–66.
2. Zhang Y, Zhang M, Ma Z, Wu S. Hypothermic machine perfusion reduces the incidences of early allograft dysfunction and biliary complications and improves 1-year graft survival after human liver transplantation: a meta-analysis. Medicine (Baltimore). 2019;98(23):e16033.
3. Henry SD, Nachber E, Tulipan J, Stone J, Bae C, Reznik L, et al. Hypothermic machine preservation reduces molecular markers of ischemia/reperfusion injury in human liver transplantation. Am J Transplant. 2012;12(9):2477–86.
4. van Leeuwen OB, Bodewes SB, Lantinga VA, Haring MPD, Thorne AM, Brüggenwirth IMA, et al. Sequential hypothermic and normothermic machine perfusion enables safe transplantation of high-risk donor livers. Am J Transplant. 2022;22(6):1658–70.
5. Ravikumar R, Leuvenink H, Friend PJ. Normothermic liver preservation: a new paradigm? Transpl Int. 2015;28(6):690–9.
6. van Leeuwen OB, de Vries Y, Fujiyoshi M, Nijsten MWN, Ubbink R, Pelgrim GJ, et al. Transplantation of high-risk donor livers after ex situ resuscitation and assessment using combined hypo- and normothermic machine perfusion: a prospective clinical trial. Ann Surg. 2019;270(5):906–14.
7. Bishop GA, Ierino FL, Sharland AF, Hall BM, Alexander SI, Sandrin MS, et al. Approaching the promise of operational tolerance in clinical transplantation. Transplantation. 2011;91(10):1065–74.
8. Demetris AJ, Isse K. Tissue biopsy monitoring of operational tolerance in liver allograft recipients. Curr Opin Organ Transplant. 2013;18(3):345–53.
9. Wu SL, Pan CE. Tolerance and chimerism and allogeneic bone marrow/stem cell transplantation in liver transplantation. World J Gastroenterol. 2013;19(36):5981–7.
10. Demetris AJ, Minervini MI, Nalesnik MA, Randhawa P, Sasatomi E. Histopathology of liver transplantation. In: Busuttil RW, Klintmalm GK, editors. Transplantation of the liver. 3rd ed. Philadelphia, PA: Elsevier/Saunders; 2015. p. 1112–70.
11. Demetris AJ, Crawford JM, Isse K, Minervini MI, Nalesnik MA, Rubin E, et al. Pathology of liver and hematopoietic stem cell transplantation. In: Odze RD, Goldblum JR, editors. Surgical pathology of the GI tract, liver, biliary tract and pancreas. 3rd ed. Philadelphia, PA: Elsevier/Saunders; 2015. p. 1408–61.
12. Demetris AJ, Bellamy C, Hubscher SG, O'Leary J, Randhawa PS, Feng S, et al. 2016 comprehensive update of the Banff working group on liver allograft pathology: introduction of antibody-mediated rejection. Am J Transplant. 2016;16:2816.
13. Demetris AJ, Adeyi O, Bellamy CO, Clouston A, Charlotte F, Czaja A, et al. Liver biopsy interpretation for causes of late liver allograft dysfunction. Hepatology. 2006;44(2):489–501.
14. Demetris AJ, Adams D, Bellamy C, Blakolmer K, Clouston A, Dhillon AP, et al. Update of the international Banff schema for liver allograft rejection: working recommendations for the histopathologic staging and reporting of chronic rejection. Int Panel Hepatol. 2000;31(3):792–9.
15. anonymous. Banff schema for grading liver allograft rejection: an international consensus document. Hepatology. 1997;25(3):658–63.
16. Geramizadeh B, Malek-Hosseini SA. Role of histopathologist in liver transplantation. Int J Organ Transplant Med. 2017;8(1):1–6.
17. Rastogi A. Liver transplant biopsy interpretation: diagnostic considerations and conundrums. Indian J Pathol Microbiol. 2022;65(2):245–57.

18. Banff Working Group on Liver Allograft Pathology. Importance of liver biopsy findings in immunosuppression management: biopsy monitoring and working criteria for patients with operational tolerance. Liver Transpl. 2012;18(10):1154–70.
19. Bellamy CO, Herriot MM, Harrison DJ, Bathgate AJ. C4d immunopositivity is uncommon in ABO-compatible liver allografts, but correlates partially with lymphocytotoxic antibody status. Histopathology. 2007;50(6):739–49.
20. Kozlowski T, Rubinas T, Nickeleit V, Woosley J, Schmitz J, Collins D, et al. Liver allograft antibody-mediated rejection with demonstration of sinusoidal C4d staining and circulating donor-specific antibodies. Liver Transpl. 2011;17(4):357–68.
21. Chen JW, Chen DZ, Yang ZR. Diagnosis and differentiation of rejection after liver transplantation: report of 5 cases. Hepatobiliary Pancreat Dis Int. 2005;4(2):182–4.
22. Henson JB, Muir AJ. Evaluation of an abnormal liver panel after liver transplantation. Clin Liver Dis. 2023;27(1):103–15.
23. Anonymous. Terminology for hepatic allograft rejection. International Working Party. [Review]. Hepatology. 1995;22(2):648–54.
24. Lee BT, Fiel MI, Schiano TD. Antibody-mediated rejection of the liver allograft: an update and a clinico-pathological perspective. J Hepatol. 2021;75(5):1203–16.
25. O'Leary JG, Cai J, Freeman R, Banuelos N, Hart B, Johnson M, et al. Proposed diagnostic criteria for chronic antibody-mediated rejection in liver allografts. Am J Transplant. 2016;16(2):603–14.
26. O'Leary JG, Smith C, Cai J, Hart B, Jennings LW, Everly M, et al. Chronic AMR in liver transplant: validation of the 1-year cAMR score's ability to determine long-term outcome. Transplantation. 2017;101(9):2062–70.
27. Evans HM, Kelly DA, McKiernan PJ, Hubscher S. Progressive histological damage in liver allografts following pediatric liver transplantation. Hepatology. 2006;43(5):1109–17.
28. Feng S, Bucuvalas JC, Demetris AJ, Burrell BE, Spain KM, Kanaparthi S, et al. Evidence of chronic allograft injury in liver biopsies from long-term pediatric recipients of liver transplants. Gastroenterology. 2018;155(6):1838–51.e7.
29. Knechtle SJ, Kwun J. Unique aspects of rejection and tolerance in liver transplantation. Semin Liver Dis. 2009;29(1):91–101.
30. Yeh MM, Larson AM, Tung BY, Swanson PE, Upton MP. Endotheliitis in chronic viral hepatitis: a comparison with acute cellular rejection and non-alcoholic steatohepatitis. Am J Surg Pathol. 2006;30(6):727–33.
31. Jadlowiec CC, Morgan PE, Nehra AK, Hathcock MA, Kremers WK, Heimbach JK, et al. Not all cellular rejections are the same: differences in early and late hepatic allograft rejection. Liver Transpl. 2019;25(3):425–35.
32. Nacif LS, Pinheiro RS, Pécora RA, Ducatti L, Rocha-Santos V, Andraus W, et al. Late acute rejection in liver transplant: a systematic review. Arq Bras Cir Dig. 2015;28(3):212–5.
33. Krasinskas AM, Ruchelli ED, Rand EB, Chittams JL, Furth EE. Central venulitis in pediatric liver allografts. Hepatology. 2001;33(5):1141–7.
34. Tsamandas AC, Jain AB, Felekouras ES, Fung JJ, Demetris AJ, Lee RG. Central venulitis in the allograft liver: a clinicopathologic study. Transplantation. 1997;64(2):252–7.
35. Sanei MH, Schiano TD, Sempoux C, Fan C, Fiel MI. Acute cellular rejection resulting in sinusoidal obstruction syndrome and ascites postliver transplantation. Transplantation. 2011;92(10):1152–8.
36. Demetris AJ, Eghtesad B, Marcos A, Ruppert K, Nalesnik MA, Randhawa P, et al. Recurrent hepatitis C in liver allografts: prospective assessment of diagnostic accuracy, identification of pitfalls, and observations about pathogenesis. Am J Surg Pathol. 2004;28(5):658–69.
37. Hubscher SG. Antibody-mediated rejection in the liver allograft. Curr Opin Organ Transplant. 2012;17(3):280–6.
38. Dao M, Habès D, Taupin JL, Mussini C, Redon MJ, Suberbielle C, et al. Morphological characterization of chronic antibody-mediated rejection in ABO-identical or ABO-compatible pediatric liver graft recipients. Liver Transpl. 2018;24(7):897–907.

39. Iacob S, Cicinnati VR, Lindemann M, Heinemann FM, Radtke A, Kaiser GM, et al. Donor-specific anti-HLA antibodies and endothelial C4d deposition-association with chronic liver allograft failure. Transplantation. 2015;99(9):1869–75.
40. Egawa H, Miyagawa-Hayashino A, Haga H, Teramukai S, Yoshizawa A, Ogawa K, et al. Non-inflammatory centrilobular sinusoidal fibrosis in pediatric liver transplant recipients under tacrolimus withdrawal. Hepatol Res. 2012;42(9):895–903.
41. Miyagawa-Hayashino A, Yoshizawa A, Uchida Y, Egawa H, Yurugi K, Masuda S, et al. Progressive graft fibrosis and donor-specific human leukocyte antigen antibodies in pediatric late liver allografts. Liver Transpl. 2012;18(11):1333–42.
42. Fiel MI, Schiano TD. Plasma cell hepatitis (de-novo autoimmune hepatitis) developing post liver transplantation. Curr Opin Organ Transplant. 2012;17(3):287–92.
43. Demetris AJ, Sebagh M. Plasma cell hepatitis in liver allografts: variant of rejection or autoimmune hepatitis? Liver Transpl. 2008;14(6):750–5.
44. Walter T, Dumortier J, Guillaud O, Hervieu V, Paliard P, Scoazec JY, et al. Rejection under alpha interferon therapy in liver transplant recipients. Am J Transplant. 2007;7(1):177–84.
45. Pappo O, Ramos H, Starzl TE, Fung JJ, Demetris AJ. Structural integrity and identification of causes of liver allograft dysfunction occurring more than 5 years after transplantation. Am J Surg Pathol. 1995;19(2):192–206.
46. Mells G, Mann C, Hubscher S, Neuberger J. Late protocol liver biopsies in the liver allograft: a neglected investigation? Liver Transpl. 2009;15(8):931–8.
47. Gane E, Sallie R, Saleh M, Portmann B, Williams R. Clinical recurrence of hepatitis a following liver transplantation for acute liver failure. J Med Virol. 1995;45(1):35–9.
48. Starzl TE, Demetris AJ. Liver transplantation: a 31-year perspective. Part I. Curr Probl Surg. 1990;27(2):55–116.
49. Starzl TE, Demetris AJ. Liver transplantation: a 31-year perspective. Part II. Curr Probl Surg. 1990;27(3):123–78.
50. Starzl TE, Demetris AJ. Liver transplantation: a 31-year perspective. Part III. Curr Probl Surg. 1990;27(4):187–240.
51. Huang J. Ethical and legislative perspectives on liver transplantation in the People's Republic of China. Liver Transpl. 2007;13(2):193–6.
52. Charlton MR, Thompson A, Veldt BJ, Watt K, Tillmann H, Poterucha JJ, et al. Interleukin-28B polymorphisms are associated with histological recurrence and treatment response following liver transplantation in patients with hepatitis C virus infection. Hepatology. 2011;53(1):317–24.
53. Sebagh M, Yilmaz F, Kounis I, Saliba F, Feray C, Taupin JL, et al. Evidence for alloimmune sinusoidal injury in. Transpl Int. 2023;36:11306.

Early and Late Complications of Liver Transplantation

23

Alyssa Justus and James J. Pomposelli

Introduction

Liver transplantation (LT) continues to evolve and remains the standard treatment for liver failure, and patients have enjoyed decreasing morbidity and mortality over the last several decades. Post-transplant survival has reached rates of up to 96% at 1 year and 71% at 10 years, respectively [1]. Transplant survival benefit for recipients of deceased donors and living donors is well over a decade, respectively [2, 3]. Despite improvements in surgical technique and postoperative care, complications after liver transplant still occur at rates between 26% and 50% [4].

With advent of direct-acting antiviral agents (DAA), hepatitis C (HCV) is no longer the main indication for LT globally. In many countries, HCV continues to decline as an indication for LT and is being surpassed by metabolic-associated steatohepatitis (MASH) (previously known as nonalcoholic steatohepatitis or NASH) [5, 6]. In the United States, cirrhosis secondary to MASH is the second most common indication for LT [7]. During COVID, alcohol related liver disease has increased dramatically, especially in younger individuals. Obesity continues to be a major health issue and a major source of morbidity and mortality not only after liver transplant but in general [8]. Obese patients with a body mass index (BMI) over 30 undergoing LT suffer an increased rate of cardiopulmonary complications, and those with morbid obesity (BMI ≥ 40) have increased mortality risk [9].

In this chapter, we will review common early and late complications often seen after liver transplantation and strategies for treatment. As with any surgical

A. Justus
Department of Surgery, University of New Mexico School of Medicine, Albuquerque, NM, USA

J. J. Pomposelli (✉)
Tufts Medical Center, Boston, MA, USA

B. Eghtesad et al. (eds.), *Liver Transplantation*,
https://doi.org/10.1007/978-3-032-07072-2_23

procedure, a favorable outcome requires sound judgment, technical acumen, and attention to detail.

Donor Selection and Procurement Injuries

The number of candidates for liver transplantation added to the wait-list each year continues to grow as more patients with chronic liver disease are identified and evaluated. There has been a gradual increase in donor organ supply over the last decade, but this growth has not been able to "close the gap" between supply and demand. Living donor liver transplantation (LDLT) has remained somewhat stagnant over the last decade and provides about 5% of the liver grafts in the United States per year. Much of the growth in organ availability has been from a dramatic increase in the number of donation after cardiac death (DCD) donors. In these cases, the donor is not brain dead but has suffered irreversible brain injury and recovery is not anticipated. The family consents to the removal of supportive measures, and the donor is allowed to die "naturally." After cessation of all cardiac function for at least 5 min, the patient is declared dead, and organ retrieval can then take place. In some hospitals and countries, an additional "standoff" period between 5 and 20 min is required before organ retrieval can commence. Because of these protracted time periods without blood flow, DCD donors have historically been considered inferior to donation after brain death (DBD) or LDLT. Despite the dramatic increase in DCD donors nationally, only about 12.1% of all LT in the United States come from DCD donors [10]. However, newer data suggest that carefully selected younger DCD donors may have better LT outcomes than older DBD donors [10]. Recent advances in both in vivo and ex vivo organ perfusion technology with normothermic regional perfusion (NRP) and normothermic machine perfusion (NMP) have improved the outcomes comparable to DBD donation [10, 11].

The obesity epidemic has not only increased the rate of cirrhosis from MASH but has also affected the quality of liver grafts from eligible donors. Donor liver steatosis encountered during procurement continues to be a common indication for declining a liver graft [7]. However, given the growing mismatch in supply and demand, there have been ongoing efforts to expand acceptance of livers with steatosis. Steatosis can be classified as microvesicular (MiS) or macrovesicular (MaS), with only MaS shown to significantly impact graft survival [12]. Grafts with mild MaS (<30%) have been demonstrated to have comparable outcomes to non-steatotic grafts with no increase in complications [13]. However, increased levels of MaS have been associated with early allograft dysfunction (EAD), primary graft nonfunction (PNF), biliary complications, and increased graft loss at 1 year [12]. Organs with more advanced degrees of MaS (>30%) can be used safely when baseline liver function tests are normal, whereas abnormal liver function tests in the setting of less steatosis may be problematic. The decision to use a particular organ depends on the status of the recipient and medical urgency at the time. While "perfect" organs are desirable for more severely ill, high MELD patients, compromise on donor quality may be justified in urgent settings. Current studies are underway to determine if livers with more advanced steatosis can be "defatted" with perfusion technologies, making them more usable.

Once the decision is made to procure the organ for a particular patient, the liver procurement team dictates the conduct of the dissection below the diaphragm, while the cardiac and thoracic teams are responsible for activity above the diaphragm. When the procurement is occurring in a DCD donor, use of perfusion technologies such as NRP and NMP is becoming standard to reduce early graft dysfunction and postoperative ischemic cholangiopathy which were more common after DCD donation using static cold storage alone. When thoracic and abdominal organs are being procured from a DCD donor, thoracoabdominal NRP (TA-NRP) is used with cannulas placed in the chest to revitalize the lungs and the heart in addition to abdominal organs. Alternatively, if abdominal organs alone are to be recovered, abdominal NRP with cannulas placed in the lower aorta and vena cava is used. The use of TA-NRP remains controversial in that there is an ethical concern about possible reanimation of the brain with re-establishment of perfusion. Current guidelines from the American Society of Transplant Surgeons (ASTS) recommend ligation or division of major head vessels to prevent perfusion of the brain during NRP [14, 15]. Since the donor is declared dead during the DCD donation process with cessation of heart rhythm and absence of pulses for at least 10–25 min with the standoff periods, many of these theoretical concerns seem unwarranted but are under current study.

Regardless of the type of donor being used (DBD or DCD), good communication and operative planning between the organ bank staff and operative teams are required to minimize ischemia time for all organs being procured. However, if a donor becomes unstable, dissection can be expedited with subsequent rapid organ recovery. This can lead to missed identification of anatomy and increases the likelihood of technical errors, which usually involve cutting important vascular structures that need to be reconstructed later before implantation. Procurement-related liver injury (PRLI) occurs in roughly 10–20% of procurements, with variant anatomy increasing the risk [16, 17]. Injuries can occur to the parenchyma, vasculature, or biliary system. Hepatic arterial anatomic variation occurs in approximately 28% of liver grafts [18]. Injury to the aberrant hepatic arteries occurs by failure to recognize the variation or unintentional division. If an arterial injury occurs before cross-clamping and flushing of the organs, it can be serious due to a lack of perfusion to that portion of the graft. Injuries occurring after cross-clamp and flushing of the organs is less serious but in both cases and requires back table reconstruction. Accessory or replaced right hepatic arteries requiring reconstruction have a higher rate of hepatic artery thrombosis (HAT), and injured right hepatic arteries requiring reconstruction have an even higher rate of HAT (14.3%) [19]. Parenchymal injuries are the most common form of minor liver injury during graft removal that can occur during implantation as well. These can increase operative time and blood loss, but are easily treated with hemostatic agents, cautery, or sutures without an impact on graft function [20]. Biliary injuries occur less frequently, often due to stripping of the vascular supply or transecting the duct too short for anastomosis. Roux-en-Y biliary reconstruction can often manage these injuries with similar outcomes and without graft loss [21, 22].

Total warm (WIT) and cold ischemia (CIT) times become significant risk factors for graft function and survival. There is no absolute consensus on CIT, but recent studies show adverse outcomes after 10 h and that problems can be observed with even shorter times [23, 24]. Generally, CIT greater than 12 h is associated with primary nonfunction, HAT, biliary complications, and mortality, and should be avoided [24]. WIT includes both procurement time (during DCDs) prior to cooling and during implantation. Prolonged WIT has been associated with poor outcomes and increased recipient mortality [25]. With the advent of NRP and NMP, programs are pushing the limits of acceptable WIT since there is an opportunity for resuscitation of graft after the initial ischemic event.

To increase the donor pool, surgical innovations have been developed for deceased donor grafts and include split-liver grafts in deceased donors and LDLT using living donors. Because these operations required splitting of the liver parenchyma, higher complication rates and inferior outcomes for recipients were seen during early experience and included bile leaks, hepatic artery thrombosis (HAT), unplanned re-exploration, portal vein thrombosis, and patient and graft loss [26, 27]. However, as experience in this area has increased, outcomes have improved and are similar to or better than deceased donor liver transplantation (DDLT). [27] Yet, recipients of split-liver grafts are at risk of small-for-size syndrome (SFSS), which occurs when the liver graft is unable to meet metabolic demands of the recipient [28]. This clinically presents as postoperative coagulopathy, prolonged cholestasis, liver dysfunction, hyperbilirubinemia, and encephalopathy. SFSS is a bit of misnomer since the syndrome is more accurately characterized by portal hyperperfusion with allograft dysfunction and may be seen with larger grafts in small recipients. For this reason, early allograft dysfunction (EAD) rather than SFSS may be a more accurate descriptive term [29]. Generally, graft size should be at least 0.8 graft weight to body weight ratio (GW/BW) and smaller grafts <0.8 GW.BW can have worse outcomes, especially in high MELD patients with severe portal hypertension [28]. Split liver grafts from both deceased and living donors generally have higher rates of biliary complications, and improved outcomes can be observed with careful donor selection, recipient matching, and surgical skill [30, 31].

Coagulopathy and Bleeding

The coagulopathies of end-stage liver disease (ESLD) often require aggressive management in the perioperative LT period. These patients are prone to both hypercoagulability and thrombotic complications, as well as bleeding diathesis, likely secondary to increased portal and splanchnic pressures [32]. However, transfusion of >2 units of blood products has been independently associated with increased mortality following LT [33]. For this reason, efforts to reduce overall blood product administration using viscoelastic testing (VET) to help guide resuscitation in the perioperative period are gaining popularity [34].

Intraoperative bleeding is often treated with blood product administration using VET guidance, antifibrinolytics, volume restriction, topical hemostatic agents, cautery, and prothrombin complex concentrate (PCC) [33]. Bleeding leading to hemorrhagic shock can also be managed with vasopressors. All of these modalities come with their own associated risks and complications. If coagulopathy is not able to be controlled, laparotomy packs can be placed to tamponade bleeding with planned returned to the operating room in 24–48 h. Failure to identify and correct ongoing coagulopathy can result in unplanned return to the operating room and worse outcomes.

Vascular Complications

Occlusive Arterial Complications

Occlusive arterial complications include hepatic artery thrombosis (HAT) and hepatic artery stenosis (HAS). HAT is the most common and most serious vascular complication following LT and frequently leads to hepatic failure, biliary strictures, ischemic cholangiopathy, and graft loss. Occasionally, HAT can be clinically silent and the recipient can be watched expectantly. More often, HAT requires retransplantation, especially when diagnosed early after transplant and the liver is irreparably harmed. HAT has an incidence of about 2–9% and is associated with ~50% retransplantation or mortality [35]. Operative risk factors include surgical technique, number of anastomoses, use of conduits, vessel kinking, and small vessel size. Nonoperative risk factors include donor age >60, long CIT, preservation damage, lack of blood group compatibility, cytomegalovirus (CMV) positive donor, hypercoagulable state, recipient cigarette smoking, rejection, and primary sclerosing cholangitis [35]. Since the biliary duct epithelium is supplied solely by the hepatic artery, thrombotic complications often lead to biliary complications such as strictures, leaks, or bilomas, even if early repair is performed [36].

The early diagnosis and treatment of HAT is crucial to prevent graft necrosis. Routine Doppler ultrasound (US) should be used at any suspicion of HAT, especially in the first 2 postoperative weeks. US may show no arterial signal within the liver parenchyma or non-visualization of the hepatic artery. Patent hepatic artery with nonflow within the liver is compatible with HAT, as arterial flow can go retrograde down the gastroduodenal artery and result in a false positive result. Confirmation can be made with contrast-enhanced US, computed tomography, magnetic resonance imaging, or conventional angiography [36].

HAT can be divided into early and late. United Network for Organ Sharing (UNOS) defines early HAT in adult recipients as less than 7 days, AST greater than 3000, and international normalized ratio (INR) greater than 2.5 or acidosis (arterial PH <7.3 or lactate >4), and these patients qualify for relisting as status 1A. If the adult recipient does not meet these criteria, but HAT occurs within 14 days, they will be relisted with a MELD score of 40 [37]. Revascularization should be attempted, and if successful, can help mitigate the need for retransplantation.

Minimally invasive revascularization can be done with catheter-directed thrombolysis or thrombectomy. Thrombolysis has been associated with up to a 75% success rate but has known hemorrhagic complications, while thrombectomy has been associated with up to a 100% success rate in smaller studies; however, if the HAT is related to arterial dissection, surgical repair is required [38, 39]. Stents may be placed after either procedure across the arterial stenosis and carry a high rate of re-occlusion [38]. Alternatively, revascularization can be attempted surgically through a variety of techniques such as surgical thrombectomy or arterial reconstruction. Unfortunately, many HATs occur due to arterial dissection, making reconstruction more difficult or impossible if it occurs within the graft itself. Due to transient ischemia to the biliary system, biliary complications can present in a delayed fashion following revascularization [39].

Late HAT can present with fever, elevation in alkaline phosphatase, jaundice, hepatic abscesses, biliary leaks, and bilomas. Some late HAT cases have demonstrated arterial collateralization, and asymptomatic recipients can often be observed for biliary complications. However, many patients still develop ischemic cholangiopathy (IC) and require retransplantation [40, 41].

Hepatic artery stricture (HAS) can develop within 3–6 months of transplantation and is often seen on radiographic imaging. If there is good arterial flow within the liver and adequate liver function, we typically refrain from treating an image with interventional procedures. When HAS is combined with questionable liver function, interventional procedures may be of benefit and late cases after 6 months may not benefit from angioplasty [42].

Nonocclusive Arterial Complications

Nonocclusive arterial complications include arteriovenous fistula, dissection, inadequate hepatic flow, pseudoaneurysms, and arterial ruptures and represent less than 5% of arterial complications [42]. Recipient arterial dissection can occur and is often identified intraoperatively and reconstructed using donor iliac allograft, recipient saphenous vein, or synthetic conduit. Very rarely is this complication not recognized in the operating room. However, if missed, dissection can be asymptomatic or present with continuous pain, increasing false lumen, aneurysmal dilatation, and rupture [43]. Pursuing endovascular management is appropriate if the patient is hemodynamically stable [43].

While hepatic artery pseudoaneurysms (HAP) are rare, graft loss and excessive mortality can be observed [42]. Intrahepatic HAP are often due to iatrogenic injury and can often be managed with observation. However, if they are large, symptomatic, or progressing, percutaneous embolization can be considered. Extrahepatic HAP can be due iatrogenic injury such as endovascular procedures or surgical technique or due to localized infection causing arteritis. These must be managed urgently with a stent to avoid rupture. However, these still often require surgical debridement of the infection and carry a high mortality [42].

Portal Vein Complications

Portal vein thrombosis (PVT) occurs at a rate of about 5–26% and up to 31% of those are identified intra-operatively. While PVT is no longer an absolute contraindication to LT, preoperative anticoagulation often paired with intraoperative thrombectomy is required for proper portal vein anastomosis during LT [44]. Early identification (<6 months) and treatment with anticoagulation is associated with a higher recanalization rate [44]. A PVT scoring system was proposed by Yerdel et al. in which grade 1 is less than 50% PVT, grade 2 is greater than 50% with minimal superior mesenteric vein (SMV) obstruction, grade 3 is 100% PVT, and grade 4 is 100% PVT with SMV thrombosis [45]. During LT, lower Yerdel PVT (grades 1–3) can often be managed with thrombectomy or jump grafts. A very high Yerdel PVT (grade 4) is a relative contraindication to LT. Complicated vascular reconstruction to tenuous inflow during LT requires major planning and is often unsatisfying [44].

Postoperative PVT occurs at a rate of about 3%, and is independently associated with increased postoperative blood transfusion of erythrocytes and platelets, and is associated with pre-operative PVT. [46] Though rare, postoperative PVT can be serious with about 50% of patients requiring retransplantation if urgent revascularization cannot be achieved [46]. Reoperation, thrombectomy, and systemic anticoagulation are appropriate for early PVT. If the PVT is nonocclusive, this can be managed more conservatively with anticoagulation and serial US. To prevent fibrotic changes with progressive or chronic PVT, percutaneous balloon angioplasty and stent placement may be appropriate [47].

Portal vein stenosis (PVS) occurs in less than 5% of cases and is more common in split liver transplantation (LDLT and pediatrics) and in the setting of prior radiation [48]. PVS is often asymptomatic but can present with portal hypertension, ascites, and progressive graft failure. Liver function tests (LFTs) may remain normal and may be found on routine ultrasound or imaging studies [48].

Venous Outflow Obstruction

Venous outflow obstruction occurs at a rate of 1–6%, and is mostly observed within the first few weeks postoperatively. Persistent ascites, renal dysfunction, venous congestion on biopsy, increased pressure gradient across the outflow anastomosis without parenchymal gradient on pressure measurements suggest outflow obstruction. Outflow obstruction can be caused by kinking, stenosis, or thrombosis [48]. Historically, bi-caval reconstruction after LT is used where the inferior vena cava (IVC) of the graft was anastomosed to both supra- and infra-hepatic vena cava in the recipient. To reduce blood loss, warm ischemia time, and acute kidney injury, the piggyback technique has become more commonly used, in which the donor suprahepatic IVC is anastomosed to the recipient middle and left hepatic vein confluence [49]. Though, some studies report higher stenosis with the piggyback approach. Endovascular interventions with balloon dilatation have a high success rate for stenosis; in some instances, surgical intervention is required [1]. In a single-center study, 25–36.3% of LDLT recipients with venous outflow obstruction had recurrence after balloon angioplasty [50]. Kinking and intrahepatic stenoses are more likely to require stent placement, while anastomotic stricture can often be treated with balloon angioplasty alone [51]. For this reason, some surgeons prefer bi-caval reconstruction.

Non-occlusive IVC thrombus can often be treated conservatively with systemic anticoagulation. For more persistent cases, catheter-directed thrombectomy or thrombolysis can be used [52]. Surgical thrombectomy is an option, though has poorer outcomes compared to percutaneous interventions [52].

A recent systematic review concluded that either venous outflow reconstruction can be used with similar outcomes and should be based on surgeon preference and center experience with consideration to the individual patient and circumstance [53]. If outflow obstruction results in significant graft dysfunction, retransplantation may be needed [48]. Transjugular intrahepatic portosystemic shunt (TIPS) can be used as a bridge for those awaiting retransplantation, and it is associated with accelerated decline in liver function [54].

Biliary Complications

The biliary tree blood supply is by the hepatic artery, and even transient decreases in arterial flow can result in biliary complications. Biliary complications occur more frequently than vascular complications (up to 25% of recipients), but often have a better prognosis [55]. Early biliary complications are predominantly centered around leaks and, less frequently, anastomotic disruptions. Late biliary strictures are debilitating to the patient and can occur within the liver as seen with ischemic cholangiopathy or in the common bile duct, usually at the site of the anastomosis.

Biliary Leaks

Biliary leaks have an incidence of approximately 10% and usually occur within the first days or weeks after transplantation [1]. Biliary leaks can occur at the site of anastomosis or the cystic duct stump. During live donor procedures, cut surface leaks are also possible. Biliary leaks can range from asymptomatic to fever and abdominal pain [1]. Many leaks can be treated expectantly and may resolve spontaneously. A brief interval of observation often rewards the clinician and the patient. Persistent, high-volume leaks require intervention with endoscopic retrograde cholangiopancreatography (ERCP) or surgical revision. Choledochocholedocostomy (duct to duct) has a lower incidence of leak than choledochojejunostomy, which can be associated with a risk of enteric contamination [1].

Larger leaks and those associated with ischemic necrosis require surgical revision with Roux-en-Y hepaticojejunostomy. The development of early postoperative leaks is associated with late stricture formation, and lifelong surveillance by the surgeon is warranted.

Biliary Strictures

Biliary strictures account for about 40% of all biliary complications and occur at a higher frequency after DCD and LDLT [55]. Obstructive LFTs can be seen, but strictures often present as a shaking chill and high fever even in the setting of normal LFTs. Any recipient who complains of high fever after a rigor should be initially treated with antibiotics and can be assessed with magnetic resonance cholangiopancreatography (MRCP). Recurrent fevers warrant intervention with ERCP or percutaneous transhepatic cholangiogram (PTC) for diagnosis and intervention. Occasionally, biliary strictures can present with abdominal pain, fever, and jaundice consistent with acute cholangitis. Strictures can occur at the site of the anastomosis or be non-anastomotic, within the liver parenchyma. Anastomotic strictures are mainly due to ischemic insult. Non-anastomotic strictures are more often multiple, longer, complex strictures and may be related to ischemic cholangiopathy or recurrent disease such as primary sclerosing cholangitis. Additionally, non-anastomotic strictures often require more aggressive management as these strictures are more complex and treatment carries a higher risk of graft loss and the need for retransplantation [55].

Anastomotic strictures can be treated with ERCP dilation and stenting or surgical revision [55]. Early stenosis, within the first 2 months after LT, often requires fewer interventions than late stenosis. If ERCP is chosen as the therapeutic management for late stenosis, it may require multiple sessions of dilation while subsequently increasing stent diameter. More than 80% of biliary strictures can be successfully treated with endoscopic procedures [55]. The American Society for Gastrointestinal Endoscopy recommends ERCP as the initial intervention and covered self-expandable metal stents (cSEMSs) as the stent of choice. Antibiotics should be administered during ERCP if biliary drainage cannot be ensured [56]. If endoscopic efforts fail, surgical revision may be warranted with Roux-en-Y reconstruction.

Ischemic Cholangiopathy

Ischemic cholangiopathy (IC) is a severe outcome on the spectrum of non-anastomotic biliary strictures (NAS). It is associated with HAT, biliary salt toxicity, ischemia-reperfusion, and immune-mediated injury [57]. IC occurs at a rate between 1–10% and 10–30% in DBD and DCD donors, respectively [57]. IC can be subclinical or clinical and has been described as four distinct imaging patterns, including diffuse necrosis, multifocal progressive, confluence dominant, and minor form [58]. IC can be diffuse within the biliary tree, multifocal, and resistant to therapy. Severe IC can lead to ductal wall necrosis and breakdown and can require urgent or delayed retransplantation. Attempted stricture treatment of mild IC may afford additional graft survival, though there is still a marked reduction of graft survival at 5 years [59]. The associated cholestasis may result in gallstones, biliary sludge, and debris, and these patients may develop bilomas or intrahepatic abscesses [52]. Avoiding IC altogether is the best strategy.

Early Graft Dysfunction

Early graft dysfunction (EAD) is a spectrum that can range from mild to severe and can result in acute liver failure and graft loss. Thought to be caused by ischemia-reperfusion injury (IRI), graft dysfunction is also associated with acute kidney injury. Signs are often nonspecific, including liver enzyme abnormalities, and trending lab values remain the mainstay of monitoring [60]. Proposed definitions include bilirubin >10 mg/dL, INR >1.6, and ALT/AST >2000 IU/L within postoperative day (POD) 7 and is associated with increased graft loss within 90 days [60]. Any rise in or non-normalization of serum bilirubin or INR postoperatively should prompt suspicion.

Incidence of EAD ranges from 5.2% to 36.3%, and it is associated with older donors, grafts with steatosis, and prolonged ischemia time (warm and cold). Dysfunction has been associated with left lobe grafts, split grafts, lower graft weight, higher pre-operative bilirubin, higher portal reperfusion pressure, higher donor age, and higher donor BMI [61]. Mild forms can be completely reversible in up to 28 days. Despite this, graft dysfunction has been associated with inferior long-term outcomes and worse patient survival [60]. The model for early allograft function (MEAF) is a clinical tool that can be done within 3 days after transplantation to grade severity of dysfunction and predict short- and long-term survival. After exclusion of other causes of graft dysfunction (HAT, biliary complications, etc.), care is supportive. In the era of normothermic regional perfusion (NRP) and normothermic machine perfusion (NMP), updated definitions of EAD need to be developed, as the conventional definition listed above does not predict graft loss at the same rate.

Primary Graft Nonfunction

Primary graft nonfunction (PGF) is the most severe form of graft dysfunction. Unfortunately, there is no universal definition of primary graft nonfunction, but clinically it presents with extremely elevated liver enzymes (usually within 48 h post-transplant), severe coagulopathy, little to no bile production, lactic acidosis, hypoglycemia, and acute progressive liver failure with multiorgan failure [60]. Though PGF is more rare than early graft dysfunction, ranging from 0.9% to 7.2%, PGF is a fatal condition and requires urgent retransplantation for salvage [60].

Machine perfusion strategies have helped to mitigate the occurrence of PGF after both deceased donor and DCD donation [62]. Early identification, aggressive medical management, excluding other identifiable causes of graft dysfunction, and urgent relisting are required. Aggressive medical management of acute liver failure (coagulopathy, acid-base status, urine output, fluid shifts, etc.) also helps to optimize the patient if retransplantation is required [62]. Even after retransplantation, mortality risk remains very high.

Rejection

While rejection can occur at any time following transplantation, this chapter will cover the acute postoperative period, mainly acute cellular rejection. T-cell mediated rejection (TCMR) often occurs within the first 6 weeks after LT with host lymphocytes recognizing antigens from the donor liver with the major histocompatibility complex (MHC) playing a large role [63]. These changes include a mixed inflammatory cell infiltrate, predominantly lymphocytes, that involves the portal triads and disrupts the biliary, hepatic artery, and portal venous endothelia [64]. Incidence of acute rejection can be as high as 20–40% and early rejection episodes do not significantly impair long-term graft success or patient outcomes [65]. Many patients are asymptomatic, a variety of clinical signs and symptoms may develop that include fever, abdominal pain, malaise, fatigue, and poor appetite. Elevated serum bilirubin level, and a modest increase in alkaline phosphatase and transaminase levels may be seen. However, confident diagnosis of rejection requires liver biopsy, as routine laboratory tests and biomarkers have not proven sufficient alone [63]. Histologic diagnosis and grading is made using the Banff Working Group classification [66].

TCMR severity is graded using the rejection activity index (RAI). Mild rejection (RAI <4) can be treated with increasing calcineurin inhibitor, but moderate (RAI 4–6) and severe (RAI >7) RAI should be treated with high-dose pulse corticosteroids, which are successful in approximately 80–90% of cases [63, 67].

Antibody-mediated rejection (AMR) is rare (incidence <1%) and treatment protocols include steroids, plasmapheresis, and B-cell depletion. The Banff histologic characteristics include portal microvascular endothelial cell hypertrophy, capillary dilation, mixed portal microvasculitis, and portal edema [63]. Because AMR is often associated with a component of TCMR, typical first-line therapies include switching to tacrolimus, optimization of trough levels, and steroid boluses. Several days of plasmapheresis to reduce antibody levels followed by B-cell depletion medication such as Rituximab is indicated [63].

Repeated episodes of TCMR, inadequately treated episodes of TCMR, or a severe episode of AMR can result in chronic rejection, with an incidence of <5% in adults [63]. Chronic ductopenic rejection rarely occurs in the first 2 months after LT, and is defined as loss of bile ducts in more than 50% of portal tracts, when 20 or more portal tracts are available for evaluation, and is diagnosed on the basis of histologic criteria [68]. The only effective treatment is retransplantation.

Hyperacute rejection is a very aggressive, immediate form of rejection that occurs after incompatible ABO LT, now rarely seen with modern pre-transplant screening [63]. Successful transplant with ABO incompatible pairs is possible with aggressive immunosuppression protocols.

Infection

With necessary immunosuppression, infectious risk is increased in transplant recipients. There is always a balance between too little immunosuppression with increased incidence of rejection and too much immunosuppression with increased incidence of infection. Bacterial infection after LT is a major cause of morbidity with a four- to fivefold increase in mortality. In fact, infection is the leading cause of death following LT [69]. Most patients will be overwhelmingly worried about rejection, whereas infection is their biggest risk for a poor outcome. Bacterial infections occur in approximately 14–75% of recipients in the first 3 months [70]. Up to 80% of LT recipients will develop an infection in the first year following transplantation [71]. The clinical presentation of infection is often subtle in individuals on immunosuppression, and prompt identification and treatment are needed to avoid devastating consequences [71]. A high rate of suspicion is warranted as both rejection and infection can appear similarly. Changes in mental status are often a sign of early infection.

Risk factors for postoperative infection after LT include those incurred from the donor, recipient, or intraoperative course. Donor and recipient viral status, underlying medical comorbidities, and nutritional status can all contribute. Prolonged surgery with massive blood loss, prolonged ischemia time, and violation of the gastrointestinal (GI) tract are also risk factors for nosocomial infection. Patients with a pre-transplant infection are more likely to develop a post-transplant infection [70]. Pre-operative infections can include spontaneous bacterial peritonitis (SBP), urinary tract infection (UTI), surgical site infection (SSI), pneumonia, and *Clostridioides difficile*. Common bacterial pathogens include gram-negative organisms found in the bile (Escherichia coli, Enterobacter, and Pseudomonas spp.) and gram-positive organisms (Staphylococcus aureus, coagulase-negative staphylococci, group D streptococci). Rarely, S. aureus can result in the development of toxic shock syndrome in the early postoperative period. Listeria, Nocardia, and Legionella are uncommon but significant pathogens.

Viral infections are common in immunocompromised patients after transplantation, the most important of which is cytomegalovirus (CMV). While CMV is often asymptomatic in the general population, its course can be more severe in transplant recipients. Symptoms onset about 30–50 days after LT and include fever, malaise, arthralgia, leukopenia and thrombocytopenia, hepatitis, interstitial pneumonitis, enterocolitis, and disseminated disease. Incidence of CMV infection after LT ranges from 23% to 80% [72]. About half of patients with CMV infection (positive culture, biopsy, etc.) go on to develop CMV disease (CMV infection plus organ-invasive symptoms). The biggest risk factor for CMV disease is recipient CMV-seronegative status [73]. Other risk factors include donor CMV-seropositive status, higher doses of immunosuppression, use of lymphocyte-depleting antibodies (alemtuzuman, muromonab-CD3, anti-thymocyte globulins), donor and/or recipient advanced age, HLA mismatch, immediate graft rejection by itself, impaired humoral immunity and coinfection with other herpes viruses (HSV 6 and 7) [73]. Diagnosis is made with polymerase chain reaction (PCR), though liver biopsy may be warranted [73]. Prolonged CMV infection increases the risk of chronic rejection [72].

CMV prophylaxis with oral valganciclovir or intravenous ganciclovir is warranted in seronegative recipients who receive a liver from a seropositive donor. Similarly, treatment with the above medications should begin as soon as CMV viremia (>threefold increase in serum CMV PCR) is detected and should be continued for at least 2 weeks until a documented negative CMV PCR [73]. Intravenous therapy is recommended for severe disease. Additionally, immunosuppression should be decreased if possible. Foscarnet and cidofovir are second-line agents.

Herpes simplex virus (HSV) seropositivity is present in most patients (about 75%) undergoing LT. HSV infection postoperatively is usually related to immunosuppression-induced reactivation and occurs in about 8.9% of recipients with seropositivity [74]. HSV infection usually manifests as a mild mucocutaneous oral or genital disease that responds to acyclovir treatment. However, prompt recognition is important to prevent progression to lethal disseminated disease or fulminant hepatitis with coagulopathy, disseminated intravascular coagulation, and death. Graft involvement is diagnosed by liver biopsy.

Epstein-Barr virus (EBV) infection in a transplant patient is characterized by a mononucleosis-like syndrome that differs from that observed in the normal host by the absence of a heterophil antibody response and the infrequency of pharyngitis or splenomegaly. More than 95% of patients show a previous infection pattern [75]. The clinical significance of EBV infection in an LT patient is related to its role in the pathogenesis of post-transplant lymphoproliferative diseases (PTLD), the development of which is thought to reflect the unrestricted proliferation of B cells stimulated by EBV infection. PTLD is a general term for lymphoproliferative disease and lymphoma that develops after LT and can range from benign to malignant.

Opportunistic invasive fungal infections have a cumulative incidence of 5–42% with mortality of 25–80% [69]. Host risk factors include prior colonization, a breach in mucosal barriers, and comorbid conditions such as diabetes, malnutrition, cirrhosis, or chronic kidney injury [69]. The most common fungal infections in LT recipients are in order candidiasis, aspergillosis, and cryptococcosis [69]. While studies have shown a reduction in fungal infections with prophylactic treatment with no risk of graft function, there is ongoing debate regarding resistance and side effect profile. The more common approach is to prophylactically treat high-risk recipients.

Other rare, but potentially still severe, opportunistic infections include Cryptococcus neoformans, coccidiomycosis, and Pneumocystis jirovecii. Cryptococcus can present many years after LT with altered mental status, headache, and fever. Coccidiomycosis is endemic to the southwestern United States, and individuals from this area should begin lifelong fluconazole prophylaxis. Pneumocystis jirovecii incidence has decreased since routine prophylaxis with daily low-dose oral trimethoprim/ sulfamethoxazole (TMP/SMX) for 6–12 months following LT.

Recurrent Disease

As alcohol-associated liver disease (ALD) has become a more common indication for LT in the US, especially during the COVID pandemic, there is increasing concern about allocation of organs and potential relapse. Survival after LT in patients with ALD is comparable to other indications for LT, indicating that the selection process is appropriately selective [76]. However, about 50% of those recipients return to alcohol consumption to some degree.

Primary biliary cholangitis (PBC), primary sclerosing cholangitis (PSC), and autoimmune Hepatitis (AIH) recur after LT at rates of 10.9–53%, 8.2–44.7%, and 7–42%, respectively [77]. Recurrent PSC often requires retransplantation, and the allocation policy has shifted to provide additional urgency status for patients with symptomatic recurrent PSC.

With the advent of potent nucleoside or nucleotide analogues and hepatitis B immunoglobulin (HBIG), recurrent hepatitis B virus (HBV) infection now only occurs in about 1% of recipients [78]. Recurrent hepatitis C virus (HCV) infection occurs universally after LT. About 60% have mild hepatitis, while 30% develop a more severe pattern. In patients with severe recurrent HCV, cirrhosis develops in 20% within 5 years if untreated. The advent of improved HCV medications, with almost 100% cure rates, has significantly improved the outlook for patients with HCV infection who are waiting for or have received an LT.

Conclusion

LT is a lifesaving treatment modality for patients with ESLD. The wide range of comorbidities that develop preoperatively contributes significantly to the development of postoperative complications. Aggressive use of immunosuppression is successful in preventing rejection in many cases, but therapy can be complicated by the development of life-threatening neoplasms and infections. Remarkably, no major breakthroughs in immunosuppression medications have been made over the last several decades.

Positive outcomes after LT require a multidisciplinary team approach that includes surgeons, transplant coordinators, hepatologists, and internists to maintain constant surveillance for the inevitable complications that arise. Early diagnosis with rapid treatment provides the best opportunity for disease-free survival.

References

1. Agostini C, et al. Complications in post-liver transplant patients. J Clin Med. 2023;12(19)
2. Malamon JS, et al. Reassessing the survival benefit of deceased donor liver transplantation: retrospective cohort study. Int J Surg. 2023;109(9):2714–20.
3. Jackson WE, et al. Survival benefit of living-donor liver transplant. JAMA Surg. 2022;157(10):926–32.

4. Moreno R, Berenguer M. Post-liver transplantation medical complications. Ann Hepatol. 2006;5(2):77–85.
5. Durand F, Francoz C. The future of liver transplantation for viral hepatitis. Liver Int. 2017;37(Suppl 1):130–5.
6. Brancaccio G, et al. Changing indications for liver transplant: slow decline of hepatitis viruses in Italy. Infect Dis (Lond). 2020;52(8):557–62.
7. Linares I, et al. Steatosis in liver transplantation: current limitations and future strategies. Transplantation. 2019;103(1):78–90.
8. Alqahtan SA, Brown RS. Management and risks before, during, and after liver transplant in individuals with obesity. Gastroenterol Hepatol (N Y). 2023;19(1):20–9.
9. Barone M, et al. Systematic review with meta-analysis: post-operative complications and mortality risk in liver transplant candidates with obesity. Aliment Pharmacol Ther. 2017;46(3):236–45.
10. Haque OJ, et al. Long-term outcomes of early experience in donation after circulatory death liver transplantation: outcomes at 10 years. Ann Transplant. 2021;26:e930243.
11. Morrissey PE, Monaco AP. Donation after circulatory death: current practices, ongoing challenges, and potential improvements. Transplantation. 2014;97(3):258–64.
12. Steggerda JA, et al. Higher thresholds for the utilization of steatotic allografts in liver transplantation: analysis from a U.S. national database. PLoS One. 2020;15(4):e0230995.
13. Kwon CH, et al. Safety of donors with fatty liver in liver transplantation. Transplant Proc. 2006;38(7):2106–7.
14. Croome KP, et al. American Society of Transplant Surgeons recommendations on best practices in donation after circulatory death organ procurement. Am J Transplant. 2023;23(2):171–9.
15. Hoffman JRH, et al. Consensus statement: technical standards for thoracoabdominal normothermic regional perfusion. Ann Thorac Surg. 2024;118(4):778–91.
16. Lam HD, et al. Certification training and liver transplant experience improves liver procurement outcomes: the Dutch approach. Transplantation. 2024;108(10):2093–9.
17. Walcott J, et al. Procurement-related liver injury for transplantation: an analysis of the risk factors and consequences in an Australian transplant centre. ANZ J Surg. 2021;91(12):2669–74.
18. Karakoyun R, et al. Impact of hepatic artery variations and reconstructions on the outcome of orthotopic liver transplantation. World J Surg. 2020;44(6):1954–65.
19. Ausania F, et al. Clinical impact of right accessory hepatic artery injury in deceased donor livers. J Hepatobiliary Pancreat Sci. 2012;19(6):656–60.
20. Soliman T, et al. Parenchymal liver injury in orthotopic liver transplantation. Transplantation. 2000;69(10):2079–84.
21. Shamsaeefar A, et al. Biliary reconstruction in liver transplant patients with primary sclerosing cholangitis, duct-to-duct or Roux-en-Y? Clin Transpl. 2017;31(6)
22. Nijkamp DM, et al. Surgical injuries of postmortem donor livers: incidence and impact on outcome after adult liver transplantation. Liver Transpl. 2006;12(9):1365–70.
23. Paterno F, et al. Clinical implications of donor warm and cold ischemia time in donor after circulatory death liver transplantation. Liver Transpl. 2019;25(9):1342–52.
24. Cesaretti M, et al. Cold ischemia time in liver transplantation: an overview. World J Hepatol. 2024;16(6):883–90.
25. Al-Kurd A, et al. Short recipient warm ischemia time improves outcomes in deceased donor liver transplantation. Transpl Int. 2021;34(8):1422–32.
26. Freise CE, et al. Recipient morbidity after living and deceased donor liver transplantation: findings from the A2ALL Retrospective Cohort Study. Am J Transplant. 2008;8(12):2569–79.
27. Olthoff KM, et al. Defining long-term outcomes with living donor liver transplantation in North America. Ann Surg. 2015;262(3):465–75; discussion 473–5
28. Ma KW, et al. Impact of small-for-size liver grafts on medium-term and long-term graft survival in living donor liver transplantation: a meta-analysis. World J Gastroenterol. 2019;25(36):5559–68.
29. Govil S, Reddy MS, Rela M. Has "small-for-size" reached its "sell-by" date. Transplantation. 2016;100(11):e119.

30. Matsushima H, et al. Biliary complications following split liver transplantation in adult recipients: a matched pair analysis on single-center experience. Liver Transpl. 2023;29(3):279–89.
31. Moussaoui D, et al. Early complications after liver transplantation in children and adults: are split grafts equal to each other and equal to whole livers? Pediatr Transplant. 2017;21(4)
32. Allison MG, Shanholtz CB, Sachdeva A. Hematological issues in liver disease. Crit Care Clin. 2016;32(3):385–96.
33. Saracoglu A, Saracoglu KT. Coagulopathy during liver transplantation. J Anaesthesiol Clin Pharmacol. 2018;34(3):289–95.
34. Stewart E, et al. Viscoelastic management of coagulopathy during the perioperative period of liver transplantation. Semin Thromb Hemost. 2023;49(2):119–33.
35. Algarni AA, Mourad MM, Bramhall SR. Anticoagulation and antiplatelets as prophylaxis for hepatic artery thrombosis after liver transplantation. World J Hepatol. 2015;7(9):1238–43.
36. Craig EV, Heller MT. Complications of liver transplant. Abdom Radiol (NY). 2021;46(1):43–67.
37. Kim HB. Urgent revascularization for hepatic artery thrombosis: maybe good for the few, definitely good for the many. Liver Transpl. 2010;16(7):812–4.
38. Lynch JM, et al. Hepatic artery thrombectomy after orthotopic liver transplantation: a stent retriever and/or aspiration-guided catheter approach. J Vasc Interv Radiol. 2024;35(10):1519–24.
39. Li T, et al. Intra-arterial thrombolysis for early hepatic artery thrombosis after liver transplantation. World J Clin Cases. 2021;9(7):1592–9.
40. Buchholz BM, et al. Retransplantation in late hepatic artery thrombosis: graft access and transplant outcome. Transplant Direct. 2017;3(8):e186.
41. Mourad MM, et al. Etiology and management of hepatic artery thrombosis after adult liver transplantation. Liver Transpl. 2014;20(6):713–23.
42. Cizman Z, Saad W. Transplant hepatic artery complications. Tech Vasc Interv Radiol. 2023;26(4):100923.
43. Miranda LE, et al. Dissection of the hepatic artery: a rare cause of late ischemia after liver transplant. Exp Clin Transplant. 2020;18(5):641–4.
44. Bhangui P, et al. Current management of portal vein thrombosis in liver transplantation. Int J Surg. 2020;82S:122–7.
45. Yerdel MA, et al. Portal vein thrombosis in adults undergoing liver transplantation: risk factors, screening, management, and outcome. Transplantation. 2000;69(9):1873–81.
46. Xue Z, et al. Analysis of portal vein thrombosis after liver transplantation. ANZ J Surg. 2019;89(9):1075–9.
47. Kim KS, et al. Stent insertion and balloon angioplasty for portal vein stenosis after liver transplantation: long-term follow-up results. Diagn Interv Radiol. 2019;25(3):231–7.
48. Piardi T, et al. Vascular complications following liver transplantation: a literature review of advances in 2015. World J Hepatol. 2016;8(1):36–57.
49. Schmitz V, et al. Different cava reconstruction techniques in liver transplantation: piggyback versus cava resection. Hepatobiliary Pancreat Dis Int. 2014;13(3):242–9.
50. Koc S, et al. Hepatic venous outflow obstruction after living-donor liver transplant: single center experience. Exp Clin Transplant. 2021;19(8):832–41.
51. Sambommatsu Y, et al. Hepatic venous outflow obstruction after adult living donor liver transplantation. Liver Transpl. 2023;29(12):1292–303.
52. Naidu SG, et al. Interventional radiology management of adult liver transplant complications. Radiographics. 2022;42(6):1705–23.
53. Shaker TM, et al. Which cava anastomotic techniques are optimal regarding immediate and short-term outcomes after liver transplantation: a systematic review of the literature and expert panel recommendations. Clin Transpl. 2022;36(10):e14681.
54. Bonnel AR, Bunchorntavakul C, Rajender Reddy K. Transjugular intrahepatic portosystemic shunts in liver transplant recipients. Liver Transpl. 2014;20(2):130–9.
55. Gheorghe, G., et al., Biliary and vascular complications after liver transplantation-from diagnosis to treatment. Medicina (Kaunas), 2023. 59(5).

56. Kohli DR, et al. American Society for Gastrointestinal Endoscopy guideline on management of post-liver transplant biliary strictures: summary and recommendations. Gastrointest Endosc. 2023;97(4):607–14.
57. de Vries Y, von Meijenfeldt FA, Porte RJ. Post-transplant cholangiopathy: classification, pathogenesis, and preventive strategies. Biochim Biophys Acta Mol basis Dis. 2018;1864(4 Pt B):1507–15.
58. Zulfiqar M, et al. Imaging of ischemic cholangiopathy following donation after circulatory death liver transplant. Radiographics. 2024;44(11):e240031.
59. Giesbrandt KJ, et al. Radiologic characterization of ischemic cholangiopathy in donation-after-cardiac-death liver transplants and correlation with clinical outcomes. AJR Am J Roentgenol. 2015;205(5):976–84.
60. Kok B, Dong V, Karvellas CJ. Graft dysfunction and management in liver transplantation. Crit Care Clin. 2019;35(1):117–33.
61. Pomposelli JJ, et al. Patterns of early allograft dysfunction in adult live donor liver transplantation: the A2ALL experience. Transplantation. 2016;100(7):1490–9.
62. Hartog H, Hann A, Perera M. Primary nonfunction of the liver allograft. Transplantation. 2022;106(1):117–28.
63. Montano-Loza AJ, et al. Liver transplantation immunology: immunosuppression, rejection, and immunomodulation. J Hepatol. 2023;78(6):1199–215.
64. Esquivel CO, et al. Liver rejection and its differentiation from other causes of graft dysfunction. Semin Liver Dis. 1985;5(4):369–74.
65. Dogan N, et al. Acute allograft rejection in liver transplant recipients: incidence, risk factors, treatment success, and impact on graft failure. J Int Med Res. 2018;46(9):3979–90.
66. Charlton M, et al. International liver transplantation society consensus statement on immunosuppression in liver transplant recipients. Transplantation. 2018;102(5):727–43.
67. Calne RY. Immunosuppression in liver transplantation. N Engl J Med. 1994;331(17):1154–5.
68. Demetris AJ, et al. The liver allograft, chronic (ductopenic) rejection, and microchimerism: what can they teach us? Transplant Proc. 1995;27(1):67–70.
69. Senoner T, et al. Invasive fungal infections after liver transplantation. J Clin Med. 2023;12(9)
70. Heldman MR, et al. Pre- and post-transplant bacterial infections in liver transplant recipients. Transpl Infect Dis. 2019;21(5):e13152.
71. Ayvazoglu Soy EH, et al. Early postoperative infections after liver transplant. Exp Clin Transplant. 2018;16 Suppl 1:145–8.
72. Oldakowska-Jedynak U, et al. Cytomegalovirus infection as a common complication following liver transplantation. Transplant Proc. 2003;35(6):2295–7.
73. Lizaola-Mayo BC, Rodriguez EA. Cytomegalovirus infection after liver transplantation. World J Transplant. 2020;10(7):183–90.
74. Arana C, et al. Primary herpes simplex virus type 1 infection with acute liver failure in solid organ transplantation: report of three cases and review. IDCases. 2022;28:e01485.
75. Okamoto T, et al. Management of Epstein-Barr virus infection and post-transplant lymphoproliferative disorder in pediatric liver transplantation. J Clin Med. 2022;11(8)
76. Terrault NA, et al. Liver transplantation 2023: status report, current and future challenges. Clin Gastroenterol Hepatol. 2023;21(8):2150–66.
77. Tanaka A, et al. Recurrence of disease following organ transplantation in autoimmune liver disease and systemic lupus erythematosus. Cell Immunol. 2020;347:104021.
78. Li MS, et al. The strategy and efficacy of prophylaxis against hepatitis B virus recurrence after liver transplantation for HBV-related diseases in the era of potent nucleos(t)ide analogues: a meta-analysis. J Dig Dis. 2021;22(2):91–101.

Infection After Liver Transplantation

24

Anita R. Modi and Christine E. Koval

Introduction

Infections are a leading cause of morbidity and mortality following liver transplantation (LT), affecting over 45% of recipients in the first year with 20–50% attributable mortality [1–3]. The post-transplantation timeline of infection risk incorporates early postoperative factors, anatomic complications, intensity of immunosuppression, and epidemiologic exposures (Table 24.1) [4]. Early consultation with Transplant Infectious Diseases specialists improves outcomes and optimizes antimicrobial use [5, 6]. Table 24.2 highlights an approach to diagnosis and management of suspected infections in the early, intermediate, and late post-LT periods. Table 24.3 provides a summary of common pathogens responsible for infections in liver transplant recipients (LTRs).

A. R. Modi · C. E. Koval (✉)
Cleveland Clinic Foundation, Cleveland, OH, USA
e-mail: modia@ccf.org; KOVALC@ccf.org

B. Eghtesad et al. (eds.), *Liver Transplantation*,
https://doi.org/10.1007/978-3-032-07072-2_24

Table 24.1 Timeline of infectious considerations and complications in the pre- and post-liver transplantation settings

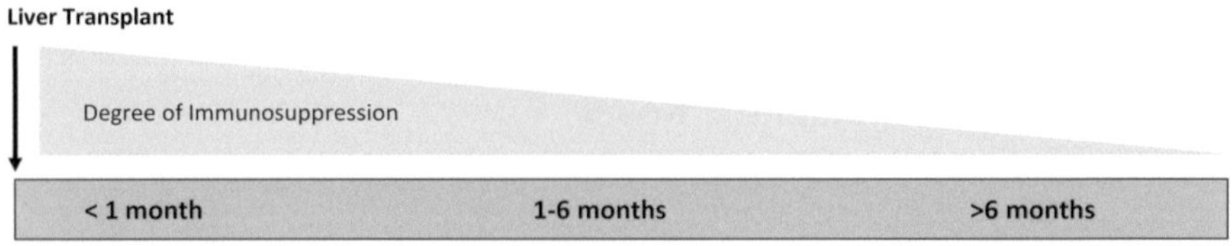

Early Post-OLT	Intermediate Post-OLT	Late Post-OLT
Nosocomial infections Line infection Pneumonia Urinary tract infection *Clostridium difficile* **Surgical infections** Anastomotic leaks Abdominal wounds **Organisms:** *Candida* spp. Gram negative bacilli *Enterococcus* spp. *Staphylococcus* spp. **Donor-derived infections**	**Persisting biliary complications** *Candida* spp., Enteric gram negatives, *Enterococcus* spp. **Opportunistic infections** Nocardiosis Listeriosis Aspergillosis Cryptococcosis Endemic fungal mycoses *Pneumocystis jirovecii* pneumonia (PJP) Strongyloidiasis Toxoplasmosis **Reactivation of latent infections** Herpes viruses: CMV, HSV, VZV, EBV, HHV6/7 Adenovirus Tuberculosis Chagas	**Community-acquired infections** Pneumonia Respiratory viral infection Sexually transmitted disease Urinary tract infection **Environmental fungal infections** Aspergillosis Cryptococcosis Endemic fungal mycoses **Late reactivation of viral infections** CMV Polyoma viruses (JC) **Recurrent disease-related infections** Cholangitis, HBV **Splenectomy-related infections** Pneumococcus, Meningococcus Haemophilus

Adapted from "Infection in the Renal Transplant Recipient" [4]

Table 24.2 Approach to the liver transplant recipient with suspected infection, stratified by period of risk

	Early Post-OLT	Intermediate Post-OLT	Late Post-OLT
History and physical exam data	Pre-transplantation recipient exposures, infections, immunosuppression Operative course Induction immunosuppression agent Evaluation of catheters, drains Evaluation of surgical incision	Experiences with rejection and augmented immunosuppression Ongoing antibiotic prophylaxis Biliary complications Post-discharge exposures	Experiences with rejection and augmented immunosuppression Ongoing antibiotic prophylaxis Complications of disease recurrence Updated vaccine history Environmental exposures
Microbiological data	Pre-transplantation recipient serologies and colonization Blood, urine, respiratory specimen culture data *Clostridioides difficile* toxin PCR and EIA testing Donor serologies and culture data	CMV DNA PCR Specimen collection tailored to suspected syndrome, potentially meriting invasive procedure (ie. bronchoscopy, colonoscopy)	CMV DNA PCR Specimen collection tailored to suspected syndrome (ie. nasopharyngeal swab to obtain respiratory pathogen panel)

(continued)

Table 24.2 (continued)

	Early Post-OLT	Intermediate Post-OLT	Late Post-OLT
Imaging data	Abdominal ultrasound to assess hepatic vasculature Abdominal computed tomography Chest computed tomography	Imaging tailored to suspected syndrome (ie. chest x-ray)	Imaging tailored to suspected syndrome (ie. chest x-ray)
Empiric antibiotic selection	Coverage of intraabdominal pathogens (*Streptococcus* spp., *Enterococcus* spp., gram-negative and anaerobic flora), *Candida* spp., and skin flora including *Staphylococcus aureus*	Coverage of pathogens tailored to suspected syndrome and recipient colonization history	Coverage of community-acquired pathogens tailored to suspected syndrome (ie. *Streptococcus pneumoniae*, *Haemophilus influenzae*, atypical bacteria with respiratory tract disease)

Table 24.3 Common pathogens responsible for infection in the liver transplant recipient

	Onset Post-LT Period	Manifestations	Diagnosis	Treatment	Risk/Prevention
Bacteria					
Clostridioides difficile	Early	Diarrhea Leukocytosis Toxic megacolon	Stool C. difficile PCR and/ or toxin by EIA Colonoscopy: pseudomembranous colitis	Oral vancomycin Fidaxomicin Metronidazole	Proper hand hygiene Contact precautions Minimizing unneeded antibiotics
Diarrheal bacteria Salmonella spp., Shigella spp., E. coli, Campylobacter spp., Yersinia spp., Listeria spp.	Late	Diarrhea Vomiting Abdominal pain Rare toxin-mediated angiopathy	Stool culture or PCR	Varies by organism	Avoid unpasteurized dairy, raw or undercooked foods, deli meats
Enterococcus E. faecalis E. faecium (VRE)	Early Intermediate	Abdominal: post-op, bile leak, stricture Blood Urine	Culture of fluid collections Blood cultures	E. faecalis: ampicillin E. faecium: daptomycin, linezolid, vancomycin	Perioperative antibiotics If VRE colonized or risk: Daptomycin or linezolid
Gram negative bacilli Enteric: E. coli, Klebsiella spp., Enterobacter spp., Citrobacter spp. Non-enteric: Pseudomonas spp., Acinetobacter spp., Stenotrophomonas spp.	Early	Abdominal: post-op, bile leak Blood: any source (abdomen), CVCs Lungs: pneumonia Urine	Culture of fluid collections Blood cultures Urine cultures Respiratory cultures	Empiric: beta-lactam, cephalosporin Targeted: ESBL, CRE, CRAB, MDR Pseudomonas spp., Stenotrophomonas spp.	Perioperative antibiotics: coverage for enteric organisms Target drug resistance if colonized (ESBL, CRE)

Table 24.3 (continued)

	Onset Post-LT Period	Manifestations	Diagnosis	Treatment	Risk/Prevention
Nocardia N. brasiliensis N. asteroides	Intermediate Late	Respiratory symptoms Lung nodules, cavities, consolidations Brain abscess(es) Skin lesions	Respiratory cultures Blood cultures Tissue biopsy	Empiric: TMP/SMX 10–20 mg/kg daily +1–2 additional drugs	Wear gloves in soil Avoid outdoor dust, decaying vegetation
Tuberculosis	Early (DD) Intermediate	Cavitary, nodular lung consolidations Lymphadenopathy, adenitis Granulomatous liver disease Meningitis, CNS tuberculomas Disseminated, miliary disease, marrow	Respiratory samples: AFB stain, culture, PCR AFB blood cultures Tissue stains, culture, PCR	Traditional four-drug therapy, including cautious use of rifamycin with CNIs	Recipient screening: risk factors, PPD, or TB interferon gamma release assay Donor risk assessment
Fungi (mold, yeast)					
Aspergillus A. fumigatus, A.niger, A. terreus, A. calidoustus, A. versicolor	Early Intermediate Late	Lung nodules, cavities, consolidation Brain lesions Skin lesions Sinusitis Angioinvasive hemorrhagic lesions	Respiratory samples: Culture, Galactomannan, PCR Serum galactomannan Tissue biopsy: fungal stain	Drug of choice: Voriconazole Others: Isavuconazole Posaconazole Amphotericin	Minimize exposure to construction sites, marijuana, gardening/landscaping, farming (grain storage), decomposing vegetation (compost)

(continued)

Table 24.3 (continued)

	Onset Post-LT Period	Manifestations	Diagnosis	Treatment	Risk/Prevention
Candida C. auris, C. albicans, C. glabrata C. krusei, C. lusitaniae C. parapsilosis, C. tropicalis	Early Intermediate	Abdominal- post-op, bile leak, stricture Blood- central venous catheters	Culture of fluid collections Blood cultures	Empiric: Echinocandin If sensitive: Fluconazole Drainage, washout Remove CVC	Prophylaxis high risk: Post-LT dialysis, op time >10 h, retransplant, return OR, PRBCs> 20 units, bile leak Echinocandin or azole
Cryptococcus C. neoformans C. gattii	Early (DD) Intermediate	Respiratory symptoms Lung nodules or infiltrates Meningitis: headache, altered sensorium Skin lesions, cellulitis	Serum cryptococcal antigen CSF cryptococcal antigen CSF opening pressure	CNS: Amphotericin + 5FC Disseminated: Amphotericin Localized: Fluconazole	Minimize exposure to bird droppings, soil, decaying wood
Endemic molds Blastomyces spp. (midwest) Coccidioides spp. (desert southwest) Histoplasma spp. (Great Lakes, Ohio and St Lawrence River Valleys)	Early (DD) Intermediate Late	Febrile illness Acute pneumonia, lung nodules Skin lesions Organ involvement Subacute meningitis	Serum, urine antigen (histo, blasto) Tissue biopsy (fungal stain) Blood cultures Serologies (coccidiomycosis)	Disseminated: amphotericin Localized: itraconazole, posaconazole fluconazole (coccidioides)	Minimize exposure to dusty soil with bird or bat droppings, construction sites, landscaping, cleaning chicken coops, caving
Pneumocystis jirovecii (PJP)	Intermediate Late	Cough, shortness of breath, hypoxia Diffuse ground glass opacities	Respiratory samples PJP PCR Fungal stain	Drug of choice: TMP/SMX 10–20 mg/kg daily	Prophylaxis: 6–12 m TMP/SMX DS MWF or SS daily (alternatives: inhaled pentamidine, atovaquone, dapsone)

Table 24.3 (continued)

	Onset Post-LT Period	Manifestations	Diagnosis	Treatment	Risk/Prevention
Viral					
CMV (Cytomegalovirus) HR:HighRiskCMVD+/R- IR: Intermediate Risk CMV R+ LR:LowriskCMVD-/R-	Intermediate Late	Fever, flu like illness Neutropenia Hepatitis, colitis, pneumonitis	Serum/blood CMV DNA Tissue biopsy: viral inclusions, immunohistochemical stain	Drug of Choice: Valganciclovir Ganciclovir Others: Foscarnet, Maribavir Letermovir	Prophylaxis Valganciclovir, then CMV DNA monitoring Preemptive CMV DNA weekly, treat at threshold
EBV (Ebstein Barr virus) HR:HighRiskEBVD+/R- IR: Intermediate Risk EBV R+ LR:LowriskEBVD-/R-	Intermediate Late	Symptoms of lymphoproliferative disorder Fever, lymphadenopathy, pleural effusions, mass lesions (Mononucleosis in low risk recipients)	Tissue biopsy EBV DNA may be supportive	Oncology referral Chemotherapy Rituximab	Monitor EBV DNA, reduce immunosuppression
HSV (Herpes simplex virus 1&2)	Intermediate Late	Vesicular skin lesions Oral lesions/ulcers Rarely disseminated disease: hepatitis, encephalitis, meningitis Rarely donor derived: hepatitis	Lesion: HSV PCR Blood, CSF: HSV PCR Tissue biopsy: inclusions, immunohistochemical stain	Valacyclovir Famciclovir Intravenous acyclovir	Prevention Acyclovir if not receiving valganciclovir for CMV

(continued)

Table 24.3 (continued)

	Onset Post-LT Period	Manifestations	Diagnosis	Treatment	Risk/Prevention
VZV (Varicella zoster virus)	Intermediate	Dermatomal rash Often with lesions outside dermatome Rare: Encephalitis, pneumonitis, hepatitis	VZV PCR from lesion VZV PCR blood CSF: VZV PCR or IgG	Valacyclovir Famciclovir Intravenous acyclovir	Screen LT candidates: VZV IgG VZV IgG negative: Zostavax VZV IgG positive: Shingrix
Respiratory viruses Adenovirus, Influenza, RSV SARS-CoV2, Parainfluenza Human metapneumovirus Rhinovirus	Early (DD) Intermediate Late	Fever Headache, myalgias Diarrhea Lobar or diffuse ground glass opacities ARDS	Nasal, sputum, BAL: PCR Blood: adenovirus PCR	Influenza: Oseltamavir SARS-CoV-2: Remdesivir Molnupiravir (Paxlovid caution) RSV: rarely ribavirin	Hand hygiene, masking, distance SARS-CoV-2 vaccine Influenza vaccine; seasonal RSV vaccine (over age 60 years)
Parasites					
Toxoplasma gondii	Early (DD) Intermediate	Fevers Granulomatous liver disease Cystic brain lesions Pulmonary infiltrates	Serum toxoplasma PCR CSF toxoplasma PCR Tissue biopsy	Pyrimethamine + Sulfadiazine Or TMP/SMX	TMP/SMX (as PJP prophylaxis) Avoid cat litter (or change daily) Ensure fully cooked meat (pork)
Strongyloides	Early (DD) Intermediate	Hyperinfestation syndrome Abdominal pain Pulmonary infiltrates Enteric gram negative bacteremia	Serum: Strongyloides IgG Stool: ova, parasite stain BAL cytology Tissue stain	Ivermectin	Screen donors and recipients pre-transplant: Strongyloides IgG

PCR polymerase chain reaction, *EIA* enzyme immunoassay, *VRE* vancomycin-resistant *Enterococcus*, *CVC* central venous catheter, *ESBL* extended-spectrum beta-lactamase, *CRE* carbapenem-resistant enterobacteriaceae, *CRAB* carbapenem-resistant Acinetobacter baumannii, *MDR* multidrug resistant, *BAL* bronchoalveolar lavage, *TMP/SMX* trimethoprim-sulfamethoxazole, *DD* donor-derived, *CNS* central nervous system, *AFB* acid-fast bacilli, *TB* tuberculosis, *LT* liver transplantation, *OR* operating room, *pRBCs* packed red blood cells, *DS* double strength, *SS* single strength, *MWF* Monday/Wednesday/Friday, *D* donor, *R* recipient, *CSF* cerebrospinal fluid, *RSV* respiratory syncytial virus, *ARDS* acute respiratory distress syndrome

Early Post-transplantation Infections (First 30 Days)

Early infections are predominantly mediated by bacteria and fungi related to donor or recipient colonization or nosocomial acquisition.

Risk Factors for Early Post-transplantation Infections

Pre-transplantation cirrhosis results in renal impairment, frequent hospitalizations, and intensive care which increase infection risk and exposure to multidrug-resistant (MDR) organisms [1, 7]. Though rare, early cryptococcosis and aspergillosis can present early post-transplantation in LTRs with advanced cirrhosis or with pre-LT immunosuppression [8, 9].

Glucocorticoids affect innate immunity, glucose control, and wound healing. Lymphocyte-depleting therapies such as anti-thymocyte globulin limit steroid exposure and delay calcineurin inhibitors (CNIs) and increase risk for viral and other opportunistic infections [10].

Nosocomial Infections

Early bacterial infections occur in 30–45% of LTRs, mostly attributable to biliary and intestinal manipulation and invasive procedures related to hospitalization [11, 12]. Bloodstream infections (BSIs) occur in 12–25% of LTRs, primarily due to intra-abdominal sources, followed by central venous catheters, pulmonary, and urinary sources [13–15]. The most common organisms are *Enterobacteriaceae*, *Enterococcus,* and *Staphylococcus* spp., which may indicate their source [13–15].

Pneumonia occurs in up to 15–25% of LTRs, with risk factors including prolonged mechanical ventilation, noninfectious pulmonary issues (atelectasis, effusion), and re-transplantation. Most are due to nosocomial and enteric gram-negative bacteria [16–18]. Early urinary tract infections (UTIs) affect less than 10% of LTRs and are associated with female sex, diabetes, older age, and urinary catheters [11, 19]. *Clostridium difficile* colitis occurs in 3–7% of LTRs, three-fold greater than in the general hospitalized population, and is associated with increased septic shock and mortality [20–22].

Surgical Site Infections

Surgical infections, primarily mediated by bacteria and *Candida* spp., affect 7–27% of LTRs, with variability attributed to surgical practice [23]. Perioperative antibiotics, post-operative prophylaxis, and early corrective interventions mitigate this risk.

Cholangitis and bilomas emerge from biliary anastomotic leaks, strictures, stent occlusions, or ischemic cholangiopathy related to hepatic artery thrombosis and stenosis. Living donor LT (LDLT) requires smaller ductal and vascular anastomoses, posing a greater risk for these complications [24]. Most biliary infections are due to

Enterococcus spp., enteric gram-negative bacteria, and *Candida* spp. MDR isolates account for over half of cholangitis-related BSIs [25, 26]. Non-*albicans Candida* spp. remains highly prevalent post-LT, meriting empiric echinocandins when candidiasis is suspected [27, 28]. Other intra-abdominal infections, including peritonitis, abscesses, and infected hematomas, may represent extensions of biliary complications, operative contamination, or consequences of pre-LT peritonitis.

Incisional infections manifest with erythema, induration, and drainage and can involve enteric or skin flora. While local debridement and antibiotics usually suffice, extension into the underlying fascia and peritoneum should be considered in those with bacteremia [26].

Donor-Derived Infections

Most donor-derived infections (DDIs) are predicted by routine donor screening and are successfully managed with recipient treatment and prevention protocols. These include infections such as syphilis, cytomegalovirus (CMV), hepatitis, and certain parasites [29, 30]. Unanticipated DDIs occur in 0.1–0.2%, are mostly bacterial or fungal and less commonly viruses or parasites [30]. Unexplained fevers, altered sensorium, or other signs of occult infection should prompt review of donor history and data [31]. When DDI is highly suspected or diagnosed, the organ procurement organization should be notified expediently.

Intermediate Post-transplantation Infections (Months 1–6)

The intermediate post-transplantation period is characterized by impaired cell-mediated immunity. Infections are usually due to environmental and opportunistic pathogens to which the LTR is exposed following the index hospitalization, or which reactivate in the context of immunosuppression.

Risk Factors for Intermediate Post-transplantation Infections

Treatment of allograft rejection leads to additional immunosuppression, including reinduction with steroids and lymphodepleting agents, or augmentation of maintenance agents. Ongoing mechanical and ischemic biliary complications extend the risk for bacterial and yeast infections. Later donor-derived infections may manifest in this period.

Atypical Bacterial Infections

Nocardia

Nocardiosis occurs in less than 1–3.5% of LTRs, mostly within the first year [33–35]. Nocardia is a soil-borne organism introduced by inhalation of dust or direct inoculation through the skin. Infection with *Nocardia* spp. usually manifests with respiratory disease, though 15–30% of patients face dissemination to skin, brain, or other sites [33, 34]. Risk factors include high-dose prednisone, high median CNI level in 30 days, and recent CMV disease [34]. Trimethoprim-sulfamethoxazole (TMP/SMX) is the preferred treatment and does not reliably prevent nocardiosis at prophylactic doses [34–36]. Attributable 12-month mortality ranges from 11% to 17%; most cases are effectively cured [34, 37].

Fungal Infections

Invasive Aspergillosis

Less than 1% of LTRs face aspergillosis, with median presentation in the intermediate period [38–42]. It presents with pulmonary disease and disseminates to the central nervous system (CNS) in up to 42% of LTRs [38, 39]. Fever may be absent [32]. Chest imaging may display ground glass opacities, nodules, cavitary, or mass-like consolidations and is less likely to feature the "halo" or "air-crescent" signs seen in stem cell transplant recipients [38]. A presumptive diagnosis is made with culture, galactomannan antigen >1.0, or Aspergillus polymerase chain reaction (PCR) detection of respiratory specimens with supportive imaging findings. A definitive diagnosis is made with characteristic pathology on tissue biopsy with culture or Aspergillus PCR detection [43]. Risk factors include recent CMV or respiratory viral infection (RVI), fulminant hepatitis, re-transplantation, and post-LT dialysis [38, 42]. Voriconazole is the drug of choice, though alternatives include posaconazole, isavuconazole, and amphotericin [41, 42, 44]. All azoles will inhibit CNI metabolism, meriting empiric CNI dose adjustments and monitoring [41]. Overall survival has improved in the extended spectrum azole era [39]. However, early onset disease and CNS involvement are associated with increased mortality [38, 39].

Cryptococcus

Cryptococcosis occurs in less than 1–2.8% of LTRs and is the most common cause of meningitis in this population [45]. Inhalation of spores leads to pneumonia or pulmonary nodules with dissemination, primarily to the CNS, in over 50% of cases [8, 45]. Skin findings, including papules, nodules, cellulitis, or ulcers, represent disseminated disease in 70% of cases [46]. Meningitis often presents subacutely with headache, fever, and altered sensorium [47]. A likely diagnosis can be made with a serum cryptococcal antigen, and a lumbar puncture (LP) is required for definitive diagnosis and to measure and manage intracranial pressure. LTRs with cryptococcosis at other sites merit LP to assess for occult CNS involvement [48]. Amphotericin is indicated for disseminated infection. Fluconazole is indicated for subsequent maintenance therapy and for mild to moderate pulmonary disease [45, 48]. Reduction of immunosuppression can lead to immune reconstitution effects resembling worsening infection.

Endemic Mycoses

Endemic mycoses (*Histoplasma*, *Blastomyces*, and *Coccidioides* spp.) typically present as pulmonary disease with potential dissemination to other organs, including skin and CNS, following inhalation of airborne conidia [49]. These infections are uncommon, with most linked to environmental exposures, even in endemic areas [50, 51]. Granulomas seen on histopathology may be absent or poorly formed in solid organ transplant recipients (SOTRs), though characteristic yeast may be identified on stain. While mild or localized infection may be treated with azoles, severe disease merits amphotericin followed by prolonged azole therapy [49].

Histoplasmosis typically occurs around the Ohio, Mississippi, and St. Lawrence River Basins [52]. Acute infection can present as a community-acquired pneumonia, and pulmonary findings may be subtle with nodules, cavities, or lymphadenitis. Disseminated disease occurs in over 80% of cases and presents with fever, fungemia, and involvement of almost any organ, namely, bone marrow, liver, lymph nodes, skin, and spleen [49, 53]. Detection of *Histoplasma* antigen in urine or blood is a sensitive diagnostic method [49, 53].

Blastomycosis is endemic to the Great Lakes, the South Central states, and the upper Midwest [52]. It presents with pneumonia, cavitary disease, or even acute respiratory distress syndrome [54]. Disseminated disease involving the skin and bone occurs in up to 40% of SOTRs [49, 54]. Characteristic skin findings include often painful, verrucous, irregular, and violaceous lesions. Detection of urine or serum *Blastomyces* antigen may be diagnostic and cross-reacts with *Histoplasma* antigen [49].

Coccidiomycosis is endemic to arid climates of the southwestern US and parts of Central America, manifesting with a range of acute or chronic pulmonary pathologies with dissemination to skin, bone, joints, or CNS. Risk factors include pre-transplantation infection, positive *Coccidioides* spp. serologies, and augmented immunosuppression [55, 56]. Post-LT prophylaxis is merited in those residing in endemic regions, lengthened in those with evidence of latent infection on screening [57]. False-negative serologic tests may obscure the diagnosis in SOTRs, though sensitivity improves with the use of multiple tests serially. Sputum, blood, and urine fungal cultures, nucleic acid testing, or tissue staining may help establish a diagnosis [49].

Pneumocystis jirovecii

With prophylaxis, *Pneumocystis jirovecii* pneumonia (PJP) is rare. Prophylaxis is recommended for 6–12 months in LTRs [58]. Early PJP is often due to prophylaxis non-adherence and late PJP to CMV infection, age >65 years, and rejection [59–61]. Alternatives to TMP/SMX for patients with sulfa allergies include inhaled pentamidine, atovaquone, or dapsone. Dapsone can cause methemoglobinemia and hemolytic anemia in SOTRs even with normal G6PD levels [62, 63].

PJP presents with fever, hypoxia, shortness of breath, dry cough, and interstitial pulmonary infiltrates. SOTRs demonstrate low organism burden, greater acuity, and higher mortality than patients with acquired immunodeficiency syndrome (AIDS) [61, 64]. TMP/SMX is the recommended treatment. Desensitization or rechallenge may be appropriate for those with morbilliform rash or other intolerances [65]. However, those with a history of a severe T-cell-mediated reaction (i.e., Stevens–Johnson syndrome) require alternative agents. Adjunctive glucocorticoids in SOTRs with PJP remain controversial and without clear benefit [58, 60].

Viral Infections

Herpes Viruses

Herpes viruses (i.e., herpes simplex virus [HSV], varicella zoster virus [VZV], Epstein-Barr virus [EBV], and CMV) remain latent in host cells after primary infection. Reactivated or de novo herpes virus infections occur within months of LT and can have immunomodulatory effects leading to increased risk for other infections and malignancy [66–68].

CMV presents as an asymptomatic viremia, flu-like syndrome, or tissue-invasive disease (mostly hepatitis or colitis) in LTRs. CMV risk is highest in CMV seronegative recipients of a CMV seropositive donor (CMV IgG D+/R−). Recipients with existing immunologic control (CMV IgG R+) are at lower risk of CMV, primarily from reactivation. Preventive strategies include antiviral prophylaxis during peak immunosuppression and preemptive molecular monitoring with antiviral initiation at a serum or blood CMV DNA cutoff [69]. The preemptive strategy can be equally effective at CMV prevention compared to prophylaxis in CMV D+/R- LTRs [70]. A hybrid approach involving molecular monitoring after an initial period of prophylaxis is commonly used [67, 71]. CMV management includes antiviral therapy and reasonable reductions of immunosuppression. Ganciclovir and its prodrug valganciclovir are first line choices for viremia and disease, but risk cytopenias. Maribavir is effective in two-thirds of those with ganciclovir resistant and refractory CMV [72].

Other reactivated herpesviruses, such as HSV and VZV, frequently manifest with limited, local vesicular lesions and rarely result in hepatitis of the allograft and/or fatal, disseminated disease [73, 74]. VZV vaccination and antivirals are recommended to prevent and treat the disease [75]. EBV DNA monitoring of high-risk LTRs screens for lymphoproliferative disorders.

Late Post-transplantation Infections (After 6 Months)

If free of rejection, maintenance immunosuppression is typically reduced in the late post-LT period. Most programs stop PJP prophylaxis at 6–12 months, and most LTRs will have developed effective immunologic control of CMV and other herpes viruses. Vaccinations, deferred during earlier periods, can be resumed.

Risk Factors for Late Post-transplantation Infections

The incidence of infection in this period is markedly diminished compared to earlier periods [76]. Infections in the late period are generally attributed to new exposures in the community, through travel, outdoor activities, animal contacts, or dietary indiscretions [10].

Patients with persisting or enhanced need for immunosuppression, such as those with repeated episodes of rejection and those with recurrent autoimmune hepatitis of the allograft, should be closely monitored for opportunistic infection risk and may merit extended PJP prophylaxis and CMV monitoring [10, 77].

LDLT recipients may undergo splenectomy to manage small-for-size grafts, leading to risk for infections with encapsulated organisms (i.e., pneumococcus and meningococcus) and certain parasitic infections (i.e., babesiosis). Vaccinations against encapsulated organisms and tick prevention in regions endemic for *Babesia* spp. should be recommended.

Bacterial Infections

Community-acquired and aspiration-related pneumonias account for about 25% of late infections in SOTRs, typically due to *Streptococcus pneumoniae*, *Hemophilus influenzae*, and *Staphylococcus aureus*, atypical bacteria (i.e., *Legionella* spp., *Mycoplasma* spp.), or enteric flora [76].

Urinary tract, skin/soft tissue, and abdominal infections are the next most frequent [76]. Enteritis due to *Salmonella* spp. and *Escherichia coli* may arise from unpasteurized milk, raw flour, and undercooked eggs.

Cholangitis or infected bilomas may occur following recurrence of cholestatic liver diseases or residual cholangiopathy [78–80]. Elevated hepatobiliary enzymes may indicate cholangitis, warranting imaging studies, cholangiograms, and directed antibiotics.

Fungal Infections

All previously described fungal infections may present in the late post-LT period, depending on exposure risk, inoculum, and degree of immunosuppression. Presentation of community-acquired pneumonia or undifferentiated febrile illness should elicit evaluation for fungal exposure (gardening, farming, cleaning chicken coops, demolition or construction work, caving).

Viral Infections

Community-Acquired Respiratory Viruses

RVIs may present in any period and are commonly community-acquired and occur after the index hospitalization. Some RVIs have a predilection for winter months (influenza, RSV), while others manifest throughout the year (coronaviruses, human metapneumovirus, parainfluenza, adenovirus, rhinovirus). Some RVIs progress to pneumonia or bronchiolitis in SOTRs, resulting in hospitalization [81]. However, most are successfully managed with supportive care alone. Oseltamivir for influenza is recommended, ideally given within 48 h of symptom onset, and may prevent progression to intensive care [82]. Prolonged viral shedding occurs in SOTRs, and molecular detection may persist for months after the resolved infection. Seasonal influenza vaccination reduces risk for pneumonia and ICU admission [82]. In 2023, two vaccines against RSV were approved for use in older adults to prevent pneumonia, although these have not been studied in SOTRs.

Outcomes from SARS-CoV-2 infections have improved since 2020, when 28-day mortality in LTRs was 13–14% [83, 84]. Vaccination, previous infection, early treatment, and viral evolution have led to improved outcomes with more recent mortality estimates at 1% [83]. Serologic response to SARS-CoV-2 vaccination is blunted in the setting of immunosuppression; thus, LTRs merit additional doses [85, 86]. Early antiviral use of agents such as remdesivir and molnupiravir may ameliorate symptoms and improve outcomes. Nirmatrelvir/ritonavir drastically inhibits CNI metabolism and will result in CNI toxicity if dosing is not reduced [87].

Conclusion

Infections are a significant cause of morbidity and mortality after LT, with infection risk determined by epidemiological exposures and net state of immunosuppression. Understanding the original indication for transplantation, infection history, operative course, and time from transplantation, as well as the post-transplantation environment, can inform screening, prevention, and management practices. Advances have improved post-transplantation outcomes in LTRs with chronic viral infections and reduced the risk of surgical site and invasive fungal infections.

References

1. Lim S, Kim EJ, Lee TB, Choi BH, Park YM, Yang K, et al. Predictors of postoperative infectious complications in liver transplant recipients: experience of 185 consecutive cases. Korean J Intern Med. 2018;33(4):798–806.
2. Baganate F, Beal EW, Tumin D, Azoulay D, Mumtaz K, Black SM, et al. Early mortality after liver transplantation: defining the course and the cause. Surgery. 2018;164(4):694–704.
3. Serrano MT, Sabroso S, Esteban LM, Berenguer M, Fondevila C, Lorente S, et al. Mortality and causes of death after liver transplantation: analysis of sex differences in a large nationwide cohort. Transpl Int. 2022;35:10263.
4. Rubin RH, Wolfson JS, Cosimi AB, Tolkoff-Rubin NE. Infection in the renal transplant recipient. Am J Med. 1981;70(2):405–11.
5. Hamandi B, Husain S, Humar A, Papadimitropoulos EA. Impact of infectious disease consultation on the clinical and economic outcomes of solid organ transplant recipients admitted for infectious complications. Clin Infect Dis. 2014;59(8):1074–82.
6. So M, Morris AM, Nelson S, Bell CM, Husain S. Antimicrobial stewardship by academic detailing improves antimicrobial prescribing in solid organ transplant patients. Eur J Clin Microbiol Infect Dis. 2019;38(10):1915–23.
7. Gao S, Huang X, Zhou X, Dai X, Han J, Chen Y, et al. A comprehensive evaluation of risk factors for mortality, infection and colonization associated with CRGNB in adult solid organ transplant recipients: a systematic review and meta-analysis. Ann Med. 2024;56(1):2314236.
8. Singh N, Sifri CD, Silveira FP, Miller R, Gregg KS, Huprikar S, et al. Cryptococcosis in patients with cirrhosis of the liver and posttransplant outcomes. Transplantation. 2015;99(10):2132–41.

9. Prodanovic H, Cracco C, Massard J, Barrault C, Thabut D, Duguet A, et al. Invasive pulmonary aspergillosis in patients with decompensated cirrhosis: case series. BMC Gastroenterol. 2007;7(1):2.
10. Fishman JA. Infection in organ transplantation. Am J Transplant. 2017;17(4):856–79.
11. Leibovici-Weissman Y, Anchel N, Nesher E, Leshno M, Shlomai A. Early post-liver transplantation infections and their effect on long-term survival. Transpl Infect Dis. 2021;23(4):e13673.
12. Heldman MR, Ngo S, Dorschner PB, Helfrich M, Ison MG. Pre- and post-transplant bacterial infections in liver transplant recipients. Transpl Infect Dis. 2019;21(5):e13152.
13. Neofytos D, Stampf S, Hoessly LD, D'Asaro M, Tang GN, Boggian K, et al. Bacteremia during the first year after solid organ transplantation: an epidemiological update. Open Forum Infect Dis. 2023;10(6):ofad247.
14. Kim SH, Mun SJ, Ko JH, Huh K, Cho SY, Kang CI, et al. Poor outcomes of early recurrent post-transplant bloodstream infection in living-donor liver transplant recipients. Eur J Clin Microbiol Infect Dis. 2021;40(4):771–8.
15. Bert F, Larroque B, Paugam-Burtz C, Janny S, Durand F, Dondero F, et al. Microbial epidemiology and outcome of bloodstream infections in liver transplant recipients: an analysis of 259 episodes: bloodstream infection and liver transplantation. Liver Transpl. 2010;16(3):393–401.
16. Golfieri R, Giampalma E, Morselli Labate AM, d'Arienzo P, Jovine E, Grazi GL, et al. Pulmonary complications of liver transplantation: radiological appearance and statistical evaluation of risk factors in 300 cases. Eur Radiol. 2000;10(7):1169–83.
17. Levesque E, Hoti E, Azoulay D, Honore I, Guignard B, Vibert E, et al. Pulmonary complications after elective liver transplantation—incidence, risk factors, and outcome. Transplantation. 2012;94(5):532–8.
18. Weiss E, Dahmani S, Bert F, Janny S, Sommacale D, Dondero F, et al. Early-onset pneumonia after liver transplantation: microbiological findings and therapeutic consequences. Liver Transpl. 2010;16(10):1178–85.
19. Vidal E, Torre-Cisneros J, Blanes M, Montejo M, Cervera C, Aguado JM, et al. Bacterial urinary tract infection after solid organ transplantation in the RESITRA cohort. Transpl Infect Dis. 2012;14(6):595–603.
20. Wijarnpreecha K, Aby ES, Kim D, Ungprasert P, Cheungpasitporn W, Thongprayoon C, et al. The burden of Clostridioides difficile infection in patients with history of liver transplant and during index admission. Eur J Gastroenterol Hepatol. 2021;33(6):894–8.
21. Dudzicz-Gojowy S, Więcek A, Adamczak M. Clostridioides difficile infection in patients after organ transplantation—a narrative overview. J Clin Med. 2022;11(15):4365.
22. Ali H, Patel P, Pamarthy R, Fatakhova K, Bolick NL, Satapathy SK. Comparative analysis and trends in liver transplant hospitalizations with *Clostridium difficile* infections: a 10-year national cross-sectional study. Transpl Infect Dis. 2022;24(6):e13985.
23. Hellinger WC, Heckman MG, Crook JE, Taner CB, Willingham DL, Diehl NN, et al. Association of surgeon with surgical site infection after liver transplantation. Am J Transplant. 2011;11(9):1877–84.
24. Miller CM, Quintini C, Dhawan A, Durand F, Heimbach JK, Kim-Schluger HL, et al. The international liver transplantation society living donor liver transplant recipient guideline. Transplantation. 2017;101(5):938–44.
25. Van Delden C. Bacterial biliary tract infections in liver transplant recipients. Curr Opin Organ Transplant. 2014;19(3):223–8.
26. Viehman JA, Clancy CJ, Clarke L, Shields RK, Silveira FP, Kwak EJ, et al. Surgical site infections after liver transplantation: emergence of multidrug-resistant bacteria and implications for prophylaxis and treatment strategies. Transplantation. 2016;100(10):2107–14.
27. Bassetti M, Peghin M, Carnelutti A, Righi E, Merelli M, Ansaldi F, et al. Invasive Candida infections in liver transplant recipients: clinical features and risk factors for mortality. Transplant Direct. 2017;3(5):e156.
28. Husain S, Tollemar J, Dominguez EA, Baumgarten K, Humar A, Paterson DL, et al. Changes in the spectrum and risk factors for invasive candidiasis in liver transplant recipients: prospective, multicenter, case-controlled study1. Transplantation. 2003;75(12):2023–9.

29. Nam H, Nilles KM, Levitsky J, Ison MG. Donor-derived viral infections in liver transplantation. Transplantation. 2018;102(11):1824–36.
30. Kaul DR, Vece G, Blumberg E, La Hoz RM, Ison MG, Green M, et al. Ten years of donor-derived disease: a report of the disease transmission advisory committee. Am J Transplant. 2021;21(2):689–702.
31. Wolfe CR, Ison MG, Practice the AIDC of. Donor-derived infections: guidelines from the American Society of Transplantation Infectious Diseases Community of Practice. Clin Transpl. 2019;33(9):e13547.
32. Chang FY, Singh N, Gayowski T, Wagener MM, Marino IR. Fever in liver transplant recipients: changing spectrum of etiologic agents. Clin Infect Dis. 1998;26(1):59–65.
33. Restrepo A, Clark NM, Transplantation on behalf of the IDC of P of the AS of. Nocardia infections in solid organ transplantation: guidelines from the Infectious Diseases Community of Practice of the American Society of Transplantation. Clin Transpl. 2019;33(9):e13509.
34. Peleg AY, Husain S, Qureshi ZA, Silveira FP, Sarumi M, Shutt KA, et al. Risk factors, clinical characteristics, and outcome of Nocardia infection in organ transplant recipients: a matched case-control study. Clin Infect Dis. 2007;44(10):1307–14.
35. Coussement J, Lebeaux D, van Delden C, Guillot H, Freund R, Marbus S, et al. Nocardia infection in solid organ transplant recipients: a multicenter European case-control study. Clin Infect Dis. 2016;63(3):338–45.
36. Majeed A, Beatty N, Iftikhar A, Mushtaq A, Fisher J, Gaynor P, et al. A 20-year experience with nocardiosis in solid organ transplant (SOT) recipients in the southwestern United States: a single-center study. Transpl Infect Dis. 2018;20(4):e12904.
37. Yetmar ZA, Challener DW, Seville MT, Bosch W, Beam E. Outcomes of Nocardiosis and treatment of disseminated infection in solid organ transplant recipients. Transplantation. 2023;107(3):782–91.
38. Neofytos D, Chatzis O, Nasioudis D, Boely Janke E, Doco Lecompte T, Garzoni C, et al. Epidemiology, risk factors and outcomes of invasive aspergillosis in solid organ transplant recipients in the Swiss Transplant Cohort Study. Transpl Infect Dis. 2018;20(4):e12898.
39. Barchiesi F, Mazzocato S, Mazzanti S, Gesuita R, Skrami E, Fiorentini A, et al. Invasive aspergillosis in liver transplant recipients: epidemiology, clinical characteristics, treatment, and outcomes in 116 cases. Liver Transpl. 2015;21(2):204–12.
40. Steinbach WJ, Marr KA, Anaissie EJ, Azie N, Quan SP, Meier-Kriesche HU, et al. Clinical epidemiology of 960 patients with invasive aspergillosis from the PATH Alliance registry. J Infect. 2012;65(5):453–64.
41. Husain S, Camargo JF. Invasive Aspergillosis in solid-organ transplant recipients: guidelines from the American Society of Transplantation Infectious Diseases Community of Practice. Clin Transpl. 2019;33(9):e13544.
42. Gioia F, Filigheddu E, Corbella L, Fernández-Ruiz M, López-Medrano F, Pérez-Ayala A, et al. Invasive aspergillosis in solid organ transplantation: diagnostic challenges and differences in outcome in a Spanish national cohort (Diaspersot study). Mycoses. 2021;64(11):1334–45.
43. Donnelly JP, Chen SC, Kauffman CA, Steinbach WJ, Baddley JW, Verweij PE, et al. Revision and update of the consensus definitions of invasive fungal disease from the European Organization for Research and Treatment of Cancer and the Mycoses Study Group Education and Research Consortium. Clin Infect Dis. 2020;71(6):1367–76.
44. Maertens JA, Rahav G, Lee DG, Ponce-de-León A, Ramírez Sánchez IC, Klimko N, et al. Posaconazole versus voriconazole for primary treatment of invasive aspergillosis: a phase 3, randomised, controlled, non-inferiority trial. Lancet. 2021;397(10273):499–509.
45. Baddley JW, Forrest GN, the AST Infectious Diseases Community of Practice. Cryptococcosis in solid organ transplantation—guidelines from the American Society of Transplantation Infectious Diseases Community of Practice. Clin Transpl. 2019;33(9):e13543.
46. Sun HY, Alexander BD, Lortholary O, Dromer F, Forrest GN, Lyon GM, et al. Cutaneous cryptococcosis in solid organ transplant recipients. Med Mycol. 2010;48(6):785–91.
47. Jabbour N, Reyes J, Kusne S, Martin M, Fung J. Cryptococcal meningitis after liver transplantation. Transplantation. 1996;61(1):146.

48. Perfect JR, Dismukes WE, Dromer F, Goldman DL, Graybill JR, Hamill RJ, et al. Clinical practice guidelines for the Management of Cryptococcal Disease: 2010 update by the Infectious Diseases Society of America. Clin Infect Dis Off Publ Infect Dis Soc Am. 2010;50(3):291–322.
49. Miller R, Assi M, Practice the AIDC of. Endemic fungal infections in solid organ transplant recipients—guidelines from the American Society of Transplantation Infectious Diseases Community of Practice. Clin Transpl. 2019;33(9):e13553.
50. Cuellar-Rodriguez J, Avery RK, Lard M, Budev M, Gordon SM, Shrestha NK, et al. Histoplasmosis in solid organ transplant recipients: 10 years of experience at a large transplant Center in an Endemic Area. Clin Infect Dis. 2009;49(5):710–6.
51. Kauffman CA, Freifeld AG, Andes DR, Baddley JW, Herwaldt L, Walker RC, et al. Endemic fungal infections in solid organ and hematopoietic cell transplant recipients enrolled in the Transplant-Associated Infection Surveillance Network (TRANSNET). Transpl Infect Dis Off J Transplant Soc. 2014;16(2):213–24.
52. Mazi PB, Sahrmann JM, Olsen MA, Coler-Reilly A, Rauseo AM, Pullen M, et al. The geographic distribution of dimorphic mycoses in the United States for the modern era. Clin Infect Dis Off Publ Infect Dis Soc Am. 2022;76(7):1295–301.
53. Assi M, Martin S, Wheat LJ, Hage C, Freifeld A, Avery R, et al. Histoplasmosis after solid organ transplant. Clin Infect Dis Off Publ Infect Dis Soc Am. 2013;57(11):1542–9.
54. Mehta TI, Kurman J, Dolan S, Gill H, Thapa B. Blastomycosis in solid organ transplant recipients-A retrospective series from southeastern Wisconsin. Transpl Infect Dis Off J Transplant Soc. 2021;23(4):e13671.
55. Blair JE. Coccidioidomycosis in liver transplantation. Liver Transpl. 2006;12(1):31–9.
56. Holt CD, Winston DJ, Kubak B, Imagawa DK, Martin P, Goldstein L, et al. Coccidioidomycosis in liver transplant patients. Clin Infect Dis Off Publ Infect Dis Soc Am. 1997;24(2):216–21.
57. Kahn A, Carey EJ, Blair JE. Universal fungal prophylaxis and risk of coccidioidomycosis in liver transplant recipients living in an endemic area. Liver Transpl. 2015;21(3):353–61.
58. Fishman JA, Gans H, Practice the AIDC of. Pneumocystis jiroveci in solid organ transplantation: guidelines from the American Society of Transplantation Infectious Diseases Community of Practice. Clin Transpl. 2019;33(9):e13587.
59. Andreasen PB, Rezahosseini O, Møller DL, Wareham NE, Thomsen MT, Houmami R, et al. Pneumocystis jirovecii pneumonia in liver transplant recipients in an era of routine prophylaxis. Immun Inflamm Dis. 2021;10(1):93–100.
60. Hosseini-Moghaddam SM, Kothari S, Humar A, Albasata H, Yetmar ZA, Razonable RR, et al. Adjunctive glucocorticoid therapy for pneumocystis jirovecii pneumonia in solid organ transplant recipients: a multicenter cohort, 2015-2020. Am J Transplant. 2023;S1600613523008584
61. Neofytos D, Hirzel C, Boely E, Lecompte T, Khanna N, Mueller NJ, et al. Pneumocystis jirovecii pneumonia in solid organ transplant recipients: a descriptive analysis for the Swiss Transplant Cohort. Transpl Infect Dis. 2018;20(6):e12984.
62. Lum J, Echenique I, Athans V, Koval CE. Alternative pneumocystis prophylaxis in solid organ transplant recipients at two large transplant centers. Transpl Infect Dis. 2021;23(1):e13461.
63. Lee I, Barton TD, Goral S, Doyle AM, Bloom RD, Chojnowski D, et al. Complications related to Dapsone use for pneumocystis Jirovecii pneumonia prophylaxis in solid organ transplant recipients. Am J Transplant. 2005;5(11):2791–5.
64. Schmidt JJ, Lueck C, Ziesing S, Stoll M, Haller H, Gottlieb J, et al. Clinical course, treatment and outcome of pneumocystis pneumonia in immunocompromised adults: a retrospective analysis over 17 years. Crit Care. 2018;22(1):307.
65. Krantz MS, Stone CA, Abreo A, Phillips EJ. Oral challenge with trimethoprim-sulfamethoxazole in patients with "sulfa" antibiotic allergy. J Allergy Clin Immunol Pract. 2020;8(2):757–760.e4.
66. Hosseini-Moghaddam SM, Shokoohi M, Singh G, Dufresne SF, Boucher A, Jevnikar A, et al. A multicenter case-control study of the effect of acute rejection and cytomegalovirus infection on pneumocystis pneumonia in solid organ transplant recipients. Clin Infect Dis. 2019;68(8):1320–6.

67. Razonable RR, Humar A. Cytomegalovirus in solid organ transplant recipients—guidelines of the American Society of Transplantation Infectious Diseases Community of Practice. Clin Transpl. 2019;33(9):e13512.
68. Munoz-Price LS, Slifkin M, Ruthazer R, Poutsiaka DD, Hadley S, Freeman R, et al. The clinical impact of ganciclovir prophylaxis on the occurrence of bacteremia in orthotopic liver transplant recipients. Clin Infect Dis. 2004;39(9):1293–9.
69. Kotton CN, Kumar D, Caliendo AM, Huprikar S, Chou S, Danziger-Isakov L, et al. The third international consensus guidelines on the management of cytomegalovirus in solid-organ transplantation. Transplantation. 2018;102(6):900–31.
70. Singh N, Winston DJ, Razonable RR, Lyon GM, Silveira FP, Wagener MM, et al. Effect of preemptive therapy vs antiviral prophylaxis on cytomegalovirus disease in seronegative liver transplant recipients with seropositive donors: a randomized clinical trial. JAMA. 2020;323(14):1378.
71. Engelmann C, Sterneck M, Weiss KH, Templin S, Zopf S, Denk G, et al. Prevention and management of CMV infections after liver transplantation: current practice in German transplant centers. J Clin Med. 2020;9(8):2352.
72. Avery RK, Alain S, Alexander BD, Blumberg EA, Chemaly RF, Cordonnier C, et al. Maribavir for refractory cytomegalovirus infections with or without resistance post-transplant: results from a phase 3 randomized clinical trial. Clin Infect Dis Off Publ Infect Dis Soc Am. 2021;75(4):690–701.
73. Côté-Daigneault J, Carrier FM, Toledano K, Wartelle-Bladu C, Willems B. Herpes simplex hepatitis after liver transplantation: case report and literature review. Transpl Infect Dis. 2014;16(1):130–4.
74. Lee DH, Zuckerman RA, Practice on behalf of the AIDC of. Herpes simplex virus infections in solid organ transplantation: guidelines from the American Society of Transplantation Infectious Diseases Community of Practice. Clin Transpl. 2019;33(9):e13526.
75. Pergam SA, Limaye AP, Practice the AIDC of. Varicella zoster virus in solid organ transplantation: guidelines from the American Society of Transplantation Infectious Diseases Community of Practice. Clin Transpl. 2019;33(9):e13622.
76. San Juan R, Aguado J, Lumbreras C, Díaz-Pedroche C, López-Medrano F, Lizasoain M, et al. Incidence, clinical characteristics and risk factors of late infection in solid organ transplant recipients: data from the RESITRA study group. Am J Transplant. 2007;7(4):964–71.
77. Montano-Loza AJ, Ronca V, Ebadi M, Hansen BE, Hirschfield G, Elwir S, et al. Risk factors and outcomes associated with recurrent autoimmune hepatitis following liver transplantation. J Hepatol. 2022;77(1):84–97.
78. Alabraba E, Nightingale P, Gunson B, Hubscher S, Olliff S, Mirza D, et al. A re-evaluation of the risk factors for the recurrence of primary sclerosing cholangitis in liver allografts. Liver Transpl. 2009;15(3):330–40.
79. Ueda Y, Kaido T, Okajima H, Hata K, Anazawa T, Yoshizawa A, et al. Long-term prognosis and recurrence of primary sclerosing cholangitis after liver transplantation: a single-center experience. Transplant Direct. 2017;3(12):e334.
80. Silveira MG, Talwalkar JA, Lindor KD, Wiesner RH. Recurrent primary biliary cirrhosis after liver transplantation. Am J Transplant. 2010;10(4):720–6.
81. Ariza-Heredia EJ, Fishman JE, Cleary T, Smith L, Razonable RR, Abbo L. Clinical and radiological features of respiratory syncytial virus in solid organ transplant recipients: a single-center experience. Transpl Infect Dis. 2012;14(1):64–71.
82. Kumar D, Ferreira VH, Blumberg E, Silveira F, Cordero E, Perez-Romero P, et al. A 5-year prospective multicenter evaluation of influenza infection in transplant recipients. Clin Infect Dis. 2018;67(9):1322–9.
83. Okumura K, Nishida S, Dhand A. Trends in COVID-19 mortality among solid organ transplant recipients: implications for prevention. Transplantation. 2022;106(8):e380–1.
84. Heldman MR, Kates OS, Safa K, Kotton CN, Georgia SJ, Steinbrink JM, et al. Changing trends in mortality among solid organ transplant recipients hospitalized for COVID-19 during the course of the pandemic. Am J Transplant. 2022;22(1):279–88.

85. Boyarsky BJ, Werbel WA, Avery RK, Tobian AAR, Massie AB, Segev DL, et al. Antibody response to 2-dose SARS-CoV-2 mRNA vaccine series in solid organ transplant recipients. JAMA. 2021;325(21):2204.
86. Hall VG, Ferreira VH, Ku T, Ierullo M, Majchrzak-Kita B, Chaparro C, et al. Randomized trial of a third dose of mRNA-1273 vaccine in transplant recipients. N Engl J Med. 2021;385(13):1244–6.
87. Lange NW, Salerno DM, Jennings DL, Choe J, Hedvat J, Kovac D (Bley), et al. Nirmatrelvir/ritonavir use: managing clinically significant drug-drug interactions with transplant immunosuppressants. Am J Transplant. 2022;22(7):1925–6.

Role of the Interventional Radiologist in Caring for Patients with Complications After Orthotopic Liver Transplant

25

Anouva Kalra-Lall, Dhruv Patel, Anvit Kalra-Lall, and Sameer Gadani

Introduction

Liver transplant is considered definitive or curative therapy for patients with end-stage liver disease and for eligible patients with hepatocellular cancer. Maintenance of the graft is critical to long-term survival in these patients. Despite advances in surgical technique and medical management with immunosuppression and antiviral therapy, complications in this patient population can be devastating. These complications are now more frequently encountered in daily clinical practice because of the increasing rate of liver transplants performed in the United States, currently second only to kidney transplants [29].

With increased awareness of endovascular and biliary interventional techniques for liver transplant salvage, we hope to invite interdisciplinary collaboration and offer more minimally invasive, image-guided interventional radiology options to these patients. In this chapter, we describe the four anatomical categories of complications (biliary, hepatic arterial, portal, and hepatocaval venous) that can be managed by an interventional radiologist. Each of these sections includes a review of the postoperative anatomy, an overview of the clinical manifestation and diagnostic features of the complication, and a discussion of relevant catheter-based therapies with examples. In the final section, we offer a brief overview of nonvascular percutaneous interventions.

A. Kalra-Lall · D. Patel · A. Kalra-Lall · S. Gadani (✉)
Cleveland Clinic Foundation, Section of Interventional Radiology, Cleveland, OH, USA
e-mail: gadanis@ccf.org

B. Eghtesad et al. (eds.), *Liver Transplantation*,
https://doi.org/10.1007/978-3-032-07072-2_25

Section 1: Biliary Complications

Background and Postoperative Anatomy

Biliary complications such as stricture, leak, ischemic cholangiopathy, infection, and biloma are the most common post-transplant complications, occurring in 5–45% of patients [2]. Biliary complications are typically divided into anastomotic and nonanastomotic. In liver transplant procedures, the biliary anastomosis is usually the last surgical anastomosis after hepatocaval, portal, and arterial vascular anastomoses. Anatomic considerations regarding size mismatch, length of pedicle available, and possibility of direct insertion into the jejunum for an end-to-side anastomosis (hepaticojejunostomy) versus an end-to-end biliary anastomosis are intraoperative decisions that will also play a role in determining which options are available for subsequent image-guided interventions (Fig. 25.1).

Biliary complications are typically classified as early (<30 days after transplant) or late (>30 days after transplant) complications. The most common overall complication is biliary stricture. However, biliary leak is the more commonly seen entity in the early postoperative period and is more prevalent in patients with a biliary-enteric reconstruction than in those with a duct-to-duct anastomosis [2].

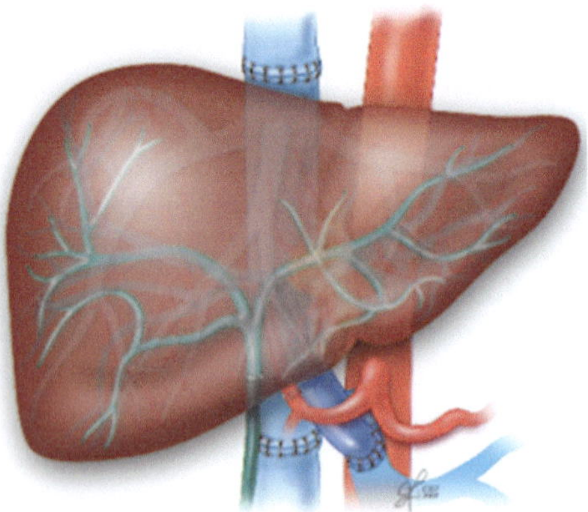

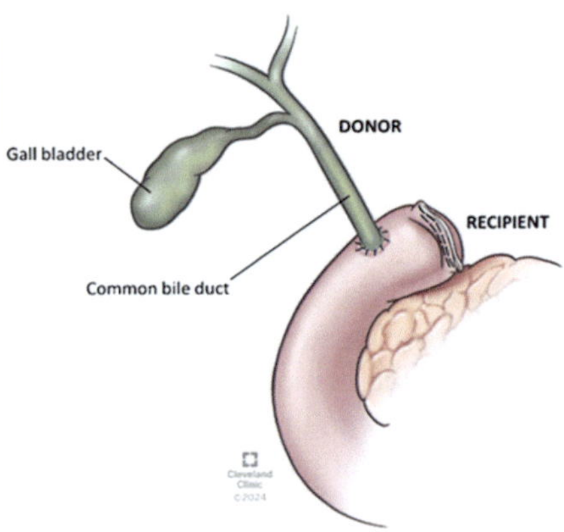

Fig. 25.1 Illustrations of common biliary anastomoses: end-to-end biliary anastomosis of the common bile duct (on the left) and an alternative, hepaticojejunostomy (on the right)

Clinical Manifestation and Diagnostic Features

Biliary Leak and Stricture

The clinical presentation of a biliary leak or stricture typically depends on etiology. Causes of biliary leak and/or stricture include, but are not limited to, surgical anastomotic technique, incomplete repair of the cystic duct stump, ischemia, thermal injury during dissection, injury related to T-tube placement or early extraction, and bile leak from the free or cut edge of a liver graft. The quickest way to identify bile leak and perhaps the most common manifestation of biliary leak in the early postoperative period is bilious output in the surgical drain. The diagnosis of bile leak can be confirmed by assessing the bilirubin level in this drain output fluid. If the leak goes undiagnosed or occurs later in the postoperative course, bilomas or intra-abdominal collections are noted on surveillance imaging or present with signs and symptoms of infection.

Biliary strictures can be differentiated from biliary leaks by measuring total and direct bilirubin levels to assess for conjugated or unconjugated hyperbilirubinemia. Often, patients with biliary stricture and direct hyperbilirubinemia may present with jaundice, pruritus, acholic stool, dark urine, nausea, or vomiting depending on the degree of impairment [48].

Imaging can also be used to distinguish between biliary strictures and biliary leaks. Biliary strictures are associated with upstream dilatation on ultrasonography (US) and computed tomography (CT), and the level or extent of dilatation is directly correlated with the severity or degree of the stricture. Magnetic resonance cholangiopancreatography (MRCP) tends to be the better study, compared to US or CT, when biliary stricture is suspected, as this modality can demonstrate the intrinsic, fluid-like T2 hyperintensity that highlights the salient biliary anatomy and stricture. MRCP can also identify biliary stones and bile leak with reproducible anatomic detail [13].

For clinicians attempting to diagnose or trace the origin of a bile leak, the use of hepatobiliary scintigraphy with hepatobiliary iminodiacetic acid (HIDA) or MRI with hepatospecific Gasoxetate Disodium contrast (Eovist or Primovist) may be useful, as the intrinsic hepatobiliary excretion of these agents enables a high degree of sensitivity in diagnosing leaks. MR imaging with hepatospecific contrast (Eovist or Primovist) is arguably superior study, in comparison to scintigraphy as the cross-sectional information obtained with this technique increases its specificity in identifying the source of the leak. Additionally, cross sectional imaging is sensitive in identifying aberrant biliary ducts and cystic duct stumps, which is a critical information for interventions [2, 13, 48].

Ischemic Cholangiopathy/Biliary Cast Syndrome

Biliary cast syndrome may be seen in the setting of ischemic insult to the hepatic arteries. This condition involves sloughed biliary mucosa, which appears on ultrasound images as isoechoic biliary debris within periportal branches. On MR imaging, the sloughed mucosa appears as filling defects with an irregular beaded appearance on T2 heavily weighted sequences. Etiologies of ischemic cholangiopathy include but are not limited to acute or chronic rejection, infection, and bile stasis [47].

Management

Biliary Leak and Stricture

The treatment techniques for biliary leak and stricture are similar but accomplish slightly different goals. For example, in patients with anastomotic biliary leak, placement of a transhepatic internal/external biliary catheter across the biliary ductal disruption should lead to reduced leakage and diversion of the bile away from the area of leakage. The catheter acts as a scaffold and promotes healing of the disrupted bile duct. Additionally, it drains the adjacent biloma, reducing the risk of infection. In patients with anastomotic biliary stricture, sequential upsizing of the transhepatic internal/external biliary catheter after balloon cholangioplasty performed serially at 6–8 weeks should lead to remodeling of the benign stricture with improvement in the luminal diameter of the stricture. However, this conventional remodeling technique for management of benign biliary stricture has a high failure rate of 15–40% [5, 17], and the use of balloon cholangioplasty with cutting balloons and placement of dual catheters has only marginally improved outcomes [14, 23].

Because of these limitations, advanced remodeling techniques such as endoluminal radiofrequency ablation and laser ablation are being studied for the management of benign biliary stricture. In these procedures, the scar tissue at the anastomotic stricture is ablated, and a large-bore catheter is then placed. This catheter acts as a scaffold for remodeling, with improvement of the luminal diameter to match that of the catheter. In a recent study of 16 patients who underwent radiofrequency ablation for benign biliary strictures, Husnain et al. [16] reported a 100% technical success rate, an 87% clinical success rate over a median follow-up of 17 months, and a 1-year patency rate of 100%. There was also a significant reduction in the median number of interventional radiology visits and drainage procedures required. In a retrospective study, Thai Binh et al. [43] reviewed the effect of endoluminal laser ablation on benign biliary strictures and reported a technical success rate of 100% and a clinical success rate of 100% with no recurrence at 6-month follow-up. Note that the studies assessing the use of radiofrequency and laser ablation for benign biliary strictures have been retrospective in nature with small sample sizes and short follow-up periods. Large multi-institutional studies with long-term follow-up are needed before these technologies can be implemented into routine clinical practice.

Ischemic Cholangiopathy

Although the management of ischemic cholangiopathy is similar to that used for biliary stricture, patients with ischemic cholangiopathy require closer follow-up in terms of imaging surveillance and shorter intervals between internal-external biliary drain exchanges. The original ischemic etiology must also be treated (see Section 2).

Choledocholithiasis can occur in patients receiving cyclosporine therapy or in patients with desquamated biliary epithelium from ischemia, infection, or cholesterol saturation. In such cases, interventional radiologists can offer electrohydraulic or laser lithotripsy under direct visualization with percutaneous cholangioscopy. With advances in percutaneous cholangioscopy techniques, the management of choledocholithiasis and potential concomitant benign stricture has become more feasible (Fig. 25.2) [28].

Even with these advances, there are cases refractory to endoscopic and/or interventional radiology percutaneous techniques. These cases, in addition to the biliary complications identified in the immediate post-operative period, are outside of the scope of interventional radiology and fit clearly within the purview of surgery. The latter situation is rare and is usually reserved for an early timepoint when a return to the operating room would be well-tolerated and in which a revised/new end-to-end or biliary-enteric anastomosis is warranted. Surgical management has two main limitations. The first is that the technique is dictated by the location of the biliary abnormality; favorable anatomy is required. Peripheral, intrahepatic ducts are not easily accessible despite the use of advanced mobilization techniques and resections of segment IV and/or the umbilical fissure. The second limitation is the overall failure rate and likelihood of biliary stricture restenosis. Failure rates can be as high as 50–60%,

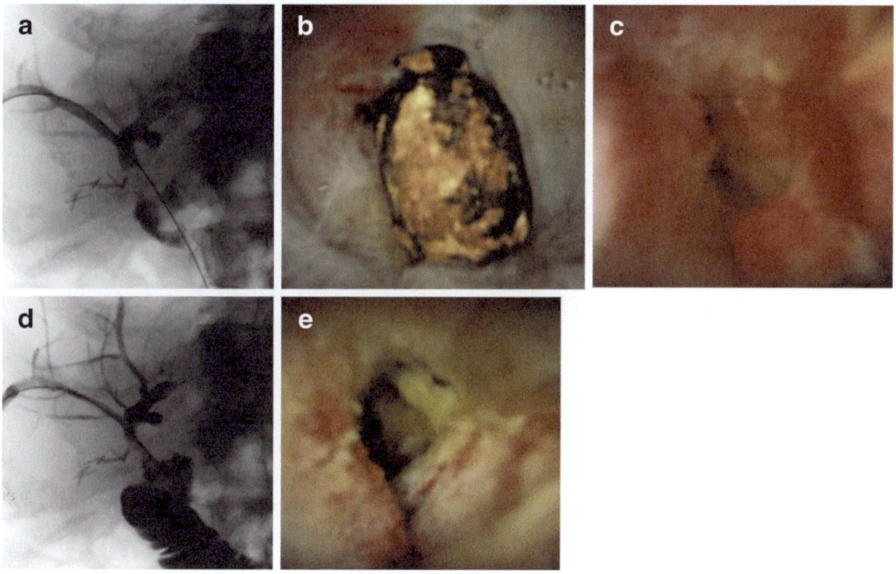

Fig. 25.2 Fluoroscopic and cholangioscopic images obtained before and after lithotripsy and radiofrequency ablation. (**a**) Initial cholangiogram shows stones and strictures. (**b**) Stone visualized with direct cholangioscopy. (**c**) Stricture after lithotripsy on cholangioscopy. (**d**) Cholangiogram obtained after ablation demonstrates improved duct patency. (**e**) Cholangioscopic view after ablation demonstrates near-complete resolution of the benign stricture

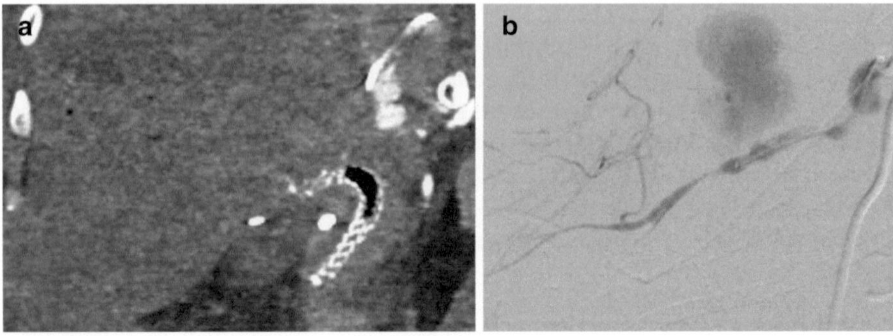

Fig. 25.3 (**a**) Coronal CT reformat centered at the porta hepatis demonstrated a biloma despite the presence of a bare metal stent and percutaneous biliary drain, with focal arterial enhancement abutting the biloma and hematoma, causing concern for a ruptured pseudoaneurysm. (**b**) A hepatic angiogram provided fluoroscopic confirmation of a ruptured mycotic pseudoaneurysm into the biloma

and complications of surgery can include not only recurrent stricture but also cholangitis, abscess, wound infections, sepsis, and biliary fistulas. Surgery also has inherent higher overall mortality and morbidity, compared to endovascular techniques, that are proportional with underlying overall health and liver dysfunction [10, 25].

An example demonstrating the role of surgery in the setting of infection is a case that ultimately also required retransplantation (Fig. 25.3). The patient in this case had a biliary leak with biloma formation at the porta hepatis, abutting the hepatic arterial vasculature. A mycotic hepatic artery pseudoaneurysm developed secondary to infection. In this case, there was no role for an interventionalist other than to ensure preoperative stability from a hemodynamic/bleeding standpoint. The biloma and bile leak were managed both endoscopically and with percutaneous techniques; however, the chronic inflammation caused rupture of the mycotic hepatic artery pseudoaneurysm and graft failure.

Section 2: Hepatic Arterial Complications

Background and Postoperative Anatomy

The second most common type of complication after liver transplant is related to hepatic arterial supply. Such complications can be particularly devastating as the hepatic arterial supply is the sole supply for the biliary system and still contributes substantially to parenchymal flow in the post-transplant liver. Similar surgical considerations regarding vessel size, length, and orientation dictate the post-transplant anatomy, and thus the potential management of these complications. Variations beyond the standard end-to-end arterial anastomosis can be seen in Fig. 25.4.

The prevalence of variant hepatic arterial anatomy has been reported to range from 10% to 48% [41, 46, 49]. The most common anastomosis is between the

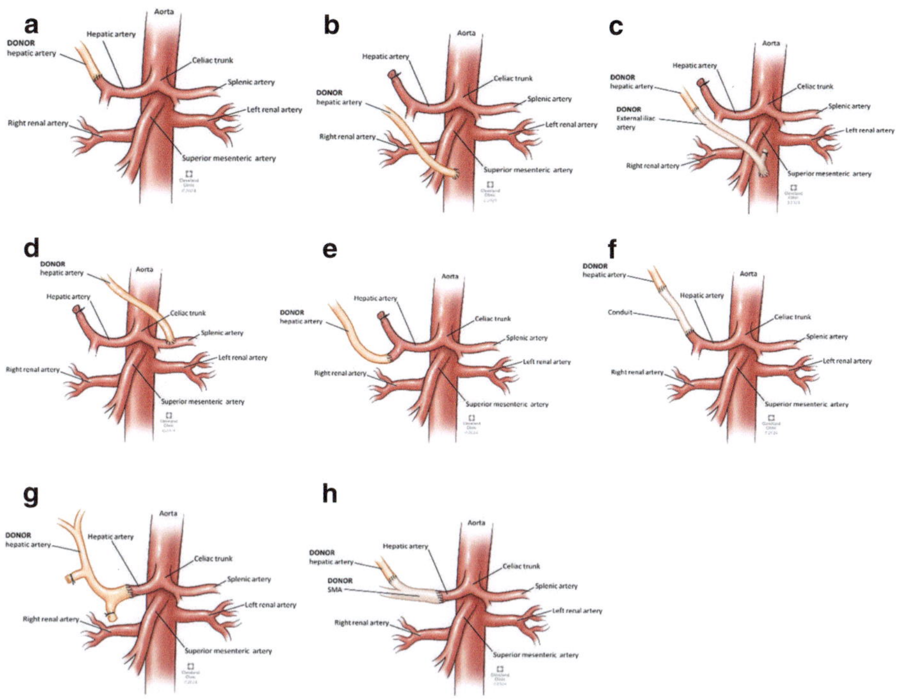

Fig. 25.4 (**a**) Typical end-to-end proper hepatic artery anastomosis. The donor hepatic artery can be directly sewn to the aorta (**b**) with or without a jump graft or external iliac artery graft (**c**). Alternative sites to anastomose are the splenic artery (**d**) or gastroduodenal artery (**e**). Size mismatch may be ameliorated with the use of a conduit (**f**). Normal anatomic variations in the donor or recipient may necessitate use of the donor's hepatic vasculature beginning at the common hepatic artery (**g**) or superior mesenteric artery (**h**)

recipient hepatic artery proper and donor common hepatic artery with ligation of the donor gastroduodenal artery. Another common anastomosis is between the donor-replaced right hepatic artery and the recipient gastroduodenal artery. In patients requiring retransplant, the use of a conduit may be more helpful than a native vessel. An understanding of postoperative anatomy is critical for post–liver transplant imaging interpretation, accurate diagnosis of complications, and management.

Clinical Manifestation and Diagnostic Features

Hepatic Artery Stenosis

Hepatic artery stenosis (HAS) is characterized by more than 50% intraluminal narrowing in the appropriate clinical context. The clinical presentation of HAS may include transaminitis and graft dysfunction and can be subclinical in up to 20% of cases [9, 11, 34]. In the liver transplant population, the incidence of HAS is reported to range from 2% to 13% [29]. Close surveillance in the immediate postoperative period is critical for prompt diagnosis. Clinical suspicion should be centered around possible pathologies affecting the arterial anastomosis, which is the most common site for HAS; these include vessel diameter mismatch, extrinsic compression, operative techniques, and preoperative microvascular injury (i.e., compromise of the vasa vasorum or previous transarterial chemoembolization) [38, 44].

HAS is classified as early (<30 days after transplant) or late (>30 days after transplant). If not appropriately treated in a timely fashion, HAS leads to hepatic artery thrombosis (HAT). These entities are closely related in pathophysiology and can lead to ischemic injury to the hepatic parenchyma. HAS and HAT can also cause biliary stricture or ischemic cholangiopathy, as stated earlier.

Early diagnosis and prompt treatment of HAS are related to improved transplant success rates [6, 38]. Doppler ultrasonography (DUS) is the predominant surveillance modality. As many cases of HAS are subclinical, DUS plays a key role in routine postoperative care and surveillance, demonstrating 100% sensitivity, 99.5% specificity, 95% positive predictive value, and 100% negative predictive value for the detection of HAS [38]. With DUS, HAS is defined as a resistive index (RI) lower than 0.5, although some authors recommend a threshold of 0.4, and a peak velocity higher than 200 cm/s [30, 33, 38]. A peak velocity of more than 200 cm/s is diagnostic for stenosis. A peak velocity higher than 400 cm/s is associated with >75% stenosis. A tardus parvus waveform, characterized by a delayed systolic acceleration time (>0.12 s) and associated diminished peak systolic velocity (<48 cm/s) distal to the site of suspected stenosis, is an essential additional parameter [30].

Limitations of DUS are that the technique is operator dependent and the entirety of the hepatic artery can be difficult to visualize secondary to postoperative air, superficial bowel gas, or depth from the skin. Alternative modalities, namely CT angiogram or MR angiogram, can be used to diagnose HAS; in such cases, the same definition of a focal, intraluminal narrowing of more than 50% is used (Fig. 25.5).

Hepatic Artery Thrombosis (HAT)

HAT or occlusion secondary to thrombosis accounts for approximately half of all hepatic arterial complications after liver transplant. It is the most common cause of primary graft nonfunction in the early postoperative period [24, 38]. HAT can lead to graft failure or death in approximately 50% of cases if not treated promptly with revascularization or retransplant [38]. Similar to HAS, HAT is also classified as early (<30 days after transplant) or late (>30 days after transplant). Again, morbidity with HAT is associated with biliary complications, as the hepatic arteries are the sole blood supply to the biliary tree.

The clinical presentation of HAT ranges from transaminitis to sepsis to fulminant graft failure. The spectrum in clinical presentation depends time of onset, postoperatively. Early HAT more often presents as graft dysfunction, whereas late HAT is associated with biliary complications. This is thought to be secondary to the

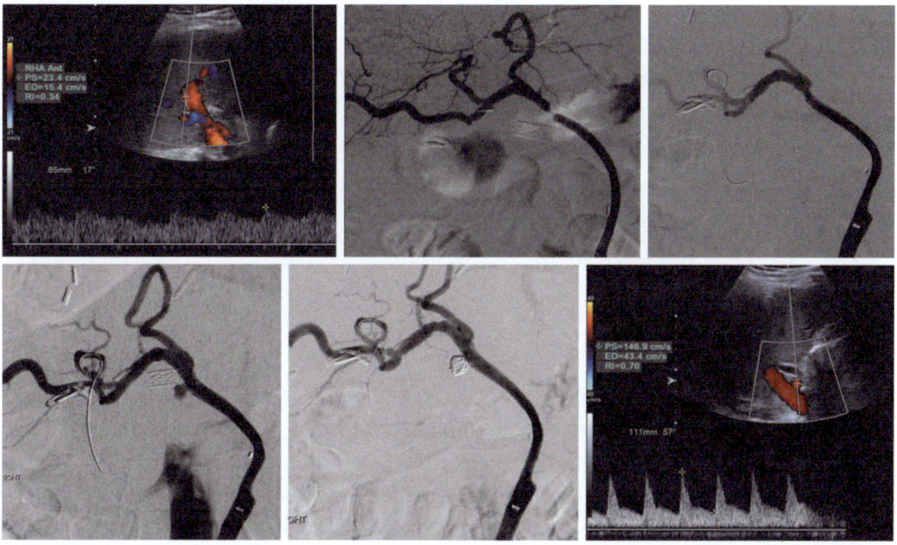

Fig. 25.5 Images from a 45-year-old woman who had undergone a liver transplant 2 years earlier and subsequently presented with abnormal findings on surveillance ultrasonography. (*Top row*) The first ultrasound image shows the classic tardus parvus waveform, low peak systolic velocity 23 cm/s and RI 0.34 indicative of poor hepatic arterial inflow. This was confirmed on angiography, which demonstrated a severe high-grade focal stenosis at the liver margin that improved with angioplasty. (*Bottom row*) Angioplasty was complicated by a traumatic pseudoaneurysm, which was subsequently coil embolized. The final ultrasound image of this area shows resolution of the abnormal tardus parvus waveform with the return of a normal hepatic arterial waveform and improved velocity as well as RI

development of collateral blood supply from the gastroduodenal artery and pancreaticoduodenal arcade [34].

Similar to HAS, early diagnosis and intervention lead to improved outcomes (decreased need for retransplantation). DUS is the gold standard modality for the diagnosis of HAT. DUS findings depend on the spectrum and timeline of the pathophysiology—slow or stagnant flow to occlusive thrombosis. Impending thrombosis appears as low-velocity, high-resistance flow (i.e., elevated RI), whereas complete thrombosis appears as the absence of flow within the hepatic artery [3, 30]. Similar to HAS, close surveillance is critical for diagnosis; therefore, some institutions offer routine screening DUS within 48 h of transplant and additional DUS 7 days after transplant [22].

Hepatic Artery Pseudoaneurysm

Hepatic artery pseudoaneurysm (HAP) is characterized by interruption of the hepatic arterial wall. Clinical acuity relates to the degree of wall tear or disruption, from rupture to contained leak or hematoma. While rare, with an estimated prevalence of 0.3% to 3%, HAP has a high mortality rate of up to 75%. Risk factors for

HAP include the presence of bacteremia, trauma, bile leak, intra-abdominal infection, and iatrogenic injury. The clinical presentation of HAP varies from asymptomatic with incidental diagnosis on routine surveillance imaging to catastrophic intra-abdominal hemorrhage. Almost all cases are diagnosed with DUS with or without cross-sectional imaging and are identified within the first month after transplant [34, 42]

Management

Hepatic Artery Stenosis

There are two main treatment avenues for HAS: endovascular and surgical revascularization. In refractory cases, retransplantation is a last resort; statistically, however, retransplantation is the most successful option and is only limited by organ availability. Early HAS can often be treated with endovascular therapy (EVT) or surgical revision. EVT is the first-line option because of overall decreased associated morbidity and mortality; however, there are higher stakes in the setting of a fresh anastomosis. Endovascular options include percutaneous transluminal angioplasty (PTA) and/or stent placement. The surgical option involves resecting the preexisting anastomosis and performing reanastomosis with the existing artery (if length is available) or using a jump/interposition graft.

The choice between primary placement of an endovascular stent and the use of PTA alone is controversial. A 2014 meta-analysis showed no significant difference in outcomes with PTA versus primary stent placement [7], but a more recent retrospective study from 2020 demonstrated higher 1-year patency with primary stent placement than with PTA alone (93.8% vs 73.5%) [50]. Le et al. demonstrated longer patency and a later timepoint for re-intervention with primary stent placement (105.8 days) than with PTA alone (51 days) [22]. Naidu et al. [26] compared placement of bare-metal stents (BMS) with placement of drug-eluting stents (DES) and found primary patency rates at 1 year to be 76% for BMS and 81% for DES. At 3-year follow-up, these rates had decreased to 46% for BMS and 71% for DES. Overall, we suggest that the decision to place a primary stent or to perform PTA alone should be based on the operator's preference and on the factors of the individual case (e.g., stenosis location, length of available stent landing zone, length of available stent, patient's suitability for dual antiplatelet therapy. It is reasonable to first use PTA alone and then offer re-intervention with stent placement, depending on the individual clinical scenario.

The overall complication rate for EVT has been reported to be approximately 7–10%, with most events related to arterial dissection, rupture, and/or access site complications [35, 50].

Hepatic Artery Thrombosis

HAT is typically managed with EVT or surgical revascularization. Retransplantation or observation are considerations depending on the time of diagnosis. Timely revascularization or retransplantation is required for cases of early HAT. The decision between EVT and surgery depends on the local institutional multidisciplinary consensus and the expertise available at the time of diagnosis. At our institute, surgical revascularization is considered first-line management in the first 1 to 2 weeks after transplant; this is consistent with the institutional protocol described by Naidu et al. (i.e., surgical revascularization within the first 7 to 10 days after transplant because of a high risk of rupture with EVT) [24]. EVT options for HAT include catheter-directed thrombolysis, mechanical thrombectomy, PTA, and stent placement.

PTA with or without stent placement is required to treat underlying HAS, which is primarily an endoluminal process. However, if there is external compression (e.g., due to hematoma), stent placement is required to maintain patency. If the underlying cause is related to surgical factors (e.g., kink or twist at the anastomosis), surgical revision is necessary. Catheter-directed thrombolysis can be performed either on the table, in a single session, or can be accomplished via slow thrombolysis overnight.

Late HAT (or late HAS) can more often be managed conservatively due to the delayed onset and chance for collateral blood supply development. However, biliary complications may need attention in such cases, as previously described.

Hepatic Artery Pseudoaneurysm

HAP is usually managed endovascularly with placement of a covered stent or embolization (possibly with balloon assistance), with the goal of excluding flow to the pseudoaneurysm. In a summary of several studies, Pardi et al. found that overall high mortality and poor graft function were associated with surgical ligation, whereas better outcomes were seen with EVT. However, the studies included in this analysis had a small sample size of patients treated with EVT [34, 38].

Section 3: Portal Vein Complications

Background and Postoperative Anatomy

Portal vein–related compromise is the second most common vascular complication after liver transplant, with a reported prevalence of 1–3%. Because the portal flow is the primary contributor to the parenchymal blood supply, issues with this flow are associated with significant morbidity and mortality and are often linked to graft failure. As with hepatic arterial complications, portal vein complications are divided into early (<30 days after transplant) and late (>30 days after transplant) complications.

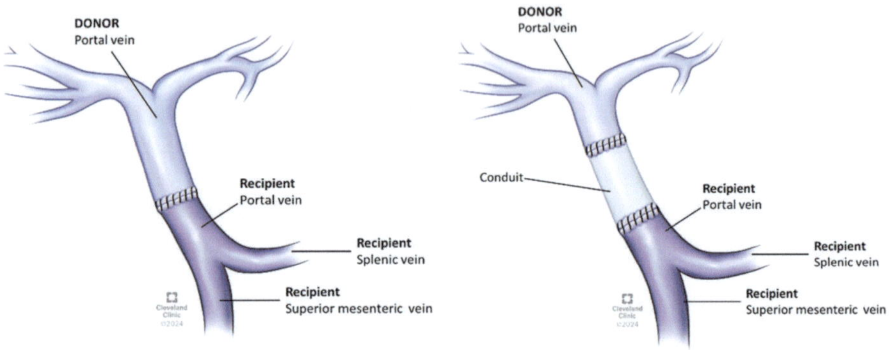

Fig. 25.6 End-to-end portal vein anastomoses between the donor and recipient portal vein vasculature (**a**) can also be altered to address length discrepancy via the use of a conduit or graft (**b**)

Portal vein size mismatch, the presence of a hypercoagulable state, and surgical technique have been described as potential underlying causes of portal vein complications. Additionally, it is thought that portal vein complications may occur more often in split liver transplants, living donor liver transplants, and pediatric transplants because of the shorter available vascular pedicle length. Again, knowledge of the underlying postoperative anatomy is critical, because most complications are seen at the anastomosis (Fig. 25.6) [9, 29, 33, 34].

The location and type of the anastomosis will vary depending on the individual patient and donor anatomy (e.g., length of the main portal vein, presence of portal vein thrombus, cavernous transformation of the recipient portal vein, presence of a transjugular intrahepatic portosystemic shunt). The most common form of portal vein anastomosis is the donor portal vein to the recipient portal vein. In cases involving portal vein thrombus or cavernous transformation, thrombectomy or recanalization may be required. Other options include placing a bypass conduit from the superior mesenteric vein or portosplenic confluence or placing an interposition graft if length is an issue.

Clinical Manifestation and Diagnostic Features

Portal Vein Stenosis

Most cases of portal vein stenosis (PVS) are asymptomatic and incidentally noted on routine DUS surveillance; symptoms arise only if the degree of stenosis is severe enough to cause portal hypertension. The etiology of PVS is typically related to surgical technique, and the incidence after liver transplant is low (<3%) [9, 29, 34]. The presentation of PVS may include upper gastrointestinal variceal bleeding or ascites. These are often diagnosed several months after transplant and are caused by scarring and/or neointimal hyperplasia. If left untreated, PVS can progress to PV thrombosis (PVT), which carries significant morbidity.

Using DUS to diagnose PVS is controversial, as DUS is considered very sensitive but not specific for diagnosis. Some authors have suggested that a peak anastomotic velocity greater than 125 cm/s and an anastomotic-to-preanastomotic velocity ratio higher than 3:1 are indicative of PVS [3, 8, 15, 40]. Such cases should subsequently undergo cross-sectional imaging with CTA or MRA to confirm the stenosis, which will appear as focal luminal narrowing at the level of the anastomosis. CTA may also show sequelae of portal hypertension. Our preference is to define PVS based on the pressure gradient between the prestenosis and poststenosis site, with a pressure gradient higher than 5 mmHg considered significant and warranting treatment [32, 37]. However, some authors consider a pressure gradient higher than 3 mmHg as diagnostic of PVS [4].

Portal Vein Thrombosis

PVT is categorized based on the time of onset: perioperative PVT occurs in the first 72 h after transplant, early PVT occurs 72 h to 30 days after transplant, and late PVT occurs more than 30 days after transplant. Early PVT presents with severe and acute liver insufficiency or graft failure. In later stages, the severity of presentation depends on the degree of available collateral circulation, and the condition is more likely to manifest as sequelae of portal hypertension.

Like PVS, PVT is more common in pediatric transplants, living donor liver transplants, and split liver transplants because of the technical complexities involved in portal vein reconstruction. The most common cause of PVT is surgical technique–related complications (e.g., venous redundancy and kinking with or without stenosis at the anastomosis). Several other risk factors have been reported for PVT, including pretransplant thrombosis requiring thrombectomy at the time of transplant, small diameter portal vein (<5 mm), use of a venous conduit for portal vein reconstruction, reduced flow through the portal vein due to previous splenectomy or portosplenic venous surgery, hypoplastic portal vein, and large portosystemic collaterals [21, 36].

DUS is the first-line imaging modality for diagnosing PVT. On DUS, an absence of flow within the portal vein or a filling defect will be seen [15, 40]. A thrombus or filling defect can also be identified on contrast-enhanced CT and MR imaging. Clots in the portal venous, splenic, or mesenteric veins can be easily identified on cross-sectional imaging. Portal venous thrombosis can also be seen on pretreatment portovenography as a filling defect, which should improve on venography after intervention (Fig. 25.7).

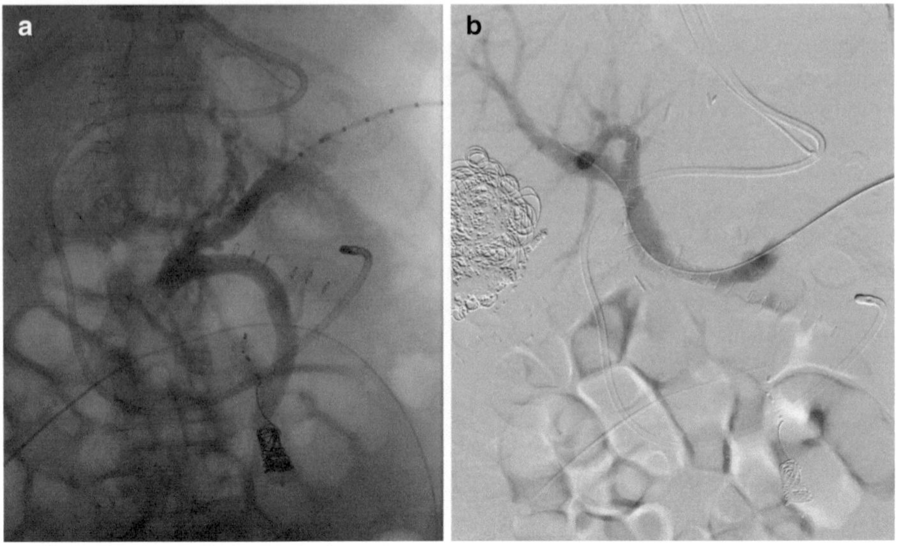

Fig. 25.7 Images from a 66-year-old woman with multiple comorbidities, including autoimmune hepatitis with cirrhosis (featuring esophageal varices, hepatic encephalopathy, and splenic vein thrombosis), who was transferred to our institution for liver transplant. The post-transplant course of this patient was complicated by a left hepatic lobe artery pseudoaneurysm, which was coil embolized and later surveillance imaging demonstrated portal vein thrombosis. (**a**) Fluoroscopic image demonstrating transsplenic access for mesenteric venogram, which opacified the superior mesenteric vein but demonstrated complete thrombosis of the portal system. (**b**) Portal venogram obtained after recanalization demonstrated restored flow

Management

Portal Vein Stenosis

The treatment plan will vary depending on the onset of PVS, the patient's clinical status (i.e., symptomatic vs asymptomatic) and liver function, and the severity of PVS. Asymptomatic cases with normal liver function and absence of portal hypertension can be managed conservatively with close monitoring. Regular surveillance (approximately every 3 to 6 months) is recommended because of the risk of progression to PVT and graft failure. There is no consensus regarding the use of anticoagulation therapy in such cases. In cases involving significant PVS on imaging or symptomatic PVS, treatment is indicated. For early PVS, surgical revision or retransplantation can be considered. However, EVT by interventional radiology is widely recognized as the first-line treatment for PVS [27, 34, 44].

EVT for PVS includes balloon venoplasty or, more rarely, stent placement. Possible approaches include transhepatic, transsplenic, or transjugular access. Depending on the patient's individual anatomy and site of stenosis, we prefer to maintain linearity of the transcatheter system during treatment and thus prefer a transsplenic or transhepatic approach. Although there is no general recommended EVT technique, several groups have reported great success with venoplasty alone. For instance, Kim et al. [18] reported an initial success rate of 85% after balloon angioplasty alone in 27 patients, and at 1, 3, and 10-year follow-up, the patency rates were 87%, 82%, and 68%, respectively. Shibata et al. [39] similarly reported a 71.4% patency rate at a mean follow-up of 24.4 months after balloon angioplasty alone in 45 patients.

In cases involving multifocal stenoses throughout the portal vein, high-grade stenosis, or refractory stenosis after venoplasty (i.e., no improvement in the pressure gradient after venoplasty or recurrence of stenosis within a few months after balloon venoplasty), stent placement is preferred, and self-expandable stents are generally recommended in this setting. A few studies with small sample sizes have described good long-term outcomes with stent placement in such cases. For instance, Ko et al. [21] reported initial technical success in 7 of 9 patients and a 100% stent primary patency rate at 66 months in 6 patients (1 patient died due to other surgical complications). Funaki et al. [12] reported 100% success with venoplasty and/or stent placement in 12 patients at a mean follow-up of 3 years, and Kim et al. [19] reported a 100% stent primary patency rate at 10 years in 8 patients. However, larger prospective studies are required for more reliable evidence.

Portal Vein Thrombosis

Treatment options for PVT include systemic anticoagulation, catheter-directed thrombolysis or thrombectomy with or without stent placement, and surgical thrombectomy or retransplantation. Perioperative PVT is associated with a high rate of graft failure (75%) [36]. Thus, surgical revision is required to correct any underlying technical issues such as kink or twist. If this fails, urgent retransplantation is required.

For cases of early PVT, EVT is considered first-line management. Such cases can be treated with percutaneous (transhepatic, transsplenic, or transjugular) thrombolysis and/or thrombectomy with or without stent placement. These individual therapies are viable options for recanalization.

For cases of late PVT, if new collaterals have formed with cavernous transformation of the portal vein and there is no liver dysfunction, conservative management with observation is reasonable. Late PVT presenting with gastroesophageal variceal bleeding or ascites requires EVT, specifically intrahepatic portosystemic shunt placement along with portal vein thrombolysis or thrombectomy for reconstruction. The shunt can be a transjugular intrahepatic portosystemic shunt from a branch of the portal vein to a hepatic vein or directly from the main portal vein to the inferior vena cava. In either case, thrombolysis or thrombectomy should be performed before the shunt graft is placed to reduce the risk of pulmonary embolism and to ensure good inflow.

Section 4: Hepatocaval Complications

Background and Postoperative Anatomy

Hepatocaval anastomotic issues are the least common vascular complication after liver transplant, noted in <2% of patients [20]. These complications can include thrombosis, anastomotic leak or bleeding, and stenosis or stricture.

There are two main approaches to caval harvest and reimplantation (Fig. 25.8). The first and more conventional method is the bicaval approach, which was originally described by Starzl. The second and more widely adopted approach is the piggyback technique, which was originally described by Tzakis [45]. This method requires one caval anastomosis on implantation and can usually be performed more quickly and with less need for intraoperative blood products when compared with the conventional technique (Fig. 25.8).

Commonly, the right hepatic vein is ligated while the right lobe of the donor liver is mobilized, and the middle hepatic and left hepatic veins are used to form a suprahepatic cuff. If the less traditional left-sided approach is used, the inverse configuration of hepatic veins may be involved. Salvaging two suprahepatic cuffs has also been described for patients undergoing retransplantation.

In the context of a living donor transplant in which both donor and recipient cavae need to be preserved, end-to-end hepatic venous anastomoses or end-to-side anastomosis to the inferior vena cava are the two most commonly used options. In adults, the donor typically keeps the middle hepatic vein, and hepatic venous reconstruction in the donor is performed using autologous veins or grafts. Overall, hepatocaval anastomoses are created based on the available venous real estate.

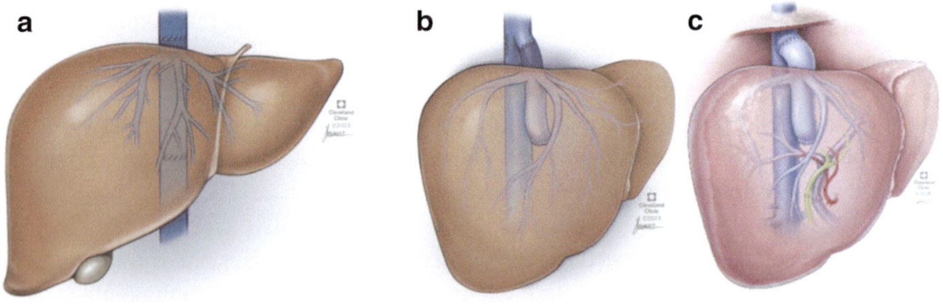

Fig. 25.8 (**a**) The bicaval technique is the conventional approach. (**b**, **c**) The piggyback approach is the more commonly practiced surgical technique

Clinical Manifestation and Diagnostic Features

Early hepatocaval complications are often clinically silent. At our institution, serial liver vascular ultrasound examinations are used for surveillance. Hepatovenous or caval complications in transplant patients are either stenotic or leak/bleed. Stenosis of the IVC can lead to its thrombosis.

Clinically, the severity of symptoms (if present) is correlated with the degree of hepatocaval integrity compromise. Bleeding at the anastomosis will manifest as tachycardia and hypotension; this is often seen only in the immediate postoperative period. A more subtle manifestation is hepatic venous outflow obstruction caused by either thrombosis or stenosis. The presentation of this condition is related to the onset of thrombosis or stenosis and can lead to congestive symptoms. Patients with hepatic venous outflow obstruction may have a combination of transaminitis, abdominal pain, ascites, pleural effusions, bilateral lower extremity edema, splenomegaly, renal dysfunction, intestinal congestion, and possibly fulminant graft dysfunction. [31]

Hepatic venous and caval outflow obstruction can also occur as a result of graft torsion or extrinsic compression secondary to postoperative fluid collection(s) (i.e., hematoma). Although the incidence of obstruction is generally low (approximately 1%), rates have been reported to be as high as 6% in the living donor liver transplant and pediatric transplant populations, likely because of the increased complexity involved in venous reconstruction in these patients. Mortality associated with hepatic venous outflow obstruction has been reported to be as high as 24% [1, 31].

DUS can be used to monitor the transplanted liver as the systemic and splanchnic circulations re-equilibrate and as post-analgesia vasoplegia diminishes in the immediate postoperative period. Ultrasonography is helpful in detecting patency with waveform/spectral Doppler and angle-corrected velocities. However, as previously mentioned, ultrasonography is limited by its operator dependence and the potential obscuration of anatomy secondary to postoperative pneumoperitoneum, depth, and skin or incisional defects, limiting placement of the ultrasound probe. On ultrasound images, the findings for outflow obstruction include monophasic venous spectrum, reversal of flow direction, and reversal of portal venous flow in extreme cases. Although a monophasic venous waveform is a sensitive finding, a venous pulsatility index lower than 0.45 is 95% specific [8]. Velocity and pressure gradients can also be assessed on ultrasound examinations. The extent and implications of the outflow obstruction to hepatic perfusion may or may not be well depicted via grayscale imaging of the liver parenchyma; contrast-enhanced CT may be better suited for this purpose.

Liver perfusion compromised by bridging vein occlusion or stenosis with focal graft venous congestion and graft torsion are both etiologies that can be better assessed with contrast-enhanced CT. Bridging vein occlusion and/or stenosis may be occult on ultrasound images due to their small caliber. In cases of graft torsion, ultrasound images may show acute venous outflow obstruction with reversal of flow in the main portal vein; however, these are nonspecific findings for torsion. CT allows for assessment and may hint at the mechanism underlying these complications, whether it be a factor of a small graft in a large hepatectomy bed or a rapidly regenerated liver compromised by extrinsic compression.

Management

Cases involving anastomotic breakdown and bleeding are best handled surgically if caught early. Regardless of the predisposing factor (i.e., redo anastomosis, caliber mismatch, adrenal vein manipulation, or concern for tissue friability in the initial operation), early bleeding concerns are best controlled surgically when the pretest probability of the expected site of bleeding is known. For cases involving gross structural complications such as caval kinking or graft torsion, only surgical manipulation is indicated. There is no role for an interventional radiologist in this setting. However, as the postoperative timeline progresses, the likelihood of success of surgical treatment is limited by extensive, prolonged lysis of adhesions and/or difficulty dissecting to possible sites of intervention. This is when EVT becomes a viable option.

For cases of hepatovenous/caval stenosis, intravascular ultrasonography and/or venography can be helpful in characterizing the degree of disease, as well as in preprocedural planning and allowing for targeted treatment with balloon angioplasty and/or stent placement. Stenosis at the caval anastomosis can be resolved with angioplasty alone in up to 100% of cases [34]. Intra-procedural, post-intervention, venous pressures should be evaluated to ensure that a gradient across the stenosis/anastomosis can be obtained to inform additional monitoring/serial dilations as needed.

Placement of a stent requires the technical consideration of preserving hepatic venous outflow; an open-cell structured stent with enhanced radial strength is therefore required (i.e., the Z-stent manufactured by Cook). Sizing this stent requires finesse to avoid either undersizing or stretching the cava. One study by Jang et al. described a 10-year patency rate of up to 88%. [31] Patency can be assessed with intravascular ultrasonography and/or venography. For long-term follow-up, DUS and CT can be used as a means of less invasive monitoring (Fig. 25.9).

In the event of hepatic vein and/or caval thrombosis after liver transplant, recanalization, thrombolysis, and/or thrombectomy can be used for management. Catheter-directed therapy offers lower morbidity rates than surgical thrombectomy and is associated with better overall outcomes than surgical management [27]. After recanalization, depending on the anatomy and the risk of re-thrombosis or stenosis, placement of a stent may also be warranted. Given the anatomy of caval reconstructions, thrombosis occurs more frequently with the piggyback technique than with the conventional technique. However, outflow obstruction is seen less often with the modified piggyback technique, in which the hepatic cuff has two or three veins for improved drainage.

Depending on the extent of thrombus and postoperative time frame, mechanical or aspiration thrombectomy or thrombolysis or a combination of the two can be pursued. There are a plethora of chemical and mechanical thrombolytic options and

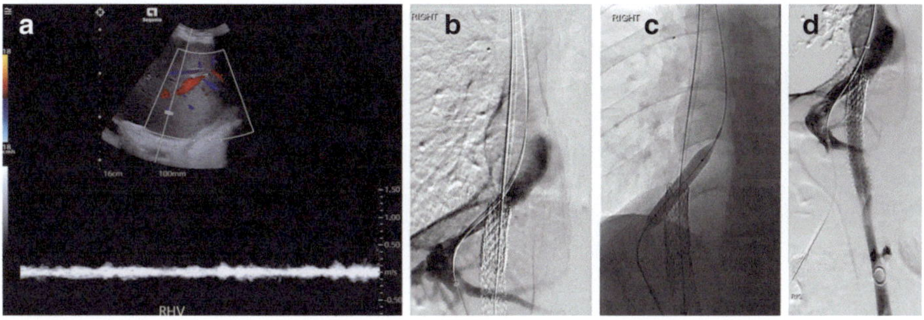

Fig. 25.9 Images from a 23-year-old man with recurrent ascites after liver transplant who also had prior caval occlusion that required stenting at an outside hospital. (**a**) Liver vascular ultrasonography was performed to evaluate for recurrent ascites. Ultrasonography demonstrated diminished phasicity within the right hepatic vein, indicating low flow. (**b**) Fluoroscopy corroborated that there was nearly no flow through the right hepatic vein, which was fortunately cannulated with a wire. (**c**) Across the wire, serial dilatation of the right hepatic vein was performed using angioplasty balloons ranging from 2 mm to 10 mm in diameter. (**d**) Venography performed after angioplasty and stenting showed greatly improved flow

thrombectomy devices that all serve a similar purpose; the choice of technique should therefore be based on operator comfort and therapeutic goal. The advantage of thrombectomy is that it often provides gross debulking of the thrombus in a single session, whereas lysis involves an ongoing drip irrigation of lytics in the vascular bed over a few hours or over multiple days with a planned return to the angiography suite to assess the status of the thrombus. The advantage of lytics is that the thrombus "melts" away from even smaller vascular branches that may be involved, whereas thrombectomy often targets larger vessels that allow for a device to be seated within the thrombus and the anatomy. There are no meaningful head-to-head comparison studies demonstrating which technique is superior; the choice of technique should therefore be made on a case-by-case basis. Long-term anticoagulation therapy is often an option for these patients, depending on the underlying pathophysiology.

Section 5: Nonvascular Percutaneous Interventions

Postoperative Collections: Seroma, Hematoma, Biloma, and Abscess

Postoperative fluid collections can cause outflow obstruction or stenosis of the hepatovenous/caval vasculature and/or biliary system as described earlier. These postoperative collections can be serous, hemorrhagic, or bilious secondary to bleeding or bile leak. Although surgical Jackson-Pratt or flat fenestrated drains are left in place to allow for assessment of bleeding or bile leaks and to drain postoperative fluid, these drains are often removed when the patient is discharged or at a postoperative follow-up appointment. Even with drains in place, if there is bleeding and/or bilious drainage, the abdominal fluid can become loculated and thus cannot be adequately drained by surgical drains. Image-guided drainage and decompression can therefore be used for these purposes, as well as to ensure functionality of the graft, to provide pain control, and to prevent superinfection. Drainage of these collections can be performed via ultrasonography, fluoroscopy, CT, or a combination of these modalities using a Seldinger-based approach or trocar/coaxial technique.

Liver Biopsy

The most frequently performed image-guided procedure after liver transplant is liver biopsy. Common indications for biopsy are abnormal hepatic serologies, inadequate immunosuppression, and/or concern for graft rejection. Image-guided biopsy can be performed via ultrasonography, fluoroscopy, or CT. If there is concern regarding concomitant hepatic venous or caval complications, a transjugular liver biopsy is indicated, as pressure measurements obtained at the time of biopsy can be useful in identifying hepatocaval stricture or venous hypertension. Otherwise, the mainstay for assessing graft rejection is the percutaneous approach, which can be performed at any point in the postoperative course.

Conclusion

As the rate of liver transplants and thus the prevalence of transplant-related complications increase, it is vital that clinicians understand when to involve an interventional radiologist in the management of post-transplant complications. Relevant catheter-based therapy options are available to minimize the morbidity and mortality of these complications and thus to improve patient outcomes.

Acknowledgment The authors acknowledge Megan Griffiths for her assistance with medical editing.

References

1. Agostini C, Buccianti S, Risaliti M, et al. Complications in post-liver transplant patients. J Clin Med. 2023;12:6173.
2. Boeva I, Karagyozov PI, Tishkov I. Post-liver transplant biliary complications: current knowledge and therapeutic advances. World J Hepatol. 2021;13:66–79.
3. Brookmeyer CE, Bhatt S, Fishman EK, et al. Multimodality imaging after liver transplant: top 10 important complications. Radiographics. 2022;42:702–21.
4. Buell JF, Funaki B, Cronin DC, et al. Long-term venous complications after full-size and segmental pediatric liver transplantation. Ann Surg. 2002;236:658–66.

5. Cantwell CP, Pena CS, Gervais DA, et al. Thirty years' experience with balloon dilation of benign postoperative biliary strictures: long-term outcomes. Radiology. 2008;249:1050–7.
6. Chen GH, Wang GY, Yang Y, et al. Single-center experience of therapeutic management of hepatic artery stenosis after orthotopic liver transplantation: Report of 20 cases. Eur Surg Res. 2009;42:21–7.
7. Chen J, Weinstein J, Black S, et al. Surgical and endovascular treatment of hepatic arterial complications following liver transplant. Clin Transplant. 2014;28:1305–12.
8. Chong WK, Beland JC, Weeks SM. Sonographic evaluation of venous obstruction in liver transplants. AJR Am J Roentgenol. 2007;188:W515–21.
9. Cizman Z, Saad W. Transplant hepatic artery complications. Tech Vasc Interv Radiol. 2023;26:100923.
10. Corvera CU, Wisneski AD. Benign biliary strictures and biliary fistulae. In: Jarnagin WR, editor. Blumgart's surgery of the liver, biliary tract and pancreas. 7th ed. Philadelphia: Elsevier; 2023.
11. da Silva RF, Raphe R, Felício HC, et al. Prevalence, treatment, and outcomes of the hepatic artery stenosis after liver transplantation. Transplant Proc. 2008;40:805–7.
12. Funaki B, Rosenblum JD, Leef JA, et al. Percutaneous treatment of portal venous stenosis in children and adolescents with segmental hepatic transplants: Long-term results. Radiology. 2000;215:147–51.
13. Girometti R, Cereser L, Bazzocchi M, et al. Magnetic resonance cholangiography in the assessment and management of biliary complications after OLT. World J Radiol. 2014;6:424–36.
14. Gwon DI, Sung KB, Ko GY, et al. Dual catheter placement technique for treatment of biliary anastomotic strictures after liver transplantation. Liver Transpl. 2011;17:159–66.
15. Huang TL, Cheng YF, Chen TY, et al. Doppler ultrasound evaluation of postoperative portal vein stenosis in adult living donor liver transplantation. Transplant Proc. 2010;42:879–81.
16. Husnain A, Aadam AA, Keswani R, et al. Outcomes of percutaneous endobiliary radiofrequency ablation in managing resistant benign biliary strictures: a retrospective analysis. Br J Radiol. 2024; https://doi.org/10.1093/bjr/tqae204.
17. Janssen JJ, van Delden OM, van Lienden KP, et al. Percutaneous balloon dilatation and long-term drainage as treatment of anastomotic and nonanastomotic benign biliary strictures. Cardiovasc Intervent Radiol. 2014;37:1559–67.
18. Kim KS, Kim JM, Lee JS, et al. Stent insertion and balloon angioplasty for portal vein stenosis after liver transplantation: long-term follow-up results. Diagn Interv Radiol. 2019;25:231–7.
19. Kim YJ, Ko GY, Yoon HK, et al. Intraoperative stent placement in the portal vein during or after liver transplantation. Liver Transpl. 2007;13:1145–52.
20. Kimura Y, Tapia Sosa R, Soto-Trujillo D, Sandoval YK, et al. Liver transplant complications radiologist can't miss. Cureus. 2020;12(6):e8465. https://doi.org/10.7759/cureus.8465.
21. Ko GY, Sung KB, Yoon HK, et al. Early posttransplantation portal vein stenosis following living donor liver transplantation: Percutaneous transhepatic primary stent placement. Liver Transpl. 2007;13:530–6.
22. Le L, Terral W, Zea N, et al. Primary stent placement for hepatic artery stenosis after liver transplantation. J Vasc Surg. 2015;62:704–9.
23. Ludwig JM, Webber GR, Knechtle SJ. Percutaneous management of benign biliary strictures with large-bore catheters: comparison between patients with and without orthotopic liver transplantation. J Vasc Interv Radiol. 2016;27:219–225.e1.
24. Magand N, Coronado JL, Drevon H, et al. Primary angioplasty or stenting for hepatic artery stenosis treatment after liver transplantation. Clin Transplant. 2019;33:e13729.
25. Mittler J, Chavin KD, Heinrich S, et al. Surgical duct-to-duct reconstruction: an alternative approach to late biliary anastomotic stricture after deceased donor liver transplantation. J Gastrointest Surg. 2021;25:708–12.
26. Naidu S, Alzubaidi S, Knuttinen G, et al. Treatment of hepatic artery stenosis in liver transplant patients using drug-eluting versus bare-metal stents. J Clin Med. 2021;10:380.
27. Naidu SG, Alzubaidi SJ, Patel IJ, et al. Interventional radiology management of adult liver transplant complications. Radiographics. 2022;42:1705–23.

28. Nam K, Lee SK, Song TJ, et al. Percutaneous transhepatic cholangioscopy for biliary complications after liver transplantation: a single center experience. J Hepatobiliary Pancreat Sci. 2016;23:650–7.
29. Organ Procurement Transplantation Network (2024) Organ Procurement Transplantation Network's national data. https://optn.transplant.hrsa.gov/data/view-data-reports/national-data/#. Accessed 12 Dec 2024.
30. Orons PD, Sheng R, Zajko AB. Hepatic artery stenosis in liver transplant recipients: prevalence and cholangiographic appearance of associated biliary complications. AJR Am J Roentgenol. 1995;165:1145–9.
31. Pandhi M, Lipnik A, Niemeyer M. Endovascular treatment of hepatic venous outflow obstruction after liver transplant. DDI. 2019;3:277–86.
32. Pareja E, Cortes M, Navarro R, et al. Vascular complications after orthotopic liver transplantation: hepatic artery thrombosis. Transplant Proc. 2010;42:2970–2.
33. Pérez-Saborido B, Pacheco-Sánchez D, Barrera-Rebollo A, et al. Incidence, management, and results of vascular complications after liver transplantation. Transplant Proc. 2011;43:749–50.
34. Piardi T, Lhuaire M, Bruno O, et al. Vascular complications following liver transplantation: a literature review of advances in 2015. World J Hepatol. 2016;8:36–57.
35. Rostambeigi N, Hunter D, Duval S, et al. Stent placement versus angioplasty for hepatic artery stenosis after liver transplant: a meta-analysis of case series. Eur Radiol. 2013;23:1323–34.
36. Saad WEA. Portal interventions in liver transplant recipients. Semin Intervent Radiol. 2012;29:99–104.
37. Saad WEA, Davies MG, Sahler L, et al. Hepatic artery stenosis in liver transplant recipients: Primary treatment with percutaneous transluminal angioplasty. J Vasc Interv Radiol. 2005;16:795–805.
38. Sabri SS, Saad WEA, Schmitt TM, et al. Endovascular therapy for hepatic artery stenosis and thrombosis following liver transplantation. Vasc Endovascular Surg. 2011;45:447–52.
39. Shibata T, Itoh K, Kubo T, et al. Percutaneous transhepatic balloon dilation of portal venous stenosis in patients with living donor liver transplantation. Radiology. 2005;235:1078–83.
40. Singh AK, Nachiappan AC, Verma HA, et al. Postoperative imaging in liver transplantation: what radiologists should know. Radiographics. 2010;30:339–51.
41. Song SY, Chung JW, Yin YH, et al. Celiac axis and common hepatic artery variations in 5002 patients: systematic analysis with spiral CT and DSA. Radiology. 2010;255:278–88.
42. St. Michel DP, Goussous N, Orr NL, Barth RN, Gray SH, La Mattina JC, et al. Hepatic artery pseudoaneurysm in the liver transplant recipient: a case series. Case Rep Transplant. 2019;2019:9108903.
43. Thai Binh N, My TT, Oanh DT, et al. Percutaneous transhepatic endoscopic thulium laser vaporesection for management of severe and focal benign biliary strictures. Clin Ter. 2023;174:360–4.
44. Thornburg B, Katariya N, Riaz A, et al. Interventional radiology in the management of the liver transplant patient. Liver Transpl. 2017;23:1328–41.
45. Tzakis A, Todo S, Starzl TE. Orthotopic liver transplantation with preservation of the inferior vena cava. Ann Surg. 1989;210(5):649–52.
46. Ugurel MS, Battal B, Bozlar U, et al. Anatomical variations of hepatic arterial system, coeliac trunk and renal arteries: an analysis with multidetector CT angiography. Br J Radiol. 2010;83:661–7.
47. Voigtländer T, Negm AA, Strassburg CP, et al. Biliary cast syndrome post-liver transplantation: risk factors and outcome. Liver Int. 2013;33:1287–92.
48. Wanjara S, Kashyap S. Bile duct stricture. Treasure Island: StatPearls Publishing; 2023.
49. Winston CB, Lee NA, Jarnagin WR, et al. CT angiography for delineation of celiac and superior mesenteric artery variants in patients undergoing hepatobiliary and pancreatic surgery. AJR Am J Roentgenol. 2007;189:W13–9.
50. Zhong J, Smith C, Walker P, et al. Imaging post liver transplantation part I: vascular complications. Clin Radiol. 2020;75:845–53.

Abdominal Imaging Post-Liver Transplantation

26

Xiaoyang Liu, Christie Cheng, Martin O'Malley, and Korosh Khalili

Introduction

Liver transplantation has become a life-saving intervention for patients with end-stage liver disease, acute liver failure, and certain malignancies. The success of liver transplantation depends not only on the surgical procedure but also on the careful monitoring of the patient postoperatively to ensure graft function and identify potential complications early. Abdominal imaging plays a crucial role in the postoperative management of liver transplant recipients, providing critical information on the structure of the transplanted liver, early detection of complications, and long-term surveillance for both recurrent disease and neoplasia. It is important to note that imaging does not detect immune disturbances/rejection, which may be assessed by biopsy when structural complications have been excluded by imaging.

This chapter will explore the indications for abdominal imaging following liver transplantation, discuss the various imaging modalities used, describe normal post-transplant findings, and review complications that can be detected through imaging.

Rationale for Abdominal Imaging After Liver Transplantation

The primary goal of post-transplant imaging is to assess graft structure, monitor for complications, and provide long-term surveillance. Imaging studies are often performed both routinely in the immediate postoperative period and selectively based on clinical symptoms or laboratory abnormalities.

The following are key indications for post-transplant imaging:

X. Liu · C. Cheng · M. O'Malley · K. Khalili (✉)
Department of Medical Imaging, University Medical Imaging Toronto, University Health Network, University of Toronto, Toronto, ON, Canada
e-mail: Korosh.khalili@uhn.ca

B. Eghtesad et al. (eds.), *Liver Transplantation*,
https://doi.org/10.1007/978-3-032-07072-2_26

- Assessment of graft perfusion: Ensuring patency of hepatic arteries, hepatic veins, portal veins, and inferior vena cava (IVC) in the immediate postoperative period.
- Evaluation of complications: Complications include vascular thrombosis, biliary leaks or stricture, and infection, as well as late complications such as rejection or recurrence of the primary liver disease.
- Long-term surveillance: Surveillance for hepatocellular carcinoma (HCC) recurrence or de novo malignancies, especially in patients with underlying hepatitis B or C infection.

Imaging Modalities for After Liver Transplant

Several imaging modalities are used in the assessment of liver transplant patients, each with unique strengths and limitations.

Ultrasound (US)

Ultrasound is the first-line imaging modality due to its accessibility, lack of radiation, and ability to provide real-time assessment of vascular flow using Doppler technology. It is commonly performed in the immediate postoperative period to assess the hepatic artery, portal vein, hepatic veins, and inferior vena cava (IVC). Doppler ultrasound can be used to detect vascular complications such as hepatic artery thrombosis or stenosis, portal vein thrombosis, and hepatic vein outflow obstruction. In addition, US can assess the biliary tree for evidence of bile duct obstruction or leaks.

- Advantages: Non-invasive, high level of patient acceptance, bedside capability, no radiation, can assess vascularity without the need for intravenous contrast. Additionally, Doppler provides information about quality of flow reflecting pressure and vascular resistance, which is not possible with CT/MRI.
- Disadvantages: Operator-dependent; quality depends on patient's ability to cooperate and their body habitus.

Computed Tomography (CT)

Contrast-enhanced CT provides detailed structural information of both the hepatic parenchyma and vasculature. It is often employed when ultrasound findings are equivocal or when a more comprehensive evaluation of complications such as vascular complications, abscesses, hematomas, or biliary complications is needed.

- Advantages: Detailed cross-sectional imaging, evaluation of both parenchymal and vascular structures, and widespread availability.
- Disadvantages: Radiation exposure and potential nephrotoxicity/allergic-like reactions from contrast agents. Lack of bedside access.

Magnetic Resonance Imaging (MRI)

MRI, particularly magnetic resonance cholangiopancreatography (MRCP), is a powerful tool for evaluating the biliary system and liver parenchyma without the need for radiation. Excretory cholangiography using hepatobiliary-specific contrast agents such as gadoxetic acid can also detect biliary leak.

- Advantages: Superior soft-tissue contrast, non-invasive biliary imaging, and no radiation.
- Disadvantages: Longer imaging times, lower patient tolerance, limited access in the immediate postoperative period, higher cost, and contraindications in patients with certain implants (e.g., pacemakers).

MRI can also detect subtle parenchymal changes that may suggest ischemia or recurrent disease, making it invaluable in long-term surveillance.

Normal Post-transplant Imaging Findings

Understanding the spectrum of normal post-transplant imaging appearances is crucial to differentiate between physiological changes and pathological findings. For a thorough and accurate evaluation, it is important to convey the post-surgical anatomy of the graft to the imaging team to understand the vascular and biliary surgical anastomoses.

Liver Morphology and Parenchyma

The contour of the transplanted whole liver or partial liver lobe should be smooth without irregularities. The liver parenchyma should appear homogeneous without focal lesions. In the early postoperative period (<1 month), perihepatic fluid pockets/collections are commonly seen and resolved over time. Persistent collections demonstrating a thick enhancing wall on CT are worrisome for infection, and sampling or drainage may be considered if there are clinical/serological signs of infection. Hematomas have a typical appearance on respective imaging modalities; however, active hemorrhage is not often detected by ultrasound and requires multiphase contrast-enhanced CT.

Vascular Anatomy and Normal Imaging Findings

The hepatic artery, portal vein, and hepatic vein demonstrate a unique normal waveform on Doppler ultrasound and should appear patent without significant narrowing on contrast-enhanced CT or MRI. The normal Doppler waveforms for each of the hepatic artery, portal vein, and hepatic vein are illustrated in Fig. 26.1.

- Hepatic artery: The hepatic artery is typically reconstructed as an end-to-end anastomosis to the recipient's hepatic artery or via a conduit. Due to the variability of location/vessels used, ultrasound does not reliably assess the arterial anastomosis. Assessment of flow in the hepatic artery is *downstream* from the anastomosis, and particularly cogent for the intrahepatic arteries. On Doppler US, a normal intrahepatic artery waveform is pulsatile with a sharp systolic upstroke, and has resistive indices (RI) in the range of 0.5–0.8 (Fig. 26.1a) [1]. Elevated peak systolic velocity (PSV) >200 cm/sec is not a rare finding immediately post-transplant surgery and can be caused by transient edema at the anastomosis. Elevated RI of 0.8–1.0 is seen in up to ½ of recipients and can be considered a normal postoperative finding. It often normalizes within a few days post-surgery. A low RI <0.5 immediately postoperative is associated with increased vascular complications and should be assessed with CT angiography, which can assess the anastomosis directly [2].
- Portal vein: The portal vein is anastomosed to the recipient's portal vein end-to-end, or via an interposition jump graft from the superior mesenteric vein (SMV). The portal vein should have continuous hepatopetal flow with mild cardiac and respiratory variations (Fig. 26.1b). Post-surgical edema may cause elevated portal vein velocity above 50 cm/s, which usually resolves within a few weeks.
- Hepatic veins and inferior vena cava (IVC): Piggyback surgical technique is typically used to create caval anastomosis in cadaveric donor transplants, where the donor IVC is anastomosed to the preserved recipient IVC. Other more complex reconstruction techniques are used in living donor liver transplant (LDLT), such as end-to-end hepatic venous anastomoses or end-to-side anastomosis to the IVC. In right hepatic lobe LDLT, the middle hepatic vein is often preserved in the donor, and maintenance of its tributaries in the graft requires reconstruction with an autologous vein or synthetic graft. On ultrasound imaging, the normal waveform of the hepatic vein is triphasic flow (Fig. 26.1c). However, because of the pliability of the hepatic veins, presence of collections and ascites, and the mobility of the liver, it is common to see flow disturbances in the hepatic veins such as monophasic flow and high velocity at their anastomoses or within the IVC at the level of the diaphragm. Therefore, further evaluation of Doppler disturbances in the hepatic veins should be balanced with other parameters of graft function.

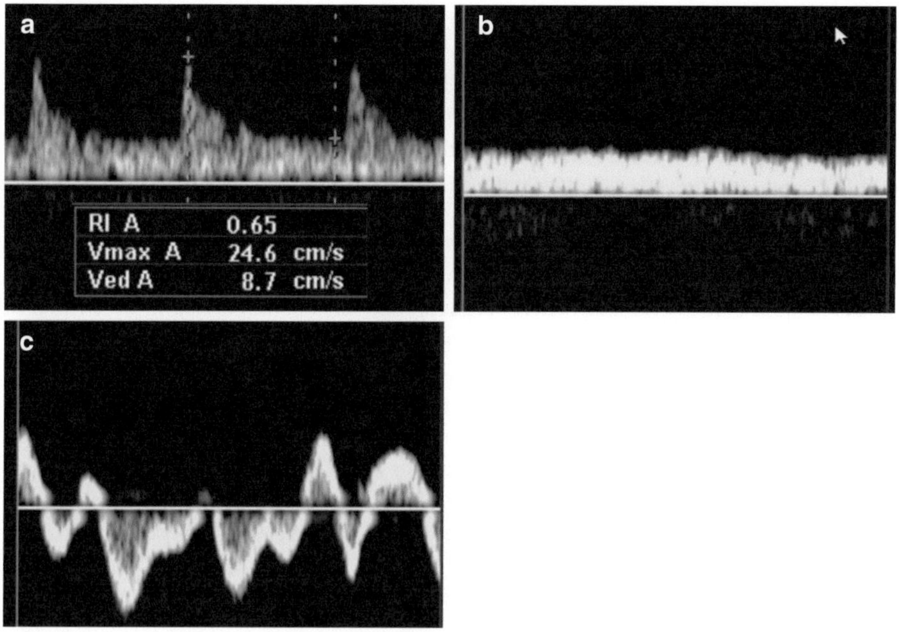

Fig. 26.1 Normal Doppler ultrasound findings of hepatic artery, hepatic vein and portal vein after liver transplant. (**a**) Normal hepatic artery waveform is pulsatile with sharp systolic upstroke, and has resistive indices (RI) in the range of 0.5–0.8. (**b**) Normal portal vein Doppler shows continuous hepatopetal flow with mild cardiac and respiratory variations. (**c**) Normal hepatic vein flow is triphasic on Doppler ultrasound

Biliary System

- Biliary reconstruction most commonly consists of two types: duct-to-duct anastomosis or bilio-enteric anastomosis, including hepatico-jejunostomy and choledocho-jejunostomy.
- Post-transplant, the bile ducts should be patent without evidence of dilatation. Persistent fluid collection adjacent to the anastomotic site with the presence of ascites should prompt suspicion for biliary leaks.

Common Complications Detected via Imaging

Despite advances in surgical techniques and immunosuppression, complications remain a significant concern after liver transplantation. Early detection through imaging is critical for effective management.

Vascular Complications

Vascular complications after liver transplant include thrombosis or stenosis of the hepatic artery, hepatic vein, or portal vein, as well as hepatic artery pseudoaneurysm. Selected examples with case demonstrations are discussed in detail, as follows.

Hepatic Artery Thrombosis/Stenosis

- Incidence: Hepatic artery thrombosis was reported to have an overall incidence of 2.9% in some series. However its incidence has been decreasing over the past decade due to the refinement of surgical techniques. It can lead to biliary necrosis, graft loss, and high mortality rate in the early postoperative period [1].
- Imaging findings: On Doppler ultrasound, absence of arterial signal in the intrahepatic arteries is often technical in nature and should prompt re-examination utilizing an experienced sonographer and/or specialized techniques such as contrast-enhanced ultrasound. If no or a low-resistance (RI < 0.5) flow is detected, the artery and the anastomosis should be evaluated by CT angiogram (CTA) (Fig. 26.2). Liver parenchymal infarct manifests as peripheral wedge-shaped nonenhancing or hypoenhancing areas on CT and areas of heterogeneity on ultrasound.

Hepatic Arterial Ischemic Cascade

A cascade of catastrophic events occurs with prolonged arterial ischemia, which leads to graft failure; due to its varying appearances during progression, it can be difficult to recognize. The most common cause of the cascade is hepatic artery thrombosis or significant stenosis, but prolonged hypoxia/hypotension can be causative or contributory as well. The cascade manifests indolently, with elevation of cholestatic liver enzymes as a result of biliary necrosis, leading eventually to significant biliary obstruction. Bilomas can then develop as a result of the biliary obstruction and infection can set it causing peribiliary abscesses. Ultimately the infection results in portal vein thrombosis and parenchymal ischemia.

- Imaging findings: Imaging findings: Early biliary findings can be insidious on imaging and should be sought after detection of low resistance HA flow (Fig. 26.3). The earliest finding is a mild but progressive dilatation of intrahepatic bile ducts in the setting of rising cholestatic liver markers such as alkaline phosphatase (ALP) and bilirubin. The dilated ducts should be followed centrally on sonographic examination, often showing echogenic filling defects representing bile duct casts. On MRI examination, the casts appear as T1 bright intraductal filling defects due the presence of bilirubinate and/or blood products. Bilomas appear as subcapsular hypoechoic/anechoic geographic lesions on ultrasound and nonenhancing areas in the liver parenchyma without a defined wall on CT and MRI (Fig. 26.3).

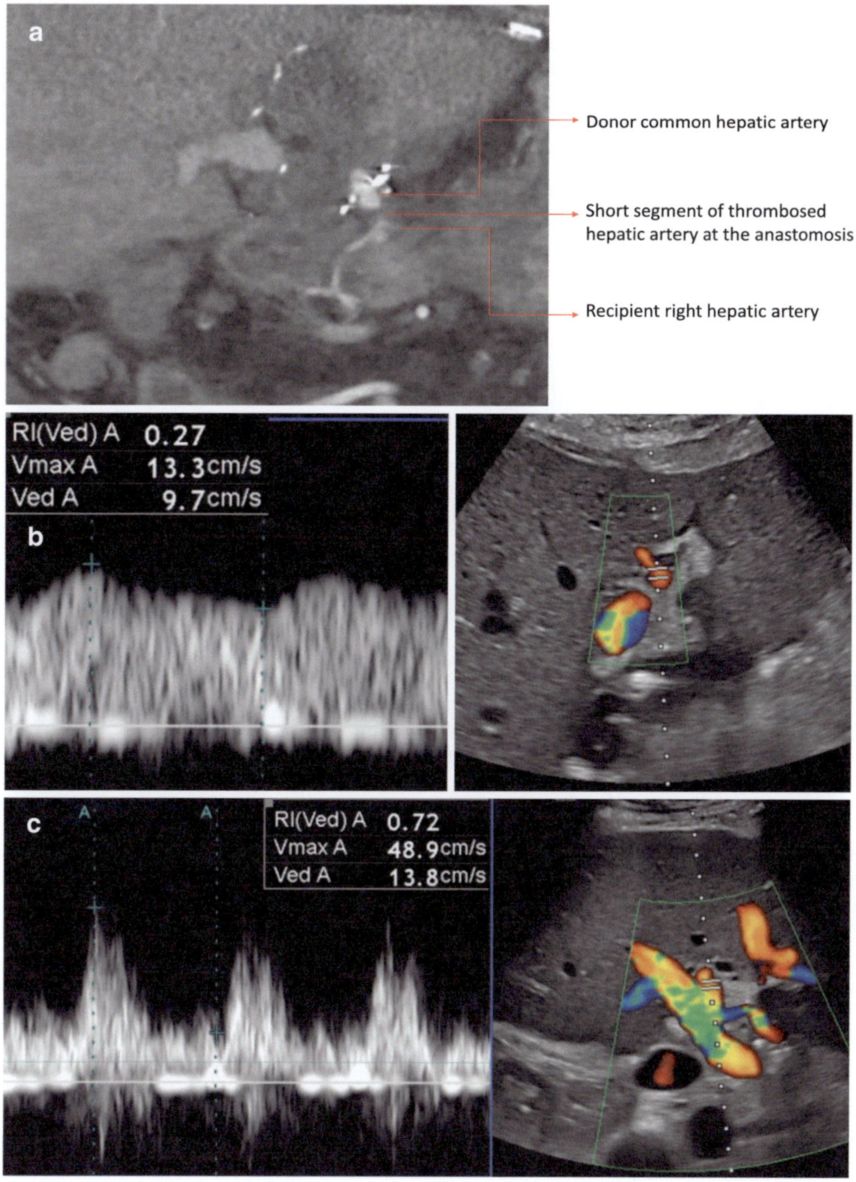

Fig. 26.2 Hepatic Artery Stenosis: A 55-year-old male patient received living donor liver transplant. Contrast-enhanced CT was performed 15 days post transplant due to patient's elevated liver enzyme and drop in hemoglobin. During the transplant, hepatic artery anastomosis was performed from the donor's common hepatic artery to recipient's replaced right hepatic artery which originated from the superior mesenteric artery (SMA). (**a**) A short segment of non-opacification was seen on CT at the hepatic artery anastomosis, representing severe arterial stenosis at the anastomosis. (**b**) On ultrasound, there is abnormally low resistive index (RI) of 0.27 in the left hepatic, with tardus-parvus waveform. Similar findings were discovered in the right hepatic artery with RI of 0.35 (not shown). Urgent hepatic artery reconstruction with saphenous vein was performed to repair the thrombosed hepatic artery. (**c**) Repeat ultrasound after surgical revision of the thrombosed hepatic artery showed normalization of hepatic artery waveform and normal RI of 0.72

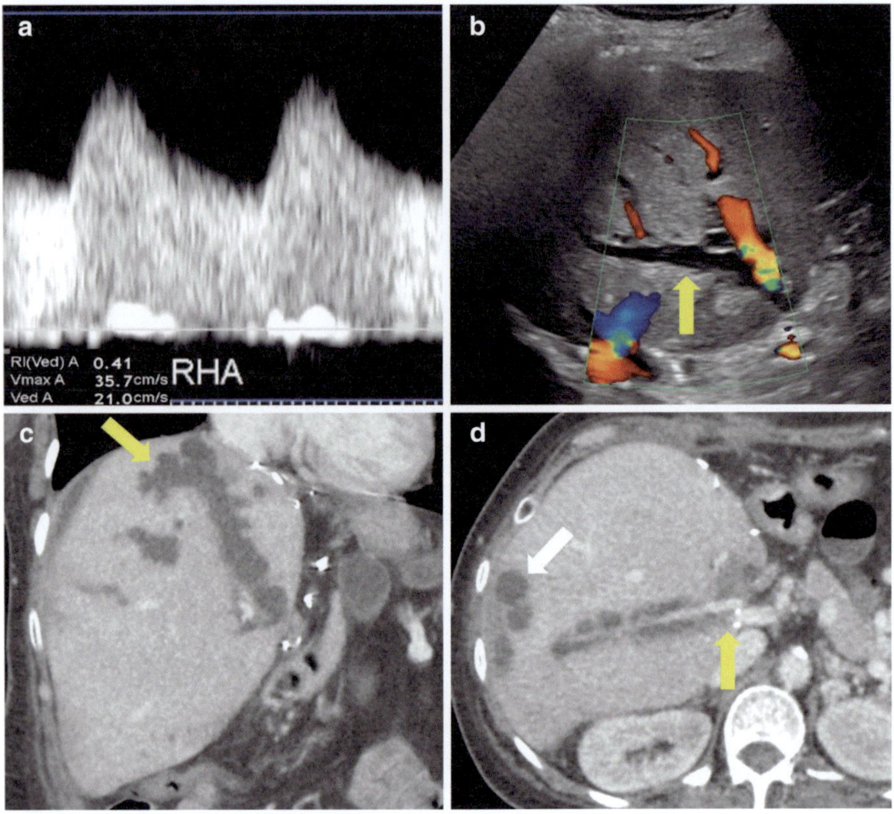

Fig. 26.3 Hepatic Arterial Ischemic Cascade: (**a**) At day 23 post right lobe living donor liver transplantation, a sudden rise in liver enzymes was noted. Ultrasound examination revealed a new tardus-parvus hepatic arterial waveform with reduced resistive index (RI) of 0.41. (**b**) Ultrasound of 10 days later depicted diffuse dilatation of in the intrahepatic biliary tree (arrow). (**c**) CT scan in the coronal plane in day 33 shows biloma about the bile ducts and confluent in the peripheral parenchyma (arrow). (**d**) CT scan at day 70 obtained because of recurrent fevers shows thrombosis of the right posterior portal vein (yellow arrow) with new cystic lesions in the subcapsular lesion showing subtle wall enhancement (white arrow). Aspiration confirmed bacterial abscess

Portal Vein Thrombosis

- Incidence: Portal vein complications have an incidence of 1% [3]. It can happen in the early or late period after transplant. And imaging plays an essential role in the diagnosis. The risk factors for portal vein thrombosis include preoperative portal vein abnormalities, a significant stenosis at the portal vein anastomosis, hypercoagulable states, and infection.
- Imaging findings:
  - US/Doppler: Absent or attenuated portal flow, presence of echogenic thrombus in the portal vein (Fig. 26.4).

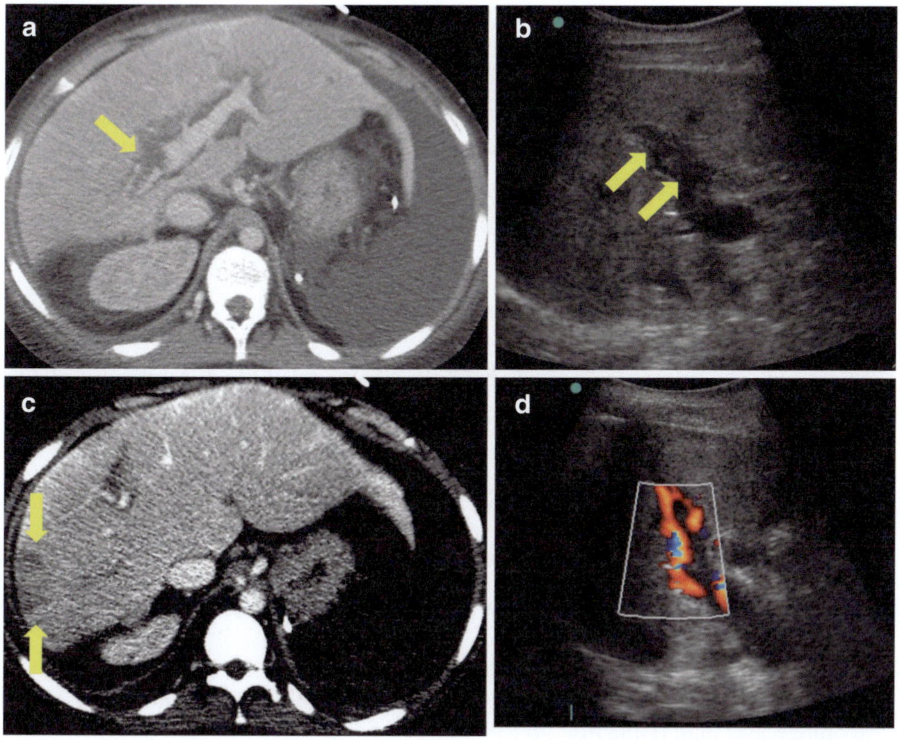

Fig. 26.4 Portal Vein Thrombosis: 23-year-old female had liver transplant for autoimmune liver disease, developed partial right portal vein thrombosis 1 month after liver transplant. (**a**) Contrast enhanced CT showed non obstructing thrombus in the right portal vein (arrow). (**b**) CT also showed wedge-shaped areas of hypoattenuation in the periphery aspect of the right lobe of the liver (arrows), in keeping with liver hypoerfusion/ischemia. (**c**) Ultrasound showed echogenic thrombus in the right portal vein (arrows). (**d**) Doppler showed partial thrombosis of the right portal vein with some flow still observed

- CT/MRI: Filling defects within the portal vein (Fig. 26.4), absence of enhancement, or partial enhancement of the portal vein. If associated liver parenchyma ischemia/infarct occurs, it will manifest as a wedge-shaped hypoattenuating area in the periphery of the transplant liver (Fig. 26.4).

Hepatic Vein Stenosis

- Incidence: True hepatic vein stenosis after liver transplant is a relatively uncommon complication, and occurs more often in living donor liver transplant [4]. It typically arises at the anastomotic site of the hepatic veins and can lead to hepatic congestion, graft dysfunction, and eventually graft failure if not promptly recognized or treated. Risk factors for hepatic vein stenosis include a size mismatch between donor and recipient veins.
- Imaging findings:

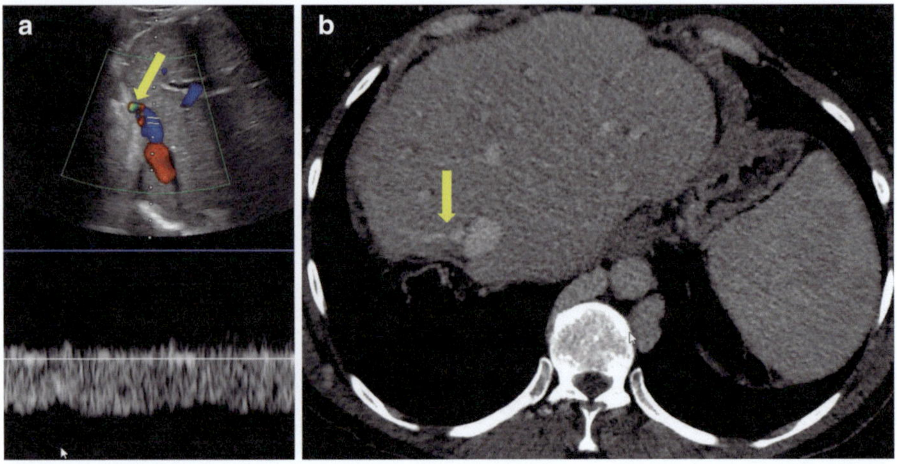

Fig. 26.5 Hepatic Vein Stenosis: 38-year-old male with liver transplant at age 8 performed for biliary atresia. Presented with elevated liver function test and was found to have right hepatic vein stenosis. (**a**) Doppler ultrasound demonstrated focal area of turbulence in the vein (arrow) with monophasic waveform with decreased pulsitility upstream in the right hepatic vein. (**b**) Contrast enhanced CT showed focal narrowing of the right hepatic vein close to the junction to the IVC (arrow)

- US/Doppler: Monophasic waveform of the hepatic veins, venous pulsatility index less than 0.45 (Fig. 26.5).
- CT/MRI: Focal narrowing of the hepatic vein (Fig. 26.5).

Biliary Complications

Biliary complications are an important cause of morbidity in the early- and late-period after liver transplants. Overall incidence of biliary complications ranges from 15% to 25%, with associated mortality of 10% [5]. The most common biliary complications include biliary leaks, strictures, and stones. Biliary leaks or strictures can happen at the anastomotic site, which are caused by a technical issue; they can also occur at non-anastomotic sites, with common causes such as ischemia or immune reaction.

Biliary Leaks

- Biliary leak is the most common biliary complication in the early post-transplant period (within a 4-week post-surgery) [6]. The reported incidence of biliary leaks ranges from 2% to 25% [5]. Anastomotic biliary leaks happen more frequently than non-anastomotic biliary leaks. Causes of biliary leak include ischemic injury, technical factors such as tension at the anastomosis, incomplete cystic stump suture, and bleeding from the cut end of the duct.
- Imaging findings:

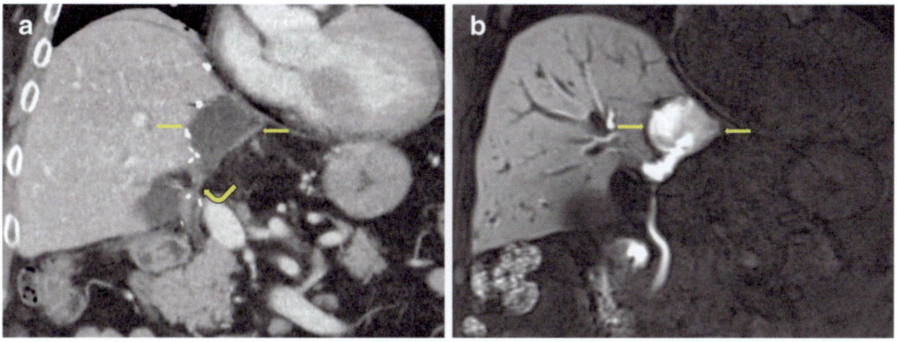

Fig. 26.6 Bile Leak: 61-year-old male who underwent liver transplant 2 months ago with persistently AST, ALT and ALP, was found to have biliary leak. (**a**) CT demonstrated a fluid collection (straight arrows) adjacent to the duct-to-duct anastomosis (curved arrow)of the biliary tree, suspicious for a biloma secondary to biliary leak at the anastomosis. (**b**) MRI using gadoxetate contrast agent at hepatobiliary phase demonstrated opacification of the biliary tree by the bright contrast, and leakage of the contrast into the collection, at the level of the biliary duct-to-duct anastomosis

- Ultrasound: In the setting of biliary leaks, the intrahepatic biliary tree generally appears normal. An anechoic collection in the porta hepatis or ascites may be observed.
- CT/MRI: A persistent or enlarging fluid collection in the vicinity of the biliary anastomosis with ascites should raise suspicion for a biliary leak (Fig. 26.6).
- Excretory MR cholangiography/ERCP: Biliary leak can be visualized on MRI using a hepatobiliary contrast agent. At the (delayed) hepatobiliary phase, the contrast will have opacified the biliary tree, and biliary leak will be visualized as progressive contrast accumulation outside of the biliary tree (Fig. 26.6). ERCP represents an invasive modality pinpointing the site of excretion.

Biliary Strictures

- Biliary stricture manifests as narrowing of the biliary ductal lumen, with obstruction or disturbance of the bile outflow. Strictures may be anastomotic or non-anastomotic.
- Anastomotic biliary stricture: It makes up 50% of biliary complications after liver transplant, most commonly at the anastomotic site, occurring mostly within the first year after transplantation. Risk factors for anastomotic biliary strictures include biliary leak, LDLT & DDLT, ABO incompatibility, advanced recipient age, prolonged ischemia, and cytomegalovirus infection [5].
  - Imaging findings: Biliary dilatation proximal to a narrowed segment of biliary ducts can be seen, most often at the level of the anastomosis (Fig. 26.7).
- Non-anastomotic biliary strictures: They happen to biliary ducts proximal to the anastomosis, and are more often longer and multiple as well as more rare compared to anastomotic strictures. Common risk factors for non-anastomotic stric-

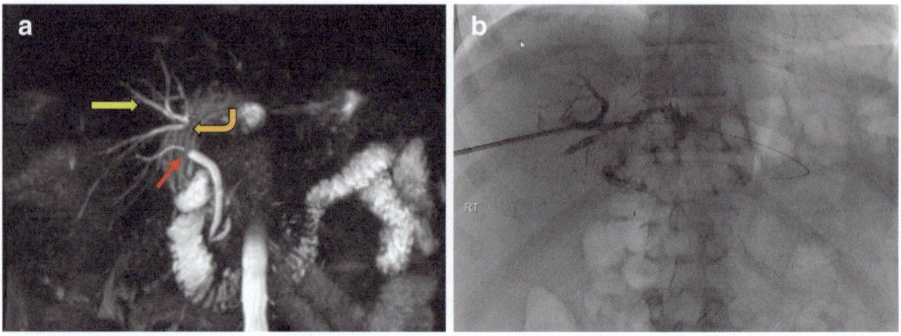

Fig. 26.7 Anastamotic biliary Stricture: 56-year-old male had liver transplant for chronic hepatitis C, presented with elevated serum bilirubin level 6 months post liver transplant, was found to have biliary stricture on imaging. (**a**) MRCP demonstrated dilation of right intrahepatic biliary duct (yellow arrow), with cut-off at the choledocho-enteric anastomosis (curved arrow) representing a biliary stricture. Segment 6 was drained through a direct anastomosis (red arrow) of the segment 6 branch with the native bile duct. Patient was treated initially with balloon dilatation of the anastomotic stricture without a response, and was subsequently treated with surgical revision of his anastomosis. Bilirubin showed significant decrease post revision. (**b**) Cholangiogram performed after revision of biliary anastomosis showed good flow from the biliary duct through the biliary enteric anastomosis and into the bowel. No evidence of stricture at the biliary-enteric anastomosis

tures include hepatic artery thrombosis/stenosis, prolonged ischemia during surgery, and primary sclerosing cholangitis (PSC) in the recipient [7].

– Imaging findings: Multifocal central strictures are seen in CT. On sonography or T1W MRI sequences, intraductal contents are seen centrally causing the strictures and represent necrotic material and bile duct casts made of cellular debris, bilirubin products, and/or blood products.

Infectious Complications

Infectious complications after liver transplantation are a leading cause of morbidity and mortality, particularly in the early postoperative period when the patients are the most immunosuppressed. The infections can be bacterial, fungal, or viral in origin. Common bacterial infections include wound infections, pneumonia, cholangitis, and other causes of septicemia, typically emerging within the first month after transplant. Fungal infections, especially those caused by Candida and Aspergillus, are more likely to occur in critically ill patients or those requiring prolonged immunosuppression, and can present as multiple small abscesses in the liver and/or spleen. The most common and clinically significant viral infection is cytomegalovirus (CMV) infection. CMV can cause a wide range of manifestations, from asymptomatic viremia to life-threatening disease involving the liver, gastrointestinal tract, or lungs. Epstein-Barr virus (EBV) infection is another important viral pathogen, due to its association with post-transplant lymphoproliferative disorder (PTLD).

Radiological imaging is useful for detecting intra-abdominal abscess formation and organ involvement by bacterial or fungal infections.

Recurrence of Malignancy and Post-transplant Lymphoproliferative Disorder

Recurrent malignancy in patients with a known or incidentally found malignancy in the explant is a significant concern. While liver transplantation offers the potential for curative treatment in patients with early-stage HCC, recurrence occurs in approximately 6–16% of cases and is associated with poor long-term survival [8]. Risk factors for recurrence include tumor characteristics such as vascular invasion, poor differentiation, and size or number of lesions exceeding criteria like the Milan criteria at the time of transplant. Surveillance imaging is used for the early detection of malignancy, typically presenting as new liver nodules, or extrahepatic metastases, often in the nodes, lungs, or bones. The imaging appearance depends on the type of malignancy. Typical enhancement pattern of HCC is similar to the primary HCC, with major features including non-peripheral arterial hyperenhancement, washout, and/or capsule at portal venous or delayed phase (Fig. 26.8).

Post-transplant lymphoproliferative disorder (PTLD) is another potentially life-threatening complication that can arise in the setting of immunosuppression following liver transplantation. PTLD is most commonly associated with Epstein-Barr virus (EBV) reactivation and can range from benign lymphoid hyperplasia to aggressive lymphomas. The risk of PTLD is highest in the first year post-transplant

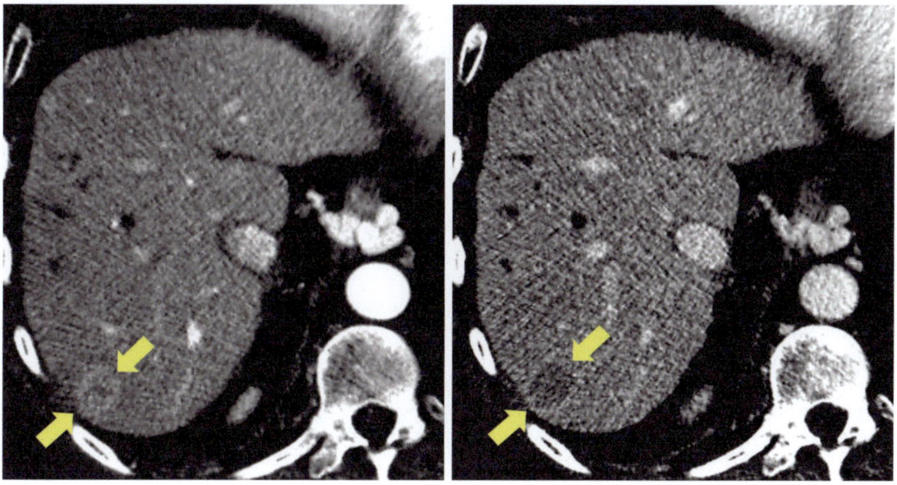

Fig. 26.8 HCC Recurrence Post Transplantation: 69-year-old male, who had liver transplant for hepatocellular carcinoma (HCC). Two years after liver transplant, patient developed recurrent HCC. On imaging, recurrent HCC manifested similar to primary HCC showing arterial hyperenhancement (**a**, arrows) and washout on portal venous phase (**b**, arrows)

and often presents with nonspecific symptoms such as fever, weight loss, and lymphadenopathy. It may involve the liver, gastrointestinal tract, or central nervous system. Imaging is not routinely used in screening for PTLD in asymptomatic patients. Radiologic findings can include lymph node enlargement, organ infiltration, or liver masses, with FDG-PET scans sometimes utilized to assess the metabolic activity of the lesions.

Conclusion

Abdominal imaging is an indispensable component of postoperative care in liver transplant recipients. It provides critical insights into graft structure, facilitates the early detection and management of complications, and plays a central role in long-term surveillance. Advances in imaging technology continue to enhance the precision and efficacy of post-transplant evaluations, ultimately contributing to improved patient outcomes and graft survival.

References

1. Brookmeyer CE, Bhatt S, Fishman EK, Sheth S. Multimodality imaging after liver transplant: top 10 important complications. Radiographics. 2022;42(3):702–21. https://doi.org/10.1148/rg.210108.
2. Uzochukwu LN, Bluth EI, Smetherman DH, et al. Early postoperative hepatic sonography as a predictor of vascular and biliary complications in adult orthotopic liver transplant patients. Am J Roentgenol. 2005;185(6):1558–70. https://doi.org/10.2214/AJR.04.1258.
3. Hu LS, Zhao Z, Li T, Li QS, Lu Y, Wang B. The management of portal vein thrombosis after adult liver transplantation: a case series and review of the literature. J Clin Med. 2022;11(16) https://doi.org/10.3390/jcm11164909.
4. Singh AK, Nachiappan AC, Verma HA, et al. Postoperative imaging in liver transplantation: what radiologists should know. Radiographics. 2010;30(2):339–51. https://doi.org/10.1148/rg.302095124.
5. Boeva I, Karagyozov PI, Tishkov I. Post-liver transplant biliary complications: current knowledge and therapeutic advances. World J Hepatol. 2021;13(1):66–79. https://doi.org/10.4254/wjh.v13.i1.66.
6. Kochhar G, Parungao JM, Hanouneh IA, Parsi MA. Biliary complications following liver transplantation. World J Gastroenterol. 2013;19(19):2841–6. https://doi.org/10.3748/wjg.v19.i19.2841.
7. Macías-Gómez C, Dumonceau JM. Endoscopic management of biliary complications after liver transplantation: an evidence-based review. World J Gastrointest Endosc. 2015;7(6):606. https://doi.org/10.4253/wjge.v7.i6.606.
8. Agarwal PD, Lucey MR. Management of hepatocellular carcinoma recurrence after liver transplantation. Ann Hepatol. 2022;27(1):100654. https://doi.org/10.1016/J.AOHEP.2021.100654.

The Role of Interventional Endoscopy Post Transplantation

27

Mohamed Tausif Siddiqui and John Vargo

Introduction

Liver transplantation (LT) is a lifesaving intervention, but it carries a significant risk of postoperative complications [1–3]. Among these, biliary complications (BC) represent the most common cause of morbidity in transplant recipients, making timely endoscopic intervention a crucial component of comprehensive postoperative management [1, 4]. The incidence rate for biliary complications has been reported to range between 5% and 20% [5–8]. The majority of postoperative biliary complications are amenable to endoscopic retrograde cholangiopancreatography (ERCP), which offers high success rates (>90%) [9, 10]. Consequently, ERCP-based interventions have become the first-line therapy for managing most biliary issues following liver transplantation [7, 10]. In this chapter, we will discuss a brief review of the role of interventional endoscopy and ERCP in LT patients, covering the common indications, procedural techniques, complication management, and new frontiers in this evolving field.

Significance of ERCP in the Post-transplant Care In the early LT era, post-LT complications such as biliary strictures and leaks were historically treated either via surgical or radiologic interventions [11–14]. Advances in endoscopic techniques and accessories have vastly improved outcomes, leading to widespread utilization of ERCP, which provides a minimally invasive approach to diagnosing and treating biliary complications simultaneously [15]. This is especially valuable in liver transplant recipients, who are typically immunosuppressed and at high risk for complications from major surgical interventions. Studies have shown that timely endoscopic

M. T. Siddiqui · J. Vargo (✉)
Department of Gastroenterology, Hepatology and Nutrition, Digestive Disease Institute,
Cleveland Clinic, Cleveland, OH, USA
e-mail: SIDDIQM5@ccf.org; vargoj@ccf.org

B. Eghtesad et al. (eds.), *Liver Transplantation*,
https://doi.org/10.1007/978-3-032-07072-2_27

management significantly reduces graft loss and patient mortality by effectively addressing biliary obstructions, bile leaks, and preventing cholangitis [16]. Notably, the overall complication rate of ERCP in liver transplant recipients (approximately 5–9%) is comparable to that of non-transplant patients, highlighting the safety of ERCP in this population [16–19]. Nonetheless, specific nuances—such as altered anatomy in some transplant patients and their immunosuppressed state—necessitate careful consideration and detailed procedural planning [20].

Indications for ERCP in Liver Transplant Patients

Major indications for ERCP in liver transplant patients include: (i) anastomotic (AS) and non-anastomotic biliary strictures (NAS); (ii) biliary leaks and bilomas; (iii) biliary obstruction due to stones or sludge; as well as, less common indications such as (iv) sphincter of Oddi dysfunction (SOD); and (v) biliary stent exchange or removals. It is important for clinicians to have a high index of suspicion for these post-LT complications, and early imaging (Ultrasound or MRI) can often guide the diagnosis; however, ERCP would generally be indicated once a treatable lesion is identified. Please see a brief discussion of each indication as follows.

Biliary Strictures (Anastomotic and Non-anastomotic)

Biliary strictures are the most common biliary complication after LT, and the overall incidence is higher in Living-donor liver transplant (28–32%) compared to after Diseased Donor Liver Transplant (5–15%) because anastomoses involving small-caliber peripheral donor ducts are more complex in LDLT [9, 11, 21]. Post-LT biliary strictures can be either anastomotic or non-anastomotic.

(i). *Anastomotic Strictures (AS)*

AS occur at the site of anastomosis between donor and recipient ducts, are usually short and singular, and typically present within the first year post-transplant [7, 9]. Incidence rate of AS ranges from 4% to 12% [7, 9]. The main causes for AS are usually technical or ischemic: surgical technique causing localized fibrosis, inadequate blood supply to the anastomosis, or scarring from prior bile leakage [11]. Patients typically present with clinical signs of biliary obstruction or a cholestatic liver pattern. ERCP is indicated as first-line therapy, has high efficacy for dilation and stenting of the stricture and success rate has been reported to range from 80% to 90%; however, it often requires multiple sessions of progressive dilation [22]. Timely intervention for AS has been reported to be associated with better outcomes and a decrease in need for multiple therapies [23]. Novel approaches include placement of multiple plastic stents and utilizing covered self-expandable metal stents (cSEMSs) to shorten the therapy duration and decrease the number of interventions [24–27].

(ii). *Non-anastomotic Strictures (NAS)*

NAS are the strictures that occur in the donor bile ducts proximal to the anastomosis. These strictures are usually longer and involve multiple sites [22, 28] NAS are usually less common but more severe, and the incidence rate ranges between 0.5% and 10% [9]. Risk factors for NAS include hepatic artery thrombosis, longer cold and warm ischemia time, longer operating time, and pre-transplant diagnoses of primary sclerosing cholangitis (PSC) and autoimmune hepatitis [29]. NAS is also associated with recurrent cholangitis and increased graft loss after LT [29]. ERCP is considered the first-line therapy as an attempt to provide bile drainage however management is more challenging and less consistently successful then AS and alternate approaches with combination of ERCP with percutaneous transhepatic (PTC) drainage and sometimes re-transplant is required for significant intrahepatic biliary disease [11, 22, 28].

Bile Leak

Bile leak is the second most common complication after LT, and the incidence rate has been reported to range between 5% and 15% and occurrences ranged from Day 1 to 6 months within the post-LT period [8, 11, 30–33]. The incidence is higher up to 24% if a T tube is used, and common sites for bile leak include the anastomotic junction, T tube insertion site, or the cut surface of the liver [11, 34]. Hepatic artery thrombosis can also cause ischemic necrosis of the bile duct and lead to leaks. Clinically, patients may have bilious output in drains, ascites with high bile content, abdominal pain, or sepsis signs if bile leaks into the peritoneum [11, 12]. Imaging can confirm the bile leak but ERCP is the preferred diagnostic and therapeutic modality [9, 11, 23]. During ERCP, a cholangiogram will typically show extravasation of contrast from the bile duct into an abnormal location (e.g., along the T-tube tract or at the anastomosis). Smaller bile leaks or those after T tube removal can close spontaneously within 24 h [35]. The endoscopic treatment aims to promote internal drainage of bile and reduce pressure across the leak site to facilitate its closure, which is usually achieved by sphincterotomy with biliary stent placement across the leaks to divert the bile away from the leak site [9, 11]. Endoscopic treatment of bile leaks has a high success rate for treatment with resolution in 90–95% of cases [9, 11, 36]. Prompt intervention for biliary leak is a key factor because unresolved biliary leak can also lead to secondary strictures over time. In addition to ERCP therapy, percutaneous drainage of the biloma is necessary to promote healing and reduce the symptoms of bile peritonitis. Biliary tube drainage is also an excellent way to gauge the success of ERCP-mediated therapy.

Choledocholithiasis and Sludge

Biliary stones, sludge, and casts can result in filling defects and biliary obstruction after LT, and the incidence has been reported to a range of 5–10% [9, 37] Biliary strictures are also noted in up to 90% patients with bile stones [11, 38]. ERCP is indicated as the therapeutic modality to clear bile duct stones and sludge in transplant patients, similar to the non-transplant setting [11]. The endoscopist should perform a biliary sphincterotomy (if not already done) to facilitate extraction. Standard stone extraction techniques are used: balloon sweeps and basket retrieval. If a stone is large or located in a tight stricture, balloon dilation of the papilla (sphincteroplasty) and/or of the stricture can assist in removing the stone. In complex cases with multiple intrahepatic stones or casts, direct cholangioscopy with electrohydraulic lithotripsy (EHL) may be employed to fragment stones [39].

Sphincter of Oddi Dysfunction

Sphincter of Oddi Dysfunction (SOD) can occur after LT which can result from denervation or disruption of normal sphincter function and the incidence rate can range between 2% and 5% [7, 12, 40, 41] Diagnosis can be challenging, and high quality magnetic resonance imaging (MRI/MRCP) should be pursued prior to ERCP to exonerate alternate etiologies. Once diagnosed, an ERCP with sphincterotomy with or without stenting has been the most acceptable treatment option for SOD, which is usually highly effective [12, 22, 42].

Stent Placement, Removal, or Exchange

Other common indications for ERCP in post-LT patients are for the management of biliary stents. A repeat ERCP is often indicated for upsizing the stent for biliary strictures, exchange of plastic stents (usually within 2–3 months to prevent complications), or to address issues of stent occlusion or stent migration [43].

Procedural Considerations and Technical Challenges

Performing ERCP in liver transplant recipients follows the fundamental principles of ERCP in any patient, but there are important technical considerations and adjustments given the surgical anatomy and immunosuppressed status.

(i) *Pre-procedural Consideration*

Prior to undertaking ERCP in a patient with LT, a thorough review of surgical history and imaging is essential. An endoscopist must know the type of biliary reconstruction. The most common type is duct-to-duct anastomosis to the native common bile duct (also known as choledochocholedochostomy), with other types being connection of the bile duct to a portion of jejunum (Roux-en-y hepatico/choledocho-jejunostomy) [12, 22, 44]. Prior imaging can be helpful to map out the biliary system and plan an endoscopic approach. Immunosuppression is usually continued, and antibiotic prophylaxis is generally indicated. The American Society of Gastrointestinal Endoscopy (ASGE) guidelines recommend that antibiotics prophylaxis be administered before ERCP in patients who have had liver transplantation or who have known or suspected biliary obstruction, where there is a possibility of incomplete biliary drainage [45–47]. It recommends that antibiotics that cover biliary flora such as enteric gram-negative organisms and enterococci should be used and continued after the procedure if biliary drainage is incomplete.

(ii) *Intraprocedural Challenges and Technique Modification*

In patients with Roux-en-Y hepaticojejunostomy, an ERCP is technically challenging [7]. A single-balloon guided ERCP has shown both diagnostic and therapeutic value [48]. For the anastomotic strictures, a sequential multiple plastic stent placement has been a traditional approach,

And alternatively, fully covered self-expandable metal stents can also be used and have shown similar efficacy and safety with fewer ERCP sessions and shorter treatment duration [49, 50].

(iii) *Use of Advanced Techniques*

Modern ERCP in LT patients increasingly employs adjunct technologies to manage complex biliary issues. The addition of intervention such as peroral cholangioscopy (POCS) to the conventional ERCP has facilitated direct visualization of the bile duct lumen, strictures, and sampling, shown improved diagnostic value, and helped guide management [51]. POCS can also allow lithotripsy of bile duct stones [11, 52]. Another advanced technique is the rendezvous method (combined percutaneous-endoscopic approach). In post-LT patients with a very tight anastomotic stricture that cannot be traversed via ERCP alone, an interventional radiologist can perform PTC to access the biliary tree through the liver [53]. The rendezvous technique has been reported to be safe and useful for post-LDLT biliary strictures that are otherwise endoscopy-resistant [11, 53]. Magnetic recanalization by magnetic compression anastomosis has emerged as an alternative non-surgical hybrid modality to create a new tract and has shown success in reestablishing continuity in the majority of attempted cases [11, 54, 55].

Role of Endoscopic Ultrasound (EUS) in Post-LT

Endoscopic ultrasound (EUS) has emerged as a valuable adjunct in patients with altered anatomy, including those with the LT, primarily as an alternative means of biliary drainage when ERCP is not feasible [56–58]. EUS-guided biliary drainage is feasible and safe but requires technical expertise and robust data for its support is still lacking particularly in patients with LT [56, 59].

Complications of ERCP and Their Management in Liver Transplant Patients

ERCP is an invasive procedure that carries certain risks, which include pancreatitis, bleeding, perforation, and infection [47]. The baseline risk profile of ERCP complications in patients with LT is generally similar to those without LT [7, 17, 60, 61]. However, special consideration due to immunosuppression, altered anatomy, and comorbidities due to sequelae of chronic liver disease is necessary [47, 60–62].

(i) *Post-ERCP Pancreatitis (PEP)*

PEP is one of the most common complications of ERCP [47]. Although mild elevation of lipase and amylase can be seen up to 75% of patients undergoing ERCP, the overall rate of PEP has been reported to be around 9.7% for the average risk patients and 14.7% for the high risk patients [47, 63] Studies have reported that the overall rate of PEP post-LT is likely similar with some studies reporting a lower rate of PEP compared to non-LT [60, 61, 64]. Risk factors for PEP include prior PEP, suspected Sphincter of Oddi dysfunction absence of chronic pancreatitis and normal bilirubin, while procedure related risk factors include difficult cannulation (>10 min), repetitive pancreatic guidewire cannulation, pancreatic sphincterotomy and pancreatic injection [47, 63]. Robust data for post-LT PEP risk factors is lacking; however, studies have reported pre-ERCP cholangitis was an independent risk factor while previous stent in the biliary tract was protective [62]. To reduce the risk of PEP, the ASGE guidelines recommend routine use of rectal NSAIDs in all patients, suggest wire-guided over contrast-assisted cannulation to minimize ductal trauma, and advise prophylactic pancreatic stent placement in high-risk cases—particularly when deep or repeated pancreatic duct access occurs [65]. While these recommendations are not specific to liver transplant recipients, they reflect general best practices for PEP prevention.

(ii) *Bleeding*

Bleeding, which can be immediate or delayed, is a serious complication of ERCP and most commonly results from endoscopic sphincterotomy [47]. While immediate bleeding occurs during or immediately after the procedure, delayed bleeding can occur up to several weeks [47]. The bleeding rate in non-LT patients have been reported to be up to 2%, while studies have reported similar or slightly higher incidence of bleeding (up to 8%) in post-LT patients [17, 47, 60, 61, 64, 66, 67]. In LT patients, coagulopathy is usually corrected by the time of transplant, but some patients (especially early post-op) might have low platelets, coagulopathy or be on anti-coagulation which requires careful consideration [68–70]. Management of post-ERCP bleeding is generally similar in LT patients, and includes steps such as fluid resuscitation, reversal of coagulopathy, transfusion as needed, and endoscopic therapies (epinephrine injection, thermal therapy, balloon tamponade, clips, or fully covered self-expandable metal stents), with angiographic embolization or surgery reserved for refractory cases [47].

(iii) *Perforation*

Risk of perforation in LT and non-LT patients is similar, overall very low, and reported to range from 0% to 0.06% [61, 64] However, if occurred, prompt management is necessary with broad-spectrum antibiotics and surgical consultation.

(iv) *Cholangitis or Infectious Complication*

While ERCP is an effective treatment for acute cholangitis, it can also lead to complications such as cholangitis and sepsis, with an incidence ranging from 0.5% to 5% [17, 62, 64]. Immunosuppressed status and LT is a known risk factor of post-ERCP cholangitis, and prophylactic antibiotics are generally recommended (discussed in an earlier section of this chapter) [47]. ASGE society guidelines also recommend making a meticulous effort to achieve complete drainage involving all segments to decrease the risk of post-ERCP cholangitis [71].

(v) *Consideration Related to Immunocompromised Status and Risk Mitigating Strategies*

In immunosuppressed LT patients, ERCP complications pose heightened risks due to slower wound healing and atypical infections, often requiring prompt management, possible adjustment of immunosuppressants, and close coordination with transplant hepatology. Risk mitigation strategies include using prophylactic measures, minimizing the number of ERCP sessions, and intervening early before complications worsen. While ERCP is generally safe post-transplant, proactive techniques and vigilant follow-up are crucial for optimal outcomes [9].

Comparative Efficacy of ERCP Versus Other Imaging and Therapeutic Modalities

In evaluating post-transplant biliary complications, clinicians often employ a combination of noninvasive imaging and invasive interventions. It is important to understand the roles and relative efficacies of ERCP compared to other modalities such as magnetic resonance cholangiopancreatography (MRCP) and percutaneous transhepatic cholangiography (PTC), both in diagnosis and in treatment.

(i) *MRCP Versus ERCP for Bile Duct Evaluation*

MRCP is an excellent diagnostic tool that provides detailed, non-invasive visualization of the biliary system, with a diagnostic yield comparable to ERCP and PTC—both of which are more invasive but offer therapeutic options [72]. Studies have shown that MRCP can achieve a sensitivity of around 95–98% and a specificity of ~91–94% for diagnosing biliary strictures with a particularly high negative predictive value (~94–98%) [71, 73]. Therefore for the suspected biliary stricture ASGE guideline currently recommends MRCP as preferred diagnostic test, which can help guide therapeutic intervention via ERCP or PTC [7, 11, 71].

(ii) *ERCP Versus PTBD (Percutaneous Transhepatic Biliary Drainage)*

In patients with LT, both ERCP and percutaneous approaches are effective for achieving biliary drainage [7, 11, 71]. The ASGE guidelines recommend ERCP as the first-line therapy whenever feasible due to its excellent success rate, safety profile, and minimally invasive technique. However, they also acknowledge that PTBD can serve as a first-line option in patients with altered anatomy or when ERCP fails to achieve adequate drainage [20, 71]. Notably, in contrast to ERCP, the PTBD has a lower risk of PEP, but carries concerns such as drain dislodgement, scar formation, and the need for periodic drain exchanges [74].

Emerging Trends and Future Directions

The field of interventional endoscopy in liver transplant patients continues to evolve, with ongoing innovations aimed at improving success rates, reducing the number of procedures, and minimizing complications.

Traditionally, benign biliary strictures (including post-liver transplant strictures) were managed with multiple plastic stents. In recent years, however, the use of covered self-expandable metal stents (cSEMS)—which reduces the need for multiple ERCPs—has increased [7, 11]. Notably, the 2023 ASGE guidelines now suggest cSEMS over multiple plastic stents as the initial therapy for post-LT anastomotic strictures, recognizing this as a conditional recommendation with emerging evidence [71]. Recently, the use of biodegradable and drug-eluting stents has been explored; however, they have not yet achieved widespread clinical adoption [75].

Managing complex biliary anatomy from 2D fluoroscopic images can be challenging; therefore, a novel concept involving 3D fluoroscopy or augmented imaging during ERCP has been explored, which allows real-time 3D reconstruction of the bile ducts [76]. Other advances, including AI-assisted ERCP and robotic-assisted endoscopy, have emerged as new frontiers garnering attention; however, more data are needed, and these avenues are not yet ready for prime time [77].

Conclusion

In conclusion, the role of interventional endoscopy, and ERCP in particular, in liver transplant patients is indispensable and continues to expand. By integrating careful diagnostic imaging, skilled endoscopic therapy, and multidisciplinary collaboration, clinicians can effectively manage the majority of post-transplant biliary complications, thereby prolonging graft survival and enhancing patient outcomes. The best practices for gastroenterologists and hepatologists are to maintain a proactive, informed approach: intervene early, use the full range of available minimally invasive techniques, and individualize the plan to each patient's anatomy and pathology. This ensures that liver transplant recipients receive the best possible care for biliary complications.

References

1. Seehofer D, Eurich D, Veltzke-Schlieker W, Neuhaus P. Biliary complications after liver transplantation: old problems and new challenges. Am J Transplant. 2013;13(2):253–65.
2. Agostini C, Buccianti S, Risaliti M, Fortuna L, Tirloni L, Tucci R, et al. Complications in post-liver transplant patients. J Clin Med. 2023;12(19)
3. Moreno R, Berenguer M. Post-liver transplantation medical complications. Ann Hepatol. 2006;5(2):77–85.
4. Maheshwari A, Maley W, Li Z, Thuluvath PJ. Biliary complications and outcomes of liver transplantation from donors after cardiac death. Liver Transpl. 2007;13(12):1645–53.
5. Gu W, Schaaf L, Hortlik H, Zeleke Y, Brol MJ, Schnitzbauer AA, et al. Epidemiology of liver transplantation and post-LT complications in Germany: nationwide study (2005–2018). Eur J Gastroenterol Hepatol. 2023;35(11):1289–97.
6. Parikh A, Washburn KW, Matsuoka L, Pandit U, Kim JE, Almeda J, et al. A multicenter study of 30 days complications after deceased donor liver transplantation in the model for end-stage liver disease score era. Liver Transpl. 2015;21(9):1160–8.
7. Magro B, Tacelli M, Mazzola A, Conti F, Celsa C. Biliary complications after liver transplantation: current perspectives and future strategies. Hepatobiliary Surg Nutr. 2021;10(1):76–92.
8. Gastaca M. Biliary complications after orthotopic liver transplantation: a review of incidence and risk factors. Transplant Proc. 2012;44(6):1545–9.
9. Moy BT, Birk JW. A review on the management of biliary complications after orthotopic liver transplantation. J Clin Transl Hepatol. 2019;7(1):61–71.
10. Tang F, Song J, Cai T, Lei Z, Huang F, Hu Y, et al. Feasibility and safety of ERCP in the treatment of biliary strictures after liver transplantation: with a report of 37 cases. Gastroenterol Res Pract. 2022;2022:4498443.
11. Lee HW, Shah NH, Lee SK. An update on endoscopic management of post-liver transplant biliary complications. Clin Endosc. 2017;50(5):451–63.
12. Kochhar G, Parungao JM, Hanouneh IA, Parsi MA. Biliary complications following liver transplantation. World J Gastroenterol. 2013;19(19):2841–6.
13. Stratta RJ, Wood RP, Langnas AN, Hollins RR, Bruder KJ, Donovan JP, et al. Diagnosis and treatment of biliary tract complications after orthotopic liver transplantation. Surgery 1989;106(4):675–83; discussion 83–4.
14. Boeva I, Karagyozov PI, Tishkov I. Post-liver transplant biliary complications: current knowledge and therapeutic advances. World J Hepatol. 2021;13(1):66–79.
15. Buechter M, Katsounas A, Saner F, Gerken G, Canbay A, Dechene A. ERCP in critically ill patients is safe and does not increase mortality. Medicine (Baltimore). 2022;101(5):e28606.

16. Rizk RS, McVicar JP, Emond MJ, Rohrmann CA Jr, Kowdley KV, Perkins J, et al. Endoscopic management of biliary strictures in liver transplant recipients: effect on patient and graft survival. Gastrointest Endosc. 1998;47(2):128–35.
17. Balderramo D, Bordas JM, Sendino O, Abraldes JG, Navasa M, Llach J, et al. Complications after ERCP in liver transplant recipients. Gastrointest Endosc. 2011;74(2):285–94.
18. Mahnke D, Chen YK, Antillon MR, Brown WR, Mattison R, Shah RJ. A prospective study of complications of endoscopic retrograde cholangiopancreatography and endoscopic ultrasound in an ambulatory endoscopy center. Clin Gastroenterol Hepatol. 2006;4(7):924–30.
19. Thuluvath PJ, Pfau PR, Kimmey MB, Ginsberg GG. Biliary complications after liver transplantation: the role of endoscopy. Endoscopy. 2005;37(9):857–63.
20. Mukund A, Choudhury A, Das S, Pamecha V, Sarin SK. Salvage PTBD in post living donor liver transplant patients with biliary complications-a single Centre retrospective study. Br J Radiol. 2020;93(1108):20191046.
21. Gomez CM, Dumonceau JM, Marcolongo M, de Santibanes E, Ciardullo M, Pekolj J, et al. Endoscopic management of biliary complications after adult living-donor versus deceased-donor liver transplantation. Transplantation. 2009;88(11):1280–5.
22. Villa NA, Harrison ME. Management of Biliary Strictures after Liver Transplantation. Gastroenterol Hepatol (N Y). 2015;11(5):316–28.
23. Verdonk RC, Buis CI, Porte RJ, van der Jagt EJ, Limburg AJ, van den Berg AP, et al. Anastomotic biliary strictures after liver transplantation: causes and consequences. Liver Transpl. 2006;12(5):726–35.
24. Tal AO, Finkelmeier F, Filmann N, Kylanpaa L, Udd M, Parzanese I, et al. Multiple plastic stents versus covered metal stent for treatment of anastomotic biliary strictures after liver transplantation: a prospective, randomized, multicenter trial. Gastrointest Endosc. 2017;86(6):1038–45.
25. Martins FP, De Paulo GA, Contini MLC, Ferrari AP. Metal versus plastic stents for anastomotic biliary strictures after liver transplantation: a randomized controlled trial. Gastrointest Endosc. 2018;87(1):131e1–e13.
26. Bordacahar B, Perdigao F, Leblanc S, Barret M, Duchmann JC, Guillaumot MA, et al. Clinical efficacy of anti-migration features in fully covered metallic stents for anastomotic biliary strictures after liver transplantation: comparison of conventional and anti-migration stents. Gastrointest Endosc. 2018;88(4):655–64.
27. Kao D, Zepeda-Gomez S, Tandon P, Bain VG. Managing the post-liver transplantation anastomotic biliary stricture: multiple plastic versus metal stents: a systematic review. Gastrointest Endosc. 2013;77(5):679–91.
28. Michael FA, Friedrich-Rust M, Erasmus HP, Graf C, Ballo O, Knabe M, et al. Treatment of non-anastomotic biliary strictures after liver transplantation: how effective is our current treatment strategy? J Clin Med. 2023;12(10)
29. Guichelaar MM, Benson JT, Malinchoc M, Krom RA, Wiesner RH, Charlton MR. Risk factors for and clinical course of non-anastomotic biliary strictures after liver transplantation. Am J Transplant. 2003;3(7):885–90.
30. Hong SY, Hu XG, Lee HY, Won JH, Kim JW, Shen XY, et al. Longterm analysis of biliary complications after duct-to-duct biliary reconstruction in living donor liver transplantations. Liver Transpl. 2018;24(8):1050–61.
31. Sendino O, Fernandez-Simon A, Law R, Abu Dayyeh B, Leise M, Chavez-Rivera K, et al. Endoscopic management of bile leaks after liver transplantation: an analysis of two high-volume transplant centers. United European Gastroenterol J. 2018;6(1):89–96.
32. Li Z, Rammohan A, Gunasekaran V, Hong S, Chih-Yi Chen I, Kim J, et al. Biliary complications after adult-to-adult living-donor liver transplantation: an international multicenter study of 3633 cases. Am J Transplant. 2024;24(7):1233–46.
33. Scatton O, Meunier B, Cherqui D, Boillot O, Sauvanet A, Boudjema K, et al. Randomized trial of choledochocholedochostomy with or without a T tube in orthotopic liver transplantation. Ann Surg. 2001;233(3):432–7.

34. Soltani E, Mehrabi Bahar A, Dehghanian P, Afzal Aghaei M, Mozaffari S. Prevention of biliary leakage after removal of T-tube in immunocompromised patients. Indian J Surg. 2015;77(Suppl 2):645–9.
35. Shuhart MC, Kowdley KV, McVicar JP, Rohrmann CA, McDonald MF, Wadland DW, et al. Predictors of bile leaks after T-tube removal in orthotopic liver transplant recipients. Liver Transpl Surg. 1998;4(1):62–70.
36. Morelli J, Mulcahy HE, Willner IR, Baliga P, Chavin KD, Patel R, et al. Endoscopic treatment of post-liver transplantation biliary leaks with stent placement across the leak site. Gastrointest Endosc. 2001;54(4):471–5.
37. Ayoub WS, Esquivel CO, Martin P. Biliary complications following liver transplantation. Dig Dis Sci. 2010;55(6):1540–6.
38. Starzl TE, Putnam CW, Hansbrough JF, Porter KA, Reid HA. Biliary complications after liver transplantation: with special reference to the biliary cast syndrome and techniques of secondary duct repair. Surgery. 1977;81(2):212–21.
39. Nandi N, Tontini GE, Scaramella L, Sorge A, Pessarelli T, Topa M, et al. Electrohydraulic lithotripsy with direct peroral cholangioscopy via double-balloon enteroscopy and endoscopic retrograde cholangiopancreatography in a liver transplant recipient. Endoscopy. 2023;55(S 01):E1049–E50.
40. Douzdjian V, Abecassis MM, Johlin FC. Sphincter of Oddi dysfunction following liver transplantation. Screening by bedside manometry and definitive manometric evaluation. Dig Dis Sci. 1994;39(2):253–6.
41. Fernandez-Simon A, Sendino O, Chavez-Rivera K, Cordova H, Colmenero J, Crespo G, et al. The presence and outcome of biliary sphincter disorders in liver-transplant recipients according to the Rome IV classification. Gastroenterol Rep (Oxf). 2021;9(4):299–305.
42. Afghani E, Lo SK, Covington PS, Cash BD, Pandol SJ. Sphincter of oddi function and risk factors for dysfunction. Front Nutr. 2017;4:1.
43. Visconti TAC, Bernardo WM, Moura DTH, Moura ETH, Goncalves CVT, Farias GF, et al. Metallic vs plastic stents to treat biliary stricture after liver transplantation: a systematic review and meta-analysis based on randomized trials. Endosc Int Open. 2018;6(8):E914–E23.
44. Wen TC, Hsieh CE, Hsu YL, Lin KH, Hung YJ, Chen YL. The role of roux-en-Y hepaticojejunostomy for the management of biliary complications after living donor liver transplantation. BMC Surg. 2023;23(1):165.
45. Committee ASoP, Khashab MA, Chithadi KV, Acosta RD, Bruining DH, Chandrasekhara V, et al. Antibiotic prophylaxis for GI endoscopy. Gastrointest Endosc. 2015;81(1):81–9.
46. Leem G, Sung MJ, Park JH, Kim SJ, Jo JH, Lee HS, et al. Randomized trial of prophylactic antibiotics for endoscopic retrograde cholangiopancreatography in patients with biliary obstruction. Am J Gastroenterol. 2024;119(1):183–90.
47. Committee ASoP, Chandrasekhara V, Khashab MA, Muthusamy VR, Acosta RD, Agrawal D, et al. Adverse events associated with ERCP. Gastrointest Endosc. 2017;85(1):32–47.
48. Saleem A, Baron TH, Gostout CJ, Topazian MD, Levy MJ, Petersen BT, et al. Endoscopic retrograde cholangiopancreatography using a single-balloon enteroscope in patients with altered Roux-en-Y anatomy. Endoscopy. 2010;42(8):656–60.
49. Sissingh NJ, de Vries BA, Inderson A, van Hoek B, van der Heide F, van Hooft JE. Intraductal fully covered self-expandable metal stent versus multiple plastic stents for treating biliary anastomotic strictures after liver transplantation. Gastrointest Endosc. 2023;97(4):704–12 e2.
50. Baraldo S, Meine GC, Santo PAE, Barbosa EC, Nau AL, Keane MG, et al. Fully covered self-expandable metal stents versus multiple plastic stents for the treatment of post-orthotopic liver transplant anastomotic biliary strictures: an updated systematic review and meta-analysis of randomized controlled trials. Surg Endosc. 2025;39(2):721–9.
51. Franzini T, De Moura EGH, Cardenas A, Slivka A, Poley J-W, Papachristou GI, et al. The role of peroral cholangioscopy in liver transplant recipients: a prospective, international series. J Liver Transplant. 2025;17:100259.

52. Nezami N, Benchetrit L, Latich I, Schlachter T. Cholangiolithiasis postliver transplantation: successful treatment utilizing percutaneous transhepatic cholangioscopy and laser lithotripsy. Radiol Case Rep. 2019;14(12):1459–66.
53. Chang JH, Lee IS, Chun HJ, Choi JY, Yoon SK, Kim DG, et al. Comparative study of rendezvous techniques in post-liver transplant biliary stricture. World J Gastroenterol. 2012;18(41):5957–64.
54. Li Y, Zhang N, Lv Y. Scientific Committee of the Third International Conference of Magnetic S. Expert consensus on magnetic recanalization technique for biliary anastomotic strictures after liver transplantation. Hepatobil Surg Nutr. 2021;10(3):401–4.
55. Jang SI, Cho JH, Lee DK. Magnetic compression anastomosis for the treatment of post-transplant biliary stricture. Clin Endosc. 2020;53(3):266–75.
56. Jamwal KD, Sharma A, Padhan RK, Sharma MK. Outcomes of endoscopic biliary drainage in postsurgical anatomy using endoscopic ultrasound and enteroscopy: a comparative study. jdigendo. 2023;14(03):127–34.
57. Siripun A, Sripongpun P, Ovartlarnporn B. Endoscopic ultrasound-guided biliary intervention in patients with surgically altered anatomy. World J Gastrointest Endosc. 2015;7(3):283–9.
58. Lisotti A, Fusaroli P, Caletti G. Role of endoscopy in the conservative management of biliary complications after deceased donor liver transplantation. World J Hepatol. 2015;7(30):2927–32.
59. Laleman W, Peiffer KH, Tischendorf M, Ullerich HJ, Praktiknjo M, Trebicka J. Role of endoscopy in hepatology. Dig Liver Dis. 2024;56(7):1185–95.
60. Sanna C, Giordanino C, Giono I, Barletti C, Ferrari A, Recchia S, et al. Safety and efficacy of endoscopic retrograde cholangiopancreatography in patients with post-liver transplant biliary complications: results of a cohort study with long-term follow-up. Gut Liver. 2011;5(3):328–34.
61. Husing A, Cicinnati VR, Maschmeier M, Schmidt HH, Wolters HH, Beckebaum S, et al. Complications after endoscopic sphincterotomy in liver transplant recipients: a retrospective single-Centre study. Arab J Gastroenterol. 2015;16(2):46–9.
62. Ambrus RB, Svendsen LB, Hillingso JG, Hansen ML, Achiam MP. Post-endoscopic retrograde cholangiopancreaticography complications in liver transplanted patients, a single-center experience. Scand J Surg. 2015;104(2):86–91.
63. Kochar B, Akshintala VS, Afghani E, Elmunzer BJ, Kim KJ, Lennon AM, et al. Incidence, severity, and mortality of post-ERCP pancreatitis: a systematic review by using randomized, controlled trials. Gastrointest Endosc. 2015;81(1):143–9 e9.
64. Sanna C, Saracco GM, Reggio D, Moro F, Ricchiuti A, Strignano P, et al. Endoscopic retrograde cholangiopancreatography in patients with biliary complications after orthotopic liver transplantation: outcomes and complications. Transplant Proc. 2009;41(4):1319–21.
65. Buxbaum JL, Freeman M, Amateau SK, Chalhoub JM, Coelho-Prabhu N, Desai M, et al. American Society for Gastrointestinal Endoscopy guideline on post-ERCP pancreatitis prevention strategies: summary and recommendations. Gastrointest Endosc. 2023;97(2):153–62.
66. Rustagi T, Jamidar PA. Endoscopic retrograde cholangiopancreatography-related adverse events: general overview. Gastrointest Endosc Clin N Am. 2015;25(1):97–106.
67. Tenca A, Pugliese D, Consonni D, Cantu P, Rossi G, Francesca Donato M, et al. Bleeding after sphincterotomy in liver transplanted patients with biliary complications. Eur J Gastroenterol Hepatol. 2011;23(9):778–81.
68. Takahashi K, Nagai S, Safwan M, Liang C, Ohkohchi N. Thrombocytopenia after liver transplantation: should we care? World J Gastroenterol. 2018;24(13):1386–97.
69. Algarni AA, Mourad MM, Bramhall SR. Anticoagulation and antiplatelets as prophylaxis for hepatic artery thrombosis after liver transplantation. World J Hepatol. 2015;7(9):1238–43.
70. Stine JG, Northup PG. Coagulopathy before and after liver transplantation: from the hepatic to the systemic circulatory systems. Clin Liver Dis. 2017;21(2):253–74.
71. Amateau SK, Kohli DR, Desai M, Chinnakotla S, Harrison ME, Chalhoub JM, et al. American Society for Gastrointestinal Endoscopy guideline on management of post-liver transplant biliary strictures: methodology and review of evidence. Gastrointest Endosc. 2023;97(4):615–37 e11.

72. Laghi A, Pavone P, Catalano C, Rossi M, Panebianco V, Alfani D, et al. MR cholangiography of late biliary complications after liver transplantation. AJR Am J Roentgenol. 1999;172(6):1541–6.
73. Boraschi P, Donati F, Gigoni R, Volpi A, Salemi S, Filipponi F, et al. MR cholangiography in orthotopic liver transplantation: sensitivity and specificity in detecting biliary complications. Clin Transpl. 2010;24(4):E82–7.
74. Pape T, von Garrel T, Hunkemoller AM, Nalbant B, Vondran FWR, Richter N, et al. Percutaneous transhepatic biliary drainage in patients with cholestasis following liver transplantation. Abdom Radiol (NY). 2025;50(4):1699–710.
75. Anderloni A, Fugazza A, Maroni L, Ormando V, Maselli R, Carrara S, et al. New biliary and pancreatic biodegradable stent placement: a single-center, prospective, pilot study (with video). Gastrointest Endosc. 2020;92(2):405–11.
76. Koh CJ, Koo CS, Doshi BK. Real-time 3D imaging of post-transplant biliary stricture: a novel application of existing technology. Am J Gastroenterol. 2021;116(10):2145–6.
77. Kim T, Kim J, Choi HS, Kim ES, Keum B, Jeen YT, et al. Artificial intelligence-assisted analysis of endoscopic retrograde cholangiopancreatography image for identifying ampulla and difficulty of selective cannulation. Sci Rep. 2021;11(1):8381.

Disease Recurrence After Liver Transplantation

28

Marina Berenguer and Marta Tejedor

Introduction

Over recent decades, a major change in the profile of waitlisted recipients has been noticeable, namely patients are older and have more advanced liver disease with concomitant comorbidities. The cause of liver disease has also evolved, with alcohol-related liver disease (ALD), metabolic-associated steatotic liver disease (MASDL), and MASLD-related hepatocellular carcinoma (HCC) being the current leading liver transplant (LT) indications in the United States compared with hepatitis C virus (HCV) a decade ago [1].

Disease recurrence of primary liver disease is a late event (>6 months post-LT) in most cases, and a major cause of graft failure and long-term patient mortality [2, 3]. Indeed, for decades, viral recurrence, particularly HCV was the number one cause of graft loss [4]; however, with the development of potent anti-viral therapy, HCV and hepatitis B virus (HBV) infected transplant recipients no longer experience graft loss and death. In contrast, recurrence of autoimmune diseases—particularly Primary Sclerosing Cholangitis (PSC)—remains a valid concern for the LT community. Strategies directed at reducing disease recurrence, including the use of preemptive ursodeoxycholic acid (UDCA) in primary biliary cholangitis (PBC) or maintenance of low-dose steroids for autoimmune hepatitis (AIH), have improved overall outcomes.

M. Berenguer (✉)
Hepatology and Liver Transplantation Unit, Hospital Universitario la Fe—IIS La Fe Valencia, CiberEHD and University of Valencia, Valencia, Spain
e-mail: marina.berenguer@uv.es

M. Tejedor
Division of Gastroenterology and Hepatology, University of Iowa Healthcare, Iowa City, IA, USA
e-mail: marta-tejedorbravo@uiowa.edu

B. Eghtesad et al. (eds.), *Liver Transplantation*,
https://doi.org/10.1007/978-3-032-07072-2_28

Hepatitis C

Recurrent hepatitis C (rHCV) infection after LT is universal in patients who are viremic at the time of transplant, and associated with an accelerated disease course [5]. Untreated, HCV leads to recurrent cirrhosis within a decade, on average, and the overall graft survival of HCV-positive LT recipients is 30% lower than uninfected controls [6]. The cholestatic variant of rHCVis is rare (5–10%) and occurs early post-LT (1–6 months), but carries a dismal prognosis in the absence of successful antiviral therapy [7, 8].

The past era of interferon-based therapies, largely unsuccessful, has led the way to treatment based on Direct Antiviral Agents (DAA), with reported sustained virological response (SVR) rates ranging from 80% to 100% [9–17]. The achievement of SVR significantly improves graft survival [18, 19] and reduces concerns regarding immunosuppression and how it may be impacting the course of HCV infection. DAA therapies allow early treatment before the development of significant graft dysfunction or fibrosis. Treatment should be undertaken after postoperative issues have resolved and immunosuppression is stable, typically within the first 3 months. Patients with fibrosing cholestatic hepatitis and those with moderate to extensive fibrosis or portal hypertension are at high risk of graft loss and require urgent antiviral therapy [20–23].

Different combinations of DAA have been used in the post-LT setting [22]. Nowadays, pan-genotypic and pan-fibrotic options are available and have greatly simplified treatment. The same regimens used in the immunocompetent patient are used post-LT with similar success rates [24]. Potential drug-to-drug interactions (DDIs) should be assessed and managed according to the DAA regimen and concomitant medications. Protease inhibitors are more likely to be associated with significant DDIs, especially with calcineurin inhibitors (CNI) and mammalian target of rapamycin inhibitors (mTORi) [25, 26]. Apart from pharmacokinetic interactions, changes in immunosuppressive drug exposure related to improvement in liver function with antiviral treatment may occur. Blood concentrations of immunosuppressive medications should be monitored, and doses adjusted if need be, regularly during DAA treatment, and after completion of treatment until SVR12 is achieved [22].

DAA therapy provides an opportunity to consider the use of allografts from HCV-viremic donors in HCV-negative recipients because iatrogenic HCV infection can be cured with retention of graft function in most cases. In this scenario, pre-emptive DAA therapy is recommended. The goal is to undertake DAA therapy as early as clinically possible to avoid the development of acute hepatitis and other complications of HCV infection [23] (Fig. 28.1).

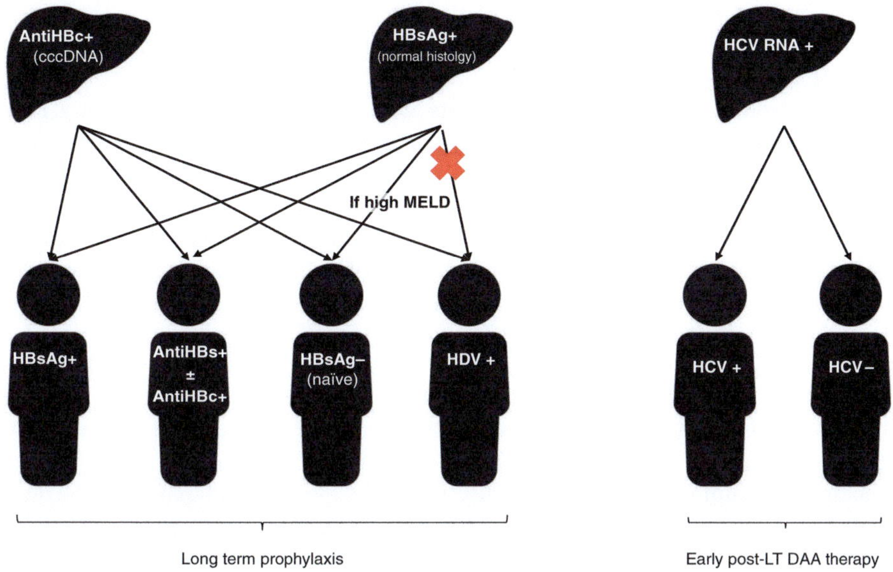

Fig. 28.1 Use of HBV and HCV positive grafts. The use of HBV positive grafts carries a risk of transmitting infection and potentially increasing HCC risk. Individual recipient assessment and informed consent should be sought, and adecuate prophylaxis and treatment started post-LT. *HBV* Hepatitis B virus, *HCV* Hepatitis C virus, *LT* liver transplant, *AntiHBc* anti Hepatitis B core antibodies, *AntiHBs* anti Hepatitis B surface antibodies, *HBsAg* Hepatitis B surface antigen, *HDV* Hepatitis Delta, *RNA* ribonucleic acid, *DAA* direct antiviral agents

Hepatitis B

HBV liver disease is a common indication for liver LT (10–15%) [27–29]. Residual HBV particles may rapidly infect the graft leading to covalently closed circular DNA formation and potentially to viral genome integration, leading to recurrent infection [30, 31]. Pre-LT serologic status and viral load confer different risks of disease recurrence and require different prophylactic approaches [32]. Prophylaxis against HBV recurrence should be tailored according to three risk groups, mainly defined by pre-LT HBV DNA levels [33–35]:

Low virological risk patients: Patients with undetectable HBV DNA pre-LT, irrespective of LT indication (cirrhosis or fulminant hepatitis). Short-term (4 weeks) combination of third-generation nucleos(t)ide analogs (NA) plus hepatitis B immunoglobulin (HBIG), or third-generation NA monotherapy can be considered as prophylactic options. Monotherapy with NA with a high genetic barrier to resistance, such as entecavir or tenofovir, has significantly improved outcomes and simplified prophylaxis [36, 37]. Entecavir is especially recommended in the case of renal failure or severe osteoporosis.

High virological risk patients: Patients with detectable HBV DNA at LT or patients with HBV reactivation resulting in HBV acute-on-chronic-liver-failure (ACLF). Combined therapy (NA + HBIG) for 1 year is advised. HBIG can be discontinued once HBV DNA is undetectable.

Special populations: In patients with HDV co-infection and those at risk of poor adherence, indefinite dual prophylaxis (NA + HBIG) remains the gold standard. HBV-HCC patients should be treated according to their virological risk.

In the LT setting, low levels of HBsAg can persist for a limited period post-LT and then spontaneously disappear, with HBsAg half-life estimated to be close to 7 days [38–40]. Most patients on NA monoprophylaxis become HBsAg negative in the first 3 months after LT, suggesting that the immune system can clear the residual HBsAg, while HBV replication is efficiently suppressed by NA. Identifying patients who develop natural anti-HBV immunity after HBIG withdrawal may open the door to further NAs withdrawal or, on the opposite, to vaccination in patients without natural HBsAb. HBV prophylaxis withdrawal should only be attempted in the setting of controlled clinical trials.

Anti-HBc positive liver grafts should be considered for all adult recipients after informed consent and be preferentially proposed to HBsAg positive recipients, as these patients have already been planned to receive HBV prophylaxis, and further to patients with detectable anti-HBs and/or anti-HBc antibodies. In HBsAg-negative recipients of an Anti-HBc-positive graft, prophylaxis should be based on NA long term. Organs from HBsAg-positive donors may be considered after assessment of risks, benefits, and patient consent. They should not be used if HDV is present (Fig. 28.1) [32].

The definition of HBV recurrence should be based on both HBsAg and HBV DNA detection/quantification, which provide complementary information and should be used together to have a full picture of the situation (Fig. 28.2) [32].

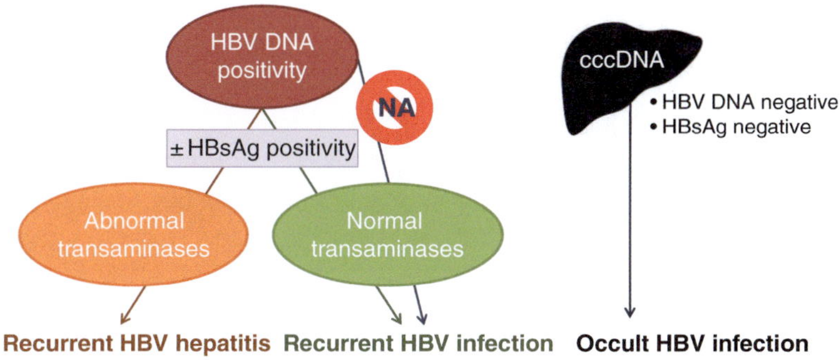

Fig. 28.2 Recurrent HBV patterns. Recurrence of HBV infection with active replication: defined by any serum HBV DNA persistence or reappearance after LT with or without detectable HBsAg and normal liver enzymes. Recurrence of HBV infection with controlled replication by NA: defined by transient or persistent detection of HBsAg and undetectable HBV DNA on NA. Recurrence of HBV hepatitis: defined by serum HBV DNA positivity with or without HBsAg detection and abnormal liver enzymes and compatible histology (liver inflammation). Occult infection: this pattern combines the detection of cccDNA in the liver with no detection of HBsAg nor HBV DNA in the serum. It should be distinguished from trueHBs Ag/HBV clearance. HBV: hepatitis B. DNA: deoxiribonucleic acid. *HBsAg* surface HBV antigen, *cccDNA* covalently closed circular DNA, *NA* nucleoside analogues

Autoimmune Hepatitis

Recurrent AIH (rAIH) occurs in 20–30% of recipients at 5 years [41–43] and is diagnosed similarly to AIH pre-LT [42, 44, 45] (Table 28.1). rAIH has been found on protocol biopsies in the absence of abnormal liver tests. It can be difficult to distinguish from alloimmune rejection, though the features typical for rejection, including endotheliitis and bile duct damage, are usually not present [45]. rAIH is associated with decreased graft and patient survival [42]. Several risk factors for rAIH have been reported, including younger age, greater inflammation pre-LT, and donor–recipient sex mismatch [42].

The most appropriate post-LT immunosuppressive regimen is still debated. Immunosuppressive regimens are centered on CNI, often combined with low-dose steroids, with or without the addition of antimetabolite therapy. Whether dual versus triple immunosuppressive therapy, cyclosporine versus tacrolimus, or maintenance versus no maintenance steroids lead to better outcomes is still controversial [42, 46–48]. However, the lack of solid evidence allows for consideration of gradual withdrawal or addition of MMF or azathioprine (AZA) to facilitate steroid weaning [46, 48–54]. An individualized approach accounting for the patient's risk of recurrent disease and rejection, balanced with the effects of long-term steroids, is likely the optimal approach.

When recurrent disease develops, immunosuppression should be increased, with the reintroduction of steroids, followed by the addition of AZA or MMF if needed, while continuing CNI [45]. If there is a lack of response, the antimetabolite or CNI can be switched, and mTORi may also be used in non-responders [45, 55].

Table 28.1 Recurrence of primary liver disease

Disease	HCV	HBV	AIH	PSC	PBC	ALD
Recurrence rate	100%	100%	20-30%	20-30%	20-40%	15-50%
Risk factors for recurrence	Viremia at the time of LT	Viremia at the time of LT Failure of prophylaxis	Younger recipient age Greater inflammation pre-LT Donor-recipient sex mismatch	Presence of IBD CC before LT Increasing donor age Episodes of ACR MELD score	Male donor Donor-recipient sex mismatch Younger age	Male sex Short duration of abstinence pre-LT Social instability Psychiatric comorbidities Poly-substance abuse Poor adherence to medical care Younger age
Recurrent disease treatment	Compensated: Sofosbuvir/ velpatasvir for 12 weeks Glecaprevir/ pibrentasvir for 12 weeks. Decompensated: Sofosbuvir/ velpatasvir with ribavirin for 12 weeks Sofosbuvir/ velpatasvir for 24 weeks without ribavirin	High genetic barrier nucleos(t)ide analogues: Entecavir Tenofovir	Increase in IS: Continue CNI and add steroids ± antimetabolites	Re-transplantation	UDCA	Multidisciplinary approach: CBT Medication Counselling

Recommended immunosuppression	Standard	Standard	CNI alone Double IS: CNI + steroids CNI + antimetabolites Triple IS: CNI + steroids + antimetabolites	Triple IS: CNI + steroids + antimetabolites	Standard High doses or prolonged use of steroids may be needed	Standard Minimization CNI alone
Special considerations	Fibrosing cholestatic hepatitis is the most severe complication	Prophylaxis reduces risk of recurrence: NA ± HBIG	Increased risk of rejection	Increased risk of rejection and biliary complications	Preventive treatment with UDCA post-LT reduces risk of recurrence	Close monitoring allows for early intervention if relapse occurs

HCV hepatitis C infection, *HBV* hepatitis B infection, *AIH* autoimmune hepatitis, *PSC* primary sclerosing cholangitis, *PBC* primary biliary cholantitis, *ALD* alcohol-related liver disease, *LT* liver transplant, *IS* immunosuppression, *NA* nucleos(t)ide analogues, *HBIG* hepatitis B immune globulin, *IBD* inflammatory bowel disease, *CC* cholangiocarcinoma, *ACR* acute cellular rejection, *MELD* model for end-stage liver disease, *UDCA* ursodeoxycholic acid, *CBT* cognitive behavioural therapy

Finally, patients transplanted for AIH carry a higher risk of T-cell-mediated rejection post-LT: early rejection has decreased from 80% to 20% in recent years, thanks to improvement in immunosuppressive regimens. Late rejection fluctuates between 10% and 30%, and chronic rejection, frequently affecting younger patients, is around 15% [56]. No association between antibody-mediated rejection and autoimmune liver disease has been reported [57, 58]. The entity previously considered *de novo* AIH has recently been renamed plasma cell-rich rejection, as this appears to be a manifestation of allograft rejection [59–61], occurring in a small percentage (3–5%) of adult LT recipients with non-AIH diseases [59].

Primary Sclerosing Cholangitis

PSC accounts for 4–7% of LT activity in Europe and North America, with increasing numbers in recent years, particularly among women [62, 63]. Cholangiocarcinoma (CC) is present in a minority of cases (2–8%) [62]. Post-LT outcome is excellent in the short term (>90% within the first year), yet declines with time (80% at 5 years and 50% at 30 years) [62, 64]. Common causes of death after LT include infections, malignancies, graft failure due to rejection or recurrent PSC (rPSC), and surgical complications such as hepatic artery thrombosis (HAT) [62]. Determinants for higher mortality are the recipient's male sex, older donor and recipient age, presence of CC and rPSC [62, 65, 66]. The effect of using reduced grafts (split, living-donor LT [LDLT]) or those donated after circulatory death (DCD) on post-LT survival is controversial [62, 67–69], although some studies show a benefit of LDLT over deceased-donor LT [70].

Severe and recurrent episodes of cholangitis often damage the biliary tree, which explains the high incidence of biliary complications among PSC recipients. Indeed, non-anastomotic strictures (NAS) are not always due to rPSC and may be due to ischemic cholangiopathy, chronic ductopenic rejection, ABO incompatibility, old donors, prolonged use of vasopressors, prolonged cold and warm ischemia times, preservative injury, and DCD [71]. NAS related to immunological factors present after one year of LT [72]. Duct-to-duct anastomosis was recently recommended as the reconstructive technique of choice whenever technically feasible to avoid ascending cholangitis in Roux-en-Y hepaticojejunostomy [73].

Inflammatory bowel disease (IBD) coexists with PSC in 70–80% of the cases. Patients with ulcerative colitis (UC) are prone to develop not only CC but also colorectal cancer (CRC), both before and after LT. Annual surveillance colonoscopy including systematic pancolonic biopsies is strongly recommended pre- and post-LT [74, 75]. The clinical course of liver disease can be affected by IBD activity and vice versa [65, 69, 76–79]. The gut microbiome in PSC patients shows a marked deviation from healthy controls and is modified after LT. This could potentially contribute to rPSC, sex differences in disease susceptibility and course in patients with rPSC [76, 80, 81]. Active IBD after LT has been documented as a risk factor for rPSC, while colectomy pre-LT has proven to be a significant protective factor in many, although not all studies [65, 77–79]. Whether new anti-IBD, such as small-molecule JAK inhibitors, may modify the risk or course of rPSC is still under investigation [82].

rPSC develops in 20–30% of recipients with increasing rates with follow-ups [66, 83, 84] (Table 28.1). rPSC, particularly if early post-LT, has a negative impact on graft survival (50%), resulting in a higher need for re-transplantation [64, 77, 83, 85, 86]. When graft failure occurs, liver re-transplantation, although associated with worse outcomes, may be the only alternative to death. Recent data from the ELTR show that patients affected by rPSC benefit from re-transplantation and show a patient survival similar to that of patients without rPSC but re-transplanted for other causes [66]. Similar results come from the analysis of the UNOS/OPTN database [87].

Confirmation of rPSC can be challenging and should be based on cholangiographic findings showing intra- and/or extrahepatic biliary stricturing, beading, and irregularity >90 days post-LT or a biopsy showing fibrous cholangitis and/or fibro-obliterative lesions with or without ductopenia, biliary fibrosis, or biliary cirrhosis, in the absence of HAT/stenosis, established ductopenic rejection, anastomotic strictures alone, non-anastomotic strictures <90 days post-LT, or donor–recipient ABO incompatibility [88].

Risk factors for rPSC remain not fully elucidated [62, 65, 66, 77, 83, 85, 89]. Data from large programmes suggest that an increased inflammatory state both before but mostly after LT, manifested by recurrent cholangitis pre-LT or increased IBD activity or multiple acute cellular rejections post-LT, increases the incidence of rPSC [69].

Immunosuppression should be planned not only for the inhibition of rejection but for the control of autoimmunity. Tacrolimus is associated with better patient and graft survival rates than cyclosporine [90]. Because acute rejection is associated with rPSC, triple-immunosuppression is recommended [74].

Primary Biliary Cholangitis

LT is usually indicated for decompensated cirrhosis or HCC. Referral to a transplant center should occur at the onset of decompensation, when total bilirubin approaches 6 mg/dL or the MELD score is ≥12 [91]. Referral may also be appropriate for patients significantly affected by severe pruritus even if with low MELD scores (<15), this indication being in the rise [92]. Importantly, fatigue attributable to PBC is no longer an indication for LT, as it may not resolve post-LT [93]. The standardization of UDCA in PBC has allowed for a reduction of this disease as an indication for LT from 30% to 50% to less than 5% of the cases [94, 95]. Characteristics of patients undergoing transplantation for PBC have changed over time, whereby they are now older, have higher MELD scores, and are more likely to be male [92, 96, 97]. Among listed candidates, those with PBC appear to have higher WL mortality, particularly in the setting of ACLF [98–100].

Outcomes of LT in patients with PBC are excellent, with 5- and 20-year survival rates of 90–93% and 53–55%, respectively; for graft, slightly higher rates have been reported [101–104]. LT significantly improves quality of life, with improvements in symptoms, function, and health satisfaction [93].

Recent long-term studies have estimated recurrence rates of 21–23% at 10 years and > 43% at 15 years [103–105] (Table 28.1). Discrepancy in reports may be explained by differences in diagnostic procedures and criteria, follow-up periods, immunosuppressive regimens and whether event, rather than protocol-based, allograft biopsies were used for monitoring [43]. Median time to recurrence is 3–5.5 years, although it can be as rapid as less than 1 year after transplant. While in the short-medium term, graft loss due to recurrent PBC (rPBC) is negligible at about 1–2%, the rate of graft loss and need for re-transplantation increase in the long-term and eventually impacts graft and patient survival [94, 103, 104, 106, 107]. Diagnosing rPBC after LT can be difficult, as symptoms and biochemical liver tests are not specific and anti-mitochondrial antibodies can remain positive after transplant without recurrent disease. The diagnosis requires a liver biopsy with histological features of portal inflammatory infiltrates, lymphoid aggregates, epithelioid granulomas, and bile duct damage [108]. Studies based on protocol biopsies show that a significant proportion of these patients do not present with biochemical signs of cholestasis; therefore, performing a liver biopsy only if abnormal transaminases can clearly underestimate the recurrence rate. In this context, monitoring of serum IgM level may help in selecting candidates for histological evaluation, as this parameter is more frequently elevated than alkaline phosphatase activity at the time of diagnosis [107].

Preventive administration of UDCA (13–15 mg/kg/day) after LT is associated with a lower risk of disease recurrence, graft loss, liver-related death, and all-cause-related death, as well as with a longer time to recurrence (6.5 vs 4.9 years). Preventive UDCA also led to a survival gain of 2.26 years over a period of 20 years [103, 107, 109, 110]. Interestingly, exposure to cyclosporine rather than tacrolimus had a complementary protective effect alongside UDCA, reducing the cumulative incidence of PBC recurrence and all-cause death [103].

While many studies have addressed predictors of disease recurrence, the data are controversial. No significant difference is seen in survival for DCD versus LDLT. In one study, male donor gender was associated with adverse outcomes [111]. Using native female grafts may improve outcomes in LT for PBC, especially in female patients. In a recent multicenter international study, younger age at the time of diagnosis with PBC or at LT, use of tacrolimus, and biochemical markers of severe cholestasis (bilirubin ≥100 μmol or alkaline phosphatase >three-fold the upper limit of normal) at 6 months after LT were associated with a higher risk of PBC recurrence [104].

There are no controlled trials that have identified the optimal immunosuppression regimen in PBC patients. Although most studies suggest that cyclosporine-based treatment is preferable to tacrolimus, data are controversial [104, 112–116]. Overall, patients with PBC may need longer courses of steroid therapy or higher doses. Some patients are even kept on low doses of prednisone chronically [106, 111]. The treatment of post-LT rPBC is also unclear. Biochemical improvement can be seen with UDCA, but there is no clear evidence that it improves patient or graft survival or alters the natural history of disease recurrence [106].

Alcohol-Related Liver Disease

The incidence of ALD is increasing worldwide, particularly in vulnerable populations, young patients, and women. Until 2019, ALD was gradually rising as an indication for LT in most countries, concomitantly to the significant fall in HCV-related indications, representing about a third of all indications both in the US and Europe [117, 118]. Following the COVID-19 pandemic, many centers have described a sharper rise with ALD representing the first LT indication both in Europe and the US [117–124]. LT is the treatment of choice for decompensated alcohol-related cirrhosis [125].

The conventional requirement of 6 months of alcohol abstinence before LT has been challenged by studies focusing on early LT in patients with acute alcoholic hepatitis (AAH) not responding to steroids, as they present a very poor prognosis (6-month mortality rate of 75%) [126, 127]. LT has been found to significantly improve the survival of patients with severe AAH not responding to steroids compared to those with AAH rejected for transplantation due to psycho-social issues (83% vs 28% at 2 years). Most importantly, post-transplant survival at 2 years was found to be similar among patients transplanted for AAH and those with alcoholic cirrhosis, regardless of duration of the pre-LT abstinence period [128].

Overall, LT for ALD has yielded satisfactory outcomes comparable to other indications [129, 130]. The main concern is the risk of alcohol relapse. Indeed, sustained alcohol use post LT especially beyond 5 years is associated with increased mortality [131–133]. Causes of death include chronic rejection due to adherence problems, alcohol-related graft disease, cardiovascular events, and *de novo* cancers [133–135]. Studies have reported varying rates of alcohol relapse post-LT (15–50% within 5 years following LT) [136–140] (Table 28.1 and Fig. 28.3). The difference in rates of alcohol relapse between studies is likely related to the use of different definitions that classify drinking patterns, from "any use," "slips," or "relapse," which can be "severe" or "regular" depending on the case [137]. It is assumed that 30–50% of patients undergoing LT for ALD resume "any" drinking after

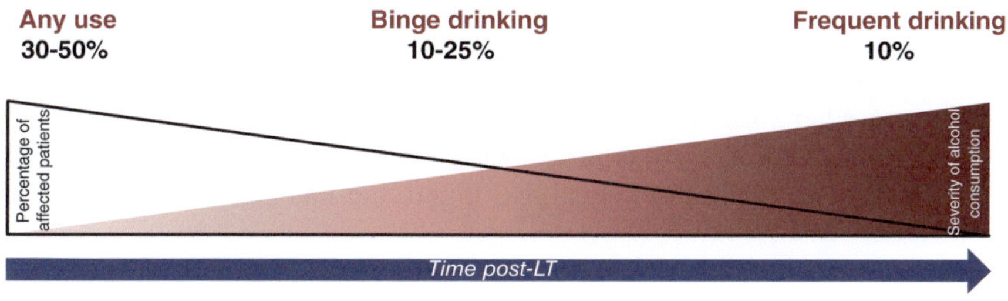

Fig. 28.3 Patterns of alcohol relapse post-LT. As many as 50% of patients had any use of alcohol by 5 years post-LT. Nearly 25% drank 6 or more standard drinks (binge drinking) by 5 years post-LT, transition to binge drinking frequently happening within 6 months from first use. Heavy alcohol use was uncommon, with only 10% of patients in this category. Those who return to alcohol use do so early, and the rates of alcohol use initiation attenuate with time. (Ref: Di Martini Liver Transplantation 2006 [137])

transplantation, but that only about 10% drink in an abusive or dependent fashion. Resumption of alcohol intake often begins within the first year after surgery but, as alcohol use disorder (AUD) is characterized by episodes of remission followed by relapse, it is not surprising to observe a progressive increase of relapse with longer follow-up times [136, 139, 141, 142]. In those transplanted for AAH, the rate is higher (10–35% within the first 2–3 years) and so is the 2-year rate of harmful alcohol intake (22%) [128, 131, 143–146]. These figures, though, are felt not to be significant enough to override the substantial survival benefit obtained by early LT in these patients.

Transplant multidisciplinary care teams, composed of transplant coordinators, hepatologists, addiction specialists, psychologists, and social workers, are fundamental to providing comprehensive care to individuals who have undergone LT and are in recovery from alcohol addiction. Regular and systematic alcohol monitoring and testing help in the early detection of any relapse or return to alcohol use. These tests can be administered randomly or on a scheduled basis, ensuring that no lapse in sobriety goes unnoticed. When relapse is identified in its early stages, healthcare providers can intervene promptly, offering timely support, counselling, and interventions to prevent the re-establishment of problematic alcohol consumption patterns. Cognitive-behavioral therapy addresses the underlying causes and triggers of alcohol addiction, empowering patients to develop healthier coping strategies and more adaptive responses to stressors, cravings, and other factors that may lead to relapse. Finally, medication-assisted therapy (naltrexone and acamprosate) is used to reduce cravings and decrease the appeal of alcohol by acting on the brain's reward system (Table 28.2) [147–155].

Vulnerable patients' pre-LT (social instability, psychiatric comorbidities, and poly-substance abuse) should be referred early to addiction programs. Additional risk factors to consider due to their association with alcohol relapse include male sex, duration of alcohol abstinence, non-compliance with medical care, and young age [147–150]. Based on these factors, several risk scores have been used to select patients for LT in the setting of AAH, including the High-Risk Alcoholism Relapse (HRAR) tool, the Stanford Integrated Psychosocial assessment for Transplantation (SIPAT), or the Sustained alcohol use post LT(SALT) scores [156, 157]. Among other items, these scores include a psychosocial assessment addressing the underlying AUD, social support, psychosocial stability, abuse of other substances, and motivation. The scores are mostly useful in determining a lower risk of relapse owing to high negative predictive value [158], but should not be used solely to determine candidacy given their low positive predictive value.

Table 28.2 Drugs for recurrent alcohol use disorder

DRUG	FDA/EMEA approval	Mechanism of action	Dose	Use in advanced liver disease	Concomitant use with immunospppressors	Hepatotoxicity	Adverse events
Disulfiram	Yes	ADH inhibitor	250–500 mg/d	No	Yes	Yes	Hepatotoxicity
Naltrexone	Yes	R-opioid antagonist	25–50 mg /d 380 mg/m IM	No	Yes	Yes	Diarrhoea Nausea Sleepiness Hepatotoxicity
Acamprosate	Yes	NMDA receptor agonist	666 mg/8h	Yes	Yes	No	Diarrhoea
Topiramate	No	Multiple receptors		Yes	Yes	Possible	Paresthesias Anorexia
Baclofen	Yes	R-GABA agonist	10 mg/8h	Yes	Yes	No	Sleepiness
Gabapentin	No	GABA transmission modulation	300–600 mg/8h	Yes	Yes	Isolated cases	Asthenia Headache Insomnia
Varenicline	No	Nicotine receptor partial agonist	2 mg/d	Yes	Yes	Isolated cases	Asthenia Nausea Sleepiness

ADH alcohol deshydrogenase, *NMDA* N-metil-D-aspartate, *GABA* γ-aminobutyric acid, *mg/d* milligrams per day, *mg/m* milligrams per month, *IM* intramuscular, References [154, 159, 160]

References

1. Tejedor M, Selzner N, Berenguer M. Are MELD and MELDNa still reliable tools to predict mortality on the liver transplant waiting list? Transplantation. 2022;106(11):2122–36.
2. Watt KD, Pedersen RA, Kremers WK, Heimbach JK, Charlton MR. Evolution of causes and risk factors for mortality post liver transplant: results of the NIDDK long term follow-up study. Am J Transplant Off J Am Soc. 2010;10(6):1420–7.
3. Rowe IA, Webb K, Gunson BK, Mehta N, Haque S, Neuberger J. The impact of disease recurrence on graft survival following liver transplantation: a single centre experience. Transpl Int. 2008;21(5):459–65.
4. Berenguer M, Agarwal K, Burra P, Manns M, Samuel D. The road map toward an hepatitis C virus-free transplant population. Am J Transplant. 2018;18(10):2409–16.
5. Berenguer M, Ferrell L, Watson J, Prieto M, Kim M, Rayón M, et al. HCV-related fibrosis progression following liver transplantation: increase in recent years. J Hepatol. 2000;32(4):673–84.
6. Forman LM, Lewis JD, Berlin JA, Feldman HI, Lucey MR. The association between hepatitis C infection and survival after orthotopic liver transplantation. Gastroenterology. 2002;122(4):889–96.
7. Taga SA, Washington MK, Terrault N, Wright TL, Somberg KA, Ferrell LD. Cholestatic hepatitis C in liver allografts. Liver Transpl Surg. 1998;4(4):304–10.
8. Verna EC, Abdelmessih R, Salomao MA, Lefkowitch J, Moreira RK, Brown RS Jr. Cholestatic hepatitis C following liver transplantation: an outcome-based histological definition, clinical predictors, and prognosis. Liver Transpl. 2013;19(1):78–88.
9. Charlton M, Gane E, Manns MP, Brown RS, Curry MP, Kwo PY, et al. Sofosbuvir and ribavirin for treatment of compensated recurrent hepatitis C virus infection after liver transplantation. Gastroenterology. 2015;148(1):108–17.
10. Fontana RJ, Hughes EA, Appelman H, Hindes R, Dimitrova D, Bifano M. Case report of successful peginterferon, ribavirin, and daclatasvir therapy for recurrent cholestatic hepatitis C after liver retransplantation. Liver Transpl. 2012;18(9):1053–9.
11. Gutierrez JA, Carrion AF, Avalos D, O'Brien C, Martin P, Bhamidimarri KR, et al. Sofosbuvir and simeprevir for treatment of hepatitis C virus infection in liver transplant recipients. Liver Transpl. 2015;21(6):823–30.
12. Alqahtani SA, Afdhal N, Zeuzem S, Gordon SC, Mangia A, Kwo P, et al. Safety and tolerability of ledipasvir/sofosbuvir with and without ribavirin in patients with chronic hepatitis C virus genotype 1 infection: analysis of phase III ION trials. Hepatology. 2015;62(1):25.
13. Pungpapong S, Aqel B, Leise M, Werner KT, Murphy JL, Henry TM, et al. Multicenter experience using simeprevir and sofosbuvir with or without ribavirin to treat hepatitis C genotype 1 after liver transplant. Hepatology. 2015;61(6):1880–6.
14. Saab S, Jimenez M, Bau S, Goo T, Zhao D, Durazo F, et al. Treating fibrosing cholestatic hepatitis C with sofosbuvir and ribavirin: a matched analysis. Clin Transpl. 2015;29(9):813–9.
15. Issa D, Eghtesad B, Zein NN, Yerian L, Cruise M, Alkhouri N, et al. Sofosbuvir and simeprevir for the treatment of recurrent hepatitis C with fibrosing cholestatic hepatitis after liver transplantation. Int J Organ Transplant Med. 2016;7(1):38–45.
16. Kim B, Trivedi A, Thung SN, Grewal P. Case report of successful treatment of fibrosing cholestatic hepatitis C with sofosbuvir and ribavirin after liver transplantation. Semin Liver Dis. 2014;34(1):108–12.
17. Pellicelli AM, Montalbano M, Lionetti R, Durand C, Ferenci P, D'Offizi G, et al. Sofosbuvir plus daclatasvir for post-transplant recurrent hepatitis C: potent antiviral activity but no clinical benefit if treatment is given late. Dig Liver Dis. 2014;46(10):923–7.
18. Picciotto FP, Tritto G, Lanza AG, Addario L, Luca MD, Costanzo GD, et al. Sustained virological response to antiviral therapy reduces mortality in HCV reinfection after liver transplantation. J Hepatol. 2007;46(3):459–65.

19. Dhanasekaran R, Sanchez W, Mounajjed T, Wiesner RH, Watt KD, Charlton MR. Impact of fibrosis progression on clinical outcome in patients treated for post-transplant hepatitis C recurrence. Liver Int. 2015;35(11):2433–41.
20. Blasco A, Forns X, Carrión JA, García-Pagán JC, Gilabert R, Rimola A, et al. Hepatic venous pressure gradient identifies patients at risk of severe hepatitis C recurrence after liver transplantation. Hepatology. 2006;43(3):492–9.
21. Neumann UP, Berg T, Bahra M, Seehofer D, Langrehr JM, Neuhaus R, et al. Fibrosis progression after liver transplantation in patients with recurrent hepatitis C. J Hepatol. 2004;41(5):830–6.
22. Terrault NA, Berenguer M, Strasser SI, Gadano A, Lilly L, Samuel D, et al. International liver transplantation society consensus statement on hepatitis C management in liver transplant recipients. Transplantation. 2017;101(5):956.
23. Hepatitis C. Guidance 2019 update: AASLD-IDSA recommendations for testing, managing, and treating hepatitis C virus infection. Hepatol Baltim Md. 2020;71(2):686–721.
24. Pawlotsky JM, Negro F, Aghemo A, Berenguer M, Dalgard O, Dusheiko G, et al. EASL recommendations on treatment of hepatitis C: final update of the series. J Hepatol. 2020;73(5):1170–218.
25. Badri PS, Parikh A, Coakley EP, Ding B, Awni WM, Dutta S, et al. Pharmacokinetics of tacrolimus and cyclosporine in liver transplant recipients receiving 3 direct-acting antivirals as treatment for hepatitis C infection. Ther Drug Monit. 2016;38(5):640.
26. Kwo PY, Badshah MB. New hepatitis C virus therapies: drug classes and metabolism, drug interactions relevant in the transplant settings, drug options in decompensated cirrhosis, and drug options in end-stage renal disease. Curr Opin Organ Transplant. 2015;20(3):235.
27. Burra P, Germani G, Adam R, Karam V, Marzano A, Lampertico P, et al. Liver transplantation for HBV-related cirrhosis in Europe: an ELTR study on evolution and outcomes. J Hepatol. 2013;58(2):287–96.
28. Flemming JA, Kim WR, Brosgart CL, Terrault NA. Reduction in liver transplant wait-listing in the era of direct-acting antiviral therapy. Hepatology. 2017;65(3):804–12.
29. Belli LS, Perricone G, Adam R, Cortesi PA, Strazzabosco M, Facchetti R, et al. Impact of DAAs on liver transplantation: major effects on the evolution of indications and results. An ELITA study based on the ELTR registry. J Hepatol. 2018;69(4):810–7.
30. Le Guerhier F, Pichoud C, Guerret S, Chevallier M, Jamard C, Hantz O, et al. Characterization of the antiviral effect of 2′,3′-dideoxy-2′, 3′-didehydro-β-l-5-fluorocytidine in the duck hepatitis B virus infection model. Antimicrob Agents Chemother. 2000;44(1):111–22.
31. Delmas J, Schorr O, Jamard C, Gibbs C, Trépo C, Hantz O, et al. Inhibitory effect of adefovir on viral DNA synthesis and covalently closed circular DNA formation in duck hepatitis B virus-infected hepatocytes in vivo and in vitro. Antimicrob Agents Chemother. 2002;46(2):425–33.
32. Duvoux C, Belli LS, Fung J, Angelico M, Buti M, Coilly A, et al. 2020 position statement and recommendations of the European liver and intestine transplantation association (ELITA): management of hepatitis B virus-related infection before and after liver transplantation. Aliment Pharmacol Ther. 2021;54(5):583–605.
33. Marzano A, Gaia S, Ghisetti V, Carenzi S, Premoli A, Debernardi-Venon W, et al. Viral load at the time of liver transplantation and risk of hepatitis B virus recurrence. Liver Transpl. 2005;11(4):402–9.
34. Zheng S, Chen Y, Liang T, Lu A, Wang W, Shen Y, et al. Prevention of hepatitis B recurrence after liver transplantation using lamivudine or lamivudine combined with hepatitis B immunoglobulin prophylaxis. Liver Transpl. 2006;12(2):253–8.
35. Shouval D, Samuel D. Hepatitis B immune globulin to prevent hepatitis B virus graft reinfection following liver transplantation: a concise review. Hepatology. 2000;32(6):1189–95.
36. Cholongitas E, Papatheodoridis GV. High genetic barrier nucleos(t)ide analogue(s) for prophylaxis from hepatitis B virus recurrence after liver transplantation: a systematic review. Am J Transplant. 2013;13(2):353–62.

37. Fung J, Wong T, Chok K, Chan A, Cheung TT, Dai JWC, et al. Long-term outcomes of entecavir monotherapy for chronic hepatitis B after liver transplantation: results up to 8 years. Hepatology. 2017;66(4):1036.
38. Loomba R, Decaris M, Li KW, Shankaran M, Mohammed H, Matthews M, et al. Discovery of half-life of circulating Hepatitis B surface antigen in patients with chronic hepatitis B infection using heavy water labeling. Clin Infect Dis. 2019;69(3):542–5.
39. Fung J. Management of chronic hepatitis B before and after liver transplantation. World J Hepatol. 2015;7(10):1421–6.
40. Fung J, Cheung C, Chan SC, Yuen MF, Chok KSH, Sharr W, et al. Entecavir monotherapy is effective in suppressing hepatitis B virus after liver transplantation. Gastroenterology. 2011;141(4):1212–9.
41. Montano-Loza AJ, Bhanji RA, Wasilenko S, Mason AL. Systematic review: recurrent autoimmune liver diseases after liver transplantation. Aliment Pharmacol Ther. 2017;45(4):485–500.
42. Montano-Loza AJ, Ronca V, Ebadi M, Hansen BE, Hirschfield G, Elwir S, et al. Risk factors and outcomes associated with recurrent autoimmune hepatitis following liver transplantation. J Hepatol. 2022;77(1):84–97.
43. Gautam M, Cheruvattath R, Balan V. Recurrence of autoimmune liver disease after liver transplantation: a systematic review. Liver Transpl. 2006;12(12):1813–24.
44. Hübscher SG. Recurrent autoimmune hepatitis after liver transplantation: diagnostic criteria, risk factors, and outcome. Liver Transpl. 2001;7(4):285–91.
45. Mack CL, Adams D, Assis DN, Kerkar N, Manns MP, Mayo MJ, et al. Diagnosis and management of autoimmune hepatitis in adults and children: 2019 practice guidance and guidelines from the American Association for the Study of Liver Diseases. Hepatology. 2020;72(2):671.
46. Montano-Loza AJ, Rodríguez-Perálvarez ML, Pageaux GP, Sanchez-Fueyo A, Feng S. Liver transplantation immunology: immunosuppression, rejection, and immunomodulation. J Hepatol. 2023;78(6):1199–215.
47. Lerut JP, Gondolesi GE. Immunosuppression in liver and intestinal transplantation. Best Pract Res Clin Gastroenterol. 2021;54–55:101767.
48. Kelly C, Zen Y, Heneghan MA. Post-Transplant Immunosuppression in Autoimmune Liver Disease. J Clin Exp Hepatol. 2023;13(2):350–9.
49. Vierling JM, Kerkar N, Czaja AJ, Mack CL, Adams D, Assis DN, et al. Immunosuppressive treatment regimens in autoimmune Hepatitis: systematic reviews and meta-analyses supporting American Association for the Study of Liver Diseases guidelines. Hepatology. 2020;72(2):753.
50. Campsen J, Zimmerman MA, Trotter JF, Wachs M, Bak T, Steinberg T, et al. Liver transplantation for autoimmune hepatitis and the success of aggressive corticosteroid withdrawal. Liver Transpl. 2008;14(9):1281–6.
51. Krishnamoorthy TL, Miezynska-Kurtycz J, Hodson J, Gunson BK, Neuberger J, Milkiewicz P, et al. Longterm corticosteroid use after liver transplantation for autoimmune hepatitis is safe and associated with a lower incidence of recurrent disease. Liver Transpl. 2016;22(1):34–41.
52. De Martin E, Londoño MC, Emamaullee J, Lerut J, Potts J, Aluvihare V, et al. The optimal immunosuppression management to prevent early rejection after liver transplantation: a systematic review of the literature and expert panel recommendations. Clin Transpl. 2022;36(10):e14614.
53. Theocharidou E, Heneghan MA. Con: steroids should not be withdrawn in transplant recipients with autoimmune hepatitis. Liver Transpl. 2018;24(8):1113.
54. Kalra A, Burton JRJ, Forman LM. Pro: steroids can be withdrawn after transplant in recipients with autoimmune hepatitis. Liver Transpl. 2018;24(8):1109.
55. Kerkar N, Dugan C, Rumbo C, Morotti RA, Gondolesi G, Shneider BL, et al. Rapamycin successfully treats post-transplant autoimmune hepatitis. Am J Transplant. 2005;5(5):1085–9.
56. Henson JB, King LY. Post-transplant management and complications of autoimmune hepatitis, primary biliary cholangitis, and primary sclerosing cholangitis including disease recurrence. Clin Liver Dis. 2024;28(1):193–207.

57. Tajima T, Hata K, Haga H, Kusakabe J, Kageyama S, Yurugi K, et al. Risk factors for antibody-mediated rejection in ABO blood-type incompatible and donor-specific antibody-positive liver transplantation. Liver Transpl. 2023;29(7):711.
58. Vandevoorde K, Ducreux S, Bosch A, Guillaud O, Hervieu V, Chambon-Augoyard C, et al. Prevalence, risk factors, and impact of donor-specific alloantibodies after adult liver transplantation. Liver Transpl. 2018;24(8):1091.
59. Demetris AJ, Bellamy C, Hübscher SG, O'Leary J, Randhawa PS, Feng S, et al. 2016 comprehensive update of the Banff working group on liver allograft pathology: introduction of antibody-mediated rejection. Am J Transplant. 2016;16(10):2816–35.
60. Harrington CR, Levitsky J. Alloimmune versus autoimmune hepatitis following liver transplantation. Clin Liver Dis. 2022;20(1):21–4.
61. Lee BT, Fiel MI, Schiano TD. Antibody-mediated rejection of the liver allograft: an update and a clinico-pathological perspective. J Hepatol. 2021;75(5):1203–16.
62. Berenguer M, Di Maira T, Baumann U, Mirza DF, Heneghan MA, Klempnauer JL, et al. Characteristics, trends, and outcomes of liver transplantation for primary sclerosing cholangitis in female versus male patients: an analysis from the European liver transplant registry. Transplantation. 2021;105(10):2255.
63. Chazouilleres O, Beuers U, Bergquist A, Karlsen TH, Levy C, Samyn M, et al. EASL clinical practice guidelines on sclerosing cholangitis. J Hepatol. 2022;77(3):761–806.
64. Graziadei IW, Wiesner RH, Marotta PJ, Porayko MK, Hay JE, Charlton MR, et al. Long-term results of patients undergoing liver transplantation for primary sclerosing cholangitis. Hepatol Baltim Md. 1999;30(5):1121–7.
65. Lindström L, Jørgensen KK, Boberg KM, Castedal M, Rasmussen A, Rostved AA, et al. Risk factors and prognosis for recurrent primary sclerosing cholangitis after liver transplantation: a Nordic multicentre study. Scand J Gastroenterol. 2018;53(3):297–304.
66. Visseren T, Erler NS, Polak WG, Adam R, Karam V, Vondran FWR, Ericzon BG, Thorburn D, IJzermans JNM, Paul A, van der Heide F, Taimr P, Nemec P, Pirenne J, Romagnoli R, Metselaar HJ, Darwish Murad S; European Liver and Intestine Transplantation Association (ELITA). Recurrence of primary sclerosing cholangitis after liver transplantation—analysing the European Liver Transplant Registry and beyond. Transpl Int. 2021;34(8):1455–67.
67. Sierra L, Barba R, Ferrigno B, Goyes D, Diaz W, Patwardhan VR, Saberi B, Bonder A. Living-donor liver transplant and improved post-transplant survival in patients with primary sclerosing cholangitis. J Clin Med. 2023;12(8):2807.
68. Trivedi PJ, Scalera I, Slaney E, Laing RW, Gunson B, Hirschfield GM, et al. Clinical outcomes of donation after circulatory death liver transplantation in primary sclerosing cholangitis. J Hepatol. 2017;67(5):957–65.
69. Visseren T, Erler NS, Heimbach JK, Eaton JE, Selzner N, Gulamhusein A, et al. Inflammatory conditions play a role in recurrence of PSC after liver transplantation: an international multicentre study. JHEP Rep Innov Hepatol. 2022;4(12):100599.
70. Sierra L, Barba R, Ferrigno B, Goyes D, Diaz W, Patwardhan VR, et al. Living-donor liver transplant and improved post-transplant survival in patients with primary sclerosing cholangitis. J Clin Med. 2023;12(8):2807.
71. Sharma S, Gurakar A, Jabbour N. Biliary strictures following liver transplantation: past, present and preventive strategies. Liver Transpl. 2008;14(6):759–69.
72. Verdonk RC, Buis CI, van der Jagt EJ, Gouw ASH, Limburg AJ, Slooff MJH, et al. Nonanastomotic biliary strictures after liver transplantation, part 2: management, outcome, and risk factors for disease progression. Liver Transplant. 2007;13(5):725–32.
73. Pandanaboyana S, Bell R, Bartlett AJ, McCall J, Hidalgo E. Meta-analysis of duct-to-duct versus Roux-en-Y biliary reconstruction following liver transplantation for primary sclerosing cholangitis. Transpl Int. 2015;28(4):485–91.
74. Carbone M, Della Penna A, Mazzarelli C, De Martin E, Villard C, Bergquist A, et al. Liver transplantation for primary sclerosing cholangitis (PSC) with or without inflammatory bowel disease (IBD)—a European Society of Organ Transplantation (ESOT) consensus statement. Transpl Int. 2023;36:11729.

75. Vannas MJ, Åberg F, Nordin A, Tukiainen E, Savikko J, Isoniemi H. Comprehensive complication index to monitor morbidity and mortality after liver transplantation in primary sclerosing cholangitis. Ann Surg. 2023;278(4):e773–9.
76. Hov JR, Karlsen TH. The microbiota and the gut-liver axis in primary sclerosing cholangitis. Nat Rev Gastroenterol Hepatol. 2023;20(3):135–54.
77. Steenstraten IC, Sebib Korkmaz K, Trivedi PJ, Inderson A, van Hoek B, Rodriguez Girondo MDM, et al. Systematic review with meta-analysis: risk factors for recurrent primary sclerosing cholangitis after liver transplantation. Aliment Pharmacol Ther. 2019;49(6):636–43.
78. Hatami B, Pasharavesh L, Sharifian A, Zali MR. Concurrent inflammatory bowel disease and primary sclerosing cholangitis: a review of pre- and post-transplant outcomes and treatment options. Gastroenterol Hepatol Bed Bench. 2023;16(3):259–69.
79. Nordenvall C, Olén O, Nilsson PJ, von Seth E, Ekbom A, Bottai M, et al. Colectomy prior to diagnosis of primary sclerosing cholangitis is associated with improved prognosis in a nationwide cohort study of 2594 PSC-IBD patients. Aliment Pharmacol Ther. 2018;47(2):238–45.
80. Visseren T, Fuhler GM, Erler NS, Nossent YRA, Metselaar HJ, IJzermans JNM, et al. Recurrence of primary sclerosing cholangitis after liver transplantation is associated with specific changes in the gut microbiome pretransplant—a pilot study. Transpl Int. 2020;33(11):1424–36.
81. Hole MJ, Jørgensen KK, Holm K, Braadland PR, Meyer-Myklestad MH, Medhus AW, et al. A shared mucosal gut microbiota signature in primary sclerosing cholangitis before and after liver transplantation. Hepatol Baltim Md. 2023;77(3):715–28.
82. Shah A, Jones MP, Callaghan G, Fairlie T, Ma X, Culver EL, et al. Efficacy and safety of biologics in primary sclerosing cholangitis with inflammatory bowel disease: a systematic review and meta-analysis. Hepatol Commun. 2024;8(1):e0347.
83. Ravikumar R, Tsochatzis E, Jose S, Allison M, Athale A, Creamer F, et al. Risk factors for recurrent primary sclerosing cholangitis after liver transplantation. J Hepatol. 2015;63(5):1139–46.
84. Gordon FD, Goldberg DS, Goodrich NP, Lok ASF, Verna EC, Selzner N, et al. Recurrent primary sclerosing cholangitis in the adult-to-adult living donor liver transplantation cohort study: comparison of risk factors between living and deceased donor recipients. Liver Transpl. 2016;22(9):1214–22.
85. Alexander J, Lord JD, Yeh MM, Cuevas C, Bakthavatsalam R, Kowdley KV. Risk factors for recurrence of primary sclerosing cholangitis after liver transplantation. Liver Transpl. 2008;14(2):245–51.
86. Fosby B, Karlsen TH, Melum E. Recurrence and rejection in liver transplantation for primary sclerosing cholangitis. World J Gastroenterol. 2012;18(1):1–15.
87. Henson JB, Patel YA, King LY, Zheng J, Chow SC, Muir AJ. Outcomes of liver retransplantation in patients with primary sclerosing cholangitis. Liver Transpl. 2017;23(6):769–80.
88. Graziadei IW, Wiesner RH, Batts KP, Marotta PJ, LaRusso NF, Porayko MK, et al. Recurrence of primary sclerosing cholangitis following liver transplantation. Hepatol Baltim Md. 1999;29(4):1050–6.
89. Henson JB, Patel YA, Wilder JM, Zheng J, Chow SC, King LY, et al. Differences in phenotypes and liver transplantation outcomes by age Group in Patients with primary sclerosing cholangitis. Dig Dis Sci. 2017;62(11):3200–9.
90. Åberg F, Sallinen V, Tuominen S, Adam R, Karam V, Mirza D, et al. Cyclosporine vs. tacrolimus after liver transplantation for primary sclerosing cholangitis—a propensity score-matched intention-to-treat analysis. J Hepatol. 2024;80(1):99–108.
91. Carey EJ, Ali AH, Lindor KD. Primary biliary cirrhosis. Lancet. 2015;386(10003):1565–75.
92. Harms MH, Janssen QP, Adam R, Duvoux C, Mirza D, Hidalgo E, et al. Trends in liver transplantation for primary biliary cholangitis in Europe over the past three decades. Aliment Pharmacol Ther. 2019;49(3):285–95.
93. Gross CR, Malinchoc M, Kim WR, Evans RW, Wiesner RH, Petz JL, et al. Quality of life before and after liver transplantation for cholestatic liver disease. Hepatol Baltim Md. 1999;29(2):356–64.

94. Nevens F. PBC-transplantation and disease recurrence. Best Pract Res Clin Gastroenterol. 2018;34–35:107–11.
95. Neuberger J. Liver transplantation for primary biliary cirrhosis: indications and risk of recurrence. J Hepatol. 2003;39(2):142–8.
96. Webb GJ, Rana A, Hodson J, Akhtar MZ, Ferguson JW, Neuberger JM, et al. Twenty-year comparative analysis of patients with autoimmune liver diseases on transplant waitlists. Clin Gastroenterol Hepatol. 2018;16(2):278–287.e7.
97. Lee J, Belanger A, Doucette JT, Stanca C, Friedman S, Bach N. Transplantation trends in primary biliary cirrhosis. Clin Gastroenterol Hepatol. 2007;5(11):1313–5.
98. Kaif M. Patients with primary biliary cirrhosis have the highest wait-list mortality. Gastroenterology. 2015;148:S.
99. Singal AK, Wong RJ, Jalan R, Asrani S, Kuo YF. Primary biliary cholangitis has the highest waitlist mortality in patients with cirrhosis and acute on chronic liver failure awaiting liver transplant. Clin Transpl. 2021;35(12):e14479.
100. Keeling SS, McDonald MF, Anand A, Goff CR, Christmann CR, Barrett SC, et al. Do patients with autoimmune conditions have less access to liver transplantation despite superior outcomes? J Pers Med. 2022;12(7):1159.
101. Adam R, Karam V, Cailliez V, O Grady JG, Mirza D, Cherqui D, et al. Annual report of the European Liver Transplant Registry (ELTR)—50-year evolution of liver transplantation. Transpl Int Off J Eur Soc Organ Transplant. 2018;31(12):1293–317.
102. Heinemann M, Adam R, Berenguer M, Mirza D, Malek-Hosseini SA, O'Grady JG, et al. Longterm survival after liver transplantation for autoimmune Hepatitis: results from the European Liver Transplant Registry. Liver Transplant. 2020;26(7):866–77.
103. Corpechot C, Chazouillères O, Belnou P, Montano-Loza AJ, Mason A, Ebadi M, et al. Long-term impact of preventive UDCA therapy after transplantation for primary biliary cholangitis. J Hepatol. 2020;73(3):559–65.
104. Montano-Loza AJ, Hansen BE, Corpechot C, Roccarina D, Thorburn D, Trivedi P, et al. Factors associated with recurrence of primary biliary cholangitis after liver transplantation and effects on graft and patient survival. Gastroenterology. 2019;156(1):96–107.e1.
105. Sylvestre PB, Batts KP, Burgart LJ, Poterucha JJ, Wiesner RH. Recurrence of primary biliary cirrhosis after liver transplantation: histologic estimate of incidence and natural history. Liver Transplant. 2003;9(10):1086–93.
106. Charatcharoenwitthaya P, Pimentel S, Talwalkar JA, Enders FT, Lindor KD, Krom RAF, et al. Long-term survival and impact of ursodeoxycholic acid treatment for recurrent primary biliary cirrhosis after liver transplantation. Liver Transplant. 2007;13(9):1236–45.
107. Bosch A, Dumortier J, Maucort-Boulch D, Scoazec JY, Wendum D, Conti F, et al. Preventive administration of UDCA after liver transplantation for primary biliary cirrhosis is associated with a lower risk of disease recurrence. J Hepatol. 2015;63(6):1449–58.
108. Hubscher SG, Elias E, Buckels JA, Mayer AD, McMaster P, Neuberger JM. Primary biliary cirrhosis. Histological evidence of disease recurrence after liver transplantation. J Hepatol. 1993;18(2):173–84.
109. Pedersen MR, Greenan G, Arora S, Murali AR, Mayo MJ. Ursodeoxycholic acid decreases incidence of primary biliary cholangitis and biliary complications after liver transplantation: a meta-analysis. Liver Transplant. 2021;27(6):866–75.
110. Jacob DA, Neumann UP, Bahra M, Klupp J, Puhl G, Neuhaus R, et al. Long-term follow-up after recurrence of primary biliary cirrhosis after liver transplantation in 100 patients. Clin Transpl. 2006;20(2):211–20.
111. Lee DU, Ponder R, Sandlow S, Yoo A, Lee KJ, Chou H, et al. The impact of recipient and donor gender-match and mismatch on the post-liver transplant outcomes of patients with primary biliary cholangitis. Dig Liver Dis. 2023;55(9):1242–52.
112. Dmitrewski J, Hubscher SG, Mayer AD, Neuberger JM. Recurrence of primary biliary cirrhosis in the liver allograft: the effect of immunosuppression. J Hepatol. 1996;24(3):253–7.

113. Liermann Garcia RF, Evangelista Garcia C, McMaster P, Neuberger J. Transplantation for primary biliary cirrhosis: retrospective analysis of 400 patients in a single center. Hepatol Baltim Md. 2001;33(1):22–7.
114. Wong PYN, Portmann B, O'Grady JG, Devlin JJ, Hegarty JE, Tan KC, et al. Recurrence of primary biliary cirrhosis after liver transplantation following FK506-based immunosuppression. J Hepatol. 1993;17(3):284–7.
115. Montano AJ, Wasilenko S, Bintner J, Mason AL. Cyclosporine a protects against primary biliary cirrhosis recurrence after liver transplantation. Am J Transplant. 2010;10(4):852–8.
116. Egawa H, Sakisaka S, Teramukai S, Sakabayashi S, Yamamoto M, Umeshita K, Uemoto S. Long-term outcomes of living-donor liver transplantation for primary biliary cirrhosis: a Japanese multicenter study. Am J Transplant. 2016;16(4):1248–57.
117. Singal AK, Arsalan A, Dunn W, Arab JP, Wong RJ, Kuo YF, et al. Alcohol-associated liver disease in the United States is associated with severe forms of disease among young, females and Hispanics. Aliment Pharmacol Ther. 2021;54(4):451–61.
118. Sandahl TD, Jepsen P, Thomsen KL, Vilstrup H. Incidence and mortality of alcoholic hepatitis in Denmark 1999–2008: a nationwide population based cohort study. J Hepatol. 2011;54(4):760–4.
119. Goldberg D, Ditah IC, Saeian K, Lalehzari M, Aronsohn A, Gorospe EC, et al. Changes in the prevalence of Hepatitis C virus infection, nonalcoholic steatohepatitis, and alcoholic liver disease among patients with cirrhosis or liver failure on the waitlist for liver transplantation. Gastroenterology. 2017;152(5):1090–1099.e1.
120. Kwong AJ, Ebel NH, Kim WR, Lake JR, Smith JM, Schladt DP, et al. OPTN/SRTR 2020 annual data report: liver. Am J Transplant. 2022;22(Suppl 2):204–309.
121. Marjot T, Eberhardt CS, Boettler T, Belli LS, Berenguer M, Buti M, et al. Impact of COVID-19 on the liver and on the care of patients with chronic liver disease, hepatobiliary cancer, and liver transplantation: an updated EASL position paper. J Hepatol. 2022;77(4):1161–97.
122. Shaheen AA, Kong K, Ma C, Doktorchik C, Coffin CS, Swain MG, et al. Impact of the COVID-19 pandemic on hospitalizations for alcoholic Hepatitis or cirrhosis in Alberta, Canada. Clin Gastroenterol Hepatol. 2022;20(5):e1170–9.
123. Cholankeril G, Goli K, Rana A, Hernaez R, Podboy A, Jalal P, et al. Impact of COVID-19 pandemic on liver transplantation and alcohol-associated liver disease in the USA. Hepatol Baltim Md. 2021;74(6):3316–29.
124. Kwong AJ, Kim WR, Lake JR, Smith JM, Schladt DP, Skeans MA, et al. OPTN/SRTR 2019 annual data report: liver. Am J Transplant. 2021;21(Suppl 2):208–315.
125. Mathurin P, Lucey MR. Liver transplantation in patients with alcohol-related liver disease: current status and future directions. Lancet Gastroenterol Hepatol. 2020;5(5):507–14.
126. Mathurin P, O'Grady J, Carithers RL, Phillips M, Louvet A, Mendenhall CL, et al. Corticosteroids improve short-term survival in patients with severe alcoholic hepatitis: meta-analysis of individual patient data. Gut. 2011;60(2):255–60.
127. Louvet A, Thursz MR, Kim DJ, Labreuche J, Atkinson SR, Sidhu SS, et al. Corticosteroids reduce risk of death within 28 days for patients with severe alcoholic Hepatitis, compared with pentoxifylline or placebo-a meta-analysis of individual data from controlled trials. Gastroenterology. 2018;155(2):458–468.e8.
128. Louvet A, Labreuche J, Moreno C, Vanlemmens C, Moirand R, Féray C, et al. Early liver transplantation for severe alcohol-related hepatitis not responding to medical treatment: a prospective controlled study. Lancet Gastroenterol Hepatol. 2022;7(5):416–25.
129. Adam R, McMaster P, O'Grady JG, Castaing D, Klempnauer JL, Jamieson N, Neuhaus P, Lerut J, Salizzoni M, Pollard S, Muhlbacher F, Rogiers X, Garcia Valdecasas JC, Berenguer J, Jaeck D, Moreno Gonzalez E, European Liver Transplant Association. Evolution of liver transplantation in Europe: report of the European Liver Transplant Registry. Liver Transpl. 2003;9(12):1231–43.
130. Mackie J, Groves K, Hoyle A, Garcia C, Garcia R, Gunson B, Neuberger J. Orthotopic liver transplantation for alcoholic liver disease: a retrospective analysis of survival, recidivism, and risk factors predisposing to recidivism. Liver Transpl. 2001;7(5):418–27.

131. Lee BP, Mehta N, Platt L, Gurakar A, Rice JP, Lucey MR, et al. Outcomes of early liver transplantation for patients with severe alcoholic hepatitis. Gastroenterology. 2018;155(2):422–430.e1.
132. Lucey MR. Liver transplantation for alcoholic liver disease. Nat Rev Gastroenterol Hepatol. 2014;11(5):300–7.
133. Faure S, Herrero A, Jung B, Duny Y, Daures JP, Mura T, et al. Excessive alcohol consumption after liver transplantation impacts on long-term survival, whatever the primary indication. J Hepatol. 2012;57(2):306–12.
134. Dumortier J, Dharancy S, Cannesson A, Lassailly G, Rolland B, Pruvot FR, et al. Recurrent alcoholic cirrhosis in severe alcoholic relapse after liver transplantation: a frequent and serious complication. Am J Gastroenterol. 2015;110(8):1160–6. quiz 1167
135. Watt KDS, Pedersen RA, Kremers WK, Heimbach JK, Sanchez W, Gores GJ. Long-term probability of and mortality from de novo malignancy after liver transplantation. Gastroenterology. 2009;137(6):2010–7.
136. Cuadrado A, Fábrega E, Casafont F, Pons-Romero F. Alcohol recidivism impairs long-term patient survival after orthotopic liver transplantation for alcoholic liver disease. Liver Transplant. 2005;11(4):420–6.
137. DiMartini A, Day N, Dew MA, Javed L, Fitzgerald MG, Jain A, et al. Alcohol consumption patterns and predictors of use following liver transplantation for alcoholic liver disease. Liver Transplant. 2006;12(5):813–20.
138. Dew MA, DiMartini AF, Steel J, De Vito DA, Myaskovsky L, Unruh M, et al. Meta-analysis of risk for relapse to substance use after transplantation of the liver or other solid organs. Liver Transplant. 2008;14(2):159–72.
139. DiMartini A, Dew MA, Day N, Fitzgerald MG, Jones BL, deVera ME, et al. Trajectories of alcohol consumption following liver transplantation. Am J Transplant. 2010;10(10):2305–12.
140. Rogal S, Shenai N, Kruckenberg K, Rosenberger E, Dew MA, DiMartini A. Post-transplant outcomes of persons receiving a liver graft for alcoholic liver disease. Alcohol Alcohol Oxf Oxfs. 2018;53(2):157–65.
141. Pageaux GP, Michel J, Coste V, Perney P, Possoz P, Perrigault PF, et al. Alcoholic cirrhosis is a good indication for liver transplantation, even for cases of recidivism. Gut. 1999;45(3):421–6.
142. De Gottardi A, Spahr L, Gelez P, Morard I, Mentha G, Guillaud O, et al. A simple score for predicting alcohol relapse after liver transplantation: results from 387 patients over 15 years. Arch Intern Med. 2007;167(11):1183–8.
143. Mathurin P, Moreno C, Samuel D, Dumortier J, Salleron J, Durand F, et al. Early liver transplantation for severe alcoholic hepatitis. N Engl J Med. 2011 Nov;365(19):1790–800.
144. Im GY, Kim-Schluger L, Shenoy A, Schubert E, Goel A, Friedman SL, et al. Early Liver Transplantation for Severe Alcoholic Hepatitis in the United States—a Single-Center Experience. Am J Transplant 2016;16(3):841–849.
145. Germani G, Angrisani D, Addolorato G, Merli M, Mazzarelli C, Tarli C, et al. Liver transplantation for severe alcoholic hepatitis: a multicenter Italian study. Am J Transplant. 2022;22(4):1191–200.
146. Weeks SR, Sun Z, McCaul ME, Zhu H, Anders RA, Philosophe B, et al. Liver transplantation for severe alcoholic hepatitis, updated lessons from the world's largest series. J Am Coll Surg. 2018;226(4):549.
147. Addolorato G, Mirijello A, Leggio L, Ferrulli A, D'Angelo C, Vassallo G, et al. Liver transplantation in alcoholic patients: impact of an alcohol addiction unit within a liver transplant center. Alcohol Clin Exp Res. 2013;37(9):1601–8.
148. Donnadieu-Rigole H, Jaubert L, Ursic-Bedoya J, Hanslik B, Mura T, Gamon L, et al. Integration of an addiction team in a liver transplantation center. Liver Transplant. 2019;25(11):1611–9.
149. Crabb DW, Im GY, Szabo G, Mellinger JL, Lucey MR. Diagnosis and treatment of alcohol-associated liver diseases: 2019 practice guidance from the American Association for the Study of Liver Diseases. Hepatol Baltim Md. 2020;71(1):306–33.

150. Schneekloth TD, Arab JP, Simonetto DA, Petterson TM, Niazi SK, Hall-Flavin DK, et al. Factors having an impact on relapse and survival in transplant recipients with alcohol-induced liver disease. Mayo Clin Proc Innov Qual Outcomes. 2021;5(6):1153–64.
151. Dom G, Peuskens H. Addiction specialist's role in liver transplantation procedures for alcoholic liver disease. World J Hepatol. 2015;7(17):2091–9.
152. Björnsson E, Olsson J, Rydell A, Fredriksson K, Eriksson C, Sjöberg C, et al. Long-term follow-up of patients with alcoholic liver disease after liver transplantation in Sweden: impact of structured management on recidivism. Scand J Gastroenterol. 2005;40(2):206–16.
153. Daniel J, Dumortier J, Del Bello A, Gamon L, Molinari N, Faure S, et al. Integrating an addiction team into the management of patients transplanted for alcohol-associated liver disease reduces the risk of severe relapse. JHEP Rep Innov Hepatol. 2023;5(10):100832.
154. Arab JP, Izzy M, Leggio L, Bataller R, Shah VH. Management of alcohol use disorder in patients with cirrhosis in the setting of liver transplantation. Nat Rev Gastroenterol Hepatol. 2022;19(1):45–59.
155. European Association for the Study of the Liver. Electronic address: easloffice@easloffice.eu; European Association for the Study of the Liver. EASL Clinical Practice Guidelines: Management of alcohol-related liver disease. J Hepatol. 2018;69(1):154–81.
156. Matthews LA, Lucey MR. Psychosocial evaluation in liver transplantation for patients with alcohol-related liver disease. Clin Liver Dis. 2022;19(1):17–20.
157. Shen NT, Shenoy A, Brown RS, Verna EC. Identifying risk of alcohol relapse after liver transplantation: what tools do we need? Liver Transplant. 2019;25(8):1133–5.
158. Lee BP, Vittinghoff E, Hsu C, Han H, Therapondos G, Fix OK, et al. Predicting low risk for sustained alcohol use after early liver transplant for acute alcoholic Hepatitis: the sustained alcohol use post-liver transplant score. Hepatol Baltim Md. 2019;69(4):1477–87.
159. Addolorato G, Leggio L, Ferrulli A, Cardone S, Vonghia L, Mirijello A, Abenavoli L, D'Angelo C, Caputo F, Zambon A, Haber PS, Gasbarrini G.Effectiveness and safety of baclofen for maintenance of alcohol abstinence in alcoholdependent patients with liver cirrhosis: randomised, double-blind controlled study. Lancet. 2007;370(9603):1915–22.
160. Chaignot C, Zureik M, Rey G, Dray-Spira R, Coste J, Weill A. Risk of hospitalisation and death related to baclofen for alcohol use disorders: Comparison with nalmefene, acamprosate, and naltrexone in a cohort study of 165 334 patients between 2009 and 2015 in France. Pharmacoepidemiol Drug Saf. 2018;27(11):1239–48.

Post-transplant Metabolic Complications: A Contemporary Overview

29

Marius Vögelin and Nazia Selzner

Introduction

The post-transplant metabolic syndrome (PTMS), including post-transplant diabetes mellitus (PTDM), hypertension, dyslipidemia, and obesity, affects approximately 50% of all liver transplant (LT) recipients and represents a significant challenge in the management of patients post-LT [1, 2]. From a broader perspective, de novo or recurrent metabolic dysfunction-associated steatotic liver disease (MASLD) should be viewed not merely as a consequence of the metabolic syndrome, rather as an independent component of it. This chapter explores risk factors, management, and emphasizes the clinical implication on long-term outcome of metabolic complications post-LT.

Risk Factors for Post-Transplant Metabolic Complications

Pre-existing Recipient Risk Factors

The aetiology of the underlying liver disease affects the risk for post-LT metabolic complications. Not surprisingly, MASLD-defined pre-existing metabolic conditions, such as obesity, insulin resistance, dyslipidemia, and hypertension, are well-established risk factors for post-LT metabolic complications [3, 4]. However, there are other pre-existing conditions that predispose for such, including though not limited to: Patients transplanted for alcohol-related liver disease (ALD) or hepatitis C virus (HCV) infection face a higher risk of developing de novo MASLD after LT [4,

M. Vögelin · N. Selzner (✉)
Department of Medicine, Division of Gastroenterology, University Health Network, University of Toronto, Toronto, ON, Canada
e-mail: marius.vogelin@uhn.ca; nazia.selzner@uhn.ca

B. Eghtesad et al. (eds.), *Liver Transplantation*,
https://doi.org/10.1007/978-3-032-07072-2_29

5]. Cryptogenic cirrhosis, often a manifestation of "burned-out" MASLD, also predisposes recipients to recurrent steatosis [6]. Genetic predisposition in both donors and recipients, such as patatin-like phospholipase domain-containing protein 3 (PNPLA3) carriers, further increases the likelihood of graft steatosis [7, 8].

Donor Factors

Donor characteristics contribute to post-LT metabolic health and should not be overlooked. For example, PNPLA3 genetic variants and high donor body mass index (BMI) are associated with an increased risk of graft steatosis [7, 9]. Furthermore, pre-existing macrovesicular steatosis in the graft negatively affects its function and survival, whereas microvesicular steatosis is thought not to have a significant impact [9, 10].

Immunosuppressive Strategy

Immunosuppression significantly influences metabolic outcomes. Corticosteroids are well known to exacerbate insulin resistance, hypertension, and weight gain, contributing to all components of the metabolic syndrome [11]. Among calcineurin inhibitors (CNIs), tacrolimus has a stronger association with PTDM, while cyclosporine is associated with a more pronounced exacerbation of hypertension [12, 13]. In contrast, antimetabolites like mycophenolate or thiopurines have no effects on metabolic parameters [14]. mTOR inhibitors (mammalian target of rapamycin inhibitors), such as sirolimus or everolimus, are associated with an increased risk of de novo MASLD and hypertriglyceridemia [15–17]. Reassuringly, however, this does not seem to impact long-term survival post-LT [17]. Table 29.1 summarizes the effect of immunosuppressive agents on metabolic risk factors.

Table 29.1 Effect of immunosuppressive agents on metabolic risk factors

Risk factor	Insulin resistance/ diabetes mellitus	Dyslipidemia/ hypertriglyceridemia	Hypertension	Weight gain
Glucocorticoids	+ to ++ (dose dependent)	+	++	+
CNI				
Tacrolimus	++	+	+	=
Cyclosporine	+	++	++	=
mTOR inhibitors	+	+++	+ (?)	=
Antimetabolites				
Mycophenolate	=	=	=	=
Azathioprine/ 6-Mercaptopurine	=	=	=	=

Clinical Implications of Metabolic Complications Post-liver Transplant

Impact on Morbidity, Graft, and Patient Survival

Both pre-existing and de novo metabolic complications significantly impact long-term outcomes. Diabetes mellitus (independent if pre-existing or PTDM) and hypertension are associated with increased long-term mortality post-LT [1]. In keeping with this, patients transplanted for MASLD experience twice the risk of cardiovascular events compared to non-MASLD recipients (60% vs. 30% at 10 years, HR 2.04, 95% CI: 1.37–3.04, $P < 0.001$) [18]. Furthermore, patients transplanted for MASLD also have a higher risk of development of chronic kidney disease (CKD) post-transplant, and this remains true after adjustment for hypertension, diabetes, and BMI [19]. CKD again is a risk factor for mortality after LT, as discussed later [1].

However, despite these associations, long-term outcomes in patients with recurrent MASLD are generally favourable and currently available data do not show any significant impact on graft or patient survival within 10 years post-liver transplant [20–22]. This seems somewhat controversial given that cardiovascular events, CKD, and liver fibrosis are all independently associated with increased mortality. Long-term outcome studies with follow-up beyond 10 years are required to assess the real impact on patient and graft survival.

Management of Metabolic Complications

Hypertension

Hypertension affects 30–60% of patients post-LT [23, 24], and remains a long term concern, with uncontrolled hypertension observed in approximately 30% at 5 years after-LT [25]. A blood pressure target of <130/80 mmHg is recommended in LT recipients [26], and further adjustments should be made according to the individual risk profile and tolerability. First-line therapy typically includes calcium channel blockers of the dihydropyridine type, which have minimal interactions with immunosuppressants [27]. Beta blockers can also be used as a second line and are equally effective as calcium channel blockers post-LT [28]. For patients with CKD and albuminuria, angiotensin-converting enzyme (ACE) inhibitors or angiotensin receptor blockers (ARBs) are preferred due to their well-established renal-protective effects [29, 30]. Due to the risk of hyperkalemia, initiation of ACE inhibitors or ARBs should be deferred until the patient is stable in the outpatient setting, with close monitoring of serum potassium levels [26]. In patients on cyclosporine and refractory hypertension, transitioning to tacrolimus can help achieve blood pressure goals [31]. Diuretics can be used with caution, in addition to other classes of antihypertensive medications, in patients with volume overload (e.g. secondary to CKD or heart failure) and to counteract potassium-retaining effects of CNIs and ACEI/

ARBs [27, 32]. Table 29.2 summarizes recommendations for managing metabolic complications in the post-LT setting.

Dyslipidemia

Dyslipidemia is prevalent in 50–70% of LT recipients, and both the risk and extent of dyslipidemia are influenced by immunosuppressive agents, particularly mTOR inhibitors (see Table 29.1) [2, 33, 34]. The latter should therefore be avoided in cases of severe and refractory dyslipidemia.

The American Association for the Study of Liver Diseases (AASLD) recommended annual fasting measurement of lipid profile in all LT patients, and statin therapy if low-density lipoprotein (LDL) is ≥2.6 mmol/l [26]. However, the individual treatment goal could be lower and should be tailored according to the patient's

Table 29.2 Recommendations on treatment of metabolic risk factors after LT

	Treatment recommendation
Assessment	Define treatment target according to individual risk profile Treat to target
Insulin resistance	Early post-transplant: Intermediate-acting insulin Long-term: GLP1 and SGLT2 inhibitors preferred (pleiotropic cardiovascular and renal benefits)
Arterial hypertension	First line: Dihydropyridine calcium channel blockers (least interactions, low risk for adverse events) Beta blocker second line (as effective as calcium channel blockers) ACE inhibitors/ARB: Preferred use in patients with CKD and proteinuria. Anticipate risk for hyperkalemia Avoid cyclosporine in refractory cases
Dyslipidemia	Statin use safe and effective, reduces mortality Cyclosporine + statin: Chose statin with least interaction and reduce dose by 50% Tacrolimus + statin: Probably safe, chose statin with least interaction, consider dose reduction Adding ezetimibe to statin: Reduces LDL by a further 15–20% Refractory: Avoid mTOR inhibitor if reasonable and consider PCSK9 inhibitor
Obesity	Office-based counselling alone mostly ineffective Consider pharmacotherapy: GLP1 agonists, GLP1/GIP agonist Simultaneous sleeve gastrectomy and liver transplant feasible and safe, outcome on weight loss comparable to available pharmacotherapies
De novo or recurrent MASLD	Treat all metabolic risk factors to target Consider GLP1 agonists, yet data emerging
CKD	ACE inhibitors/ARB and/or SGLT2 inhibitors in case of proteinuria Consider CNI sparing strategies with mTOR inhibitors and antimetabolites

ACE angiotensin converting enzyme, *ARB* angiotensin receptor blocker, *CKD* chronic kidney disease, *CNI* calcineurin inhibitor, *GIP* gastric inhibitory polypeptide, *GLP1* glucagon-like peptide 1. *LDL* low-density lipoprotein, *MASLD* metabolic dysfunction-associated steatotic liver disease, *mTOR* mammalian target of rapamycin, *PCSK9* Proprotein Convertase Subtilisin/Kexin type 9, *SGLT2* sodium-glucose cotransporter 2 risk profile. National guidelines, such as those from the American Heart Association (AHA), help determine the patient's individual risk category [34].

Regarding management, lifestyle interventions are mostly ineffective in lowering LDL after LT. On the other hand, statins are clearly underutilized in this population, despite being safe, effective, and known to improve survival [33, 35]. Statins can be safely used with some precautions with CNI. Both the AHA and the KDIGO (Kidney disease: Improving Global Outcomes) recommend pre-emptive dose reduction for statins of approx. 50% when used together with CNI, and primarily CYP 3A4 metabolized statins should be avoided [36, 37]. Statins with the least inhibition of CYP 3A4 are pravastatin or rosuvastatin [35]. Close monitoring for muscle toxicity is also warranted, in particular, in combinations with cyclosporine [38]. However, these recommendations are mostly derived from studies based on cyclosporine, and the interaction between CNI and statins differs substantially for tacrolimus compared to cyclosporine [39]. Compared to cyclosporine, tacrolimus does not alter the function of P-glycoprotein or the organic anion transporting polypeptide (OATP), and therefore does not affect statin exposure [40].

Adding ezetimibe to a statin can further lower LDL by about 15–20% and appears safe in LT patients [41]. If goals cannot be achieved with the above-mentioned measurements, a proprotein convertase subtilisin/kexin type 9 inhibitor (PCSK9i) should be evaluated by an endocrinologist. They are highly effective (lowering of plasma LDL level by 50–70%), do not interact with immunosuppressants, and are considered safe in LT patients [34].

Post-transplant Diabetes Mellitus (PTDM)

About one-third of patients have impaired glucose tolerance after transplant, and PTDM develops in approximately 15% of recipients, primarily within the first year post-LT [42]. Both CNI—in particular, tacrolimus—as well as mTOR inhibitors are associated with a greater risk for PTDM. Immediate post-transplant management often requires intermediate-acting insulin to counter the circadian effect of glucocorticoids [43, 44]. Limited data are available to guide the use of oral antidiabetics in the long-term management. All metformin, dipeptidyl-peptidase-4 inhibitors (DDP-4i), glucagon-like peptide-1 agonists (GLP1 agonists), sodium-glucose co-transporter 2 inhibitors (SGLT2i), and pioglitazone have proven to be safe in the post-transplant setting, and no relevant interactions with immunosuppressants are to be expected [44]. Both GLP1 agonists and SGLT2 inhibitors have now replaced older agents, due to their pleiotropic advantages on cardio−/cerebrovascular and renal risk factors [45]. GLP1 agonists alone or in combination with SGLT2 inhibitors have also been associated with significant weight loss, improved glycemic control, and a decrease in aminotransferase (ALT) levels in diabetic patients after liver transplant [46]. As in non-transplant patients, not only co-morbidities but also potential contraindications (e.g. severely impaired renal function) should be carefully considered when selecting the most appropriate agent.

Obesity and Weight Management

The average weight gain post-LT is 5–10 kg [47]. While some weight gain early after liver transplant is desirable when reflecting reversal of sarcopenia, about 30–60% of patients are classified as overweight (BMI > 25 kg/m^2) or obese (BMI > 30 kg/m^2) one year post-liver transplant [3, 17, 47]. Interestingly, the duration of corticosteroid use does not significantly impact the weight gain, while age > 50 years and certain modifiable risk factors are associated with a more pronounced weight gain [3, 17].

Office-based counselling for lifestyle interventions is mostly ineffective when used alone, particularly in MASLD recipients [48]. Simultaneous sleeve gastrectomy at the time of LT has been shown to be safe, and results in sustained weight loss of approx. 30% at 3 years [49]. Although feasible, data are limited on optimal timing and patient selection for bariatric surgery in the transplant setting [50]. GLP1 with or without gastric-inhibitory peptide (GIP) agonists is also considered safe in the post-transplant setting and can achieve similar or even greater weight loss compared to surgery; however, this effect is not sustained once therapy is discontinued [51].

Recurrent or De Novo MASLD

Recurrent MASLD is 5 times more frequent than de novo MASLD after LT [16]. Overall, graft steatosis occurs in approximately 30–50% of all recipients within 3 years and up to 85% of those transplanted for MASLD at 5 years [18, 52]. Notably, half of these patients develop significant fibrosis (≥F2) within 5 years, and 20% progress to advanced fibrosis (F3–F4) [53]. Post-transplant obesity or weight gain, diabetes mellitus, sirolimus use, and pre-transplant ALD or HCV are independent risk factors for the development of de novo MASLD [3, 5, 6, 52].

Of note, transaminases and gamma-glutamyl transferase are most often within normal limits and do therefore not indicate recurrence of MASLD [53]. Liver biopsy remains the gold standard for diagnosing and staging graft steatosis and fibrosis, though transient elastography can be a useful non-invasive tool even in the post-transplant setting. Liver stiffness measurements of <8 kPa reliably exclude significant fibrosis (≥F2) in MASLD recipients, although the data on cut-offs or specificity are not as robust as in the pre-transplant setting, and are known to be less reliable in obese patients [54–56]. Transient elastography values above 8 kPa should prompt further investigations, including evaluation for other potential causes of allograft damage, such as acute rejection, cholestasis, or right heart failure [56–58]. Of note, two-dimensional shear wave elastography (2D-SWE) has also proven useful in detecting advanced fibrosis in split-liver recipients, but similarly, optimal cut-offs have yet to be defined [59, 60].

Management focuses on addressing underlying metabolic risk factors. GLP1 agonists and emerging therapies such as Resmetirom show a potential for improving steatosis and fibrosis, although the data for the post-transplant setting are only recently emerging [61, 62]. Specific treatment of individual metabolic risk factors and their effect on MASLD after transplant is discussed above and is a rapidly evolving field. In the pre-transplant setting, semaglutide has been shown to improve liver and non-liver-related outcomes in MASLD patients with or without diabetes, although the effect on fibrosis regression was not statistically significant [63]. A follow-up phase 3 trial (ESSENCE trial) is focusing on assessing histologic improvement in MASLD patients with F2 and F3 fibrosis, and interim results suggest a beneficial effect. The AASLD recommends considering semaglutide for patients with MASLD when the label is met (traditionally obesity and diabetes), and semaglutide has recently been approved by the FDA in August 2025 for the indication of MASLD with moderate to severe fibrosis. The dual GLP1/GIP agonist tirzepatide has demonstrated a positive impact on reducing hepatic steatosis and fibrosis in a recently published phase 2 trial [61]. Looking ahead, new data on the management of MASLD in non-transplant patients are rapidly emerging, with novel pharmacologic targets and agents expected to expand the available therapeutic options. While it is plausible that these advances will translate to the post-transplant setting, this has yet to be conclusively demonstrated.

Additionally, there should be a low threshold for initiating statins, as they not only reduce cardiovascular risk but may also decrease mortality and, interestingly, biliary complications in MASLD recipients (see section 'dyslipidemia' above) [35].

Chronic Kidney Disease (CKD)

CKD is a strong risk factor for death after LT [1], and the metabolic complications of obesity, hypertension, and diabetes contribute to end-organ damage in the kidneys both before and after transplantation. This harm, compounded by the nephrotoxic effects of CNIs, can accelerate the decline in kidney function.

CKD management includes treating obesity, optimizing blood pressure and glycemic control, similar to approaches used in non-transplant patients [64–69]. Renal-protective therapies like SGLT2 inhibitors have been shown to slow down CKD progression and reduce renal and cardiovascular mortality in both diabetic and non-diabetic patients outside of the transplant setting [70–72]. Although the available data are very limited, the use of SGLT2 inhibitors in liver transplant patients should be taken into consideration, and is likely as safe as in the general population [73].

If the individual immunological risk profile allows, CNI-sparing regimens, incorporating mTOR inhibitors or antimetabolites, can also help mitigate nephrotoxicity [74–78].

Summary

Metabolic complications after liver transplantation impact patient morbidity and mortality. Graft steatosis occurs in up to every second LT recipient, and patients with recurrent MASLD post-LT have a higher risk for cardiovascular events, CKD, and graft fibrosis. Key strategies include early detection of individuals at highest risk, tailored immunosuppression, proactive medical management of the metabolic syndrome, and the use of renal-protective therapies. A multidisciplinary approach is essential to optimize long-term outcomes and improve the quality of life for transplant recipients.

References

1. Watt KD, Pedersen RA, Kremers WK, Heimbach JK, Charlton MR. Evolution of causes and risk factors for mortality post-liver transplant: results of the NIDDK long-term follow-up study. Am J Transplant. 2010;10(6):1420–7.
2. Watt KD, Charlton MR. Metabolic syndrome and liver transplantation: a review and guide to management. J Hepatol. 2010;53(1):199–206.
3. Dumortier J, Giostra E, Belbouab S, Morard I, Guillaud O, Spahr L, et al. Non-alcoholic fatty liver disease in liver transplant recipients: another story of "seed and soil". Am J Gastroenterol. 2010;105(3):613–20.
4. Hejlova I, Honsova E, Sticova E, Lanska V, Hucl T, Spicak J, et al. Prevalence and risk factors of steatosis after liver transplantation and patient outcomes. Liver Transpl. 2016;22(5):644–55.
5. Galvin Z, Rajakumar R, Chen E, Adeyi O, Selzner M, Grant D, et al. Predictors of De Novo nonalcoholic fatty Liver disease after Liver transplantation and associated fibrosis. Liver Transpl. 2019;25(1):56–67.
6. Losurdo G, Castellaneta A, Rendina M, Carparelli S, Leandro G, Di Leo A. Systematic review with meta-analysis: de novo non-alcoholic fatty liver disease in liver-transplanted patients. Aliment Pharmacol Ther. 2018;47(6):704–14.
7. Finkenstedt A, Auer C, Glodny B, Posch U, Steitzer H, Lanzer G, et al. Patatin-like phospholipase domain-containing protein 3 rs738409-G in recipients of liver transplants is a risk factor for graft steatosis. Clin Gastroenterol Hepatol. 2013;11(12):1667–72.
8. Trunečka P, Míková I, Dlouhá D, Hubáček JA, Honsová E, Kolesár L, et al. Donor PNPLA3 rs738409 genotype is a risk factor for graft steatosis. A post-transplant biopsy-based study. Dig Liver Dis. 2018;50(5):490–5.
9. de Graaf EL, Kench J, Dilworth P, Shackel NA, Strasser SI, Joseph D, et al. Grade of deceased donor liver macrovesicular steatosis impacts graft and recipient outcomes more than the donor risk index. J Gastroenterol Hepatol. 2012;27(3):540–6.
10. Altshuler PJ, Dang H, Frank AM, Shah AP, Glorioso J, Zhan T, et al. Evaluating outcomes related to donor and recipient metabolic environment: Macrosteatotic allografts and nonalcoholic Steatohepatitis. Liver Transpl. 2022;28(4):623–35.
11. Pham PT, Pham PC, Lipshutz GS, Wilkinson AH. New onset diabetes mellitus after solid organ transplantation. Endocrinol Metab Clin N Am. 2007;36(4):873–90. vii
12. Canzanello VJ, Textor SC, Taler SJ, Schwartz LL, Porayko MK, Wiesner RH, et al. Late hypertension after liver transplantation: a comparison of cyclosporine and tacrolimus (FK 506). Liver Transpl Surg. 1998;4(4):328–34.
13. Watt KD. Metabolic syndrome: is immunosuppression to blame? Liver Transpl. 2011;17(Suppl 3):S38–42.
14. Jardine AG, Gaston RS, Fellstrom BC, Holdaas H. Prevention of cardiovascular disease in adult recipients of kidney transplants. Lancet. 2011;378(9800):1419–27.
15. Trotter JF, Wachs ME, Trouillot TE, Bak T, Kugelmas M, Kam I, et al. Dyslipidemia during sirolimus therapy in liver transplant recipients occurs with concomitant cyclosporine but not tacrolimus. Liver Transpl. 2001;7(5):401–8.
16. Silva AC, Nogueira P, Machado MV. Hepatic steatosis after liver transplantation: a systematic review and meta-analysis. Liver Transpl. 2023;29(4):431–48.
17. Horiuchi K, Kogiso T, Sagawa T, Taniai M, Kotera Y, Egawa H, et al. Prevalence of fatty liver disease after liver transplantation and risk factors for recipients and donors. Ann Hepatol. 2022;27(2):100670.
18. Narayanan P, Mara K, Izzy M, Dierkhising R, Heimbach J, Allen AM, et al. Recurrent or De novo allograft steatosis and long-term outcomes after Liver transplantation. Transplantation. 2019;103(1):e14–21.
19. Houlihan DD, Armstrong MJ, Davidov Y, Hodson J, Nightingale P, Rowe IA, et al. Renal function in patients undergoing transplantation for nonalcoholic steatohepatitis cirrhosis: time to reconsider immunosuppression regimens? Liver Transpl. 2011;17(11):1292–8.

20. Jatana S, Krys D, Verhoeff K, Kung JY, Jogiat U, Montano-Loza AJ, et al. Liver allograft cirrhosis, Retransplant, and mortality secondary to recurrent disease after transplant for MASH: a systematic review and meta-analysis. Transplantation. 2024;109:832.
21. Yong JN, Lim WH, Ng CH, Tan DJH, Xiao J, Tay PWL, et al. Outcomes of nonalcoholic Steatohepatitis after Liver transplantation: an updated meta-analysis and systematic review. Clin Gastroenterol Hepatol. 2023;21(1):45–54.e6.
22. Madhwal S, Atreja A, Albeldawi M, Lopez R, Post A, Costa MA. Is liver transplantation a risk factor for cardiovascular disease? A meta-analysis of observational studies. Liver Transpl. 2012;18(10):1140–6.
23. Gojowy D, Adamczak M, Dudzicz S, Gazda M, Karkoszka H, Wiecek A. High frequency of arterial hypertension in patients after Liver transplantation. Transplant Proc. 2016;48(5):1721–4.
24. Hara Y, Kawagishi N, Nakanishi W, Tokodai K, Nakanishi C, Miyagi S, et al. Prevalence and risk factors of obesity, hypertension, dyslipidemia and diabetes mellitus before and after adult living donor liver transplantation. Hepatol Res. 2015;45(7):764–70.
25. Schwotzer N, Lu Y, Halfon M, Pascual M, Marques-Vidal P, Golshayan D, et al. Prevalence of hypertension and uncontrolled hypertension after solid organ transplantation: a 5-year follow-up of the Swiss transplant cohort study. J Hypertens. 2025;43(3):397–404.
26. Lucey MR, Terrault N, Ojo L, Hay JE, Neuberger J, Blumberg E, et al. Long-term management of the successful adult liver transplant: 2012 practice guideline by the American Association for the Study of Liver Diseases and the American Society of Transplantation. Liver Transpl. 2013;19(1):3–26.
27. Najeed SA, Saghir S, Hein B, Neff G, Shaheen M, Ijaz H, et al. Management of hypertension in liver transplant patients. Int J Cardiol. 2011;152(1):4–6.
28. Galioto A, Semplicini A, Zanus G, Fasolato S, Sticca A, Boccagni P, et al. Nifedipine versus carvedilol in the treatment of de novo arterial hypertension after liver transplantation: results of a controlled clinical trial. Liver Transpl. 2008;14(7):1020–8.
29. Jafar TH, Schmid CH, Landa M, Giatras I, Toto R, Remuzzi G, et al. Angiotensin-converting enzyme inhibitors and progression of nondiabetic renal disease. A meta-analysis of patient-level data. Ann Intern Med. 2001;135(2):73–87.
30. Natale P, Palmer SC, Navaneethan SD, Craig JC, Strippoli GF. Angiotensin-converting-enzyme inhibitors and angiotensin receptor blockers for preventing the progression of diabetic kidney disease. Cochrane Database Syst Rev. 2024;4(4):CD006257
31. Neal DA, Gimson AE, Gibbs P, Alexander GJ. Beneficial effects of converting liver transplant recipients from cyclosporine to tacrolimus on blood pressure, serum lipids, and weight. Liver Transpl. 2001;7(6):533–9.
32. Arab JP, Díaz LA, Baeza N, Idalsoaga F, Fuentes-López E, Arnold J, et al. Identification of optimal therapeutic window for steroid use in severe alcohol-associated hepatitis: a worldwide study. J Hepatol. 2021;75(5):1026–33.
33. Hüsing A, Kabar I, Schmidt HH. Lipids in liver transplant recipients. World J Gastroenterol. 2016;22(12):3315–24.
34. Warden BA, Duell PB. Management of dyslipidemia in adult solid organ transplant recipients. J Clin Lipidol. 2019;13(2):231–45.
35. Becchetti C, Dirchwolf M, Schropp J, Magini G, Müllhaupt B, Immer F, et al. Use of statins after liver transplantation is associated with improved survival: results of a nationwide study. Aliment Pharmacol Ther. 2022;56(7):1194–204.
36. Wiggins BS, Saseen JJ, Page RL, Reed BN, Sneed K, Kostis JB, et al. Recommendations for Management of Clinically Significant Drug-Drug Interactions with Statins and Select Agents Used in patients with cardiovascular disease: a scientific statement from the American Heart Association. Circulation. 2016;134(21):e468–e95.
37. Group KDIGOKTW. KDIGO clinical practice guideline for the care of kidney transplant recipients. Am J Transplant. 2009;9(Suppl 3):S1–155.
38. Virani SS, Newby LK, Arnold SV, Bittner V, Brewer LC, Demeter SH, et al. 2023 AHA/ACC/ACCP/ASPC/NLA/PCNA guideline for the Management of Patients with Chronic Coronary

Disease: a report of the American Heart Association/American College of Cardiology Joint Committee on clinical practice guidelines. Circulation. 2023;148(9):e9–e119.
39. Ichimaru N, Takahara S, Kokado Y, Wang JD, Hatori M, Kameoka H, et al. Changes in lipid metabolism and effect of simvastatin in renal transplant recipients induced by cyclosporine or tacrolimus. Atherosclerosis. 2001;158(2):417–23.
40. Migliozzi DR, Asal NJ. Clinical controversy in transplantation: tacrolimus versus cyclosporine in statin drug interactions. Ann Pharmacother. 2020;54(2):171–7.
41. Almutairi F, Peterson TC, Molinari M, Walsh MJ, Alwayn I, Peltekian KM. Safety and effectiveness of ezetimibe in liver transplant recipients with hypercholesterolemia. Liver Transpl. 2009;15(5):504–8.
42. Aravinthan AD, Fateen W, Doyle AC, Venkatachalapathy SV, Issachar A, Galvin Z, et al. The impact of preexisting and Post-transplant diabetes mellitus on outcomes following Liver transplantation. Transplantation. 2019;103(12):2523–30.
43. Barker HL, Morrison D, Llano A, Sainsbury CAR, Jones GC. Practical guide to glucocorticoid induced Hyperglycaemia and diabetes. Diabetes Ther. 2023;14(5):937–45.
44. Committee ADAPP. 9. Pharmacologic approaches to glycemic treatment: standards of Care in Diabetes-2025. Diabetes Care. 2025;48(Supplement_1):S181–206.
45. Ertuglu LA, Porrini E, Hornum M, Demiray A, Afsar B, Ortiz A, et al. Glucagon-like peptide-1 receptor agonists and sodium-glucose cotransporter 2 inhibitors for diabetes after solid organ transplantation. Transpl Int. 2021;34(8):1341–59.
46. Zheng K, Azhie A, You X, Naghibzadeh M, Tan E, Naimimohasses S, et al. Glucagon-like peptide-1 receptor agonists and sodium-glucose cotransporter-2 inhibitors for the treatment of diabetes mellitus in liver transplant recipients. Diabetes Obes Metab. 2024;26(10):4261–72.
47. Richards J, Gunson B, Johnson J, Neuberger J. Weight gain and obesity after liver transplantation. Transpl Int. 2005;18(4):461–6.
48. Patel SS, Siddiqui MB, Chadrakumaran A, Faridnia M, Lin FP, Hernandez Roman J, et al. Office-based weight loss counseling is ineffective in Liver transplant recipients. Dig Dis Sci. 2020;65(2):639–46.
49. Zamora-Valdes D, Watt KD, Kellogg TA, Poterucha JJ, Di Cecco SR, Francisco-Ziller NM, et al. Long-term outcomes of patients undergoing simultaneous liver transplantation and sleeve gastrectomy. Hepatology. 2018;68(2):485–95.
50. Liver EAftSot. EASL Clinical Practice Guidelines on liver transplantation. J Hepatol. 2024;81(6):1040–86.
51. Yakubu I, Spengler J, Taylor P, LaPorte M, Brown A, Sterling S, et al. Impact of glucagon-like Peptide-1 receptor agonists on metabolic health in liver transplant recipients. Transplantation. 2025;109:e501.
52. Saeed N, Glass L, Sharma P, Shannon C, Sonnenday CJ, Tincopa MA. Incidence and risks for nonalcoholic fatty Liver disease and Steatohepatitis post-liver transplant: systematic review and meta-analysis. Transplantation. 2019;103(11):e345–e54.
53. Villeret F, Dharancy S, Erard D, Abergel A, Barbier L, Besch C, et al. Inevitability of disease recurrence after liver transplantation for NAFLD cirrhosis. JHEP Rep. 2023;5(3):100668.
54. Martínez-Arenas L, Vinaixa C, Conde I, Lorente S, Díaz-Fontenla F, Marques P, et al. FibroScan compared to liver biopsy for accurately staging recurrent hepatic steatosis and fibrosis after transplantation for MASH. Liver Int. 2024;44(12):3174–82.
55. Rigamonti C, Donato MF, Fraquelli M, Agnelli F, Ronchi G, Casazza G, et al. Transient elastography predicts fibrosis progression in patients with recurrent hepatitis C after liver transplantation. Gut. 2008;57(6):821–7.
56. Winters AC, Mittal R, Schiano TD. A review of the use of transient elastography in the assessment of fibrosis and steatosis in the post-liver transplant patient. Clin Transpl. 2019;33(10):e13700.
57. Nacif LS, de Cassia Gomes C, Paranaguá-Vezozzo D, Flores Cassenote AJ, Pinheiro RS, Waisberg DR, et al. Liver elastography in acute cellular rejection after Liver transplantation. Transplant Proc. 2020;52(5):1340–3.

58. Castéra L, Foucher J, Bernard PH, Carvalho F, Allaix D, Merrouche W, et al. Pitfalls of liver stiffness measurement: a 5-year prospective study of 13,369 examinations. Hepatology. 2010;51(3):828–35.
59. Kehler T, Grothues D, Evert K, Wahlenmayer J, Knoppke B, Melter M. Elastography-the new standard in the assessment of fibrosis after pediatric Liver transplantation? Pediatr Transplant. 2024;28(6):e14832.
60. Cetinic I, de Lange C, Boström H, Ekvall N, Bennet W, Lagerstrand K, et al. Shear wave elastography and shear wave dispersion correlated to biopsy at the scheduled follow-up of pediatric liver grafts. Pediatr Transplant. 2023;27(7):e14591.
61. Loomba R, Hartman ML, Lawitz EJ, Vuppalanchi R, Boursier J, Bugianesi E, et al. Tirzepatide for metabolic dysfunction-associated Steatohepatitis with liver fibrosis. N Engl J Med. 2024;391(4):299–310.
62. Harrison SA, Bedossa P, Guy CD, Schattenberg JM, Loomba R, Taub R, et al. A phase 3, randomized, controlled trial of resmetirom in NASH with liver fibrosis. N Engl J Med. 2024;390(6):497–509.
63. Newsome PN, Sanyal AJ, Engebretsen KA, Kliers I, Østergaard L, Vanni D, et al. Semaglutide 2.4 mg in participants with metabolic dysfunction-associated Steatohepatitis: baseline characteristics and design of the Phase 3 ESSENCE trial. Aliment Pharmacol Ther. 2024;60(11–12):1525–33.
64. Rothberg AE, McEwen LN, Herman WH. Severe obesity and the impact of medical weight loss on estimated glomerular filtration rate. PLoS One. 2020;15(2):e0228984.
65. Appel LJ, Wright JT, Greene T, Agodoa LY, Astor BC, Bakris GL, et al. Intensive blood-pressure control in hypertensive chronic kidney disease. N Engl J Med. 2010;363(10):918–29.
66. Committee ADAPP. 11. Chronic kidney disease and risk management: standards of Care in Diabetes-2025. Diabetes Care. 2025;48(Supplement_1):S239–S51.
67. Chen JY, Hsu TW, Liu JH, Pan HC, Lai CF, Yang SY, et al. Kidney and cardiovascular outcomes among patients with CKD receiving GLP-1 receptor agonists: a systematic review and meta-analysis of randomized trials. Am J Kidney Dis. 2025;85:555.
68. Badve SV, Bilal A, Lee MMY, Sattar N, Gerstein HC, Ruff CT, et al. Effects of GLP-1 receptor agonists on kidney and cardiovascular disease outcomes: a meta-analysis of randomised controlled trials. Lancet Diabetes Endocrinol. 2025;13(1):15–28.
69. Colhoun HM, Lingvay I, Brown PM, Deanfield J, Brown-Frandsen K, Kahn SE, et al. Long-term kidney outcomes of semaglutide in obesity and cardiovascular disease in the SELECT trial. Nat Med. 2024;30(7):2058–66.
70. Sarafidis P, Ortiz A, Ferro CJ, Halimi JM, Kreutz R, Mallamaci F, et al. Sodium--glucose co-transporter-2 inhibitors for patients with diabetic and nondiabetic chronic kidney disease: a new era has already begun. J Hypertens. 2021;39(6):1090–7.
71. Navaneethan SD, Bansal N, Cavanaugh KL, Chang A, Crowley S, Delgado C, et al. KDOQI US commentary on the KDIGO 2024 clinical practice guideline for the evaluation and management of CKD. Am J Kidney Dis. 2025;85(2):135–76.
72. Das SR, Everett BM, Birtcher KK, Brown JM, Januzzi JL, Kalyani RR, et al. 2020 expert consensus decision pathway on novel therapies for cardiovascular risk reduction in patients with type 2 diabetes: a report of the American College of Cardiology Solution set Oversight Committee. J Am Coll Cardiol. 2020;76(9):1117–45.
73. Mreyoud H, Walter K, Wilpula E, Park JM. The efficacy and safety of sodium-glucose cotransporter-2 inhibitors in solid organ transplant recipients: a scoping review. Pharmacotherapy. 2024;44(6):444–66.
74. Moore J, Middleton L, Cockwell P, Adu D, Ball S, Little MA, et al. Calcineurin inhibitor sparing with mycophenolate in kidney transplantation: a systematic review and meta-analysis. Transplantation. 2009;87(4):591–605.
75. Hamdy AF, Bakr MA, Ghoneim MA. Long-term efficacy and safety of a calcineurin inhibitor-free regimen in live-donor renal transplant recipients. J Am Soc Nephrol. 2008;19(6):1225–32.

76. Kong Y, Wang D, Shang Y, Liang W, Ling X, Guo Z, et al. Calcineurin-inhibitor minimization in liver transplant patients with calcineurin-inhibitor-related renal dysfunction: a meta-analysis. PLoS One. 2011;6(9):e24387.
77. Buchholz BM, Ferguson JW, Schnitzbauer AA, Nightingale P, Schlitt HJ, Geissler EK, et al. Randomized Sirolimus-based early calcineurin inhibitor reduction in Liver transplantation: impact on renal function. Transplantation. 2020;104(5):1003–18.
78. Goralczyk AD, Bari N, Abu-Ajaj W, Lorf T, Ramadori G, Friede T, et al. Calcineurin inhibitor sparing with mycophenolate mofetil in liver transplantion: a systematic review of randomized controlled trials. Am J Transplant. 2012;12(10):2601–7.

Post-liver Transplant Malignancies 30

Maryam Sadat Aleali and Kymberly D. Watt

Abbreviations

CCA	Perihilar cholangiocarcinoma
CNI	Calcineurin inhibitors
CRC	Colorectal cancer
DNA	Deoxyribonucleic acid
DNM	De novo malignancy
EBV	Ebstein–Barr virus
HCC	Hepatocellular carcinoma
HHV-8	Human herpes virus-8
HPV	Human papillomavirus
IBD	Inflammatory bowel disease
LT	Liver transplantation
MASH	Metabolic dysfunction-associated steatohepatitis
MMF	Mycophenolate mofetil
PSC	Primary sclerosing cholangitis
PTLD	Post-transplant lymphoproliferative disorder
VEGF	Vascular endothelial growth factor

M. S. Aleali · K. D. Watt (✉)
Department of Internal Medicine, Division of Gastroenterology & Hepatology, Mayo Clinic, Rochester, MN, USA
e-mail: watt.kymberly@mayo.edu

B. Eghtesad et al. (eds.), *Liver Transplantation*,
https://doi.org/10.1007/978-3-032-07072-2_30

Introduction

Liver transplant recipients are more susceptible to malignancy than the general population due to improved immunosuppression and longer post-transplant survival of these transplant recipients. Malignancy is a late post-transplant complication of critical importance for its impact on long-term survival [2, 64, 83].

Recurrent Versus De Novo Malignancy: Timing of Post-transplant Cancer

To help define recurrent versus de novo malignancies (DNM), studies frequently differentiate between the two by excluding every transplant recipient with malignancies prior to the transplantation and/or excluding any emerging cancer 30 days after the transplantation. Less clear are malignancies (minus PTLD) that develop within the first 6 months after transplantation, which are of questionable origin. Given that most transplant recipients undergo a thorough evaluation for high-risk conditions that impact survival, including cancer screening, one can only assume these were malignancies that likely existed (undetected) prior to transplant and the growth was accelerated post-transplant [23, 80]. An alternative consideration would be donor-transmitted malignancy, which is addressed later in this chapter.

Epidemiology

Compared to the general population, liver transplant recipients have shown a 2–seven-fold higher incidence of developing malignancies [66].

The overall incidence of de novo malignancy reported in studies from the last three decades, regardless of the type of neoplasm, is between 1% and 16% over 8–12 years post-transplant [60, 78, 87, 93]. The reported incidence in these studies varies due to different populations and the duration of follow-up periods. However, the common finding of several studies is the escalating incidence of DNM with longer follow-up periods. Robinson et al. reported the increasing incidence of 5%, 14–20%, and 32% after 5, 10, and 20 years of follow-up intervals in one study [76]. Altieri et al. showed 2.07%, 13.30%, and 28.01% probability of de novo malignancy in 1, 5, and 10 years of intervals post-transplantation [6], and Chatrath et al. presented incidence rates of 11.7% and 24.8% after 5 and 10 years of follow-up, respectively [21].

Risk Factors

Multiple risk factors exist: some are non-modifiable, while others have a varying degree of modifiability, as outlined in Fig. 30.1.

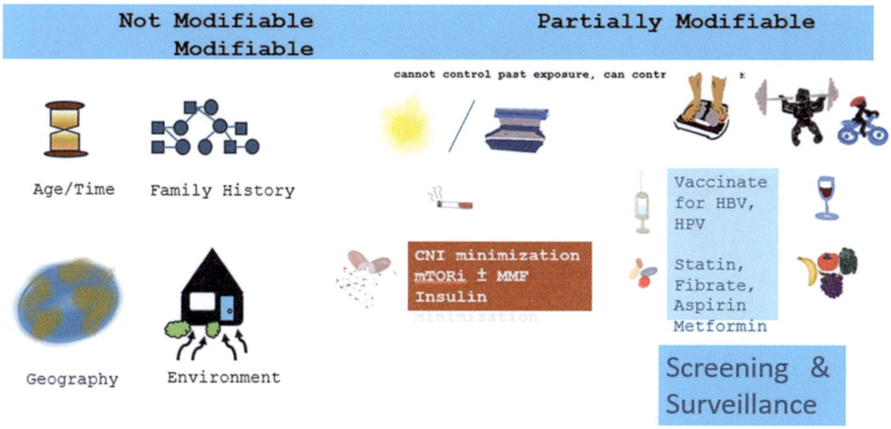

Fig. 30.1 Modifiable cancer risk

Age

Several studies have identified age as a significant risk factor in this population [6, 21, 39, 80]. Age is a well-known risk factor for malignancies in the general population, and liver transplant recipients have also shown to follow this pattern. This is a general risk factor that does not absolve younger individuals from cancer risk, as shown in studies (Fig. 30.2) that report a higher incidence of malignancy after transplantation in the younger population and incrementally higher risk than that of similar-aged individuals in the general population [70]. In the kidney transplant literature, of children who received a kidney transplant, 41% developed a cancer over 30 years of follow-up and 31% developed a second cancer within 1 year of the first [71]. Some cancer are more common in younger individuals after liver transplantation, inparticular, post-transplant lymphoproliferative disorder shows a higher incidence among younger patients, thus screening diligence is warranted [6, 51].

Gender

Male gender is recognized as one risk factor for developing cancer after liver transplantation, as demonstrated by recent large cohort studies with a 1.45–2.23 times higher risk compared to the female LT recipients [6, 80]. This finding is also notable geographically. In one study from Korea, the standardized incidence ratio (SIR) of DNM (regardless of the type of cancer) for male and female liver transplant recipients was 3.43 and 2.30, respectively [70]. In contrast, however, a cohort study in the US found gender to be of no influence in DNM incidence despite the male gender having a higher smoking rate and alcoholic liver disease as a transplant indication [21]. Data from earlier eras of transplantation will undoubtedly reflect the transplant

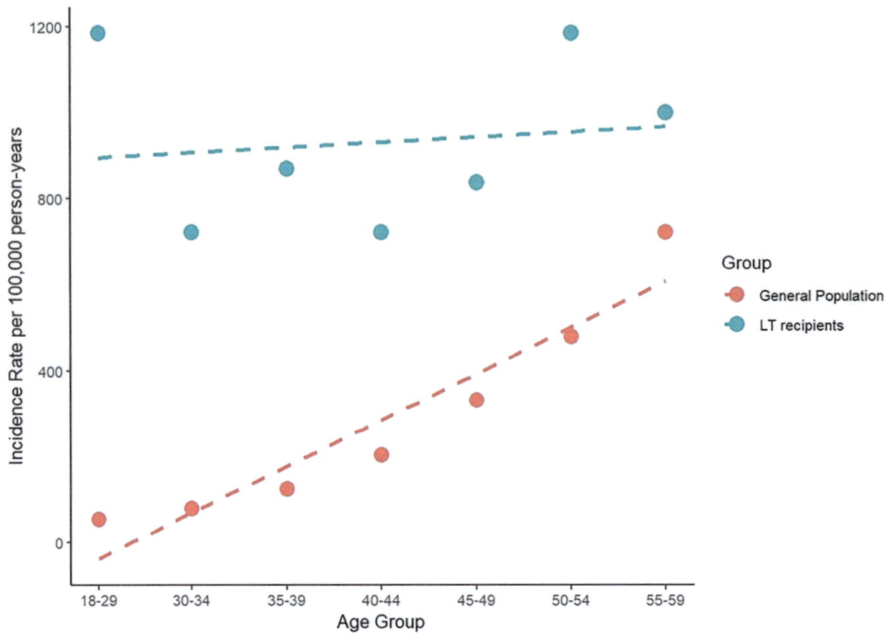

Fig. 30.2 Incidence rate of de novo malignancies in the general population compared to liver transplant recipients of different age groups. (Adapted from Taborreli et al. [84]) using R Statistical Software (version 2024.4.2.764; R Core Team [73])

population at that time, which tended to be dominated by males with both hepatitis C and alcohol-related disease and thus may not be applicable to the more contemporary era of transplant recipients.

Race/Ethnicity

Studies on race/ethnicity as a potential risk factor for DNM development in LT recipients have shown contradictory results with disparate conclusions. The study by Radmacher et al. did not find race feel free to be a risk factor for DNM in LT recipients while acknowledging their homogenous population of study, consisting mostly (95%) Caucasians, to be the limitation interpreting this result [74]. Chatrath et al. also noted that the scarcity of non-Caucasian patients in their study was an obstacle in properly evaluating race as a risk factor in their multivariate analyses. However, non-Caucasian recipients did have a significant risk for DNM development in univariate analysis, with an incidence of 17% compared to 7% in Caucasians [21].

In a large-population study in the US, when compared with Hispanic/Latino, Asian and African-American transplant recipients, white race showed a 1.45–2.04 times higher incidence for post-transplant DNM [11]. This increase is largely accounted for by the influence of non-melanoma skin cancers, which are associated with a well-established higher risk in Caucasian populations [11, 31].

Lifestyle and Behavior

Obesity is one of the independent risk factors for DNM in LT recipients and emphasizes the importance of weight management among LT recipients [18]. Tobacco use and alcohol consumption are also well-known risk factors for malignancy among the general population, and LT recipients are no exception [17, 45]. The risk of developing non-skin cancer after transplantation is 2.87 times higher for recipients with excessive alcohol use [44]. Non-smoker LT recipients are significantly less likely to develop DNM compared to active smokers or patients with a history of smoking [46]. A 10-year cumulative incidence of malignancy among smokers is approximately 6 times higher than that of non-smokers [92].

Underlying Disorders

Alcohol-related liver disease (ALD) prior to liver transplantation is noted to be an independent risk factor for cancer development after transplant in many studies with over a 2 times higher risk of DNM among those with ALD [95]. Primary sclerosing cholangitis (PSC) also appears to be associated with a higher risk of DNM and is thought to be largely related to concurrent inflammatory bowel disease, which can lead to colorectal cancer [20]. In another large-population study in Italy, primary hepatocellular carcinoma was also suggested to be a risk factor for DNM emergence in LT recipients [81]. Since LT recipients undergo immunosuppression for preventing graft rejection, they are at a greater risk of developing malignancies in case of infection with oncogenic viral agents such as HHV8, EBV, HPV, hepatitis B and C, which increase the risk of Kaposi sarcoma, nasopharyngeal carcinoma and lymphoma, genitourinary, anal and oropharyngeal cancers and de novo HCC [20].

Immunosuppression

Suppressing the immune system results in a higher risk for malignancy [66]. The immune system plays a vital role in cancer surveillance and prevention of oncogenic virus progression to cancer, amongst other mechanisms.

A single-center study from Spain assessed a change of immunosuppressive therapy for LT patients from the regimen of azathioprine, cyclosporine and steroids to higher potency mofetil mycophenolate, anti-IL2 receptor antibodies, sirolimus, and tacrolimus regimens (with an earlier cessation of steroids). Although the latter immunosuppressive regimen caused a significant decline in organ rejection, it also led to a higher incidence of de novo hematologic malignancies and an earlier presentation of de novo tumors compared to LT patients receiving the earlier regimen.

Other similar studies emphasize immunosuppression as a modifiable risk factor for DNM in LT recipients [9].

Calcineurin inhibitors and mTOR inhibitors are the most used immunosuppressive drugs after organ transplantation to prevent transplant rejection in the current era [59]. Calcineurin inhibitors interfere with the activation of T-cells by disrupting their intracellular signaling pathways and therefore lower the expression of pro-inflammatory cytokines by immune cells. Some of the explained mechanisms of these drugs' oncogenic effects are their role in inhibition of DNA repair, enhancement of angiogenesis, tumor growth, and metastasis by increasing growth factor synthesis (e.g., TGF-β, VEGF, IL-6; Table 30.1) [90, 96].

The risk of each calcineurin inhibitor in causing DNM in LT recipients has been debated with contradictory conclusions. A large-population study in France showed that liver transplant recipients who received cyclosporin-A had a 1.53 times higher incidence of developing solid organ tumors compared to those who were treated with tacrolimus [74]. This is similar to other studies that found cyclosporine to be an independent risk factor for de novo malignancy in LT recipients [88] and leading to a higher incidence of DNM in renal transplant recipients [53]. Another French study showed a clear dose effect of tacrolimus in cancer risk after transplant, where

Table 30.1 Carcinogenic effects of immunosuppression medications

IS drug class	Mechanism	Drug name	Risk of carcinogenicity in transplant recipients
Calcineurin inhibitor	Inhibit DNA repair Increase growth factor synthesis and subsequently enhance angiogenesis, tumor growth and metastasis	Cyclosporin A	Higher
		Tacrolimus	Higher
mTOR inhibitor	Disrupt tumor cell growth by inhibiting mTOR Decrease VEGF and subsequently angiogenesis	Sirolimus	Lower (monotherapy or in combination with tacrolimus)
		Everolimus	Lower
Antimetabolite	Damage DNA Accumulate DNA 6-TG in keratinocytes and increases skin sensitivity to UVA	Azathioprine	Higher (esp. squamous cell carcinoma)
	Prevent receptor-dependent dissemination of tumors	Mycophenolate mofetil	Lower (monotherapy, or lowering CNI dosing)
Steroids	Increase solid tumors' resistance to apoptosis and diminish immunosurveillance Direct pro-oncogenicity	Prednisolone Methylprednisolone	Higher

IS immunosuppressant, *mTOR* mammalian target of Rapamycin, *VEGF* vascular endothelial growth factor, *6-TG* 6-thioguanine, *CNI* calcineurin inhibitor mean tacrolimus blood concentration and consecutive drug exposure for 3 or more years increased the risk of DNM in LT recipients [16].

In contrast, studies involving kidney and liver transplant recipient found that tacrolimus led to a higher incidence of DNM compared to cyclosporine, pointing out that contradictory results on the comparative studies on these drugs were probably influenced by varied regimens, dosing and different follow-up intervals, over time [97, 98].

In a study involving renal transplant recipients, there was no association between the type of immunosuppressant drug and malignancies, except for nonmelanoma skin cancer. It was reported that Tacrolimus caused a 35% decrease and Azathioprine caused a 17% increase in skin cancer incidence in these patients. Besides the short period of follow-up (3 years) in this study, it's important to interpret the results while acknowledging that the type of immunosuppression each patient receives is based upon individual risk; a bias that can't be completely omitted without a randomized controlled trial [53]. Azathioprine is the prodrug of mercaptopurine, which, after its metabolism in the liver, turns into 6-thioguanine. DNA-6TG inhibits de novo purine synthesis and disrupts DNA replication. Although replaced by mycophenolic acid as the main anti-metabolite drug of choice, it is still used by many transplant recipients [57]. Azathioprine is recognized as a risk factor for developing de novo cancer (Table 30.1) [9]. This drug increases cancer risk via damaging DNA due to 6-TG accumulation in DNA [62, 68]. It specifically increases the risk of squamous cell carcinoma after organ transplantation by an estimated 56% [50]. Studies have observed that azathioprine increases skin sensitivity to ultraviolet light via accumulation of DNA-6TG in keratinocytes and synergistically increases both their mutagenic effects [68].

Mycophenolate mofetil is the prodrug of mycophenolic acid, which prevents proliferation of B cells and T cells by inhibiting inosine monophosphate dehydrogenase and subsequently the synthesis of purine in lymphocytes (Table 30.1) [4, 5]. The effect of mycophenolic acid in reducing cancer is hypothesized to be a result of its role in preventing receptor-dependent dissemination of tumors [56]. Aguiar et al. observed that liver transplant patients who started mycophenolate mofetil monotherapy after cessation of calcineurin inhibitors faced a lower risk of de novo malignancy [3]. In contrast, a retrospective cohort study on kidney transplant recipients showed that long-term exposure to mycophenolic acid increased the risk of DNM, especially among the female patients [34]. However, the protective effects of mycophenolic acid were further supported in a meta-analysis on mycophenolic acid by Hirunsatitpron et al., where they concluded that mycophenolic acid does not increase DNM risk in solid organ transplant recipients and could potentially reduce cancer risk likely due to calcineurin inhibitor dose reduction its use affords [48].

Sirolimus (mTOR inhibitor) and tacrolimus (calcineurin inhibitor) have the same receptor, FKBP. However, they have different actions when bound to their receptors. Sirolimus inhibits tumor cell growth by inhibiting the mammalian target of rapamycin (mTOR) and decreases VEGF production, leading to its antiangiogenic effects [79]. In an in-vitro study of hepatocellular carcinoma, administering Sirolimus alone or in combination with Tacrolimus, inhibited the cell growth [79]. Although retrospective studies demonstrated liver transplant patients with prior HCC had a lower risk of HCC recurrence and enhanced survival, the prospective randomized controlled trial (SiLVER study) [35] was unable to prove the benefit of mTOR in reducing HCC recurrence. Everolimus, another mTOR inhibitor, has been associated with decrease cancer risk in a study of kidney transplant recipients on top of increasing the survival rates of both graft and patient [49]. The reduced cancer incidence was largely attributed to reduced non-melanoma skin cancers.

Corticosteroids increase solid tumors' resistance to apoptosis and diminish immunosurveillance as well as pro-oncogenicity, which play roles in malignancy in transplant recipients [13, 38, 82]. Most transplant centers pursue early steroid minimization after transplantation now, limiting the overall influence of steroids on cancer outcomes.

Donor-Transmitted Cancer

Another rare but plausible risk factor for cancer emergence is receiving an organ from a patient with an underlying malignancy [25]. Donor-transmitted cancer is observed in approximately 3–6 cases out of every 10,000 donors, the majority of whom were not diagnosed with cancer at the time of donation [29, 30]. A Danish study reported a 1.3% chance of receiving a graft from a donor with undiagnosed cancer, and a 0.2% risk of cancer transmission to the recipient [14]. Donor-transmitted cancers have a poor prognosis and happen early (within weeks to months) after transplantation [14, 37].

Eccher et al. performed a meta-analysis on documented cases of donor-derived cancer in kidney transplant recipients; 17.1% of the donors had ongoing cancer or a history of malignancy. Evaluations were performed mostly with only clinical and lab tests, or less frequently, imaging studies with or without biopsy (only 10%). In approximately half of the recipients, the cancer was metastatic and 40% were graft-limited. The median time to cancer diagnosis was 7 months, with 68% and 84% of the recipients diagnosed within the first 12 and 24 months, respectively [30].

Screening and Surveillance

Since DNMs, especially non-skin cancers, are usually aggressive neoplasms that significantly decrease the survival of LT recipients [52], cost-effective screening programs help identify neoplasia development in this population in a timely manner that increases their chances of receiving curative treatment [42]. It is anticipated that more LT recipients with a prior history of cancer may receive a transplant closer to their cancer remission than in previous eras. In these circumstances, additional surveillance for recurrence may be warranted and expert opinion surveillance recommendations exist for these individuals [94].

Although the majority of the proposed screening and surveillance guidelines for LT recipients align with those recommended in the general population, some recommendations are modified to better address these LT recipients' notably higher risk for malignancy (de novo or recurrent) and higher mortality compared to the general population [23, 26, 94].

Skin Cancers

Squamous cell carcinoma, basal cell carcinoma, and melanoma are among the frequently observed malignancies in transplant recipients [63]. Given the incidence of melanoma is low, the survival rate after skin cancer remains intact [33, 43]. Sun exposure, fair skin type, and duration of immunosuppression are some of the risk factors of skin cancer in LT recipients [32]. It is important to be aware of the differences in skin cancer in Black populations, as the lower frequency of skin cancer compared to the white population and presentation of lesions in non-sun-exposed areas along with referral bias pattern can lead to a delay in or missing the diagnosis [1, 15]. Furthermore, it is recommended that Black LT recipients perform genital self-examination and recognize HPV infection due to the link between HPV and genital in-situ SCC [22].

In addition to skin protection against UV exposure [86], according to the ILTS-SETH Consensus Conference, annual examination of the entire body by a dermatologist is recommended and can lead to a reduction in skin cancer mortality in LT recipients. Dermatologists may increase the frequency of skin examinations in those with a prior incidence of skin cancer [23].

Non-skin Cancers

PTLD

PTLD occurs more frequently among the pediatric LT recipients and is a life-threatening condition with increasing incidence among both adult and pediatric liver transplant recipients in the recent years. Monitoring the levels of EBV-DNA in the serum can be helpful in detecting PTLD early on; however, it is only recommended in the high-risk population, which consists of seronegative patients who received a liver from a seropositive donor, for 1 year from the liver transplantation [23, 28, 36].

Lung

Screening for lung cancer is done via low-dose computed tomography scanning and can significantly reduce lung cancer mortality in high-risk populations [69].

LT recipients who actively smoke (or < 15 years since they quit smoking) with a total pack-year history of above 20 should undergo screening regardless of their age [23].

Colorectal Cancer

Based on their underlying disease, LT recipients require different intervals of CRC screening via colonoscopy. Patients with Inflammatory bowel disease and those who received liver transplantation for primary sclerosing cholangitis, even in the absence of a concomitant IBD, are at a higher risk for colorectal carcinoma than the general population [41]. Therefore, the International Liver Transplant Society (ILTS-SETH) Consensus Conference recommends a colonoscopy for LT recipients with IBD annually and those with PSC without IBD every 3–5 years [23]. According to new studies, LT recipients with underlying MASH and HCC who are above 50 years of age might benefit from a colonoscopy every 5 years; however, it is not yet strongly recommended and requires validation data [67].

Other DNM Screening Recommendations

Annual ear, nose, and throat examination is recommended for LT recipients at moderate to high risk for head and neck or oropharyngeal malignancy (i.e., active smokers or those with active HPV infection) [23, 27]. Risk of esophageal cancer increases after transplantation, especially in patients with a history of smoking and alcohol excess, which is prominent [91]. However, Renaud et al. found that endoscopic screening for esophageal cancer detection after liver transplantation was not impactful [75].

High-risk LT recipients at high risk for renal cell cancer, including those with previous renal-cell cancer, underlying chronic kidney disease and Von Hipple–Lindau or autosomal-dominant polycystic kidney disease, benefit from annual kidney ultrasonography [23]. Although bladder cancer has a higher risk and worse prognosis in LT recipients, there are no recommended screenings due to insufficient data [23, 89].

Immunosuppression increases susceptibility to human papillomavirus (HPV) infection and consequently cervical, vulvovaginal, and anal cancers [47]. Due to the higher incidence of cervical cancer in LT recipients, specific screening guidelines for female immunosuppressed populations exist. Recommendations including 3 consecutive annual pelvic, PAP test, and HPV tests. A positive test should be followed with annual HPV testing. After 3 normal test results, LT recipients can follow the general population screening plans [23, 65].

Prostate and breast cancer incidence is unaffected after transplantation; therefore, patients receive the same screenings as the general population [8, 99].

Screening plans should also be modified to take into consideration the differing incidences of DNM based on LT recipients' region of residence and race. For example, gastric cancer is one of the most common types of DNM reported in Asia in both the general population and LT recipients; Therefore, gastric cancer screening via upper endoscopy is also recommended in that region [52].

Prevention and Management

A number of strategies can be administered to mitigate the mortality rate due to malignancy in LT recipients. All patients should receive proper educational information regarding their higher risk for malignancies after transplantation and be encouraged to apply behavioral modifications necessary for reducing DNM incidence. Lifestyle modifications such as smoke cessation and abstinence from alcohol, regular sun protection, and limiting sun exposure can greatly decrease DNM risk in LT recipients [10, 23]. Increasing physical activity and maintaining a healthy diet are also inherently protective against cancer and further recommended for weight management and preventing obesity, which is another known risk factor for malignancy [7, 61].

Among other suggested protective measures against DNM in LT recipients are administration of certain drugs such as metformin (which, unlike insulin, has anticancer effects) [54, 58] and Aspirin (especially in CRC patients under 70 years) [72, 77]. Statins and fibrates are also shown to reduce cancer risk [24, 85].

As discussed, modifying the type and dose of administered immunosuppressive drug (e.g., reducing CNIs) after transplantation can impact survival rates in LT recipients [60].

Treatment

Surgical approach to management of DNM in LT recipients is similar to that of the general population. ILTS-SETH Consensus emphasizes the importance of performing required abdominal surgeries in transplant centers with the potential involvement of transplant surgeons, given the complex nature of operating on LT recipients and managing their immunosuppression [23]. Systemic therapy can be challenging due to immunosuppression use hindering the required dose-intensity maintenance and subsequently obtaining optimal therapeutic results [12, 23]. Radiotherapy can be safe depending on each individual's clinical scenario. Administration of cytotoxic chemotherapy and tyrosine kinase inhibitors in DNM management should be assessed by both an expert oncologist and transplant provider for each LT recipient individually [23]. Immune checkpoint inhibitors (ICI), however, have been associated with a higher rate of graft rejection among solid organ transplant recipients and yet improve survival in those who didn't develop graft rejection [55]. Systematic reviews include many early case reports and small case series that do not reflect the current experience utilizing these agents in transplant recipients. With a prospective, structured immunosuppression protocol, rejection risk declines, with no rejection experienced in the trial by Hanna et al. [19, 40]. Balancing and optimizing the immunosuppression with the most advantageous anti-cancer therapy should be the goal.

In summary, malignancy reduces long-term survival of liver transplant recipients, and no progress has been made in the recent decades. Pro-active lifestyle prevention techniques, optimizing immunosuppression and other medication utilization will help in reducing the risk, and diligent cancer screening will aid in identifying cancers at treatable stages. Further studies into the best balance of immunosuppression with various anti-cancer therapies can help in improving survival after a cancer diagnosis.

Financial Support and Sponsorship None

Conflicts of Interest Nothing to report

References

1. Agbai ON, Buster K, Sanchez M, Hernandez C, Kundu RV, Chiu M, Roberts WE, Draelos ZD, Bhushan R, Taylor SC. Skin cancer and photoprotection in people of color: a review and recommendations for physicians and the public. J Am Acad Dermatol. 2014;70:748–62.
2. Agostini C, Buccianti S, Risaliti M, Fortuna L, Tirloni L, Tucci R, Bartolini I, Grazi GL. Complications in post-liver transplant patients. J Clin Med. 2023;12
3. Aguiar D, Martínez-Urbistondo D, D'avola D, Iñarrairaegui M, Pardo F, Rotellar F, Sangro B, Quiroga J, Herrero JI. Conversion from calcineurin inhibitor-based immunosuppression to Mycophenolate Mofetil in monotherapy reduces risk of De novo malignancies after liver transplantation. Ann Transplant. 2017;22:141–7.
4. Allison AC. Mechanisms of action of mycophenolate mofetil. Lupus. 2005;14(Suppl 1):s2–8.
5. Allison AC, Eugui EM. Mycophenolate mofetil and its mechanisms of action. Immunopharmacology. 2000;47:85–118.
6. Altieri M, Sérée O, Lobbedez T, Segol P, Abergel A, Blaizot X, Boillot O, Boudjema K, Coilly A, Conti F, Chazouillères O, Debette-Gratien M, Dharancy S, Durand F, Duvoux C, Francoz C, Gugenheim J, Hardwigsen J, Houssel-Debry P, Kamar N, Latournerie M, Lebray P, Leroy V, Neau-Cransac M, Pageaux GP, Radenne S, Salamé E, Saliba F, Samuel D, Vanlemmens C, Besch C, Launoy G, Dumortier J. Risk factors of de novo malignancies after liver transplantation: a French national study on 11004 adult patients. Clin Res Hepatol Gastroenterol. 2021;45:101514.
7. Anderson AS, Renehan AG, Saxton JM, Bell J, Cade J, Cross AJ, King A, Riboli E, Sniehotta F, Treweek S, Martin RM. Cancer prevention through weight control-where are we in 2020? Br J Cancer. 2021;124:1049–56.
8. Becher E, Wang A, Lepor H. Prostate cancer screening and management in solid organ transplant candidates and recipients. Rev Urol. 2019;21:85–92.
9. Benlloch S, Berenguer M, Prieto M, Moreno R, San Juan F, Rayón M, Mir J, Segura A, Berenguer J. De novo internal neoplasms after liver transplantation: increased risk and aggressive behavior in recent years? Am J Transplant. 2004;4:596–604.
10. Berk C, Volk ML. Preventive care in adult liver transplant recipients. Clin Liver Dis (Hoboken). 2021;18:14–7.
11. Bhat M, Mara K, Dierkhising R, Watt KD. Gender, race and disease etiology predict De novo malignancy risk after liver transplantation: insights for future individualized cancer screening guidance. Transplantation. 2019;103:91–100.
12. Bhat M, Mara K, Dierkhising R, Watt KDS. Immunosuppression, race, and donor-related risk factors affect De novo cancer incidence across solid organ transplant recipients. Mayo Clin Proc. 2018;93:1236–46.
13. Billups K, Neal J, Salyer J. Immunosuppressant-driven De novo malignant neoplasms after solid-organ transplant. Prog Transplant. 2015;25:182–8.

14. Birkeland SA, Storm HH. Risk for tumor and other disease transmission by transplantation: a population-based study of unrecognized malignancies and other diseases in organ donors. Transplantation. 2002;74:1409–13.
15. Borik L, Balagula Y, Hinds GA, Loss MJ. Non-melanoma skin cancers in African American solid organ transplant recipients: regional bias or a real need for surveillance? Eur J Dermatol. 2017;27:530–1.
16. Carenco C, Assenat E, Faure S, Duny Y, Danan G, Bismuth M, Herrero A, Jung B, Ursic-Bedoya J, Jaber S, Larrey D, Navarro F, Pageaux GP. Tacrolimus and the risk of solid cancers after liver transplant: A dose effect relationship. Am J Transplant. 2015a;15:678–86.
17. Carenco C, Faure S, Herrero A, Assenat E, Duny Y, Danan G, Bismuth M, Chanques G, Ursic-Bedoya J, Jaber S, Larrey D, Navarro F, Pageaux G-P. Incidence of solid organ cancers after liver transplantation: comparison with regional cancer incidence rates and risk factors. Liver Int. 2015b;35:1748–55.
18. Carenco C, Faure S, Ursic-Bedoya J, Herrero A, Pageaux GP. Solid, non-skin, post-liver transplant tumors: key role of lifestyle and immunosuppression management. World J Gastroenterol. 2016;22:427–34.
19. Carroll RP, Boyer M, Gebski V, Hockley B, Johnston JK, Kireta S, Tan H, Taylor A, Wyburn K, Zalcberg JR. Immune checkpoint inhibitors in kidney transplant recipients: a multicentre, single-arm, phase 1 study. Lancet Oncol. 2022;23:1078–86.
20. Chandok N, Watt KD. Burden of de novo malignancy in the liver transplant recipient. Liver Transpl. 2012;18:1277–89.
21. Chatrath H, Berman K, Vuppalanchi R, Slaven J, Kwo P, Tector AJ, Chalasani N, Ghabril M. De novo malignancy post-liver transplantation: a single center, population controlled study. Clin Transpl. 2013;27:582–90.
22. Chung CL, Nadhan KS, Shaver CM, Ogrich LM, Abdelmalek M, Cusack CA, Malat GE, Pritchett EN, Doyle A. Comparison of posttransplant dermatologic diseases by race. JAMA Dermatol. 2017;153:552–8.
23. Colmenero J, Tabrizian P, Bhangui P, Pinato DJ, Rodríguez-Perálvarez ML, Sapisochin G, Bhoori S, Pascual S, Senzolo M, Al-Adra D, Herrero JI, Petrowsky H, Dawson LA, Hosni A, Kutzke JL, Gastaca M, Watt KD. De novo malignancy after liver transplantation: risk assessment, prevention, and management-guidelines from the ILTS-SETH consensus conference. Transplantation. 2022;106:e30–45.
24. Demierre MF, Higgins PD, Gruber SB, Hawk E, Lippman SM. Statins and cancer prevention. Nat Rev Cancer. 2005;5:930–42.
25. Desai R, Collett D, Watson CJ, Johnson P, Evans T, Neuberger J. Cancer transmission from organ donors-unavoidable but low risk. Transplantation. 2012;94:1200–7.
26. Dharia A, Boulet J, Sridhar V, Kitchlu A. Cancer screening in solid organ transplant recipients: A focus on screening liver, lung, and kidney recipients for cancers related to the transplanted organ. Transplantation, Publish Ahead of Print; 2021.
27. Dhull AK, Atri R, Dhankhar R, Chauhan AK, Kaushal V. Major risk factors in head and neck cancer: a retrospective analysis of 12-year experiences. World J Oncol. 2018;9:80–4.
28. Dierickx D, Habermann TM. Post-transplantation lymphoproliferative disorders in adults. N Engl J Med. 2018;378:549–62.
29. Domínguez-Gil B, Moench K, Watson C, Serrano MT, Hibi T, Asencio JM, Van Rosmalen M, Detry O, Heimbach J, Durand F. Prevention and management of donor-transmitted cancer after liver transplantation: guidelines from the ILTS-SETH consensus conference. Transplantation. 2022;106:106.
30. Eccher A, Girolami I, Motter JD, Marletta S, Gambaro G, Momo REN, Nacchia F, Donato P, Boschiero L, Boggi U, Lombardini L, Cardillo M, D'errico A, Neil D, Segev DL, Zaza G. Donor-transmitted cancer in kidney transplant recipients: a systematic review. J Nephrol. 2020;33:1321–32.
31. España A, Martínez-González MA, García-Granero M, Sánchez-Carpintero I, Rábago G, Herreros J. A prospective study of incident nonmelanoma skin cancer in heart transplant recipients. J Invest Dermatol. 2000;115:1158–60.

32. Euvrard S, Kanitakis J. Skin cancers after liver transplantation: what to do? J Hepatol. 2006;44:27–32.
33. Euvrard S, Kanitakis J, Claudy A. Skin cancers after organ transplantation. N Engl J Med. 2003;348:1681–91.
34. Gallagher MP, Kelly PJ, Jardine M, Perkovic V, Cass A, Craig JC, Eris J, Webster AC. Long-term cancer risk of immunosuppressive regimens after kidney transplantation. J Am Soc Nephrol. 2010;21:852–8.
35. Geissler EK, Schnitzbauer AA, Zülke C, Lamby PE, Proneth A, Duvoux C, Burra P, Jauch KW, Rentsch M, Ganten TM, Schmidt J, Settmacher U, Heise M, Rossi G, Cillo U, Kneteman N, Adam R, Van Hoek B, Bachellier P, Wolf P, Rostaing L, Bechstein WO, Rizell M, Powell J, Hidalgo E, Gugenheim J, Wolters H, Brockmann J, Roy A, Mutzbauer I, Schlitt A, Beckebaum S, Graeb C, Nadalin S, Valente U, Turrión VS, Jamieson N, Scholz T, Colledan M, Fändrich F, Becker T, Söderdahl G, Chazouillères O, Mäkisalo H, Pageaux GP, Steininger R, Soliman T, De Jong KP, Pirenne J, Margreiter R, Pratschke J, Pinna AD, Hauss J, Schreiber S, Strasser S, Klempnauer J, Troisi RI, Bhoori S, Lerut J, Bilbao I, Klein CG, Königsrainer A, Mirza DF, Otto G, Mazzaferro V, Neuhaus P, Schlitt HJ. Sirolimus use in liver transplant recipients with hepatocellular carcinoma: a randomized, multicenter, open-label phase 3 trial. Transplantation. 2016;100:116–25.
36. Green M, Michaels MG. Epstein-Barr virus infection and posttransplant lymphoproliferative disorder. Am J Transplant. 2013;13 Suppl 3:41–54. quiz 54
37. Greenhall GHB, Ibrahim M, Dutta U, Doree C, Brunskill SJ, Johnson RJ, Tomlinson LA, Callaghan CJ, Watson CJE. Donor-transmitted cancer in Orthotopic solid organ transplant recipients: a systematic review. Transpl Int. 2021;35:10092.
38. Gutierrez-Dalmau A, Campistol JM. Immunosuppressive therapy and malignancy in organ transplant recipients: a systematic review. Drugs. 2007;67:1167–98.
39. Haagsma EB, Hagens VE, Schaapveld M, Van Den Berg AP, De Vries EG, Klompmaker IJ, Slooff MJ, Jansen PL. Increased cancer risk after liver transplantation: a population-based study. J Hepatol. 2001;34:84–91.
40. Hanna GJ, Dharanesswaran H, Giobbie-Hurder A, Harran JJ, Liao Z, Pai L, Tchekmedyian V, Ruiz ES, Waldman AH, Schmults CD, Riella LV, Lizotte P, Paweletz CP, Chandraker AK, Murakami N, Silk AW. Cemiplimab for kidney transplant recipients with advanced cutaneous squamous cell carcinoma. J Clin Oncol. 2024;42:1021–30.
41. Hatami B, Pasharavesh L, Sharifian A, Zali MR. Concurrent inflammatory bowel disease and primary sclerosing cholangitis: a review of pre- and post-transplant outcomes and treatment options. Gastroenterol Hepatol Bed Bench. 2023;16:259–69.
42. Herrero JI. Screening of de novo tumors after liver transplantation. J Gastroenterol Hepatol. 2012;27:1011–6.
43. Herrero JI, España A, Quiroga J, Sangro B, Pardo F, Alvárez-Cienfuegos J, Prieto J. Nonmelanoma skin cancer after liver transplantation. Study of risk factors Liver Transpl. 2005a;11:1100–6.
44. Herrero JI, Lorenzo M, Quiroga J, Sangro B, Pardo F, Rotellar F, Alvarez-Cienfuegos J, Prieto J. De novo neoplasia after liver transplantation: an analysis of risk factors and influence on survival. Liver Transpl. 2005b;11:89–97.
45. Herrero JI, Pardo F, D'avola D, Alegre F, Rotellar F, Inarrairaegui M, Martí P, Sangro B, Quiroga J. Risk factors of lung, head and neck, esophageal, and kidney and urinary tract carcinomas after liver transplantation: the effect of smoking withdrawal. Liver Transpl. 2011a;17:402–8.
46. Herrero JI, Pardo F, D'avola D, Alegre F, Rotellar F, Iñarrairaegui M, Martí P, Sangro B, Quiroga J. Risk factors of lung, head and neck, esophageal, and kidney and urinary tract carcinomas after liver transplantation: the effect of smoking withdrawal. Liver Transpl. 2011b;17:402–8.
47. Hewavisenti RV, Arena J, Ahlenstiel CL, Sasson SC. Human papillomavirus in the setting of immunodeficiency: pathogenesis and the emergence of next-generation therapies to reduce the high associated cancer risk. Front Immunol. 2023;14:1112513.

48. Hirunsatitpron P, Hanprasertpong N, Noppakun K, Pruksakorn D, Teekachunhatean S, Koonrungsesomboon N. Mycophenolic acid and cancer risk in solid organ transplant recipients: systematic review and meta-analysis. Br J Clin Pharmacol. 2022;88:476–89.
49. Imamura R, Tanaka R, Taniguchi A, Nakazawa S, Kato T, Yamanaka K, Namba-Hamano T, Kakuta Y, Abe T, Tsutahara K, Takao T, Kishikawa H, Nonomura N. Everolimus reduces cancer incidence and improves patient and graft survival rates after kidney transplantation: A multi-center study. J Clin Med. 2022;11
50. Jiyad Z, Olsen CM, Burke MT, Isbel NM, Green AC. Azathioprine and risk of skin cancer in organ transplant recipients: systematic review and meta-analysis. Am J Transplant. 2016;16:3490–503.
51. Kamdar KY, Rooney CM, Heslop HE. Posttransplant lymphoproliferative disease following liver transplantation. Curr Opin Organ Transplant. 2011;16:274–80.
52. Kang W-H. Surveillance and management of de novo malignancy after liver transplantation. Ann Liver Transpl. 2024;4:10–5.
53. Kasiske BL, Snyder JJ, Gilbertson DT, Wang C. Cancer after kidney transplantation in the United States. Am J Transplant. 2004;4:905–13.
54. Kasznicki J, Sliwinska A, Drzewoski J. Metformin in cancer prevention and therapy. Ann Transl Med. 2014;2:57.
55. Kayali S, Pasta A, Plaz Torres MC, Jaffe A, Strazzabosco M, Marenco S, Giannini EG. Immune checkpoint inhibitors in malignancies after liver transplantation: a systematic review and pooled analysis. Liver Int. 2023;43:8–17.
56. Leckel K, Beecken WD, Jonas D, Oppermann E, Coman MC, Beck KF, Cinatl J, Hailer NP, Auth MK, Bechstein WO, Shipkova M, Blaheta RA. The immunosuppressive drug mycophenolate mofetil impairs the adhesion capacity of gastrointestinal tumour cells. Clin Exp Immunol. 2003;134:238–45.
57. Leigh IM, Proby CM, Inman GJ, Harwood CA. Azathioprine: friend or foe? Br J Dermatol. 2019;180:961–3.
58. Ma S, Zheng Y, Xiao Y, Zhou P, Tan H. Meta-analysis of studies using metformin as a reducer for liver cancer risk in diabetic patients. Medicine (Baltimore). 2017;96:e6888.
59. Malvezzi P, Rostaing L. The safety of calcineurin inhibitors for kidney-transplant patients. Expert Opin Drug Saf. 2015;14:1531–46.
60. Manzia TM, Angelico R, Gazia C, Lenci I, Milana M, Ademoyero O, Pedini D, Toti L, Spada M, Tisone G, Baiocchi L. De novo malignancies after liver transplantation: the effect of immunosuppression-personal data and review of literature. World J Gastroenterol. 2019;25:5356–75.
61. Mctiernan A, Friedenreich CM, Katzmarzyk PT, Powell KE, Macko R, Buchner D, Pescatello LS, Bloodgood B, Tennant B, Vaux-Bjerke A, George SM, Troiano RP, Piercy KL. Physical activity in cancer prevention and survival: a systematic review. Med Sci Sports Exerc. 2019;51:1252–61.
62. Melo Bisneto AVD, Oliveira LCD, Silva Fernandes A, Silva LS, Véras JH, Cardoso CG, Silva CR E, De Moraes Filho AV, Carneiro CC, Chen-Chen L. Recombinogenic, genotoxic, and cytotoxic effects of azathioprine using in vivo assays. J Toxic Environ Health A. 2021;84:261–71.
63. Mittal A, Colegio OR. Skin cancers in organ transplant recipients. Am J Transplant. 2017;17:2509–30.
64. Moreno R, Berenguer M. Post-liver transplantation medical complications. Ann Hepatol. 2006;5:77.
65. Moscicki AB, Flowers L, Huchko MJ, Long ME, Maclaughlin KL, Murphy J, Spiryda LB, Gold MA. Guidelines for cervical cancer screening in immunosuppressed women without HIV infection. J Low Genit Tract Dis. 2019;23:87–101.
66. Mukthinuthalapati PK, Gotur R, Ghabril M. Incidence, risk factors and outcomes of de novo malignancies post liver transplantation. World J Hepatol. 2016;8:533–44.
67. Nasser-Ghodsi N, Mara K, Watt KD. De novo colorectal and pancreatic cancer in liver-transplant recipients: identifying the higher-risk populations. Hepatology. 2021;74:1003–13.

68. O'donovan P, Perrett CM, Zhang X, Montaner B, Xu Y-Z, Harwood CA, Mcgregor JM, Walker SL, Hanaoka F, Karran P. Azathioprine and UVA light generate mutagenic oxidative DNA damage. Science. 2005;309:1871–4.
69. Oudkerk M, Liu S, Heuvelmans MA, Walter JE, Field JK. Lung cancer LDCT screening and mortality reduction—evidence, pitfalls and future perspectives. Nat Rev Clin Oncol. 2021;18:135–51.
70. Park B, Yoon J, Choi D, Kim HJ, Jung YK, Kwon OJ, Lee KG. De novo cancer incidence after kidney and liver transplantation: results from a nationwide population based data. Sci Rep. 2019;9:17202.
71. Ploos Van Amstel S, Vogelzang JL, Starink MV, Jager KJ, Groothoff JW. Long-term risk of cancer in survivors of pediatric ESRD. Clin J Am Soc Nephrol. 2015;10:2198–204.
72. Qiao Y, Yang T, Gan Y, Li W, Wang C, Gong Y, Lu Z. Associations between aspirin use and the risk of cancers: a meta-analysis of observational studies. BMC Cancer. 2018;18:288.
73. R Core Team. R: A language and environment for statistical computing. Vienna: R Foundation for Statistical Computing; 2024.
74. Rademacher S, Seehofer D, Eurich D, Schoening W, Neuhaus R, Oellinger R, Denecke T, Pascher A, Schott E, Sinn M, Neuhaus P, Pratschke J. The 28-year incidence of de novo malignancies after liver transplantation: a single-center analysis of risk factors and mortality in 1616 patients. Liver Transpl. 2017;23:1404–14.
75. Renaud L, Hilleret MN, Thimonier E, Guillaud O, Arbib F, Ferretti G, Jankowski A, Chambon-Augoyard C, Erard-Poinsot D, Decaens T, Boillot O, Leroy V, Dumortier J. De novo malignancies screening after liver transplantation for alcoholic liver disease: a comparative opportunistic study. Liver Transpl. 2018;24:1690–8.
76. Robinson CH, Coughlin CC, Chanchlani R, Dharnidharka VR. Post-transplant malignancies in pediatric organ transplant recipients. Pediatr Transplant. 2021;25:e13884.
77. Rothwell PM, Wilson M, Elwin CE, Norrving B, Algra A, Warlow CP, Meade TW. Long-term effect of aspirin on colorectal cancer incidence and mortality: 20-year follow-up of five randomised trials. Lancet. 2010;376:1741–50.
78. Sanaei AK, Aliakbarian M, Kazemi K, Nikeghbalian S, Shamsaeefar A, Mehdi SH, Bahreini A, Dehghani SM, Geramizadeh B, Malekhosseini SA. De novo malignancy after liver transplant. Exp Clin Transplant. 2015;13:163–6.
79. Schumacher G, Oidtmann M, Rueggeberg A, Jacob D, Jonas S, Langrehr JM, Neuhaus R, Bahra M, Neuhaus P. Sirolimus inhibits growth of human hepatoma cells alone or combined with tacrolimus, while tacrolimus promotes cell growth. World J Gastroenterol. 2005;11:1420–5.
80. Sérée O, Altieri M, Guillaume E, De Mil R, Lobbedez T, Robinson P, Segol P, Salamé E, Abergel A, Boillot O, Conti F, Chazouillères O, Debette-Gratien M, Debray D, Hery G, Dharancy S, Durand F, Duvoux C, Francoz C, Gugenheim J, Hardwigsen J, Houssel-Debry P, Jacquemin E, Kamar N, Latournerie M, Lebray P, Leroy V, Mazzola A, Neau-Cransac M, Pageaux GP, Radenne S, Saliba F, Samuel D, Vanlemmens C, Woehl-Jaegle ML, Launoy G, Dumortier J. Longterm risk of solid organ De novo malignancies after liver transplantation: A French National Study on 11,226 patients. Liver Transpl. 2018;24:1425–36.
81. Shalaby S, Taborelli M, Zanetto A, Ferrarese A, D'arcangelo F, Gambato M, Senzolo M, Russo F, Germani G, Boccagni P, Ettorre G, Baccarani U, Lauro A, Galatioto L, Rendina M, Petrara R, Rossi A, Nudo F, Toti L, Burra P. Hepatocellular carcinoma and the risk of de novo malignancies after liver transplantation. Transpl Int. 2021;34
82. Stallone G, Infante B, Grandaliano G. Management and prevention of post-transplant malignancies in kidney transplant recipients. Clin Kidney J. 2015;8:637–44.
83. Sureka B, Bansal K, Rajesh S, Mukund A, Pamecha V, Arora A. Imaging panorama in post-operative complications after liver transplantation. Gastroenterol Rep (Oxf). 2016;4:96–106.
84. Taborelli M, Piselli P, Ettorre GM, Lauro A, Galatioto L, Baccarani U, Rendina M, Shalaby S, Petrara R, Nudo F, Toti L, Sforza D, Fantola G, Cimaglia C, Agresta A, Vennarecci G, Pinna AD, Gruttadauria S, Risaliti A, Di Leo A, Burra P, Rossi M, Tisone G, Zamboni F, Serraino D. Risk of virus and non-virus related malignancies following immunosuppression in a cohort of liver transplant recipients. Italy, 1985-2014. Int J Cancer. 2018;143:1588–94.

85. Tan Y, Wang M, Yang K, Chi T, Liao Z, Wei P. PPAR-α modulators as current and potential cancer treatments. Front Oncol. 2021;11:599995.
86. Thomas BR, Barnabas A, Agarwal K, Aluvihare V, Suddle AR, Higgins EM, O'grady JG, Heaton ND, Heneghan MA. Patient perception of skin-cancer prevention and risk after liver transplantation. Clin Exp Dermatol. 2013;38:851–6.
87. Tiwari A, Saigal S, Choudhary NS, Saha S, Rastogi A, Bhangui P, Saraf N, Srinivasan T, Yadav SK, Gautam D, Nundy S, Soin AS. De novo malignancy after living donor liver transplantation: a large volume experience. J Clin Exp Hepatol. 2020;10:448–52.
88. Tjon AS, Sint Nicolaas J, Kwekkeboom J, De Man RA, Kazemier G, Tilanus HW, Hansen BE, Van Der Laan LJ, Tha-In T, Metselaar HJ. Increased incidence of early de novo cancer in liver graft recipients treated with cyclosporine: an association with C2 monitoring and recipient age. Liver Transpl. 2010;16:837–46.
89. Tomaszewski JJ, Larson JA, Smaldone MC, Hayn MH, Jackman SV. Management of bladder cancer following solid organ transplantation. Adv Urol. 2011;2011:256985.
90. Ume AC, Wenegieme T-Y, Williams CR. Calcineurin inhibitors: a double-edged sword. Am J Physiol-Renal Physiol. 2021;320:F336–41.
91. Ursic-Bedoya J, Donnadieu-Rigole H, Faure S, Pageaux G-P. Alcohol use and smoking after liver transplantation; complications and prevention. Best Pract Res Clin Gastroenterol. 2017;31:181–5.
92. Van Der Heide F, Dijkstra G, Porte RJ, Kleibeuker JH, Haagsma EB. Smoking behavior in liver transplant recipients. Liver Transpl. 2009;15:648–55.
93. Wahab MA, Abdel-Khalek EE, Elshoubary M, Yassen AM, Salah T, Sultan AM, Fathy O, Elmorshedi M, Shiha U, Elsadany M, Adly R, Samy M, Shehta A. Predictive factors of De novo malignancies after living-donor liver transplantation: a single-center experience. Transplant Proc. 2021;53:636–44.
94. Watt KD, Rolak S, Foley DP, Plichta JK, Pruthi S, Farr D, Zwald FO, Carvajal RD, Dudek AZ, Sanger CB, Rocco R, Chang GJ, Dizon DS, Langstraat CL, Teoh D, Agarwal PK, Al-Qaoud T, Eggener S, Kennedy CC, D'cunha J, Mohindra NA, Stewart S, Habermann TH, Schuster S, Lunning M, Shah NN, Gertz MA, Mehta J, Suvannasankha A, Verna E, Farr M, Blosser CD, Hammel L, Al-Adra DP. Cancer surveillance in solid organ transplant recipients with a Pretransplant history of malignancy: multidisciplinary collaborative expert opinion. Transplantation. 2024;108
95. Watt KDS, Pedersen RA, Kremers WK, Heimbach JK, Sanchez W, Gores GJ. Long-term probability of and mortality from De novo malignancy after liver transplantation. Gastroenterology. 2009;137:2010–7.
96. Weischer M, Röcken M, Berneburg M. Calcineurin inhibitors and rapamycin: cancer protection or promotion? Exp Dermatol. 2007;16:385–93.
97. Wimmer CD, Angele MK, Schwarz B, Pratschke S, Rentsch M, Khandoga A, Guba M, Jauch KW, Bruns C, Graeb C. Impact of cyclosporine versus tacrolimus on the incidence of de novo malignancy following liver transplantation: a single center experience with 609 patients. Transpl Int. 2013;26:999–1006.
98. Wimmer CD, Rentsch M, Crispin A, Illner WD, Arbogast H, Graeb C, Jauch KW, Guba M. The janus face of immunosuppression—de novo malignancy after renal transplantation: the experience of the Transplantation Center Munich. Kidney Int. 2007;71:1271–8.
99. Wong G, Au E, Badve SV, Lim WH. Breast cancer and transplantation. Am J Transplant. 2017;17:2243–53.

Index

A
Abdominal imaging
  complications, 389
    biliary complications, 394, 395
    infectious complications, 396, 397
    recurrent of malignancy and post-transplant lymphoproliferative disorder, 397, 398
    vascular complications, 390, 392–394
  findings, 387
    biliary system, 389
    liver morphology and parenchyma, 387
    vascular anatomy and normal imaging findings, 388
  post liver transplant, modalities for, 386
    computed tomography, 386, 387
    magnetic resonance imaging, 387
    ultrasound, 386
  rationale for, 385, 386
Abdominal NRP (A-NRP), 211, 212
Abscess, 381–382
Accessory or replaced right hepatic arteries, 327
Achilles heel, 187
Active pathogenic infections, 116–118
Acute antibody-mediated rejection, 292, 293
Acute coronary syndromes (ACS), 33
Acute Disease Quality Initiative (ADQI), 80, 81, 83
Acute hepatic decompensations, 116
Acute kidney injury (AKI), 24–26, 66, 71
  assessment of, 79, 80
  diagnostic criteria, 80, 81
  incidence, 79
  occurrence, 79
  pharmacologic therapy
    IV fluids, 83–84
    liver transplantation, 85
    renal replacement therapy, 84
    TIPS, 84
    vasoconstrictors, 84
  post-transplant, 39
  prevalence, 79
Acute liver failure (ALF)
  classifications, 64
  clinical prognostication, 5
  definition, 63
  etiology, 4
  indications, LT, 68, 69
  liver transplant center and ICU admission, 64
  management
    cardiovascular, 66
    coagulation, 67
    etiology, 65
    extracorporeal liver support, 68
    general, 64
    infectious, 67
    metabolic, 67
    neurology, 66
    renal, 66
    respiratory, 67
  prognosis, 64
  triage of, 4
Acute liver injury (ALI), 63, 64
Acute respiratory distress syndrome (ARDS), 67, 69
Acute T-cell-mediated rejection
  diagnosis, 290, 291
  outcomes, 291
  treatment, 291

B. Eghtesad et al. (eds.), *Liver Transplantation*,
https://doi.org/10.1007/978-3-032-07072-2

Acute-on-chronic liver failure (ACLF), 24, 116, 416
definitions, 69
grades and 28-day free-transplantation mortality, 70
ICU admission, 69
indication for liver transplantation, 73–74
prognosis, 73
supportive management
circulatory, 71
coagulation, 72
extracorporeal liver support, 72, 73
general, 70, 71
neurological, 72
nutrition, 72
renal, 71
respiratory, 72
Adherence, 156
Adult-to-adult LDLT, 175, 176, 226
Aggressive medical management, 334
Alcohol liver-related disease (ALD), 5, 6, 113, 114, 423, 424, 451
Alcohol use disorder (AUD), 424
Alcohol-associated liver disease (ALD), 139, 143, 338
Allograft, recurrent and de novo disease in, 319
Allograft dysfunction, histopathological diagnosis of
liver transplant operation/surgical intervention and factors contributing, 308
timing of causes, 309
Allograft rejection
acute antibody-mediated rejection, 292, 293
acute T-cell-mediated rejection
diagnosis, 290, 291
outcomes, 291
treatment, 291
chronic Ductopenic allograft rejection, 294
human liver allografts, long term changes in, 295
idiopathic chronic hepatitis, 295
late acute TCMR, 292
operational tolerance, 295, 296
plasma cell hepatitis/plasma-cell rich allograft rejection, 293, 294
post-transplant liver pathology, 311–312
prevention of, 289
Alloimmune injury, 253
Alpha 1 antitrypsin (A1AT) deficiency, 141, 144, 145, 147
Anastamotic biliary stricture, 395
Anastomosis, 401, 402
Anastomotic strictures (AS), 333, 400
Anhepatic phase, 178, 181–184
Ante-mortem interventions, 210
Antibody mediated rejection (AMR), 253, 256, 312, 335
post-transplant liver pathology, 314, 315
Anticoagulation, 100
Antifungal prophylaxis, 118
Aortic stenosis (AS), 36
Arginine vasopressin (AVP), 25
Arrhythmias, 35, 100, 272
Ascites, 4, 6, 7, 12, 14, 15, 79–82, 84
Aspiration-related pneumonias, 356
Atrial fibrillation (AF), 100
Atypical bacterial infections, 352–353
Autoimmune hepatitis (AIH), 338, 417, 420
Auxiliary LTX, 174
Auxiliary partial orthotopic liver transplantation (APOLT), 235–236
Azathioprine (AZA), 289, 417

B

Back-to-base model, 247
Bacterial ascending cholangitis, 283
Bacterial infections, 24, 28–29, 283, 356
Bacterial liver abscess, 283
Basal cell carcinoma, 455
Basiliximab, 289
Bicaval technique, 378
Bile leak, interventional endoscopy, 401
Biliary anastomosis, 187, 193–195
Biliary anatomy, 167
Biliary atresia, 174, 191
Biliary cast syndrome, 365–366
Biliary complications (BC), 192–194, 283, 332, 394, 399
biliary leak, 332, 394, 395
biliary strictures, 333, 395
ischemic cholangiopathy, 333
orthotopic liver transplant
biliary leak and stricture, 365
ischemic cholangiopathy/biliary cast syndrome, 365
management, 366–368
postoperative anatomy, 364
Biliary continuity, 178, 189
Biliary injuries, 327
Biliary leak, 332, 366
abdominal imaging, 394–395
orthotopic liver transplant, 365
Biliary stones, 402
Biliary strictures, 333, 366
complications, biliary complications, 395
orthotopic liver transplant, 365
Biliary system, 180, 187, 189, 193, 389
Biliary tree, 223, 226

Biloma, 351, 381–382
Blastomycosis, 354
Bleeding, 194, 328–329, 379
 ERCP, 404, 405
Body mass index (BMI), 325
Brain edema, 66
Brain oedema, 65
Bridging therapy (BT), 124, 127, 131, 132

C
C1q DSA, 259
Calcineurin inhibitor, 452
Cardiac allograft vasculopathy (CAV), 272
Cardiac arrhythmias, 33
Cardiac complications
 arrhythmias, 100
 CAD, 95, 96, 99
 CCM, 93
 HF, 93, 94
 valvular heart disease, 101–102
Cardiac magnetic resonance (CMR), 36
Cardiomyopathy, 36
Cardiopulmonary exercise testing, 94
Caregivers, 154, 155, 301
Catheter-directed therapy, 380
Caval harvest, 378
Caval kinking, 380
Caval outflow obstruction, 379
Cavoportal hemitransposition, 186
Ceruloplasmin (CPN), 145
Chimeric antigen receptors-T cells, 132
Cholangiocarcinoma (CCA), 10
 definition, 128
 iCCA, 128, 129
 perihilar, 129, 130
Cholangitis, 351, 405
Choledochocholedochostomy, 187, 193, 194
Choledochojejunostomy, 187, 193
Choledocholithiasis, 367
 interventional endoscopy, 402
Cholestatic, 281
Chronic AMR (cAMR), 314
Chronic Ductopenic allograft rejection, 294, 335
Chronic immunosuppression with calcineurin inhibitors (CNI), 99
Chronic kidney disease (CKD), 441
Chronic obstructive pulmonary disease (COPD), 36, 37
Chronic rejection, 286
Circulatory determination of death (cDCDD), 206–208, 210–213, 215
Circulatory dysfunction, 24
Cirrhosis, 23–24, 28, 51–57, 421
Cirrhotic cardiomyopathy (CCM), 26, 92, 93, 104
Classical Piggyback Technique, 184
CLIF-C ACLF score, 73
CLIF-C organ failure (OF) score, 69, 70
Clinically significant portal hypertension (CSPH), 51–56
Clostridioides difficle, 336
CMV prophylaxis, 337
Coagulopathy, 27–28, 328, 329
Coccidiomycosis, 354
Cold-ischemia time (CIT), 186, 190, 242, 266, 328
Colonization or invasive infection (IFI), 118
Colorectal cancer, 456
Colorectal liver metastasis (CRLM), 11, 130, 131, 133
Combined heart and liver transplant
 anesthesia considerations, 270
 indications, 268, 269
 patient outcomes, 272
 postoperative management, 272
 selection criteria, 270
 surgical technique, 270, 272
Combined liver and kidney transplant (CLKT), 258, 263
Combined liver and lung transplant
 indications, 272, 273
 patient outcomes, 276
 post operative management, 275, 276
 preoperative considerations, 275
 selection criteria, 273, 275
 surgical technique, 275
Combined organ transplantation, 263
 combined heart and liver transplant
  anesthesia considerations, 270
  indications, 268, 269
  patient outcomes, 272
  postoperative management, 272
  selection criteria, 270
  surgical technique, 270, 272
 combined liver and lung transplant
  indications, 272, 273
  patient outcomes, 276
  post operative management, 275, 276
  preoperative considerations, 275
  selection criteria, 273, 275
  surgical technique, 275
 combined thoracic-liver transplant, 268
 liver and kidney
  indications, 264
  outcomes, 267, 268
  postoperative management, 266, 267
  pre-transplant considerations, 265, 266
  selection criteria, 264
  surgical technique, 266
Combined thoracic-liver transplant, 268

Common bile duct (CBD), 225, 234
Common hepatic artery (CHA), 223, 234, 236
Common hepatic duct (CHD), 225
Community-acquired pneumonias, 356
Community-acquired respiratory viruses, 356–357
Complement-dependent cytotoxicity crossmatch (CDC XM) method, 254
Computed tomography (CT), 386–387
Continuous renal replacement therapy (CRRT), 65, 67
Copper (Cu) metabolism, 145
Coronary artery calcium (CAC) scoring, 35
Coronary artery disease (CAD), 33–35, 92, 94–96, 99, 100
Coronary CT angiography (CCTA), 96
Corticosteroids, 454
Couinaud segments of liver, 222
Couinaud's system, 222
Covered self-expandable metal stents (cSEMSs), 333
C-reactive protein (CRP), 116, 117
Critical patient approach, 209
Cryptococcosis, 353
Curability, 124, 133
Cystatin C, 40
Cystic fibrosis, 272
Cystic fibrosis transmembrane regulator (CFTR), 272
Cytomegalovirus (CMV), 284

D

De novo autoimmune hepatitis, 293
De novo DSAs, treatment course of, 259
De novo malignancies (DNM), 448
Deceased donor liver transplantation (DDLT), 328
Deceased organ donation
- cDCDD, 210–212
- determination of death, 207, 208
- disparities, 204
- DNDD, 209, 210
- donor coordinator, 213–215
- donor identification, 206, 207
- LT activity pmp, 204, 205
- pathway, 204, 208
- pmp and human development index, 204, 206
- uDCDD, 212, 213

Decompensated liver disease, 4, 5, 7, 8
- ascites, 6, 7
- hepatic encephalopathy, 8
- hepatorenal syndrome, 7
- variceal bleeding, 7, 8

Decompensation management, 14
De-novo MASLD, 440
Device-to-donor, 245
Digestive microbes, 28
Direct-acting antiviral agents (DAA), 114, 325, 414
Direct-acting antivirals for hepatitis C, 5
Disease recurrence, 413
- alcohol related liver disease, 423, 424
- autoimmune hepatitis, 417, 420
- hepatitis B, 415, 416
- hepatitis C, 414
- primary biliary cholangitis, 421, 422
- primary sclerosing cholangitis, 420, 421

Disseminated intravascular coagulation (DIC), 28
Distal cholangiocarcinoma (dCCA), 128
Dobutamine stress echocardiography (DSE), 34, 96
DOMINO-APOLT technique, 235
Donation after brain death (DBD), 177
Donation after cardiac death (DCD), 242, 326
Donation after circulatory death (DCD), 177, 190, 193
Donation after the circulatory determination of death (DCDD), 206
Donation after the neurological determination of death (DNDD), 205–207, 209–213, 215
Donor coordinator (DC), 206, 207, 213–215
Donor liver steatosis, 326
Donor liver transplantation, 255
Donor portal vein, 186
Donor selection and procurement injuries, 326–328
Donor transmitted cancer, 454
Donor-specific antibodies (DSAs), 253
Downstaging, 124, 125, 127, 132
Drug to drug interactions (DDIs), 414
Drug-induced liver injury, 118, 282, 319
Drugs, 285
Dual antiplatelet (DAPT) therapy, 96, 99
Dual living donor liver transplantation (LDLT), 175
Dyslipidemia, 438, 439
Dysnatremia, 66

E

Early allograft dysfunction (EAD), 210, 211, 326, 334
- primary graft nonfunction, 334

Ejection fraction (EF), 36

Elective bariatric surgery, 42
Electrohydraulic lithotripsy (EHL), 402
End stage liver disease (ESLD), 328
  patient evaluation and considerations, 97–98
Endemic mycoses, 353, 354
End-ischemic NMP, 245
Endoscopic retrograde cholangiopancreatography (ERCP), 332
  comparative efficacy of, 405
    bile duct evaluation, MRCP vs. for, 406
    vs. PTBD, 406
  complications and management, 404
    bleeding, 404, 405
    cholangitis/infectious complication, 405
    immunocompromised status and risk mitigating strategies, 405
    PEP, 404
    perforation, 405
  indications for, 400
    anastomotic strictures, 400
    biliary strictures, 400
    non-anastomotic strictures, 401
  post-transplant care, 399, 400
Endoscopic ultrasound (EUS), 403
Endoscopic variceal ligation (EVL), 54–58
Endovascular interventions, 331
End-stage liver disease (ESLD), 33, 34, 36, 41, 44, 173, 176
  bacterial infections, 28–29
  cirrhosis, 23
  extrahepatic organ/system dysfunction
    acute kidney injury, 24–26
    circulatory dysfunction, 24
    cirrhotic cardiomyopathy, 26
    coagulopathy, 27–28
    hepatic encephalopathy, 27
End-to-end portal vein anastomoses, 374
Enhanced liver fibrosis (ELF) test, 140–142
Epstein–Barr Virus (EBV), 284, 285, 337
Estimated GFR (eGFR), 32, 39, 40, 80, 85
European Association for the Study of the Liver-Chronic Liver Failure (EASL-CLIF) Consortium, 69
Eversion portal-venous thromboendarterectomy, 186
Eversion thromboendartectomy, 186
"Expanded criteria donor" (ECD), 177
Ex situ perfusion, 241
Ex situ preservation strategies, 212
Excretory MR cholangiography (ERCP), 395
Extended withdrawal period, 210
Extending life-sustaining therapies, 207
Extra-corporeal albumin dialysis systems, 72
Extracorporeal circulation, 211
Extracorporeal membrane oxygenation (ECMO), 211–213
Extrahepatic cholangiocarcinoma (eCCA), 128
Extra-hepatic malignancy screening, 43–44

F

Familial amyloid polyneuropathy (FAP), 269
Family approach, 207, 215
Fecal immunochemical test (FIT), 44
Fibrinolysis, 28
Fibrolamellar HCC, 131
Fibrosing cholestatic hepatitis, 284
Fibrosis-4 (FIB-4) Index, 140, 141
Finances, 155
Flavin mononucleotide (FMN), 242
Forced expiratory volume in one second (FEV1), 37
Fractional excretion of sodium (FENa), 83
Fractional flow reserve (FFR), 96
Frailty, 41
Functional stress tests, 34
Functional warm ischemic time (FWIT), 210
Fungal infections, 118, 285, 353–354
  cryptococcosis, 353
  endemic mycoses, 353, 354
  invasive aspergillosis, 353
  late post-transplantation infections, 356
Future liver remnant (FLR), 176

G

G6PD deficiency, 165
Gastro-duodenal artery (GDA), 223
Glomerular filtration rate (GFR), 25
Graft dysfunction, 282
Graft perfusion, 386
Graft torsion, 380
Graft-to-recipient body weight ratio (GRWR), 176

H

HCV RNA PCR, 284
Health history, 154
Heart failure (HF), 33, 36, 92–95, 100, 101, 103, 104
Hematoma, 381–382
Hemochromatosis, 94
Hemodynamic instability, 177, 181–183, 190, 192

Heparin-bonded cannulae, 182
Hepatectomy, 176, 178–181, 184, 193
Hepatic arterial complications
HAP, 371, 372
HAT, 370, 371
hepatic artery stenosis, 369–371
management, 372, 373
postoperative anatomy, 368, 369
Hepatic arterial ischemic cascade, 390–392
Hepatic artery, 388
Hepatic artery anastomosis, 369
Hepatic artery pseudoaneurysm (HAP), 330, 371–373
Hepatic artery stenosis (HAS), 190–191, 369–371
management, 372
Hepatic artery stricture (HAS), 330
Hepatic artery thrombosis (HAT), 191, 328, 370–371, 373, 390
Hepatic caval outflow obstruction, 379
Hepatic encephalopathy (HE), 4–6, 8, 14, 15, 27, 63–65, 67–69, 72, 73
Hepatic epithelioid hemangioendothelioma (HEHE), 131
Hepatic hydrothorax (HH), 39, 105
Hepatic metabolism, 118
Hepatic outflow obstruction, 192
Hepatic steatosis, 167
Hepatic vasculature, 223
Hepatic vein, 378, 388
Hepatic vein outflow obstruction (HVOO), 192, 232
Hepatic vein stenosis, 393–394
Hepatic venous outflow obstruction, 192
Hepatic venous pressure gradient (HVPG), 51, 52, 58
Hepaticojejunostomy, 178, 189
Hepatitis B, 284, 415, 416
Hepatitis B viral (HBV) infection, 5, 113–115, 125
Hepatitis C, 283, 284, 414
Hepatitis C related cirrhosis, 114
Hepatitis C virus (HCV), 125, 325
Hepatoblastoma, 131
Hepatocaval complications
clinical manifestation and diagnostic features, 379
management, 380, 381
postoperative anatomy, 378
Hepatocellular, 281
Hepatocellular carcinoma (HCC), 9, 10, 16
bridging, 127
downstaging, 125, 127
immunotherapy, 127
LT criteria, 125, 126
pre-and post-transplant period, 128
risk factors, 125
salvage transplantation, 127
transplantability, 125
Hepato-pulmonary syndrome (HPS), 12, 16, 37, 38, 104–105
Hepatorenal syndrome (HRS), 7, 15, 264
Hepatorenal syndrome associated with AKI (HRS-AKI)
diagnostic criteria, 80, 81
pathophysiology, 81–82
pharmacologic therapy
IV fluids, 83–84
liver transplantation, 85
renal replacement therapy, 84
TIPS, 84
vasoconstrictors, 84
prevention of, 82
Hepatovenous/caval stenosis, 380
Hereditary hemochromatosis (HH), 143, 144
Herpes simplex virus (HSV), 337
Heterotopic LTX, 174
High-resolution computed tomography (HRCT), 36
Hilar cholangiocarcinoma (hCCA), 10, 11
HIV infected candidates, 114
HIV infection, 114
HLA-DQ, 254
Human leukocyte antigen (HLA), 253
Human liver allografts, long term changes in, 295
Hyperacute rejection, 335
Hyperammonemia, 66
Hyperglycemia, 67
Hypertension, 437, 438
Hypertrophic cardiomyopathy (HCM), 94
Hyponatremia, 40
Hypoperfusion, 272
Hypothermic reoxygenation, 244
Hypothermic-oxygenated perfusion (HOPE), 241, 242, 244
Hypoxemia, 67

I

Iatrogenic Budd–Chiari syndrome, 192
Idiopathic chronic hepatitis, 295
Imaging, 365
Immune checkpoint inhibitors (ICIs), 127, 128
Immunocompromised status, 405
Immunosuppression, 289, 421, 451–454
Immunotherapy, 127, 132
Immunotolerance, 267

In situ machine perfusion, 241
Inborn errors of metabolism (IEM), 9
Incisional infections, 352
Indications, liver transplantation, 68, 69
acute-on-chronic liver failure, 73–74
acute liver failure
clinical prognostication, 5
etiology, 4
triage of, 4
chronic liver disease, systemic complications of, 12–13
decompensated liver disease, 5
ascites, 6, 7
hepatic encephalopathy, 8
hepatorenal syndrome, 7
variceal bleeding, 7, 8
metabolic liver diseases, 9
oncologic indications
hepatocellular carcinoma, 9, 10
hilar cholangiocarcinoma, 10
intrahepatic cholangiocarcinoma, 10, 11
metastatic colorectal cancer, 11
metastatic neuroendocrine tumor, 11
severe acute alcoholic hepatitis, 13
timing and referral, 3, 4, 14
Induction immunosuppression, 290
Infection, 336, 337
intermediate post-transplantation infections
atypical bacterial infections, 352
fungal infections, 353, 354
risk factors for, 352
viral infections, 355
late post-transplantation infections, 355
bacterial infections, 356
fungal infections, 356
risk factors for, 355, 356
viral infections, 356, 357
after liver transplantation
donor-derived infections, 352
early post-transplantation infections, 351
nosocomial infections, 351
risk factors, for early post-transplantation infections, 351
surgical site infections, 351, 352
Infectious complication, 405
abdominal imaging, 396, 397
Infectious screening testing pre-LT, 114, 115
Inferior right hepatic veins (IRHV), 224, 228
Inferior vena cava (IVC), 388
Infiltrative, 281
Intensive care to facilitate organ donation (ICOD), 207, 214
Interleukin-6 (IL-6), 25
International Club of Ascites (ICA), 80, 81, 83
International Liver Transplant Society (ILTS), 289
Interposition/jump venous grafts, 186
Interventional endoscopy, 399
bile leak, 401
choledocholithiasis and sludge, 402
endoscopic ultrasound, 403
ERCP, 405
bile duct evaluation, MRCP vs. for, 406
vs. PTBD, 406
ERCP complications and management, 404
bleeding, 404, 405
cholangitis/infectious complication, 405
immunocompromised status and risk mitigating strategies, 405
PEP, 404
perforation, 405
ERCP, indications for, 400
anastomotic strictures, 400
biliary strictures, 400
non-anastomotic strictures, 401
post-transplant care, ERCP significance in, 399, 400
procedural consideration and technical challenges, 402
advanced techniques, 403
intraprocedural challenges and technique modification, 403
pre procedural consideration, 402, 403
sphincter of Oddi Dysfunction, 402
stent placement, removal or exchange, 402
trends and future directions, 406
Intrahepatic cholangiocarcinoma (iCCA), 10, 11, 128, 129, 133
Intrahepatic shunts, 23
Intraoperative bleeding, 329
Intravascular ultrasonography, 380
Intravenous ganciclovir, 337
Invasive aspergillosis, 353
Invasive coronary angiography (ICA), 34, 35, 96
Inverted Y or Mercedes incision, 178
Invisibly, liver injury, 244
Ischemia-free liver transplantation (IFLT), 246
Ischemia-reperfusion injury, 244
Ischemic cholangiopathy (IC), 330, 333, 365–368
Isolated liver tests, 282

K

Keyser-Flescher (KF) rings, 145

Kidney after liver transplant (KALT), 264
Kidney delayed graft function (K-DGF), 267
Kings College Criteria (KCC), 5, 68
Klatskin tumor, 10
Küpffer cells, 24, 253

L

Large volume paracentesis (LVP), 58
Late acute TCMR, 292
Late liver allograft dysfunction, 318, 319
Latent tuberculosis, 119
Left hepatic duct (LHD), 225, 234, 236
Left hepatic vein (LHV), 224, 225, 228, 229, 234, 235
Left lateral segment (LLS) graft, 221, 226–228, 230, 233–235
Left lobe (LL) grafts, 221, 226, 228, 234
Left portal vein (LPV), 223, 224, 234, 235
Left ventricular ejection fraction (LVEF), 94
Liver allograft, 256
Liver anatomy, 222–226
Liver biopsy, 382
Liver grafts, 242
Liver morphology, 387
Liver perfusion, 379
Liver sinusoidal endothelial cells, 253
Liver transplantation (LT), 253, 325, 363
  blood work after, 281
    cytomegalovirus, 284
    drugs, 285
    early after transplant, 283
    EBV, 284, 285
    fungal infections, 285
    hepatitis B, 284
    hepatitis C, 283, 284
    infections, 283
    recurrent disease, 286
    rejection, 285, 286
    viral infections, 283
  candidate evaluation, tests at the time, 255
  clinical transplant coordinator in
    acceptance, 303
    after discharge, 304
    allocation process works, 304
    deferred status, 304
    denial, 303, 304
    live donor liver transplantation discussion and option, 302, 303
    living donor coordinator responsibilities, 300
    MELD score components, 300, 301
    post-transplant coordinator responsibilities, 300
    pre-transplant coordinator responsibilities, 299
    procedure, 304
    referral, 300
    required testing, 302
    transition to home, 305
    transplant evaluation, 301
    wait-list coordinator responsibilities, 299
  combined liver-kidney transplant recipient, de novo Class II DSA in, 258
  early and late complications of, 325
    biliary complications, 332, 333
    coagulopathy and bleeding, 328, 329
    donor selection and procurement injuries, 326–328
    early graft dysfunction, 334
    infection, 336, 337
    nonocclusive arterial complications, 330
    portal vein thrombosis, 331
    recurrent disease, 338
    rejection, 335
    vascular complications, 329, 330
    venous outflow obstruction, 331, 332
  hypothermic-oxygenated perfusion, 242, 244
  infection after
    donor-derived infections, 352
    early post-transplantation infections, 351
    intermediate post-transplantation infections, 352–355
    late post-transplantation infections, 355–357
    nosocomial infections, 351
    risk factors, for early post-transplantation infections, 351
    surgical site infections, 351, 352
  liver enzyme elevations after, 282
  living donor liver transplant, preformed DSA in, 257
  normothermic machine perfusion, 245, 246
  normothermic regional perfusion, 247, 248
  posttransplantation testing, 254, 256, 257
  safety net prioritization for, 265
  sequential perfusion, 246, 247
  testing at the time, 255, 256
  tests for combined transplantation with organs, 256
Liver transplantation (LT) candidate evaluation
  age, 41
  cardiovascular evaluation, 33
    arrhythmias, 35

cardiomyopathy and heart failure, 36
cardiovascular risk stratification, 34–35
coronary artery disease, 35
valvular heart disease, 35, 36
extra-hepatic malignancy screening, 43–44
frailty, 41
hyponatremia, 40
infectious disease screening, 42, 43
liver anatomic evaluation, 31–33
nutritional status, 41
obesity, 42
oral health, 42
psychosocial considerations, 44
pulmonary function evaluation, 36
HPS, 37
POPH, 38
renal evaluation, 39–40
variceal screening, 38–39
Liver volume, 167
Liver-specific frailty index (FrAI LT), 41
Living donor liver retrieval, 227, 228, 231
Living donor liver transplant, preformed DSA in, 257
Living donor liver transplantation (LDLT), 11, 130, 132, 175, 176, 226, 326
donor anatomic considerations, 166–167
biliary anatomy, 167
liver volume, 167
parenchymal evaluation, 167
vascular anatomy, 166, 167
donor characteristics, 165–166
donor selection, 226, 227
donor workup, 164, 165
exclusion, 168
graft retrieval, surgical principles of, 227–231
multidisciplinary team development, 163, 164
portal inflow modulation, 231–232
psychosocial consideration, 167, 168
Lung cancers, 455

M

Machine perfusion, 241
Machine perfusion strategies, 334
Macrovesicular (MaS), 326
Magnetic resonance cholangiopancreatography (MRCP), 193, 333
vs. ERCP, 406
Magnetic resonance imaging (MRI), 387, 395
Main portal vein (MPV), 223, 224, 234, 235
Major adverse cardiac and cerebrovascular event (MACE), 36
Mammalian target of rapamycin (mTOR) inhibitors, 99, 414
Median arcuate ligament syndrome, 187
Medical assistance in dying (MAiD), 206, 210
Medication coverage, 152, 154, 158, 159
Melanoma, 455
Mental health, 156
Metabolic associated steatohepatitis (MASH), 325
Metabolic associated steatotic liver disease (MASLD), 5
Metabolic dysfunction with alcohol-associated steatotic liver disease (MetALD), 139
Metabolic dysfunction-associated liver disease, 81
Metabolic dysfunction–associated steatotic liver disease (MASLD), 33, 113, 114, 125, 139–144
Metabolic liver disease, 9
A1AT deficiency, 144, 145
hereditary hemochromatosis, 143–144
LT evaluation, 146
MASLD, 139–143
prevalence and diagnostic testing, 147
Wilson's disease, 145, 146
Metastatic neuroendocrine tumor (NET), 11
Microbiota, 23, 24, 27, 28
Microvesicular (MiS), 326
Middle hepatic vein (MHV), 222, 224, 226, 228, 229, 234, 235
Milan criteria (MC), 125, 127
Mitral stenosis (MS), 101
Mixed HCC-CCA, 131
Model for early allograft function (MEAF), 334
Model for end-stage liver disease (MELD), 4, 5, 7, 11–16, 103, 104, 146, 264, 300
Modified neoadjuvant chemoradiation protocol, 129
Motivation, 157
Motor-driven bypass system, 182
mTOR inhibitors, 452
Multi-drug resistant organisms (MDRO), 115, 116
Mycophenolate mofetil, 453

N

N-acetyl cysteine (NAC) therapy, 65, 71
Neoadjuvant chemoradiation, 129, 131
Neuroendocrine tumor liver metastasis (NETLM), 131–133

Neutrophil gelatinase-associated lipocalin (uNGAL), 83
Nocardia, 352–353
Nonalcoholic fatty liver disease (NAFLD), 125, 139
Non-anastomotic biliary strictures (NAS), 333, 395, 396
Non-cirrhotic metabolic liver diseases (NCMLD), 235
Nonocclusive arterial complications, 330
Non-occlusive IVC thrombus, 332
Non-selective beta-blockers (NSBBs), 52–58
Non-skin cancers
  colorectal cancer, 456
  lung, 455
  PTLD, 455
Non-transplant and post-transplant, 281
Nonvascular percutaneous interventions
  liver biopsy, 382
  seroma, hematoma, biloma and abscess, 381, 382
Norepinephrine (NE), 66, 71, 73
Normothermic machine perfusion (NMP), 241, 245, 246, 326, 334
Normothermic regional perfusion (NRP), 208, 211–213, 215, 247, 248, 326, 334
No-touch period, 210

O

Obesity, 42, 326
  and weight management, 440
Occlusive arterial complications, 329–330
Operability, 124
Operational tolerance, 295, 296
Opportunistic invasive fungal infections, 337
Opt-out system, 204
Organ procurement organization (OPO), 207, 215, 248
Organ transplantation, 244
Organoid transplantation, 132
Orthotopic liver transplantation (OLT), 11, 281
  anhepatic phase, 181–184
  auxiliary, 174
  biliary complications, 192–194
    biliary leak and stricture, 365
    ischemic cholangiopathy/biliary cast syndrome, 365
    management, 366–368
    postoperative anatomy, 364
  biliary complications, 192–194
  bleeding, 194
  complications, 189
  donor considerations, 176–178
  hepatectomy, 178–181
  hepatic artery stenosis/thrombosis, 190–191
  hepatic arterial complications
    HAP, 371, 372
    HAT, 370, 371
    hepatic artery stenosis, 369–371
    management, 372, 373
    postoperative anatomy, 368, 369
  hepatocaval complications
    clinical manifestation and diagnostic features, 379
    management, 380, 381
    postoperative anatomy, 378
  hepatic venous outflow obstruction, 192
  heterotopic, 174
  history, 174–175
  implantation, 185–189
  interventional radiologist with complications after, 363
  LDLT, 175
  nonvascular percutaneous interventions
    biopsy, 382
    seroma, hematoma, biloma and abscess, 381, 382
  portal vein complications
    management, 376, 377
    portal vein stenosis, 374, 375
    postoperative anatomy, 373, 374
    PVT, 375, 376
  portal vein stenosis/thrombosis, 191, 192
  primary nonfunction, 190
  primary non-function, 190
  recipient operation, 178
  SALT survey, 194–196
  segmental, 174

P

Panel-reactive antibody (PRA), 255
Parenchyma, 387
Parenchymal evaluation, 167
Partial liver (PL) grafts, 221
Partial liver transplantation (PLT), 222, 223
  APOLT, 235, 236
  LDLT, 226
    donor selection, 226, 227
    graft retrieval, surgical principles of, 227–231
    portal inflow modulation, 231–232
  liver anatomy, 222–226
  SLT, 232
    donor selection, 233
    surgical principles of, 233, 235

Partial portacaval shunt (PPCS), 232
Pathogen-associated molecular patterns (PAMPs), 25
Pathogens, for infection, 346–350
Pattern recognition receptors (PPR), 25, 26
People living with Human Immunodeficiency Virus (PLWH), 114
Percutaneous coronary intervention (PCI), 96
Percutaneous transhepatic biliary drainage (PTBD), 406
Percutaneous transhepatic cholangiogram (PTC), 333
Perforation, 405
Perfusion, types, 243
Perihilar cholangiocarcinoma (pCCA), 128–130, 133
Piggyback technique, 183, 192
Plasma cell hepatitis/plasma-cell rich allograft rejection, 293, 294
Plasma cell-rich rejection, post-transplant liver pathology, 316, 317
Platypnea-orthodeoxia, 12
Pneumocystis jirovecii, 337
Pneumonia, 351
Portal hypertension (PH), 23–29, 177, 179, 180, 184, 190
  clinical decompensation, 51
  definition, 51
  HVPG, 51
  management of
    endoscopy/endoscopic ligation, 53, 54
    non-selective beta-blockers, 52–53
    systemic vasoconstrictors, 53
    TIPS, 53
  in specific patient populations
    compensated and decompensated cirrhosis, 54–55
    hemorrhage control, 56–57
    recurrent variceal hemorrhage, 57–58
    variceal hemorrhage, prevention of, 55–56
    with refractory ascites, 58–59
Portal inflow modulation (PIM), 231, 232
Portal revascularization, 33
Portal triad, 223
Portal vein, 388
Portal vein complications
  management, 376, 377
  portal vein stenosis, 374, 375
  postoperative anatomy, 373, 374
  PVT, 375, 376
Portal vein dissection, 180
Portal vein stenosis (PVS), 191, 192, 331
  clinical manifestation and diagnostic features, 374, 375
  management, 376–377
Portal vein thrombosis (PVT), 33, 179, 180, 186, 191, 192, 331, 392–393
  clinical manifestation and diagnostic features, 375–376
  management, 377
Portal-venous blood flow, 174
Portal-venous insufficiency, 192
Portopulmonary hypertension (POPH), 12, 13, 16, 38
  definition, 102
  management, 103
  pathophysiology, 103
  prognosis, 104
  screening, 103
Portosystemic collateral circulation, 23
Positive end-expiratory pressure (PEEP), 67, 72
Post ERCP pancreatitis (PEP), 404
Post liver transplant malignancies, 448
  de novo malignancies, incidence rate of, 450
  DNM screening recommendations, 456
  epidemiology, 448
  immunosuppression medications, carcinogenic effects of, 452
  modifiable cancer risk, 449
  non-skin cancers
    colorectal cancer, 456
    lung, 455
    PTLD, 455
  prevention and management, 457
  recurrent vs de novo malignancy, 448
  risk factors, 448
    age, 449
    donor transmitted cancer, 454
    gender, 449, 450
    immunosuppression, 451–454
    lifestyle and behavior, 451
    race/ethnicity, 450, 451
    underlying disorders, 451
  screening and surveillance, 454, 455
  skin cancers, 455
  treatment, 457, 458
Post liver transplant, modalities for
  computed tomography, 386, 387
  magnetic resonance imaging, 387
  ultrasound, 386
Post transplant diabetes mellitus (PTDM), 439
Post-operative day (POD), 334
Postoperative hemorrhage, 194
Post-reperfusion syndrome (PRS), 185, 242

Post-transplant biopsies, 311
Post-transplant liver pathology
- allograft dysfunction, histopathological diagnosis of
  - allograft rejection, 311, 312
  - antibody-mediated rejection, 314, 315
  - biopsies, 311
  - chronic rejection, 317
  - drug-induced liver injury and toxic injury, 319
  - late liver allograft dysfunction and protocol biopsies, 318, 319
  - liver transplant operation/surgical intervention and factors contributing, 308
  - plasma cell-rich rejection, 316
  - recurrent and de novo disease in, 319
  - T-cell-mediated rejection, 312, 313
  - timing of causes, 309
- complications, 308
- liver transplantation, changing trends in, 307, 308

Post-transplant lymphoproliferative disorder (PTLD), 397, 398, 455
Post-transplant metabolic syndrome (PTMS), 435
- clinical implications of
  - chronic kidney disease, 441
  - dyslipidemia, 438, 439
  - hypertension, 437, 438
  - morbidity, graft and patient survival, 437
  - obesity and weight management, 440
  - post transplant diabetes mellitus, 439
  - recurrent/de novo MASLD, 440, 441
- metabolic risk factors, treatment of, 438
- risk factors for
  - donor factors, 436
  - immunosuppressive strategy, 436
  - pre-existing recipient risk factors, 435, 436

Post-transplant survival, 325
Posttransplantation testing, 256, 257
Pre liver transplant work-up, 32–33
PREDESCI trial, 54
Preformed DSA, in living donor liver transplant recipient, 258
Pre-LT kidney function, 39
Pressure gradients, 379
Presumed consent, 204
Pre-transplant coordinator (PTC), 303
Pretransplant malignancy (PTM), 43
Pretransplantation tests, 254
Primary biliary cholangitis (PBC), 338, 421, 422
Primary graft nonfunction (PGF), 334
Primary non-function (PNF), 190, 210, 211, 213
Primary sclerosing cholangitis (PSC), 338, 413, 420, 421
Procalcitonin (PCT), 116, 117
Prognostic scoring systems, 5
Prothrombin complex concentrate (PCC), 329
Prozone effect, 255
Psychoeducation, 158
Psychosocial assessment, 151–159
Psychosocial Assessment of Candidates for Transplantation (PACT), 158
Psychosocial considerations, 163, 167, 168
Pulmonary arterial hypertension (PAH), 38, 102–104
Pulmonary artery systolic pressure (PASP), 38
Pulmonary complications
- hepatic hydrothorax, 105
- hepato-pulmonary syndrome, 104–105
- POPH
  - definition, 102
  - management, 103
  - pathophysiology, 103
  - prognosis, 104
  - screening, 103

Pulmonary disorders, 36
Pulmonary function evaluation, 36
- HPS, 37
- POPH, 38

Q

QuantiFERON Test, 42

R

Recipient portal vein, 177, 178, 185, 186
Recipient portomesenteric venous system, 186
Recurrent AIH (rAIH), 417
Recurrent disease, 286
Recurrent hepatitis C (rHCV), 414
Recurrent malignancy
- abdominal imaging, 397, 398
- vs de novo, 448

Recurrent MASLD, 440
Recurrent/de novo MASLD, 440, 441
Refractory hepatic hydrothorax, 39
Reimplantation, 378
Rejection, 285, 286, 335
Rejection activity index (RAI), 335
Relative adrenal insufficiency, 66, 71

Renal dysfunction, 264
Renal function, assessment of, 79, 80
Renal replacement therapy (RRT), 79, 84, 85
Renin-angiotensin-aldosterone system (RAAS), 25
Resectability, 124, 129
Resource navigation, 158
Right anterior sectoral ducts (RASD), 225
Right hepatic duct (RHD), 225, 228
Right hepatic vein (RHV), 224, 234
Right portal vein (RPV), 223, 236
Right posterior sectoral ducts (RPSD), 225
Right ventricular systolic pressure (RVSP), 38
Rotational thromboelastometry (ROTEM), 72
Roux-en-Y choledochojejunostomy, 189
Roux-en-Y hepaticojejunostomy, 403
Roux-en-Y reconstruction, 333

S
SAB test, 256
Salvage transplantation, 127
Sarcopenia, 41
Segmental LTX, 174
Seldinger-based approach, 382
Sepsis, 25, 79
Sequential perfusion, 241, 246, 247
Seroma, 381–382
Serum cystatin C (CysC), 80, 83
Severe acute alcoholic hepatitis (SAH), 13
Sickle cell disease, 165
Side-to-side cavo-cavoplasty, 192
Simultaneous liver-kidney transplantation (SLK), 39, 40, 79, 265
Sirolimus, 453
6-Minute Walk Test (6MWT), 41
6-month rule, 13
Skeletal muscle index (SMI), 41
Skin cancers, 455
Sleeve gastrectomy, 42
Sludge, 402
Small for size syndrome (SFSS), 166, 167, 190, 328
Social support, 154–155
Social workers
  interventions, 159
    psychoeducation, 158
    resource navigation, 158
    supportive counselling, 157–158
  psychosocial assessment, 151
    adherence, 156
    considerations, 152
    finances and medication coverage, 155
    health history, 154
    mental health, 156
    motivation, 157
    social support, 154–155
    substance use/misuse, 156
    transplant knowledge, 154
  standardized assessment tools, 158
  on transplant team, 159
Sphincter of Oddi Dysfunction (SOD), 402
Splenectomy, 232, 356
Split liver transplantation (SLT), 174, 175, 232
  APOLT, 235, 236
  donor selection, 233
  surgical principles of, 233, 235
Spontaneous bacterial peritonitis (SBP), 79, 82, 116, 117
Squamous cell carcinoma, 455
Standard orthotopic liver transplant, 178
Standardized assessment tools, 158
Stanford Integrated Psychosocial Assessment for Transplant (SIPAT), 158
Static-Cold Storage (SCS), 242
Statin therapy, 99
Steatotic liver disease (SLD), 139
Stenosis, 380
Stent placement, 402
Subclinical LV dysfunction, 94
Superior mesenteric vein, 186, 187, 192
Supportive counselling, 157–158
Suprahepatic cava anastomosis, 192
Surgical aortic valve replacement (SAVR), 101
Survey on Adult Liver Transplantation (SALT), 194, 195
Sympathetic nervous system (SNS), 25
Systemic inflammatory response syndrome (SIRS), 26
Systemic vasoconstrictors, 53

T
T tube, 187, 189, 195
Tacrolimus, 289, 453
T-cell mediated rejection (TCMR), 253, 285, 312, 335
  post-transplant liver pathology, 312–314
  severity, 335
TeleMedicine, 303
Temporary portacaval shunt, 185
Terlipressin, 39
Therapeutic thoracocentesis, 39
Thoraco-abdominal NRP (TA-NRP), 212, 327
Thrombectomy devices, 381
Thrombocytopenia, 27
Thromboelastography, 72
Thrombolysis, 330

Thrombosis of fepatic artery, 282
Toll-like receptor 4 (TLR4), 26
Total warm (WIT), 328
Toxic injury, 319–321
Transcatheter aortic valve replacement (TAVR), 36, 101
Transjugular intrahepatic portosystemic shunt (TIPS), 4, 6–8, 14, 15, 39, 53, 57–59, 84, 266
Translocation, 25
Transmissible infectious diseases, 165
Transplant center referral, 146
Transplant knowledge, 154
Transplant multidisciplinary care teams, 424
Transplant oncology, 124–125, 132, 133
Transplantability, 124, 125, 133
Transthoracic echocardiography (TTE), 32, 34, 94, 95, 101, 103, 104
Tricuspid regurgitation (TR), 36, 101
Trocar/coaxial technique, 382
Tuberculosis, 114
Tumor necrosis factor-α (TNF-α), 24, 25
Type 1 gastro-esophageal varices (GOV-1), 57
Tyrosine-kinase inhibitors, 132

U

Ultrasound (US), 379, 386
Ultrasound-based shear wave elastography (SWE), 140, 141
Umbilical fissural vein (UFV), 225
Uncontrolled donation after the circulatory determination of death (uDCDD), 206, 211–213, 215
Undifferentiated embryonal cell sarcoma, 131
Unilobar disease, 11
United Network for Organ Sharing (UNOS), 329
Urea cycle disorders (UCD), 9
UV exposure, 455

V

Vaccinations, 114–115, 132
Valganciclovir, 337
Valsalva dimensions, 36
Valvular heart disease (VHD), 35, 101–102
  recommendations and management, 102
Variant hepatic arterial anatomyial anatomy, 166
Variant hepatic venous anatomy, 166
Variant portal vein anatomy, 166
Variceal bleeding, 4, 6, 8, 14, 15
Variceal hemorrhage
  patient presentation, 56–57
  prevention of, 55–56
  recurrent, 57–58
Vascular complications, 390
  hepatic arterial ischemic cascade, 390
  hepatic vein stenosis, 393, 394
  nonocclusive arterial complications, 330
  occlusive arterial complications, 329, 330
  portal vein thrombosis, 331, 392, 393
  venous outflow obstruction, 331, 332
Vasodilation theory, 25
Velocity, 379
Venous outflow obstruction, 192, 331–332
Veno-venous bypass, 179, 181–184
Vibration-controlled elastography (VCTE), 140, 141
Viral hepatitis, 42
Viral infections, 283, 336
  late post-transplantation infections, 356–357

W

"Wadell–Calne" biliary reconstruction, 189
Waiting list (WL), 117
Wait-list transplant coordinator (WLTC), 303
Wilson's disease (WD), 9, 14, 145, 146
Withdraw life-sustaining therapies (WLST), 206–208, 210

X

Xenotransplantation, 132

Z

Z-stent, 380

MIX
Papier aus verantwortungsvollen Quellen
Paper from responsible sources
FSC® C105338

If you have any concerns about our products,
you can contact us on
ProductSafety@springernature.com

In case Publisher is established outside the EU,
the EU authorized representative is:
Springer Nature Customer Service Center GmbH
Europaplatz 3, 69115 Heidelberg, Germany

Printed by Libri Plureos GmbH
in Hamburg, Germany